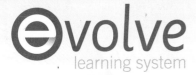

To access the free Evolve Resources, visit:

http://evolve.elsevier.com/Shankman/orthopedic/

Students, make your study time more efficient using the Evolve Student Resources for Shankman and Manske: Fundamental Orthopedic Management for the Physical Therapist Assistant, *Third Edition. Highlights of the available resources include:*

- **Reference lists linked to Medline abstracts:** References from each chapter are linked, when available, to their citation on Medline.
- **Critical thinking applications:** These activities bring critical thinking together with chapter content.
- **Essay questions:** Essay questions help reinforce new concepts.
- **Review questions:** Multiple choice questions help prepare you for exams.
- **Archie animations:** These short, often narrated, film clips help explain or reinforce key ideas.
- **Video clips:** These video clips, originally from Brotzman & Manske: Clinical Orthopaedic Rehabilitation, Third Edition, help explain or reinforce key ideas.

Instructors, make your classroom preparation easier with the Evolve Instructor Resources for Shankman and Manske: Fundamental Orthopedic Management for the Physical Therapist Assistant, *Third Edition. Highlights of the available resources include:*

- **PowerPoint Slides:** Enhance your lectures with slides created from the book's content.
- **Test bank questions:** Multiple choice questions, including answers and answer rationales, will help you prepare for exams.
- **Image collection:** Electronic access to all images from the text will help clarify concepts presented in lecture.
- **Case studies:** Access a collection of case studies to help explain new concepts.

ELSEVIER
MOSBY

FUNDAMENTAL ORTHOPEDIC MANAGEMENT

FOR THE

PHYSICAL THERAPIST ASSISTANT

Gary A. Shankman, PTA
Heritage Healthcare
Knoxville, Tennessee
Hillcrest South
Knoxville, Tennessee

Robert C. Manske PT, DPT, MEd, SCS, ATC, CSCS
Associate Professor
Department of Physical Therapy
Wichita State University
Via Christi Orthopedic and Sports Therapy
Wichita, Kansas

Third Edition

ELSEVIER
MOSBY

3251 Riverport Lane
St. Louis, Missouri 63043

Fundamental Orthopedic Management for the Physical Therapist Assistant, Third Edition

Copyright © 2011, 2004, 1997 by Mosby, Inc., an affiliate of Elsevier Inc.

ISBN: 978-0-323-05669-4

Notice

Knowledge and best practice in this field are constantly changing. As new research and experience broaden our understanding, changes in research methods, professional practices, or medical treatment may become necessary.

Practitioners and researchers must always rely on their own experience and knowledge in evaluating and using any information, methods, compounds, or experiments described herein. In using such information or methods they should be mindful of their own safety and the safety of others, including parties for whom they have a professional responsibility.

With respect to any drug or pharmaceutical products identified, readers are advised to check the most current information provided (i) on procedures featured or (ii) by the manufacturer of each product to be administered, to verify the recommended dose or formula, the method and duration of administration, and contraindications. It is the responsibility of practitioners, relying on their own experience and knowledge of their patients, to make diagnoses, to determine dosages and the best treatment for each individual patient, and to take all appropriate safety precautions.

To the fullest extent of the law, neither the Publisher nor the authors, contributors, or editors, assume any liability for any injury and/or damage to persons or property as a matter of products liability, negligence or otherwise, or from any use or operation of any methods, products, instructions, or ideas contained in the material herein.

Library of Congress Cataloging-in-Publication Data

Fundamental orthopedic management for the physical therapist assistant / [edited by] Gary A. Shankman, Robert C. Manske. — 3rd ed.
      p. ; cm.
Includes bibliographical references and index.
ISBN 978-0-323-05669-4 (pbk. : alk. paper)
1. Orthopedics. 2. Physical therapy. 3. Physical therapy assistants. I. Shankman, Gary A. II. Manske, Robert C.
[DNLM: 1. Orthopedic Procedures. 2. Allied Health Personnel. 3. Physical Therapy Modalities. WE 168]
RD731.S5513 2011
616.7—dc22

2010033423

Executive Editor: Kathy Falk
Developmental Editor: Megan Fennell
Publishing Services Manager: Julie Eddy
Senior Project Manager: Laura Loveall
Design Direction: Margaret Reid
Cover Designer: Margaret Reid

Printed in the United States

Last digit is the print number: 9 8 7 6 5 4 3 2

To my sons
Kyle, Tyler, and Jordan

To my grandson
Trevor

To my extended family
Clark, Mandy, and Payne

To my wife
Pebbles, "my rib"

-Gary A. Shankman

To my daughters
Rachael and Halle

To my son (my best friend)
Tyler

To my wife
Julie
Thank you all for letting me do what I love to do!

-Robert C. Manske

Erik P. Meira, PT, SCS, CSCS
Black Diamond Physical Therapy
Portland, Oregon

Jaime C. Paz, PT, DPT, MS
Clinical Associate Professor
Division of Physical Therapy
Walsh University
North Canton, Ohio

Michael P. Reiman, PT, DPT, OCS, SCS, ATC, FAAOMPT, CSCS
Assistant Professor
Department of Physical Therapy
Wichita State University
Wichita, Kansas

Bryan L. Riemann, PhD, ATC
Associate Professor, Sports Medicine
Coordinator, Sports Medicine Program
Director, Biodynamics Center
Department of Health Sciences
Armstrong Atlantic State University
Savannah, Georgia

Justin Rohrberg, DPT, ATC
Adjunct Faculty
Department of Physical Therapy
Wichita State University
Wichita, Kansas

Justin Rossetter
Steadman Hawkins Clinic
Denver, Colorado

Barbara Smith, PhD, PT
Professor
Wichita State University
Department of Physical Therapy
Wichita, Kansas

Matthew Smith
Steadman Hawkins Clinic
Denver, Colorado

Cheryl Sparks, PT, DPT
Assistant Professor
Department of Physical Therapy and Health Science
Bradley University
Peoria, Illinois

Terry Trundle, PTA, ATC, LAT
Owner
Athletic Rehab Institute
Acworth, Georgia

Harvey W. Wallmann, PT, DSc, SCS, LAT, ATC, CSCS
Chair and Associate Professor
University of Nevada, Las Vegas
Las Vegas, Nevada

D.S. Blaise Williams III, PhD, MPT
Director
Human Movement Research Laboratory
Department of Physical Therapy
East Carolina University
Greenville, North Carolina

John D. Willson, PhD, PT
Physical Therapy Program
Department of Health Professions
University of Wisconsin-La Crosse
La Crosse, Wisconsin

Preface

As it has been 8 years since the last edition of *Fundamental Orthopedic Management for the Physical Therapist Assistant*, we hope that you will feel that the third edition was worth the wait! As with most updates and revisions, this text is in evolution. A large part of the evolution is the movement from a single author to co-editors managing multiple contributors who are experts in their respective areas. Robert Manske has joined Gary in this new edition as a co-editor. Robert is well respected in the field of orthopedic and sports physical therapy, and he has written and edited textbooks, book chapters, and scientific papers. He is an associate professor at the Wichita State University Doctoral Physical Therapy Program where he has taught orthopedic courses for 13 years. Robert continues to practice, treating orthopedic patients on a weekly basis, as he has for the past 16 years.

As the field of orthopedic physical rehabilitation continues to change (sometimes on what seems to be a weekly basis), this new edition of *Fundamental Orthopedic Management for the Physical Therapist Assistant* is committed to bringing those fundamental orthopedic management changes to the education of physical therapist assistants (PTAs). It is certainly the intent of this text to remain entrenched within the scope of the PTA, rather than that of general orthopedic physical therapy. The focus of this third edition is largely on the critical thinking and application of physical therapy examination, development of treatment plans, and interventions that can be used by PTAs during clinical practice. Although an ability to thoroughly evaluate the orthopedic patient is not within the scope of the PTA's practice, we feel that it is necessary for the PTA to understand the basic evaluation components and tests and measures that are used in the evaluation and differential diagnosis process. Having a basic understanding of these procedures, in addition to understanding differential diagnosis and the various diseases and pathologies progression, will allow the PTA to notice even subtle changes earlier in the disease progression. Each chapter in the third edition has been extensively updated to reflect changes in practice patterns. This includes the use and descriptions of evidence-based treatments when available. As such, this text continues to be the "one-stop" for all things orthopedic and should be used by both PTA students and practicing PTAs.

During the tenure of this text, several external reviews of content were performed by faculty members from accredited PTA programs across the United States. Feedback was both honest and constructive. Following those reviews, the prior modalities chapter was removed based on the feedback that a large number of programs utilize other texts that provide more depth and detail for the various forms and usage of modalities. With loss, however, sometimes comes gain; removal of the modalities chapter allowed us to add three new chapters: Chapter 24, Rheumatic Disorders, by Steven Elliott, which describes rheumatic diseases processes; Chapter 25, Pain, by Michelle H. Cameron, in which she has done an excellent job describing types of pain, pain mechanisms, measurement, and management; and Chapter 26, Introduction to Orthotics and Prosthetics. In this chapter, Leslie K. King has described materials and uses of braces, orthoses, and prostheses.

The addition of regional experts has greatly enhanced the third edition of *Fundamental Orthopedic Management for the Physical Therapist Assistant*. Although a noble effort by Gary on the first two editions, it is almost impossible for any single person to be an expert in all areas of physical rehabilitation. By allowing regional experts in various subject areas to contribute chapters, we have significantly elevated the depth and breadth of the entire text. Although numerous contributors have helped us reach this goal, we would like to highlight just a few. Harvey W. Wallmann has recently published numerous research articles, manuscripts, and home study courses on issues pertaining to flexibility. In Chapter 4, Flexibility and Stretching, he discusses the differences between range of motion, flexibility, and stretching. He also emphasizes recent research related to ballistic versus static stretching and physical performance. Bryan Riemann from Armstrong Atlantic State University is an academician who has already written prolifically on aspects of balance and coordination. In Chapter 6, Balance and Coordination, he succinctly describes principles of balance tasks in orthopedics and further details ways to enhance balance and coordination in upper and lower extremities. Pharmacist LaDonna S. Hale has completely updated Chapter 13, Orthopedic Pharmacology, utilizing an easy-to-read approach that makes difficult concepts easy to understand. She has removed discussion points that are no longer relevant and added detail where it was lacking; creating an excellent chapter that will allow the PTA to more thoroughly understand basic pharmacology concepts. This is just a brief sampling of the excitement that awaits you in this third edition.

We know that you will continue to rely on the third edition as you have the past editions for your fundamental orthopedic management needs. We appreciate any feedback you may have regarding this text. Constructive criticism is what allows us to develop the exact textbook that fits your educational needs. If you have recommendations or additions that you think we should consider in the fourth edition, please send an email to: Robert.manske@wichita.edu. All emails will be accepted and given the highest priority.

Gary A. Shankman
Robert C. Manske

Acknowledgments

Several years ago, an impulse propagated into the text, *Fundamental Orthopedic Management for the Physical Therapist Assistant*. The concept was, in fact, simple—write a textbook specifically addressing the needs of the physical therapist assistant (PTA) that addressed basic, foundational information on orthopedic management. Prior to this, I would spend hours reviewing my own textbooks searching for information on various orthopedic pathologies. I would "ferret-out" and distill information from textbooks that were written by physical therapists for physical therapists, or by physicians for physicians. The need was obvious for a condensed, yet not simplified, text to equip entry-level PTA students with essential and practical information concerning orthopedics written from the perspective, training, and experience of a PTA for PTAs.

Years have passed. The second edition brought new information, new chapter additions, and expansion on many fronts. This third edition bears absolutely no resemblance to the first. In keeping with this fact, this project has grown much beyond me. Therefore, I am very thankful, grateful, and indebted to Robert Manske, a friend and colleague who is well respected, eminently qualified, and infinitely more capable than I to handle the vast and ever-changing landscape of sharing orthopedic knowledge. Rob has developed this text from its humble beginnings into a multi-authored unity of various orthopedic topics, addressing a wide range of issues and pathologies with substantial depth to challenge the student and practicing clinician alike. Under Rob's capable guidance and while maintaining a rigorous teaching schedule, clinical practice, and family life, he put together a list of contributors that reads like a "Who's Who" in physical therapy. To each and every contributor, I say thank you for your time, expertise, and willingness to share your wisdom, talents, and gifts.

To the three new chapter contributors, I
and personal thank you. To Steven Elliot
King, thank you for your tolerance, patie
and friendship during this long and see
journey. To Michelle Cameron, I thank
your expertise.

Naturally, there are numerous indiv
who enabled a project of this magnit
To each of these, I say thank you. T
on this project, Megan Fennell and
essarily and justifiably are deservi
praise for their efforts. They both
my unreasonable and often
and convoluted attempts at m
of artistic control. Through th
Rob, Megan, and Laura, I was
self-estimation. In so doing,

At this point, I call your a
ments in the second editi
organization that I menti
individuals may not be
influence my life today.
that I say thank you ag

It is necessary at t
a new direction in r
all of the patients,
that I have had th
great delight, hu
found gratitude
journey of learr

Finally, any
regarding this
contributor,
deficiencies

Preface

As it has been 8 years since the last edition of *Fundamental Orthopedic Management for the Physical Therapist Assistant*, we hope that you will feel that the third edition was worth the wait! As with most updates and revisions, this text is in evolution. A large part of the evolution is the movement from a single author to co-editors managing multiple contributors who are experts in their respective areas. Robert Manske has joined Gary in this new edition as a co-editor. Robert is well respected in the field of orthopedic and sports physical therapy, and he has written and edited textbooks, book chapters, and scientific papers. He is an associate professor at the Wichita State University Doctoral Physical Therapy Program where he has taught orthopedic courses for 13 years. Robert continues to practice, treating orthopedic patients on a weekly basis, as he has for the past 16 years.

As the field of orthopedic physical rehabilitation continues to change (sometimes on what seems to be a weekly basis), this new edition of *Fundamental Orthopedic Management for the Physical Therapist Assistant* is committed to bringing those fundamental orthopedic management changes to the education of physical therapist assistants (PTAs). It is certainly the intent of this text to remain entrenched within the scope of the PTA, rather than that of general orthopedic physical therapy. The focus of this third edition is largely on the critical thinking and application of physical therapy examination, development of treatment plans, and interventions that can be used by PTAs during clinical practice. Although an ability to thoroughly evaluate the orthopedic patient is not within the scope of the PTA's practice, we feel that it is necessary for the PTA to understand the basic evaluation components and tests and measures that are used in the evaluation and differential diagnosis process. Having a basic understanding of these procedures, in addition to understanding differential diagnosis and the various diseases and pathologies progression, will allow the PTA to notice even subtle changes earlier in the disease progression. Each chapter in the third edition has been extensively updated to reflect changes in practice patterns. This includes the use and descriptions of evidence-based treatments when available. As such, this text continues to be the "one-stop" for all things orthopedic and should be used by both PTA students and practicing PTAs.

During the tenure of this text, several external reviews of content were performed by faculty members from accredited PTA programs across the United States. Feedback was both honest and constructive. Following those reviews, the prior modalities chapter was removed based on the feedback that a large number of programs utilize other texts that provide more depth and detail for the various forms and usage of modalities. With loss, however, sometimes comes gain; removal of the modalities chapter allowed us to add three new chapters: Chapter 24, Rheumatic Disorders, by Steven Elliott, which describes rheumatic diseases processes; Chapter 25, Pain, by Michelle H. Cameron, in which she has done an excellent job describing types of pain, pain mechanisms, measurement, and management; and Chapter 26, Introduction to Orthotics and Prosthetics. In this chapter, Leslie K. King has described materials and uses of braces, orthoses, and prostheses.

The addition of regional experts has greatly enhanced the third edition of *Fundamental Orthopedic Management for the Physical Therapist Assistant*. Although a noble effort by Gary on the first two editions, it is almost impossible for any single person to be an expert in all areas of physical rehabilitation. By allowing regional experts in various subject areas to contribute chapters, we have significantly elevated the depth and breadth of the entire text. Although numerous contributors have helped us reach this goal, we would like to highlight just a few. Harvey W. Wallmann has recently published numerous research articles, manuscripts, and home study courses on issues pertaining to flexibility. In Chapter 4, Flexibility and Stretching, he discusses the differences between range of motion, flexibility, and stretching. He also emphasizes recent research related to ballistic versus static stretching and physical performance. Bryan Riemann from Armstrong Atlantic State University is an academician who has already written prolifically on aspects of balance and coordination. In Chapter 6, Balance and Coordination, he succinctly describes principles of balance tasks in orthopedics and further details ways to enhance balance and coordination in upper and lower extremities. Pharmacist LaDonna S. Hale has completely updated Chapter 13, Orthopedic Pharmacology, utilizing an easy-to-read approach that makes difficult concepts easy to understand. She has removed discussion points that are no longer relevant and added detail where it was lacking; creating an excellent chapter that will allow the PTA to more thoroughly understand basic pharmacology concepts. This is just a brief sampling of the excitement that awaits you in this third edition.

We know that you will continue to rely on the third edition as you have the past editions for your fundamental orthopedic management needs. We appreciate any feedback you may have regarding this text. Constructive criticism is what allows us to develop the exact textbook that fits your educational needs. If you have recommendations or additions that you think we should consider in the fourth edition, please send an email to: Robert.manske@wichita.edu. All emails will be accepted and given the highest priority.

Gary A. Shankman
Robert C. Manske

Acknowledgments

Several years ago, an impulse propagated into the text, *Fundamental Orthopedic Management for the Physical Therapist Assistant.* The concept was, in fact, simple—write a textbook specifically addressing the needs of the physical therapist assistant (PTA) that addressed basic, foundational information on orthopedic management. Prior to this, I would spend hours reviewing my own textbooks searching for information on various orthopedic pathologies. I would "ferret-out" and distill information from textbooks that were written by physical therapists for physical therapists, or by physicians for physicians. The need was obvious for a condensed, yet not simplified, text to equip entry-level PTA students with essential and practical information concerning orthopedics written from the perspective, training, and experience of a PTA for PTAs.

Years have passed. The second edition brought new information, new chapter additions, and expansion on many fronts. This third edition bears absolutely no resemblance to the first. In keeping with this fact, this project has grown much beyond me. Therefore, I am very thankful, grateful, and indebted to Robert Manske, a friend and colleague who is well respected, eminently qualified, and infinitely more capable than I to handle the vast and ever-changing landscape of sharing orthopedic knowledge. Rob has developed this text from its humble beginnings into a multi-authored unity of various orthopedic topics, addressing a wide range of issues and pathologies with substantial depth to challenge the student and practicing clinician alike. Under Rob's capable guidance and while maintaining a rigorous teaching schedule, clinical practice, and family life, he put together a list of contributors that reads like a "Who's Who" in physical therapy. To each and every contributor, I say thank you for your time, expertise, and willingness to share your wisdom, talents, and gifts.

To the three new chapter contributors, I offer a deep and personal thank you. To Steven Elliott and Leslie King, thank you for your tolerance, patience, kindness, and friendship during this long and seemingly endless journey. To Michelle Cameron, I thank you for sharing your expertise.

Naturally, there are numerous individuals at Elsevier who enabled a project of this magnitude to take shape. To each of these, I say thank you. The leadership team on this project, Megan Fennell and Laura Loveall, necessarily and justifiably are deserving of recognition and praise for their efforts. They both tolerated and endured my unreasonable and often misplaced, disjointed, and convoluted attempts at maintaining some degree of artistic control. Through the gentleness and skill of Rob, Megan, and Laura, I was shown to "grow-down" in self-estimation. In so doing, the text is better in all areas.

At this point, I call your attention to the Acknowledgments in the second edition. Each person, agency, and organization that I mentioned then, I echo now. These individuals may not be aware, but they all continue to influence my life today. It is with great joy and gratitude that I say thank you again.

It is necessary at this point for me to acknowledge a new direction in my life. Before moving on, I honor all of the patients, therapists, physicians, and educators that I have had the privilege to learn from. It is with great delight, humility, deep appreciation, and profound gratitude that I say thank you for this remarkable journey of learning and sharing.

Finally, any and all commendation and recognition regarding this text are due to Robert Manske and each contributor, while any and all errors, omissions, and deficiencies are traced to me alone.

Gary A. Shankman

Contents

xiii

PART I

BASIC CONCEPTS OF ORTHOPEDIC MANAGEMENT

The foundations for the appropriate application of skills and therapeutic techniques related to orthopedic physical therapy are based on the interdependence of basic science principles and the relationships between the patient, the supervising physical therapist (PT), and the physical therapist assistant (PTA). The PTA, although responsible for proper patient supervision and clinical observation during treatment, is frequently guided and directed to modify or adjust selected interventions in consultation with the supervising PT based on specific physiologic responses from the patient. Keen observation skills, properly directed patient supervision techniques, and a thorough understanding of physiologic and therapeutic adaptations to exercise techniques, help the PTA to effectively and skillfully apply selected interventions under the direction and supervision of the supervising PT.

Therefore, this section introduces basic orthopedic physical therapy components of patient supervision; the role of the PTA in physical assessment and problem solving with specific reference to the *Guide to Physical Therapist Practice*, second edition,[1] the problem-solving algorithm used by PTAs in patient or client intervention, and related key elements of systems review and a systems approach to physical assessment; physical agents used in treatment of musculoskeletal conditions, flexibility and soft tissue management, and muscular strength, power, and plyometrics; unique characteristics of strength and adaptation in young and elderly patients; closed kinetic chain exercise; neuromuscular fatigue; and balance, coordination, and the enhancement of the afferent neural input system related to orthopedic physical therapy management.

The focus and specific intent of this section is to provide a sound, practical, and purposeful introduction to the principles of basic orthopedic management, as well as the therapeutic application of these critical components related to specific tissue healing constraints, immobilization, and postsurgical recovery after orthopedic surgery.

---

1. American Physical Therapy Association: *Guide to physical therapist practice*, ed 2, Alexandria, Va., 2001, APTA: 9-746.

1 Patient Supervision and Observation During Treatment

Candy Bahner

SUPERVISING THE PATIENT DURING TREATMENT

Among the many challenges for the physical therapist assistant (PTA) are supervising the patient during selected interventions, solving problems effectively, and making appropriate decisions. The PTA must recognize that interpersonal **communication** skills, patient supervision methods, data collection skills, effective problem solving, and responsive clinical decision making must be learned, practiced, and demonstrated to function efficiently and effectively.

Initial contact with a patient establishes a framework of rapport and sets the stage for all future interactions with that individual. The PTA has the opportunity to convey confidence, capability, and sensitivity during the initial introductions by the supervising physical therapist (PT). This leads the patient to trust the PTA and minimizes fear and anxiety in the patient.

The PTA is responsible for carrying out prescribed selected interventions, patient supervision, data collection, and appropriate problem solving and clinical decision making. The American Physical Therapy Association's Department of Education, Accreditation, and Practice developed the "Problem-Solving Algorithm Utilized by PTAs in Patient/Client Intervention,"[1] which reflects current policies and positions on the problem-solving processes to be utilized by PTAs in the provision of selected interventions (Fig. 1-1). For proper care to be given, the PTA must monitor the patient's response to selected interventions and accurately and swiftly report changes to the supervising PT. This involves constant patient interaction, observation, data collection, reassessment of initial data, problem solving, and responsive action to clarify and enhance the effectiveness of prescribed selected interventions. Changes in the patient's status, both positive and negative, can occur throughout the treatment program, whether during a single visit or over the span of multiple treatments. Some of these changes are subtle and require keen awareness of the initial objective data and acute sensitivity to the patient's subjective reports. Other changes are profound and sudden. In either situation, the PTA observes the patient and collects appropriate data, such as range of motion, strength, pain, balance, coordination, swelling, endurance, or gait deviations. When reported to the supervising PT, these changes dictate and can significantly affect the course of treatment.

Components of Patient Supervision

Clinical patient supervision can be viewed as a process with the following purposes:
■ To gather relevant information and data
■ To establish and enhance rapport, trust, and confidence
■ To facilitate understanding of the PTA's concept of the patient's problem as outlined, described, and initially determined by the supervising PT
■ To assist in the management of the patient
■ To provide a conduit or therapeutic outlet for the patient to voice concerns about his or her problem

Clearly gathering information from the patient and interpreting those data during the initial evaluation are the responsibility of the PT. However, the PTA may need to assist the PT in helping the patient understand the problem throughout the course of rehabilitation. The PTA must recognize how difficult it is for patients to grasp all the components of the situation well enough to fully appreciate the rationale for the prescribed treatment. Therefore the PTA may be asked, when appropriate, to help the patient understand the disorder being treated, the supervising PT's plan of care, and the selected interventions to be provided. In so doing, the PTA must be keenly aware of and sensitive to subtle or overt signs of patient apprehension, fear, and anxiety.

Although direct patient supervision is frequently the task of one individual, responsibility for the patient's care is shared by the entire rehabilitation team. In addition, the patient must be actively involved in the treatment and accept shared responsibility for his or her own care.

While providing selected interventions, the PTA makes observations of the patient, collects relevant data, and develops an objective assessment using appropriate scales of measurement (Box 1-1). Using applicable questioning techniques ensures that the patient is actively involved. This interactive approach to supervision, as well as the skills of the PTA to seek, understand, and accurately relay information related to the patient's status distinguishes the PTA from an on-the-job trained aide.[5]

Patient Supervision by the Rehabilitation Team

The PTA must be aware of the key members of the rehabilitation team. The PT and PTA are involved with direct patient care on a daily basis and may be assisted by supportive personal, such as physical therapy aides or technicians. The occupational therapist and occupational therapy assistant, along with the speech language pathologist, audiologist, rehabilitation counselor, nurse, respiratory therapist, psychologist, and dietitian, play significant roles in daily patient care. These rehabilitation specialists seek to maximize recovery for each patient and always must be regarded as resources to meet specific patient needs as they are identified by any member of the team. Thus the PTA charged with direct patient care and supervision is only one vital member of the team, and he or she can take comfort in knowing that every member of the team is prepared to provide appropriate skills so that the patient can achieve the highest functional gains in recovery. Developing a team mindset helps the PTA to be responsible and accountable to the other members of the team for his or her own contribution and to reach out to others when their expertise is needed.[7]

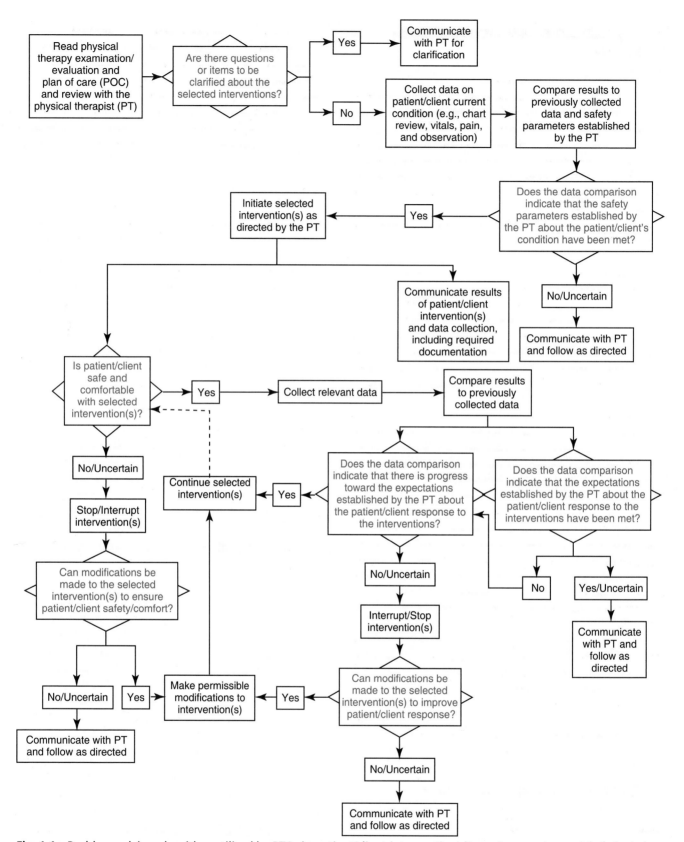

Fig. 1-1　Problem-solving algorithm utilized by PTAs in patient/client intervention. (From *A normative model of physical therapist assistant education,* version 2007, Baltimore, 2007, APTA.)

BOX 1-1

General Scales of Measurement

STRENGTH: MANUAL MUSCLE TESTING
-5/5 Normal: Full resistance against gravity
-4/5 Good: Some resistance against gravity
-3/5 Fair: No resistance against gravity
-2/5 Poor: No movement against gravity
-1/5 Trace: Slight contraction, no movement
-0/5 Zero: No contraction

PAIN: ANALOG SCALE
Graded from 0 to 10 (0 absent, 10 severe)

SWELLING: GENERALLY MEASURED BY
Circumferential measurement
Water displacement

VITAL SIGNS
Blood pressure: 120/80 mm Hg normal; use sphygmomanometer and stethoscope
Pulse: Average 72 BPM. Pulse can be lower (e.g., 55) for trained athletes
Respirations: Average 12 to 16/min
Temperature: normal range 96.8°F to 99.5°F
Oxygen saturation: normal ranges from 95% to 98%

COORDINATION
Tapping foot or hand
Finger to nose
Heel to shin
Coordination activities are tested first with eyes open, then with eyes closed. All events are described as degrees of rhythmic, symmetric, even, and consistent.

STRETCH REFLEX (DTR)
0 = Areflexia
1 to 3 = Average
3 + to 4 = Hyperreflexia

RANGE OF MOTION: STANDARD GONIOMETRY
Shoulder
Flexion 1° to 180°
Extension 0° to 60°
Abduction 0° to 180°
Internal rotation 0° to 70°
External rotation 0° to 90°
Hip
Flexion 0° to 120°
Extension 0° to 30°
Abduction 0° to 45°
Adduction 0° to 30°
External rotation 0° to 45°
Internal rotation 0° to 45°
Ankle
Dorsiflexion 0° to 20°
Plantar flexion 0° to 50°
Inversion 0° to 35°
Eversion 0° to 15°
Knee
Flexion 0° to 135°
Elbow
Flexion 0° to 150°

Effective communication is the hallmark of a great team and should be maximized. To effectively supervise and provide the best care for the patient, the PTA must learn to communicate openly and freely, with honesty and respect, and in a professional manner with every member of the team.[7] He or she must differentiate between the language used for communicating among peers and that used to define and explain injury, disease, and physical therapy interventions to a patient. The PTA must employ appropriate and professional medical terminology to outline and describe an orthopedic problem to a PT and must be able to use familiar terms to describe the same pathologic condition to a patient or family member. If the PTA uses medical jargon inappropriately, the patient or family member might perceive the PTA as insensitive, aloof, and impersonal. Generally use of language appropriate to the patient's comprehension conveys understanding, sensitivity, **warmth**, and reassurance and removes uncomfortable and unnecessary barriers to communication.[2]

The PTA also must be aware that **listening** is an effective communication tool. Listening demonstrates interest and provides the opportunity for a better understanding of the patient's concept of the problem.[4] By active listening, the PTA is better able to integrate verbal and nonverbal messages that the patient may have received.[4] In addition, patients may be more comfortable and trusting with a good listener and be more willing to provide information.[4]

Supervision of patients by the PTA must be done systematically and reliably with an emphasis on **accountability** and effective and efficient patient care. Appropriate and responsible investigative questioning of the patient during selected interventions helps the PTA focus on the areas to probe, findings to quantify, and objective changes to assess. As indicated in the "Problem-Solving Algorithm Utilized by PTAs in Patient/Client Intervention,"[1] PTAs are responsible for reporting all findings to the supervising PT so that modifications can be made in accordance with changes in patient status.

Basic Patient Supervision Skills

Communication Skills

The PTA can be most effective if he or she develops an understanding of human behavior and adopts a proactive role in supervising patients. In a proactive role, the PTA does not wait to be placed in a reactive position. Use of appropriate **probing questions** is a proactive method to use during patient supervision. Questioning patients during treatment can be insightful, rewarding, and helpful for both the supervising PT and the PTA. The format of asking probing questions is critical and strongly influences the responses received (Fig. 1-2). Using open-ended questions invites the patient to share feelings, thoughts, concerns, and opinions.[9] Examples are as follows:

- "Tell me about your pain."
- "How does that feel?"
- "What do you think about this exercise?"

These types of questions are generally not answered by "yes" or "no." They open discussions and prompt the patient to express a wide range of views and opinions.[9] Open-ended questions for patients have been described as "a good medium for facilitating rapport and, as such, are particularly useful...."[4] Using open-ended questions promotes personal interactions between the PTA and patient, may allow the patient to give a more in-depth explanation of the problem, and may lead to discussions of what the patient identifies as important. Although this type of questioning does not enable the patient to give precise, clear answers, it is appropriate in situations that require compassion and empathy from the PTA and shared feelings between the PTA and patient.

Closed-ended questions are directed toward finding facts, obtaining specific responses, and filling in details. They can be very helpful in focusing and clarifying essential details of the patient's condition.[9] By asking the patient questions such as, "Where is your pain?" "When does your knee feel unstable?" or "Does your back hurt when you bend forward?" the PTA proactively directs the discussion and sequence of questions instead of sifting out pertinent information from among all the data gathered in open-ended questioning.

Summary-type statements check understanding, help the patient clarify thinking, and provide direction for the PTA. Examples include the following: "So your back hurts only at night?" and "Then your knee doesn't hurt with this exercise." Using precise closed-ended questions with summary statements elicits information that can lead to an objective assessment of the patient. The approach the PTA takes influences the balance of questioning between open-ended and closed-ended questions.

Behavior

The behavior of the PTA during patient supervision can either reassure the patient and demonstrate appropriate responsive professional care or create a sense of indifference. Four broad categories of behavior are **dominance, submission, hostility,** and warmth.[2] Buzzotta and Lefton[2] define these four categories as follows:

Dominance

Dominance can be defined as exercising control or influence. People who show dominant behavior are forceful, dynamic, and assertive. They push their ideas forward or try to sway the way other people think or behave. They take charge, guide, lead, and move other people to action.

Submission

Submission can be defined as being passive. People who show submissive behavior are willing to take a back seat. They are ready to comply, quick to give in, and reluctant to try to exert influence.

Hostility

Hostility can be defined as being unresponsive or insensitive to others and their needs. People showing hostile behavior tend to care only about themselves; they lack regard for other people's feelings and ideas. Although anger is a form of hostility, people can be hostile while showing no open anger.

Warmth

Warmth can be defined as being responsive and sensitive to others and their needs. People who show warm behavior are open and caring and have a high regard for other people's ideas and feelings. This does not mean they automatically gush with affection. A person can be warm without being openly affectionate.

These four categories of behavior are used to describe the extremes of the **basic dimensional model** (Fig. 1-3, A). Quadrants (Q) are formed and certain patterns of behavior exist when two dimensions are combined, as described in the following:

- Q1: Dominant hostile
- Q2: Submissive hostile
- Q3: Submissive warm
- Q4: Dominant warm

Four patterns, or types, of human behavior come from this (Fig. 1-3, B).

Dominance	Active behavior: leading, controlling, making things happen
Submission	Passive behavior: following, letting things happen, reacting
Hostility	A lack of concern or regard, and unresponsiveness for other people and their position/ideas
Warmth	Concern, regard, and responsiveness for other people and their position/ideas

Probe	Definition	Objectives	Characteristics	Examples
Open-ended questions	A question or statement that invites a wide-ranging response, often asks for ideas, opinions, or views.	• Open up discussion • Invite broad response • Give other freedom to talk • Gets involvement	• Can't be answered "yes" or "no" • Gets at feelings, opinions, thoughts	• "What do you think about...?" • "Tell me about..." • "Why do you feel...?" • "What's your opinion?"
Pause	An intentional, purposeful period of silence.	• Give other a chance to think and respond • Slow down pace • Draw out other	• Usually follows open-ended question • Deliberate	• "Why do you say that?" (silence) • "Tell me more." (silence)
Reflective	A statement that describes and reflects a feeling or emotion (without implying agreement or disagreement).	• Identify emotions • Show you understand • Vent interfering emotions	• Names a feeling or emotion • Usually uses the word "you" or "you're" • May state cause of the emotion	• "You're pretty mad about it." • "You seem reluctant to talk about it." • "Sounds like you're excited."
Neutral phrase or question	A question or statement that encourages other to elaborate.	• Get other to tell more about a subject	• Few words • About subject under discussion	• "Tell me more." • "Please elaborate." • "Explain that." • "Amplify on that."
Brief assertion	A short statement, sound, or gesture, which shows involvement.	• Encourage other to continue • Increase receptivity	• Elicits additional information • Occurs automatically	• "Oh, okay." • "Yes, sure." • "I see." • Nodding your head.
Summary statements	A brief statement, in your own words, of the content of what was said.	• Check understanding • Prove you're listening • Give structure and direction • Help other clarify thinking • Invite other to comment or expand	• Summarizes content, not feelings • Restatement of essential ideas • In own words	• "So you disagree about..." • "The way you see it is..." • "You prefer working overtime..." • "Let me summarize how I..."
Close-ended questions	A question that limits the answer by requesting specific facts, or a "yes" or "no" answer.	• Find out details, specifics • Check understanding • Direct the discussion • Get other to take a stand	• Often starts with "Who," "Which," "When," "Where," "How many," etc. • Can sometimes be answered with a simple "yes" or "no"	• "Who is...?" • "Which order...?" • "When will you...?" • "Do you think...?"
Leading questions	A question that implies only one answer, or a rhetorical question—no answer is needed.	• Pin down positions or agreements • Can verify assumptions • Can be threatening	• The question gives the answer • No answer is required	• "Shouldn't we discuss...?" • "This is the best way to go, isn't it?"

Fig. 1-2 Probes and probing questions: The use of questions, statements, and pauses to elicit information, thoughts, and opinions. The type of question used elicits a characteristic response. (From Buzzotta VR, Lefton RE: *Dimensional management training*, St Louis, 1989, Psychological Associates.)

Applying this model when asking **open-ended** and **closed-ended questions** shows such questions to be equally balanced within Quadrant 4 (Q4). The goal of the PTA during supervision of the patient is to consistently demonstrate those qualities found in Q4; for example, being appropriately friendly, attentive, responsive, involved, exploring, analytical, and task oriented.

While supervising patients according to the Q4 model, the PTA must understand the differences between **prompting** and **cueing** a patient to perform a specific task. Prompting a patient to perform a task can be viewed as the presentation of a question. For example, when instructing a patient to ambulate with a standard walker, the assistant should prompt the patient by asking, "After you move the walker, what foot do you move next?" Prompting allows patients to decipher information, solve problems, and provide solutions to activities they must overcome during recovery. Cueing can be viewed as a direction. An example is, "After you move the walker, move your injured leg." Although the solution is provided for the patient, he or she must still demonstrate appropriate follow-through and proper understanding of the command.

MODIFICATIONS DURING TREATMENT

Using attentive Q4 behavior with balanced open-ended and closed-ended questioning of the patient helps the PTA identify and quantify changes in the patient's condition. After consulting the supervising PT and receiving direction, the PTA can effectively modify a specific intervention in accordance with changes in patient status.

The following example helps to clarify the scope of treatment modifications during postoperative rehabilitation after anterior cruciate ligament (ACL) reconstruction.

Swelling (joint effusion) after knee surgery is common and occurs in about 13% of cases after knee ligament surgery.[8] Usually the effusion is a hemarthrosis (blood within the joint, which can impair voluntary muscle contraction). In such a case the supervising PT provides baseline evaluation data about the degree of swelling present by making comparative circumferential measurements at midpatella, 2 inches superior to the midpatella, and 2 inches inferior to the midpatella. The PTA maintains daily records of the three comparative circumferential measurements. Because re-education and strengthening of muscle is influenced negatively by postoperative swelling, any increase or decrease in swelling necessitates a modification in the initial program outlined by the supervising PT. Thus the degree of swelling documented influences the adjustment made in the exercise prescription.

As the PTA identifies objective changes in the patient's status each day, the concept of visual, nonresponsive, and noninteractive supervision is altered to one of appropriate, responsive, and accountable supervision.

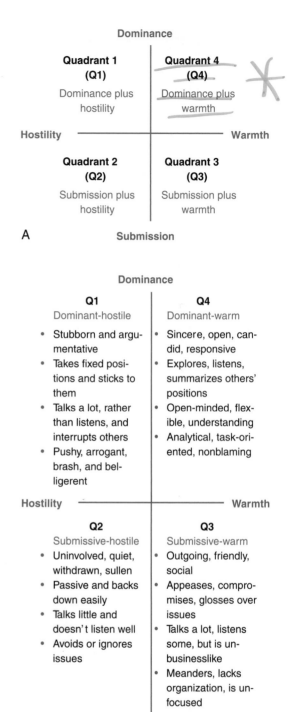

Fig. 1-3 A, The dimensional model: A tool to size up behavior. The model applies to subordinates, peers and superiors. Quadrants are formed among dominance, submission, hostility, and warmth that create certain patterns of behavior. **B,** Four distinct patterns and characteristics are formed between the four quadrants. (From Buzzotta VR, Lefton RE: *Dimensional management training*, St Louis, 1989, Psychological Associates.)

BOX 1-2

Knee Extension: Isotonic Exercise Modifications

If pain and swelling develop during full range of motion isotonic knee extension:

- Adjust the resistance. Reduce the amount of weight being used.
- Adjust the range of motion to limit full knee flexion: Example: Begin knee extension exercises from 45° of flexion or less instead of 90° or greater. Note: Some acute, chronic, and postsurgical conditions prohibit terminal knee extension (0°). In this case, limit full extension to −10° or greater.
- Adjust the speed or velocity of the performance of the exercise. Closely observe the speed of the exercise. Perform slow, controlled, nonballistic exercise.
- Adjust the volume of exercise.
  - Reduce the number of repetitions being performed.
  - Reduce the number of sets being performed.
  - Reduce the number of days per week performing the exercise.
- Change the performance of exercise.
  - Perform only isometric holds followed by eccentric loads. No concentric lifting.

Isometric exercises generally are used early in the rehabilitation of acute postoperative knee injuries. Concentric and eccentric exercises are introduced as rehabilitation proceeds. Concentric and eccentric exercises are defined as dynamic, producing work, and creating changes in joint angles and muscle length.[6] The progression from isometric to dynamic exercise produces an increase in force generated, increases muscle soreness, and causes greater articular stresses.[3] If swelling and pain increase as the patient progresses from isometric to concentric and eccentric contractions, the PTA, with direction and input from the supervising PT, can adjust or modify the program back to isometrics or reduce the amount of resistance, joint angle of exercise, volume of exercise, or velocity of movement. The specific sequence or combination of these modifications depends on the patient's specific needs, the surgical procedure, and the patient's tolerance to exercise. Usually it is prudent to begin with the least drastic change in exercise prescription and then progress (Box 1-2).

The clinical decision-making process used by the PTA involves recognizing that a problem exists, then taking orderly and specific steps to notify the supervising PT and adjust the program accordingly. Thus the PTA takes an active, participatory role while supervising patients, using his or her training and skills to the fullest extent.

Note that the recognition of changes in patient status does not imply interpretation of objective, measurable data by the PTA. The PTA's task is to provide information to the supervising PT on a daily basis, keep the supervising PT informed concerning patient status, and provide insightful and meaningful suggestions for modifications.

The objective data supplied to the supervising PT by the PTA may include but is not limited to goniometric measurements, circumferential measurements, manual muscle testing, endurance grading, heart rate, blood pressure, respirations, dynamic balance, and coordination measurements, according to the scope of the assistant's training.

UNDERSTANDING DIFFERENT PHILOSOPHIES OF PHYSICAL THERAPISTS

Fundamental differences exist among PTs concerning the methods, protocols, and directives they use to treat patients. In addition, just as the PTA is directed by the supervising PT, the PT may at times be directed by the physician. Within a hospital physical therapy department, the PTA may have contact with many supervising PTs, each with different backgrounds, experiences, and education. The PTA sees PTs use various protocols to manage the same pathologic condition. It is not the role of the PTA to change or modify treatment plans or protocols without the supervising PT's direction and approval. Opinions and controversies exist concerning how best to manage various orthopedic pathologic conditions. Changes in surgery and physical therapy occur because of advanced technology and rigorous research in rehabilitation medicine and orthopedic surgery. New procedures in arthroscopic ACL surgery allow a more rapid return to function, motion, and strength than ever before. Although ideally we presume all surgical procedures and rehabilitation techniques to be universally accepted, in fact the specialties of orthopedics and physical therapy are both art and science; therefore diversity is accepted.

The PTA can be placed in frustrating and confusing situations when dealing with various supervising PTs with different backgrounds and opinions concerning the management of patients. To minimize the confusing array of treatment protocols, the PTA must effectively and efficiently communicate with the supervising PT to clarify differences in patient care, always remembering that the PT has ultimate **responsibility** for the physical therapy interventions provided. The PTA does not divest interest in the care of any patient because of a disagreement in strategy with the supervising PT. The PTA's role requires a broader perspective and understanding that there are many ways to effectively manage the same pathology.

Having strong opinions on how to care for orthopedic patients is appropriate and shows passion, interest, and confidence in a certain method or protocol that has demonstrated good results. However, particular experience with the successful management of patients by one supervising PT may in fact conflict with the course of treatment prescribed by another. On the surface this situation may seem particularly frustrating and stressful. To better understand this difference the PTA must identify the key elements of disagreement and seek an appropriate explanation from the supervising PT. This gives each supervising PT the opportunity to teach and explain the rationale for the particular treatment and exposes the PTA to new information. The PTA then can observe and learn new methods that may actually prove equally or more successful than the previous plan of care.

Fully understanding the rationale and purpose of each selected intervention allows for improved delivery of service to the patient. During direct patient supervision the PTA can provide any selected interventions the supervising PT directs him or her to perform so long as allowed by law, and the safety and welfare of the patient are not compromised.

The well-adapted PTA views any apparent roadblocks as learning opportunities. The PTA is advised to take advantage of the broad knowledge and experience of many PTs, constantly inquire about the rationale and scientific basis for a particular program, and establish himself or herself as an eager learning participant who is open to innovative ways of managing various pathologic conditions.

❖ GLOSSARY

Accountability: Systematic, reliable, and appropriate investigative questioning, listening, and active participation at all levels of patient care.

Basic dimensional model: Two-dimensional model that consists of four behaviors (dominance, submission, hostility, and warmth), which fall into four quadrants. Q1 = dominance-hostility; Q2 = submission-hostility; Q3 = submission-warmth; and Q4 = dominance-warmth.

Closed-ended questions: Technique that requires a "yes" or "no" answer. This method effectively directs specific responses aimed at details of the patient's condition.

Communication: The exchange of information between people. To gather information relevant to the patient's problem; to establish rapport and to provide confidence. To facilitate understanding of the patient's problem to assist in comprehensive patient management.

Cueing: Can be viewed as a direction; although a solution is provided, appropriate follow-through and proper understanding of the direction(s) must be demonstrated.

Dominance: Exercising control or influence; being assertive; and putting one's idea forward.

Hostility: Defined as self-centered, unresponsive, and insensitive.

Listening: An effective communication tool. Demonstrates interest and concern for the patient and his or her individual needs.

Open-ended questions: Allows patients the opportunity to provide substantial information concerning their care. A technique to facilitate rapport and lets the patient see that the PTA is effectively listening.

Proactive: By using probing questions and appropriate communications skills, accountability, listening, and responsibility, the patient avoids being placed in a reactive position.

Probing questions: Techniques of questioning patients leading to insightful, rewarding, and responsive care.

Prompting: The presentation of a question; allows patients to decipher information, solve problems, and provide solutions to activities.

Responsibility: A component of active involvement of all areas of patient care.

Submission: Defined as following the lead of others, being passive and quick to comply.

Warmth: Defined as open-minded, responsive and sensitive.

REFERENCES

1. American Physical Therapy Association: *A normative model of physical therapist assistant education: version 2007*, Alexandria, Va, 2007, American Physical Therapy Association.
2. Buzzotta VR, Lefton RE: *Dimensional management training*, St Louis, 1989, Psychological Associates.
3. Kisner C, Colby LA: *Therapeutic exercise foundations and techniques*, ed 5, Philadelphia, 2007, FA Davis Company.
4. Lombardo P, Stolberg S: Interviewing and communication skills. In Ballweg R, Stolberg S, Sullivan EM, editors: *Physician assistant: a guide to clinical practice*, ed 4, Philadelphia, 2008, Saunders, pp258–274.
5. Lupi-Williams FA: The PTA, role and function: an analysis in three parts. Part I. Education, *Clin Manage Phys Ther* 3(3):35–38, 1983.
6. Nordin M, Frankel L: *Basic biomechanics of the musculoskeletal system*, ed 3, Baltimore, 2001, Lippincott Williams & Wilkins.
7. Payne M: *Teamwork in multiprofessional care*, Chicago, 2000, Lyceum.
8. Sacks RA, et al: Complications of knee ligament surgery. In Daniel D, Akeson W, O'Connor J, editors: *Knee ligaments structure: function, surgery and repair*, New York, 1990, Raven Press.
9. Servellen GV: *Communication skills for the health care professional: concepts, practice, and evidence*, ed 2, Sudbury, Mass, 2009, Jones and Bartlett.

REVIEW QUESTIONS

Short Answer

1. List five components of patient supervision.
2. Identify six members of the rehabilitation team who also may be involved with patient supervision.
3. Effective _____ is the hallmark of a great team and should be maximized.
4. Appropriate medical language used with the patient and his or her family helps to convey four things. What are they?
5. The PTA also must be aware that _____ is an effective communication tool.
6. Which type of probing question invites the patient to share feelings, thoughts, and opinions?

7. Which type of probing question is directed toward finding facts, obtaining specific responses, and filling in details?
8. Give three examples of open-ended probing questions that may be appropriate during the course of patient observation and interactive supervision.
9. Give three examples of closed-ended probing questions that may be appropriate during the course of patient observation and interactive supervision.
11. Give two examples of summary-type statements.
12. In the following figure, label and identify the components of the dimensional model and the quadrants formed by combining two dimensions.

13. Applying the dimensional model to the use of open-ended and closed-ended probing questions, which quadrant represents the behavioral goal of the PTA during patient supervision?

14. Give an example of prompting a patient to attempt a specific task.
15. Give an example of cueing a patient to attempt a specific task.

2 The Role of the Physical Therapist Assistant in Physical Assessment

Candy Bahner

LEARNING OBJECTIVES

1. Apply the language of the *Guide to Physical Therapist Practice* to physical assessment procedures.
2. Identify the common elements of examination, evaluation, and assessment.
3. Describe the role of the physical therapist assistant in the performance of physical assessment based on the physical therapy plan of care.
4. Discuss the role of the physical therapist assistant in data collection.
5. Explain methods of modifying the physical therapy plan of care or actions to be taken in response to physical assessment of the patient.
6. Identify critical elements to include with documentation of physical assessment.
7. Relate physical assessment to goals and outcomes of a physical therapy plan of care.

KEY TERMS

Centralization	Judgment	Trigger points
Evaluation	Peripheralization	Visceral pain
Examination	Referred pain	

CHAPTER OUTLINE

Thank you to Leigh Anne Boggs for her help in the writing of this chapter, which is based on work by Sandra Eskew Capps.

As any prospective or current student in the field of physical therapy is aware, changes in the profession are emerging rapidly. In an effort to bring physical therapy professionals to the "health care table" for discussion of legislative, regulatory, and reimbursement issues, the leaders of our profession are striving for standardization of terminology and recognition and application of evidence-based practice.[4] Needless to say, controversy or at least animated debate occurs among interested parties any time such an in-depth self-scrutiny of a profession takes place. One significant element of this debate in physical therapy revolves around the physical therapist assistant's (PTA's) role in the profession, including how the PTA participates in the administration of the physical therapy plan of care, including selected interventions, data collection techniques, and the terminology associated with the PTA's role. The purpose of this chapter is to summarize available standards and guidelines associated with the PTA's role in physical therapy treatments and to discuss techniques and implications of selected interventions and their associated data collection techniques to be utilized for the patient with a musculoskeletal condition.

AMERICAN PHYSICAL THERAPY ASSOCIATION GUIDING DOCUMENTS

Guide to Physical Therapist Practice, Second Edition

The *Guide to Physical Therapist Practice*, second edition (the *Guide*) is a tool that was developed by the American Physical Therapy Association in part to "…describe physical therapist practice in general; …standardize terminology used in and related to physical therapist practice; …delineate preferred practice patterns that will help physical therapists…promote appropriate utilization of health care services; [and] increase efficiency and reduce unwarranted variation in the provision of services…."[4] The stated purpose of the *Guide* reads, in part, that it is: "…a resource not only for physical therapist clinicians, educators, researchers, and students, but [for] health care policy makers, administrators, managed care providers, third-party payers,

and other professionals."[4] According to the *Guide*, the definition of the PTA is: "A technically educated health care provider who assists the physical therapist in the provision of selected physical therapy interventions."[4] **Assessment** is defined as "The measurement or quantification of a variable or the placement of a value on something."[4] Further, the *Guide* states, "Assessment should not be confused with examination or evaluation."[4] **Examination** involves preliminary gathering of data and performing various screens, tests, and measures to obtain a comprehensive base from which to make decisions about physical therapy needs for each individual patient, including the possibility of referral to another health care provider. **Evaluation** is the specific process reserved solely for the physical therapist (PT), in which clinical **judgments** are made from this base of data obtained during the examination.[4]

Standards of Ethical Conduct for the Physical Therapist Assistant

The Standards of Ethical Conduct for the Physical Therapist Assistant is a tool developed by the American Physical Therapy Association to delineate the ethical obligations of all PTAs.[7] There are eight standards of ethical conduct for the PTA and they can be found in the "Membership and Leadership" section on APTA website (www.apta.org).

Professionalism in Physical Therapy: Core Values

The American Physical Therapy Association has also developed a list of values, known as *core values*, which reflect what one would call a professional in physical therapy. The core values include: accountability, altruism, compassion/caring, excellence, integrity, professional duty, and social responsibility.[3] Each core value, along with its corresponding definition as defined by the APTA, can be found in the "Practice" section on the APTA website.

The Clinical Performance Instrument

The Clinical Performance Instrument (CPI), a uniform clinical education grading tool developed by the American Physical Therapy Association,[5] includes the following criteria related to the PTA's role in clinical problem solving and judgments, data collection, and assessment techniques:

- "Participates in patient status judgments* within the clinical environment based on the plan of care established by the physical therapist." (criterion #9)
- "Obtains accurate information by performing selected data collection† consistent with the plan of care established by the physical therapist." (criterion #10)
- "Discusses the need for modifications to the plan of care established by the physical therapist." (criterion #11)

A Normative Model of Physical Therapist Assistant Education: Version 2007 *Capte*

A Normative Model of Physical Therapist Assistant Education: Version 2007[2] (the *Model*) is a consensus-based document developed by the American Physical Therapy Association. Briefly, the *Model* was designed to provide a representation of all of the elements that provide the foundation for the development and evaluation of educational programs preparing PTAs.[2] According to the *Model*, PTAs, "...implement selected components of patient/client interventions and obtain data related to that intervention; make modifications in selected interventions either to progress the patient/client as directed by the physical therapist or to ensure patient/client safety and comfort."[2]

Interestingly, the *Model* includes the following five physical therapy performance expectation themes:

1. Interventions — Therex, ultra
2. Communication— Affected behaviors, Communication style
3. Education — understanding PT Journal
4. Resource Management— Don't waist stuff
5. Career Development[2] — interview skills, Resume

The Interventions physical therapy performance expectation theme is subdivided into the following seven sections:

- Plan of Care Review
- Provision of Procedural Interventions
- Patient/Client Instruction
- Patient/Client Progression
- Data Collection
- Documentation
- Emergency Response[2]

---

*The following definition for the term *judgments* is offered in the glossary of the CPI: "Decisions made within the clinical environment that are based on the established physical therapy plan of care. With consideration toward safety, a problem-solving process is applied that includes decision rules (e.g., codes, protocols), thinking, data collection, and interpretation."[5]

†*Data collection skills* are defined as "those processes/procedures used to gather information through observation, measurement, subjective, objective, and functional findings; progression toward goals; and interpretive processes/procedures applied to formulate a judgment/decision within the plan of care established by the physical therapist." The definition also states that [data collection skills] "must be integrated to achieve the most effective interventions and optimal outcomes."[5]

Each performance expectation theme includes educational outcomes, terminal behavioral objectives, and instructional objectives to be achieved in the classroom and clinic.

Frequently, the response to the question about the difference between PTs and PTAs is simply, "PTAs don't do evaluations." Considering the elements of judgment and decision making involved with evaluation and from the preceding discussion, does this imply that the PTA does not exercise judgment or make decisions? Of course not. However, the judgments and subsequent decisions of the PTA are made within the context of the existing physical therapy plan of care, established by the supervising PT through the examination and evaluation process. This process occurs on an ongoing basis.[23] Without effective data collection and reporting by the PTA, the PT would lack key information on which this data management process relies.[23]

It may be helpful to consider the functions of data collection and patient management as integral parts of managing a patient's physical therapy case, which is a dynamic process as illustrated in the APTA's "Problem-Solving Algorithm Utilized by PTAs in Patient/Client Intervention" (see Figure 1-1).[2]

This discussion of specific assessment techniques and issues begins with two conditions frequently encountered among patients with musculoskeletal involvement: inflammation and pain.

INFLAMMATION

What Is Inflammation?

Inflammation is a living organism's first response to injury or disruption of normal processes. It is a normal response, and actually can be considered the body's immediate trigger for healing. Inflammation involves the responses of several body constituents, including vascular components, fluid and semifluid (humoral) substances, and neurologic and cellular reactions. Inflammation that does not resolve within expected time frames may develop into a chronic state (as a result of either abnormality in the individual's immune or inflammatory response or as a result of prolonged, continuous, or repeated exposure to the injurious agent). Chronic inflammation (considered a pathologic condition) may result in secondary complications or permanent changes in the makeup of the involved tissue, including scarring or granulomatosis. Two important factors must be kept in mind: that inflammation is a normal and necessary response to trigger tissue healing, and that unresolved (chronic) inflammation may lead to permanent and undesired tissue changes. Therefore it is imperative for the PTA to monitor changes in the inflammatory response of the area being treated. In addition, extreme changes in the appearance of inflammation may signal the onset of serious complications, necessitating further evaluation by the PT or, in some cases, referral to the physician for immediate medical evaluation.

As discussed elsewhere in this book, certain physical agents are employed to control (but not eliminate) the acute inflammatory response or accelerate it, thus moving the healing process along. Depending on the degree of inflammation present, certain physical agents may be contraindicated. So how does the PTA differentiate between normal inflammation and an inflammatory reaction indicating the potential for contraindicated procedures or serious complications?

The commonly accepted and normal (cardinal) signs and symptoms of inflammation are localized heat, redness, swelling, and pain with a resultant loss of function in the injured area. Temperature and redness are discussed here in relation to the PTA's role in collecting data and communicating concerns appropriately to the PT. The discussion of the assessment of edema and pain are discussed in separate sections.

— w/ TheraEx, shouldn't cause (need to back off)

General Contraindications and Precautions with Inflammation

In general, remember that inflammation is a reaction to tissue trauma or injury; the increased inflammatory reactions after exercise or other interventions may indicate that the intervention is too aggressive or contraindicated, resulting in new trauma or injury to healing tissues. Furthermore, responses to interventions between visits must also be assessed; a patient may report signs of increased inflammation up to 48 hours after an injury or intervention, particularly after administration of exercise or manual stretching techniques.[19]

Acute versus Chronic

Under normal circumstances, signs of acute inflammation persist for 4 to 6 days, assuming the precipitating condition, agent, or event is removed. In the initial 48 hours after tissue injury, the observable signs of inflammation are associated with the normal inflammatory vascular response to trauma.[19] An important distinction to make is the definition of acute versus chronic in relation to the actual cause of injury or trauma. It is common for sources to refer to these tissue states in terms of time frames only, with the acute phase lasting 4 to 6 days and the chronic phase lasting 6 months to 1 year.[19] A more useful way to consider inflammation incorporates the concept of whether there is real or impending tissue damage present. The significance of this designation relates to the PTA's role in determining whether, based on the stage of inflammation present, certain interventions may be implemented or are contraindicated.[28] If an intervention normally results in an inflammatory reaction, it is contraindicated when the tissue is in an acute inflammatory state that indicates ongoing tissue damage. For example, in the presence of acute inflammation (indicating an active state of injury, tissue damage, or early tissue healing), dynamic resistance exercises are contraindicated.[19] However, the PTA also may proceed with interventions included in the plan of care that accelerate the inflammatory process if it has been determined that the original causal agent or condition no longer results in ongoing tissue damage. Contraindications related to specific diagnoses or associated with the application of specific physical agents are discussed elsewhere in this book.

During interventions involving range of motion (ROM) activities, the PTA also may note that the patient reports pain before tissue resistance is felt (before end ROM); this is an indication of acute inflammation.[19] Pain reported at the same time end ROM is reached is indicative of a subacute inflammatory state, and pain reported as a stretching sensation at the limit of ROM is a sign of inflammation in the chronic state.[19] If the PTA determines that the established plan of care includes interventions that are not appropriate for the apparent stage of inflammation, the PT must be consulted to adjust goals, time frames, or possibly the plan itself to ensure that the treatment does not contribute to a prolonged or abnormal state of inflammation.

TEMPERATURE

The PTA must be able to differentiate between expected temperature responses in a normal inflammatory response versus abnormal responses. A normal increase in temperature is local and initially mild to moderate (compared with the contralateral anatomic region) versus a more pervasive change, which may manifest as significant either as compared with the contralateral side or as a systemic increase in temperature (fever). In the former case joint effusion may be present; the latter may represent a systemic response to the injury (e.g., infection) or an unrelated condition, such as an acute disease process (e.g., flu). Either of these situations warrants action on the part of the PTA. In the presence of systemic infection, the patient's ability to participate in the physical therapy plan is affected. Because of the exclusive one-on-one time traditionally associated with physical therapy care, it is not uncommon for the PTA to be the member of the health care team who provides important pieces to the puzzle of the patient's total health or illness picture.

Both the degree of temperature elevation and duration of fever are relevant to diagnostic processes when elevated body temperature is evident. During the initial examination and evaluation, any abnormality in temperature, either locally or systemically, should be noted. The PTA's role is then to note deviations from the examination findings, determine the length of time the fever has been present (through patient interview) and note other possible related signs and symptoms: rash, cough, complaints of sore throat, and so on. Also it should be noted if the patient reports any pattern of temperature changes, because this may have diagnostic implications for the PT or physician. Immediate implications include whether or not exercise or other interventions may be contraindicated and to what extent infection control issues must be addressed. Normal adult body temperature (oral measurement) ranges from 96.8° F to 99.5° F (36° C to 37.5° C).[26] Temperature is affected by factors including age, time of day, emotions/stress, exercise, menstrual cycle, pregnancy, external environment, measurement site, and ingestion of warm or cold foods.[26] Clinical signs and symptoms of fever vary based on the underlying cause and stage and may include general malaise, headache, increased pulse and respiratory rates, general chills, shivering, piloerection, loss of appetite, pale skin, nausea, irritability, restlessness, constipation, sweating, thirst, coated tongue, decreased urinary output, insomnia, and weakness.[26] In the case of the presence of fever, the PTA must gather the related data, document it, and report it to the supervising PT. The data and report should include adequate information to enable the PT to respond appropriately, either in terms of immediate modification to the physical therapy plan of care or consultation with the medical team.

Fever and Infection Control

As always, the PTA must attend to his or her responsibility of exercising appropriate precautions for both the patient and himself or herself. The importance of hand washing by the caregiver and patient cannot be overstated as an effective means of controlling the transmission of infectious agents. In addition, treatment areas should be properly cleaned and disinfected as a routine procedure, not only in the case of patients with obvious infectious conditions. (Detailed information and guidelines for handwashing in the health care setting can be found on the website of the Centers for Disease Control and Prevention).

Fever and Exercise

In terms of exercise precautions, discretionary caution should be applied with any patient with a fever, because of stresses on the cardiopulmonary and immune systems and the possible further complications related to dehydration.[14] The PTA must be familiar with specific exercise techniques (e.g., aquatic exercise) contraindicated in the presence of diseases transmitted via water or air.

Fever and Lymph Nodes

Another condition that may become readily apparent to the PTA in the course of carrying out elements of the physical therapy plan of care is tenderness or exquisite pain in particular regions of the body. The presence of tender or enlarged lymph nodes is of particular concern to the PTA who is performing soft-tissue interventions on a patient with an elevated body temperature (or otherwise). Figure 2-1 provides a visual reference for the location of lymph nodes. PTAs using hands-on techniques such as soft-tissue massage and manual stretching are incidentally afforded the opportunity during the course of treatment to assess for the presence of unusual conditions in areas of lymph node clusters (e.g., in the neck and axilla). Because these symptoms can signify the presence of potentially serious pathologic conditions, the presence of pain, tenderness or enlargement of lymph nodes are situations in which the PTA must consult with the supervising PT to pursue medical follow-up for definitive diagnosis.[14] In addition, certain interventions are considered contraindicated if the patient has an underlying pathology related to changes in the lymph nodes.

REDNESS AND SKIN COLOR CHANGES

Redness (erythema) is a normal component of the inflammatory reaction. The PTA must be alert to abnormal or unexpected changes in skin color, which may indicate the presence of secondary complications or underlying pathologies. Redness may be considered normal when it is noted in the immediate area of injury and is associated with local temperature changes. Depending on the patient's pigmentation, color changes may appear in tones other than red.

Unexpected findings in terms of changes in skin color should be reported to the supervising PT for further evaluation. These changes include rashes or redness that appear as a streak originating from the site of injury. Red streaks may indicate an acute inflammation caused by a bacterial infection (streptococci, staphylococci, or both), resulting in acute inflammation of the lymph vessels.[14] Redness along with superficial tenderness and hardness (induration) of the area may be a sign of superficial thrombophlebitis.[14] These findings should be reported to the supervising PT because they may be a precursor to more serious conditions. A loss of skin color (paleness or pallor) associated with temperature changes, edema, or pain may be indicative of an occlusion in a blood vessel and warrants immediate medical referral. A commonly used quick assessment technique to rule out the presence of a deep vein thrombosis (DVT) is Homans' sign, performed by gentle passive stretching of the ankle into full dorsiflexion and assessing for pain in the calf. Some clinicians also incorporate a gentle squeezing of calf musculature during the passive dorsiflexion to assess for tenderness. Other structures that are stretched during this test include the calf muscles and the Achilles tendon; thus a positive Homans' sign may be noted in error if a patient has tightness or inflammation of these

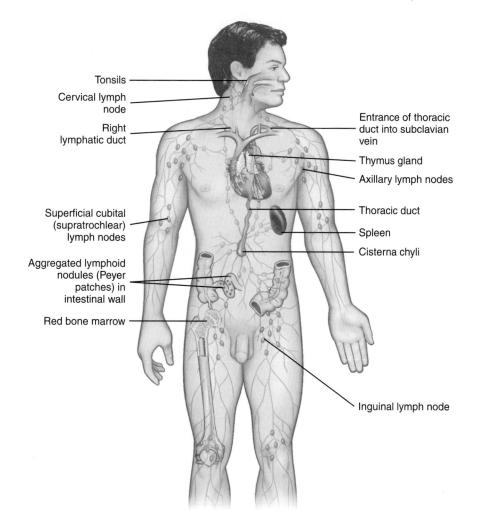

Tonsils

Cervical lymph node

Right lymphatic duct

Superficial cubital (supratrochlear) lymph nodes

Aggregated lymphoid nodules (Peyer patches) in intestinal wall

Red bone marrow

Entrance of thoracic duct into subclavian vein

Thymus gland

Axillary lymph nodes

Thoracic duct

Spleen

Cisterna chyli

Inguinal lymph node

Fig. 2-1 Location of lymph vessels and nodes. Note clusters of nodes in axilla and groin areas. (From Patton KT, Thibodeau GA: *Anatomy and physiology*, ed 7, St Louis, 2010, Mosby.)

structures. Although Homans' sign is still commonly assessed, it is considered an insensitive and nonspecific test, and is present in less than one third of all patients with a documented DVT, and more than 50% of patients with a positive Homans' sign do not have evidence of venous thrombosis.[14] Furthermore, a serious potential complication of a DVT is that a piece of the coagulated blood (the clot) may break free from the inside of the vessel wall as a result of the test (or otherwise) and travel through the bloodstream, lodging in a pulmonary artery, causing a life-threatening condition (pulmonary embolism). Therefore it is recommended that the PTA refrain from conducting the Homans' test and be alert to the risk factors and the clinical signs and symptoms of a DVT as outlined in Box 2-1 and report these findings to the supervising PT for further investigation and possible immediate medical referral. The PTA should note that signs and symptoms are the same for a PE and a DVT.

Furthermore, the PTA should be aware of differences in superficial skin changes based on the patient's skin color.

In other words, these findings in individuals with darkly pigmented skin may be less obvious and do not manifest as the same changes in skin tones as with light-skinned individuals. A critical element to be included in the lab practice and skill development of the PTA student is exposure to a number of normal subjects of different body types, skin tones, and so on (often represented within a classroom population of adult learners). By observing and practicing on different subjects, the PTA student develops an awareness of normal variations, which will subsequently enhance his or her ability to recognize differences or abnormalities in a patient population.

EDEMA

Because edema and its management have significant implications in the practice of physical therapy, the entry-level PTA should develop the ability to recognize the signs and symptoms of edema, and to effectively and efficiently measure and document it.

BOX 2-1

Risk Factors and Clinical Signs and Symptoms for Deep Venous Thrombosis (DVT)

RISK FACTORS
Previous personal/family history of thromboembolism
Congestive heart failure
Age (older than 50 years)
Oral contraceptive use
Blood Stasis
Immobilization or inactivity
■ Burns
■ Obstetric/gynecologic conditions
■ Obesity
■ Spinal cord injured, stroke
Endothelial Injury
Neoplasm
Recent surgical procedures
Trauma or fracture of the legs or pelvis
Blood disorders (e.g., hypercoagulable state, clotting abnormalities)
History of infection, diabetes mellitus
Oral contraceptive use

CLINICAL SIGNS AND SYMPTOMS
Superficial Venous Thrombosis
Subcutaneous venous distention
Palpable cord
Warmth, redness
Indurated (hard)
Deep Venous Thrombosis
Unilateral tenderness or leg pain
Unilateral swelling (difference in leg circumference)
Warmth
Discoloration
Pain with placement of blood pressure cuff around calf inflated to 160 mm Hg to 180 mm Hg

From Goodman CC, Snyder TE: *Differential diagnosis for physical therapists screening for referral*, St. Louis, 2007, Saunders Elsevier, p. 312.

For purposes of this text, the focus is on localized edema, resulting from injury or trauma to musculoskeletal tissue or structures. Other terms and conditions are defined or discussed in relation to the PTA's responsibility in the event unrelated or unexpected conditions are discovered.

Edema refers to excessive pooling of fluid in the spaces between tissues (interstitial spaces).[14] In relation to patients with orthopedic injuries or conditions, the main consideration for assessment by the PTA is measurement of the edematous part or extremity. Typically, the technique used to measure edema in an extremity is straightforward—use of a tape measure to obtain circumferential dimensions of the involved part. The data must be reliable and the measurement reproducible, regardless of who is conducting the assessment. To ensure this level of consistency, the PTA must use precisely the same landmarks as the evaluating PT. Specifically, palpable bony landmarks must be used as the starting standard reference point; then circumferential measurements can be taken at determined distances from that point. For example, to measure the lower leg, circumference measured with the tape measure at the inferior pole of the patella may be used as a reference point, with measurements then taken every 2 inches distally and at the ankle. One note of caution, the PTA must be careful to not pull the tape measure too tight when performing this skill. The skin should not have an indention if performing correctly. An example of a flow chart for recording

Table 2-1	Sample Format for Documenting Edema	
UE	**Right**	**Left**
Axilla	_____inches	_____inches
4″ above elbow	_____inches	_____inches
2″ above elbow	_____inches	_____inches
Elbow*	_____inches	_____inches
2″ below elbow	_____inches	_____inches
4″ below elbow	_____inches	_____inches
Wrist*	_____inches	_____inches

*A standard for elbow could be from the cubital fossa around the elbow, crossing the olecranon process; a standard for wrist could be just distal to the radial and ulnar styloid processes.

circumferential measurements of the upper extremity is provided in Table 2-1.

A figure-of-eight technique may be used at the ankle to ascertain a gross estimate of generalized ankle edema.[12,22,31] Refer to Box 2-2 for the steps involved in this procedure.

Another technique used to obtain a quantitative measure of edema in a limb involves immersing the limb into a specially designed container of fluid (a volumeter) and measuring the amount of water displaced.[20] Karges and colleagues[17] established correlations between different techniques of volumetric measurement but also emphasized the importance of ensuring reliability of the data

BOX 2-2

Technique for Figure-of-Eight Edema Measurement of Ankle

1. Position the patient in a long sitting position so that the lower leg is supported and the ankle is in a neutral position.
2. Mark the following landmarks with a skin pencil: tuberosity of the navicular (palpable projection on the anteromedial aspect of the hindfoot); base of the fifth metatarsal; distal tip of the medial malleolus; distal tip of the lateral malleolus; and tibialis anterior tendon.
3. Place the (0) edge of the tape measure midway between the tibialis anterior tendon and the lateral malleolus.
4. Wrap the tape medially across the instep (bottom surface of the foot), and place just distal to the navicular tuberosity.
5. Draw the tape across the arch of the foot, winding it back to the dorsum of the foot just proximal to the tuberosity (base) of the fifth metatarsal.
6. Cross back over the tibialis anterior tendon.
7. Wrap the tape measure around the ankle, drawing it just distal to the tip of the medial malleolus, crossing the calcaneal (Achilles) tendon and drawing the tape measure just distal to the lateral malleolus, back to the starting point.
8. For consistency, it is recommended that this process be repeated three times, with the average of the three measurements recorded.

Adapted from Magee DJ: *Orthopedic physical assessment*, ed 5, St. Louis, 2008, Saunders Elsevier; Tatro-Adams D, McGann S, Carbone W: Reliability of the figure-of-eight method on subjects with ankle joint swelling, *J Orthop Sports Phys Ther* 22(4):161-163, 1995; Esterson PS: Measurement of ankle joint swelling using a figure of 8, *J Orthop Sports Phys Ther* 1(1):51-52, 1979.

for a given patient, in terms of employing a consistent technique for edema measurement of the same patient. In other words, as stated, the PTA must use the method of measurement, employing the same technique chosen by the evaluating PT.[17,20]

In addition to a quantitative measurement of edema through circumferential measurement or volumetrics, data relating to the quality of edema should be collected and documented by the PTA. Characteristics of edema that may be observed are described as *brawny* or *pitting*. Brawny edema refers to edema that feels hard, tough, or thick and leathery. This indurated quality is frequently associated with chronic inflammation or systemic pathologies involving fluid shift abnormalities (e.g., congestive heart failure [CHF]). Pitting edema is characterized by the formation of a sustained indentation when the swollen area is compressed.[9,16] Pitting

Table 2-2	Scale for Rating Pitting Edema
Rating	**Characteristics**
1+	Barely perceptible depression
2+	Easily identified depression; depression takes +15 seconds for tissue to rebound
3+	Depression takes 15 to 30 seconds to rebound
4+	Depression lasts for 30 seconds or more

From Kloth L, McCulloch J: *Wound healing: alternatives in management*, Philadelphia, 2002, FA Davis.

edema may be further quantified according to the scale in Table 2-2.

Unlike transient inflammatory reactions that may normally occur in response to certain physical therapy interventions, a significant increase in edema should be regarded as abnormal and reported accordingly. Upon first noticing edema in the extremity being treated, the PTA must determine if the swelling is confined to the involved extremity or if the contralateral extremity is also involved. If the opposite extremity is also edematous, this finding could indicate a systemic pathologic condition.[14] For example, bilateral pitting edema of the distal lower extremities is a common manifestation in CHF, a relatively common diagnosis encountered among individuals with cardiac disease and those older than 65 years of age. Because this pathology is common among a significant population and it develops gradually, the PTA may play an important role in the diagnostic process via astute recognition of signs and symptoms associated with the onset of CHF. In addition to bilateral lower extremity pitting edema, the PTA also may note a decrease in tolerance to exercise (fatigue, shortness of breath, and muscle weakness). The presence of this clinical response necessitates prompt consultation with the supervising PT for medical diagnostic workup and possible subsequent modifications to the physical therapy plan of care.

A potentially serious condition involving edema is compartment syndrome. This condition occurs in anatomic compartments (of the calf or, less frequently, the antebrachium) as a result of increased fluids in an area tightly bound by fascia. Because fascia does not "give" to allow more space to accommodate this fluid buildup, this edema can compress nerves and blood vessels as they course through the compartment, leading to ischemia and possible nerve damage. Because the edema is contained within the compartment, the PTA should be alert to other associated signs and symptoms: history of blunt trauma, crush injury, or unaccustomed exercise; severe, persistent leg pain that is intensified when a stretch is applied to the involved muscles; swelling, severe tenderness, and palpable tension of the involved structures; paresthesia, paresis, and pulselessness.[8] Immediate consultation with the supervising PT and possibly immediate medical referral are warranted if the signs and symptoms are noted.

PAIN

An important skill that novice clinicians must develop along the path to entry-level competence is to attend to the patient as a whole being, with the various elements being assessed working together to produce full function. It is crucial for the PTA to collect data about the patient's pain responses and behaviors throughout each patient interaction. A common behavior of a novice clinician performing basic assessment and data collection skills is for the clinician to focus only on the involved body part and overlook the overall response of the patient to specific procedures. For example, a patient may exhibit strength of the quadriceps muscle group that measures 4+/5. However, if the student PTA performing the assessment of strength fails to observe that the patient is grimacing in pain during the resisted isometric test, he or she is overlooking an important determinant of true function of the muscle group. Likewise, other components of function, such as ROM and flexibility, must include pain-free performance to be wholly functional. Ideally the PTA student will make the transition from focusing only on the involved body part during assessment procedures and interventions, to performing assessments that include comprehensive observation of the patient's responses and behaviors.

Pain is considered subjective, but because there are multiple internal factors that determine a patient's perception of pain, complaints of pain always should be addressed as legitimate or "real." The PTA's role in assessing pain is to gather data that present a clear picture of the following:

■ Changes in pain since last physical therapy visit or examination
■ Responses of the patient in terms of how interventions to date or at present affect pain
■ Patterns of pain (e.g., physical or temporal)
■ Modalities, types, or characteristics of pain (e.g., sharp or burning)

Several standardized instruments are available to record findings of pain assessment. As with all assessment and data collection techniques, the PTA must use the same instrument or same technique for recording data related to a patient's pain complaints as was used by the supervising PT during the initial examination. Simple and commonly used tools are pain rating scales and visual analog scales that can be seen in Figures 2-2, 2-3, and 2-4.

During the course of carrying out elements of the supervising PT's plan of care, the PTA may notice a change in the quality of a patient's pain from more acute to chronic pain. As described in the section on inflammation, a chronic state is one in which the symptoms (pain in this case) persist for a period of time longer than expected, based on physiologic principles of tissue healing. Chronic pain has been described as that which lasts more than 3 months.[24] Recall also that one descriptive feature of a chronic condition relates to the lack of real, ongoing, or pending tissue damage. In regard to pain, this circumstance also often coincides with complaints of pain that are nonspecific, diffuse, or indirectly proportional to the physical appearance or presentation of the patient.

In this case the PTA's documentation or other interaction with the supervising PT may assist the therapist in making appropriate changes in the goals and plan of care to address the pain by incorporating interventions that will attend to the more complex issues involved with chronic pain. Specifically, depression and a cycle involving decreased activity levels and associated decreased tolerance to activity often ensues with chronic pain. The PTA may ask the supervising PT about the possible inclusion of relaxation exercises and a comprehensive gradual conditioning program in this case. Furthermore, when the PTA notices that a patient is exhibiting signs and symptoms of chronic pain, further diagnostic workup may be indicated by the supervising PT, because the presence of chronic pain may signal involvement of systems or factors other than musculoskeletal structures (e.g., depression).

Certain changes that occur in complaints of pain in response to therapeutic interventions are expected. **Peripheralization** may indicate a worsening or progressive condition. A typical example of this occurs with a progressively herniating spinal disk, indicating increasing compression of the associated nerve root. **Centralization** of pain symptoms may indicate improvement of the condition, such as in the case of decreasing compression on a nerve root as a disk herniation is reduced.

The PTA must establish the location of pain when the patient reports changes in pain symptoms associated with certain positions or movements. For example, the patient with a primary diagnosis of low back pain secondary to herniated nucleus pulposus may complain of pain when lying prone. The PTA must not assume that the pain is in the area of the disk lesion, which is a positive indication of centralization and a desired response. If, on further questioning, it is determined that the pain is referred to the lower extremity along the neural distribution for the involved spinal segment, then this is a sign of peripheralization of the symptoms, indicating that the prone position is not appropriate at this time. Thus the importance of understanding neuromuscular anatomy and function cannot be overlooked. The PTA student must become familiar with these anatomic relationships to fully understand the implications of data collected during pain assessment.

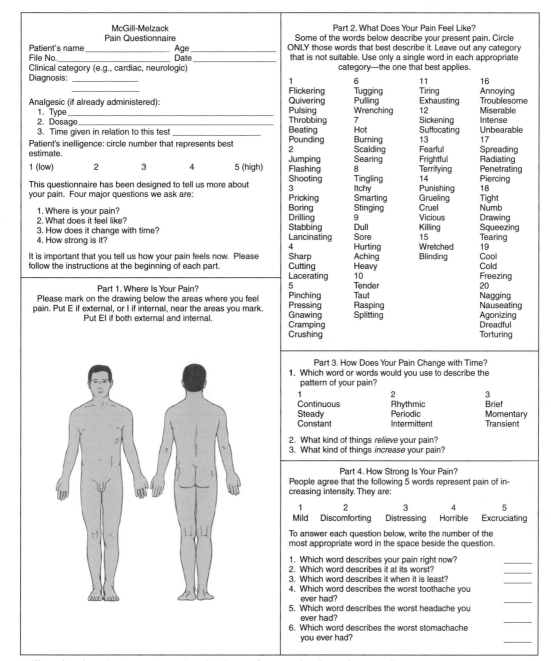

McGill-Melzack
Pain Questionnaire

Patient's name _____ Age _____
File No. _____ Date _____
Clinical category (e.g., cardiac, neurologic)
Diagnosis: _____

_____

Analgesic (if already administered):
　1. Type _____
　2. Dosage _____
　3. Time given in relation to this test _____

Patient's inelligence: circle number that represents best
estimate.

1 (low)　　　　2　　　　3　　　　4　　　　5 (high)

This questionnaire has been designed to tell us more about
your pain. Four major questions we ask are:

　1. Where is your pain?
　2. What does it feel like?
　3. How does it change with time?
　4. How strong is it?

It is important that you tell us how your pain feels now. Please
follow the instructions at the beginning of each part.

Part 1. Where Is Your Pain?
Please mark on the drawing below the areas where you feel
pain. Put E if external, or I if internal, near the areas you mark.
Put EI if both external and internal.

Part 2. What Does Your Pain Feel Like?
Some of the words below describe your present pain. Circle
ONLY those words that best describe it. Leave out any category
that is not suitable. Use only a single word in each appropriate
category—the one that best applies.

1	6	11	16
Flickering	Tugging	Tiring	Annoying
Quivering	Pulling	Exhausting	Troublesome
Pulsing	Wrenching	12	Miserable
Throbbing	7	Sickening	Intense
Beating	Hot	Suffocating	Unbearable
Pounding	Burning	13	17
2	Scalding	Fearful	Spreading
Jumping	Searing	Frightful	Radiating
Flashing	8	Terrifying	Penetrating
Shooting	Tingling	14	Piercing
3	Itchy	Punishing	18
Pricking	Smarting	Grueling	Tight
Boring	Stinging	Cruel	Numb
Drilling	9	Vicious	Drawing
Stabbing	Dull	Killing	Squeezing
Lancinating	Sore	15	Tearing
4	Hurting	Wretched	19
Sharp	Aching	Blinding	Cool
Cutting	Heavy		Cold
Lacerating	10		Freezing
5	Tender		20
Pinching	Taut		Nagging
Pressing	Rasping		Nauseating
Gnawing	Splitting		Agonizing
Cramping			Dreadful
Crushing			Torturing

Part 3. How Does Your Pain Change with Time?
1. Which word or words would you use to describe the
　 pattern of your pain?

1	2	3
Continuous	Rhythmic	Brief
Steady	Periodic	Momentary
Constant	Intermittent	Transient

2. What kind of things *relieve* your pain?
3. What kind of things *increase* your pain?

Part 4. How Strong Is Your Pain?
People agree that the following 5 words represent pain of increasing intensity. They are:

1	2	3	4	5
Mild	Discomforting	Distressing	Horrible	Excruciating

To answer each question below, write the number of the
most appropriate word in the space beside the question.

1. Which word describes your pain right now? _____
2. Which word describes it at its worst? _____
3. Which word describes it when it is least? _____
4. Which word describes the worst toothache you
　 ever had? _____
5. Which word describes the worst headache you
　 ever had? _____
6. Which word describes the worst stomachache
　 you ever had? _____

Fig. 2-2 **McGill-Melzack Pain Questionnaire.** (Redrawn from Melzack R: The McGill Pain Questionnaire: major properties and scoring methods, *Pain* 1:277, 1975. In Clayton BD: *Basic pharmacology for nurses,* ed 15, St Louis, 2010, Mosby.)

"Red Flag" Pain Symptoms

The PTA must also be keenly aware of pain that sends a "red flag" signal. In this case, the PTA should not proceed with any interventions or data collection techniques that are potentially contraindicated and should immediately report the findings to the supervising PT. Table 2-3 presents a summary of red flag or potentially serious pain conditions and the possible associated pathology or body system.

In addition to knowing the red flag symptoms described here, the PTA working with any client must be alert to signs and symptoms of myocardial infarction (MI, heart attack). Certain patterns of pain have been identified as early warning signs of a heart attack (Fig. 2-5). The PTA working with a patient exhibiting any of these patterns of pain should consult with the supervising PT right away for possible immediate medical referral. Concurrent symptoms of MI may include nausea, pallor, and profuse perspiration. Myocardial infarction may occur over a period of time and may be experienced while the patient is undergoing exertion or even at rest.

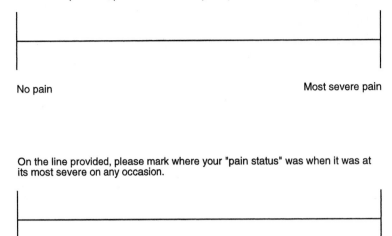

On the line provided, please mark where your "pain status" is today.

No pain   Most severe pain

On the line provided, please mark where your "pain status" was when it was at its most severe on any occasion.

No pain   Most severe pain

Fig. 2-3 Visual analog scales for pain. (From Magee DJ: *Orthopedic physical assessment*, ed 4, Philadelphia, 2002, Saunders.)

Instructions:
Below is a thermometer with various grades of pain on it from "No pain at all" to "The pain is almost unbearable." Put an × by the words that describe your pain best. Mark how bad your pain is AT THIS MOMENT IN TIME.

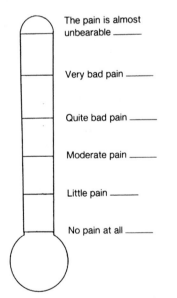

The pain is almost unbearable _____

Very bad pain _____

Quite bad pain _____

Moderate pain _____

Little pain _____

No pain at all _____

Fig. 2-4 Thermometer pain rating scale. (From Brodie DJ, Burnett JV, Walker JM, et al: Evaluation of low back pain by patient questionnaires and therapeutic assessment, *J Orthop Sports Phys Ther* 11:528, 1990.)

Table 2-3	*Red Flag Pain Symptoms*
Pathology or Body System	**Pain Complaint or Symptom**
Cardiovascular	Pain or feeling of heaviness in the chest
	Pulsating pain anywhere in the body
	Constant and severe pain in lower leg
Cancer	Persistent pain at night or pain that awakens patient
	Constant pain unrelieved by change in position or activity
Gastrointestinal	Frequent or severe abdominal pain
Neurologic	Frequent or severe headaches

Adapted from Magee DJ: *Orthopedic physical assessment*, ed 5, St. Louis, 2008, Saunders; Stith JS, Sahrmann SA, Dixon KK, et al: Curriculum to prepare diagnosticians in physical therapy, *J Phys Ther Educ* 9:50, 1995.

Intermittent Claudication

Another distinct pattern or type of pain that may manifest coincidentally with musculoskeletal symptoms or conditions is that of intermittent claudication, which is the term used to describe activity-related discomfort associated with peripheral arterial disease (PAD). Intermittent claudication is typically described as aching or cramping that is localized in the region affected by the impaired circulation.[14] Because it involves a systemic condition, it typically manifests bilaterally and usually involves the calves, thighs, or buttocks, areas that are often symptomatic with musculoskeletal pathologies.[14] Once the aggravating activity is discontinued, it is characteristic for the symptoms of claudication (pain or cramping) to improve rapidly.

The assessment for intermittent claudication consists of determining what is referred to as *claudication time*. The basic protocols involve assessing maximal treadmill

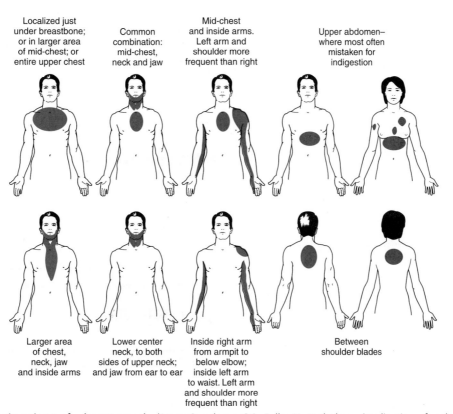

Localized just under breastbone; or in larger area of mid-chest; or entire upper chest

Common combination: mid-chest, neck and jaw

Mid-chest and inside arms. Left arm and shoulder more frequent than right

Upper abdomen— where most often mistaken for indigestion

Larger area of chest, neck, jaw and inside arms

Lower center neck, to both sides of upper neck; and jaw from ear to ear

Inside right arm from armpit to below elbow; inside left arm to waist. Left arm and shoulder more frequent than right

Between shoulder blades

Fig. 2-5 Early warning signs of a heart attack. (From Goodman CC, Fuller K: *Pathology: implications for the physical therapist,* ed 3, St Louis, 2009, Saunders.)

walking time, pain-free walking time, and walking time to severe claudication.[11] As with other standardized tests and measures, the data collection technique employed by the PTA must be the same technique used by the supervising PT.

It is also possible that the PTA may be the first clinician to recognize the symptoms associated with undiagnosed peripheral arterial occlusive vascular disease in terms of the nature, characteristics, and location of symptoms as described. Other signs and symptoms that are consistent with PAD include pallor, decrease in peripheral pulses, sensory changes, and weakness of the involved area (distal to the site of blocked circulation).[14] Diabetes mellitus and nonhealing wounds on the feet also are frequently associated with PAD.[14] Obviously observation of the signs of undiagnosed PAD should be reported to the supervising PT immediately.

Referred Pain

Referred pain is defined as pain that is "felt in an area far from the site of the lesion, but supplied by the same or adjacent neural segments."[14] Referred pain can originate from any cutaneous, somatic, or visceral source and is commonly associated with problems of the musculoskeletal system. It is usually well localized but with indistinct boundaries, tends to be felt deeply, and radiates segmentally without crossing the midline.[22] No objective sensory deficits (paresthesia, numbness, or weakness) are associated with referred pain.[14,22]

Visceral Pain

The term **visceral pain** refers to pain that originates from a body organ. The primary concerns for the PTA related to this type of pain are for the PTA to be aware of how visceral pain may manifest, and to report suspicious pain symptoms to the supervising PT. Often disease processes involving specific or multiple organs reveal themselves through a variety of symptoms and not just pain. However, it is quite possible for a patient to have more than one pathologic condition at the same time. In other words a patient with a confirmed diagnosis of herniated disc in the lumbar spine also could have some type of developing abdominal pathology. Pain of a visceral origin may present as musculoskeletal symptoms because of the innervation pattern of the involved organ. Visceral pain is not well localized secondary to viscera innervation being multisegmental. Additionally, isolation of visceral pain is difficult due to its correspondence to dermatomes from which the problem organ receives its innervation. Figure 2-6 provides a visual representation of innervation to major internal organs in terms of spinal levels of nerve supply. Note that the organs are supplied via plexuses or ganglia, resulting in innervation from multiple segmental levels. For this reason organ pain may be diffuse and difficult for the patient to localize,

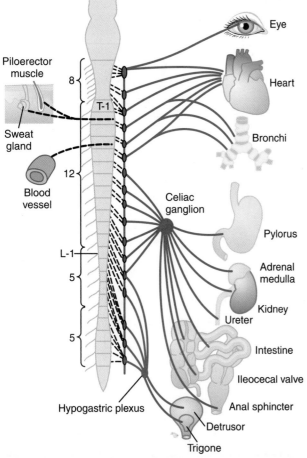

Fig. 2-6 Diagram of the autonomic nervous system. The visceral afferent fibers mediating pain travel with the sympathetic nerves, except for those from the pelvic organs, which follow the parasympathetics of the pelvic nerve. (From Guyton AC, Hall JE: *Textbook of medical physiology*, ed 9, Philadelphia, 1996, Saunders.)

appearing as nonspecific musculoskeletal discomfort. In the case of disease processes that develop over time, the PTA must be alert to changes in the patient's complaints of pain and reports from the patient of patterns that are not consistent with musculoskeletal conditions.

Trigger Points

"**Trigger points** are small, localized tender areas found within skeletal muscles, fascia, tendons, ligaments, periosteum, and pericapsular areas."[30] Trigger points are associated with musculoskeletal conditions such as temporomandibular joint dysfunction, cervical strain, fibromyalgia, and myofascial pain syndrome. The pain produced by trigger points is characterized by tenderness and a referred pattern of pain to palpation, usually in upper quarter or pelvic girdle muscles. According to an article in *American Family Physician*,[1] "Palpation of a hypersensitive bundle or nodule of muscle fiber of harder than normal consistency is the physical finding typically associated with a trigger point. Palpation of

the trigger point will elicit pain directly over the affected area or cause radiation of pain toward a zone of reference and a local twitch response." If, during the process of applying hands-on soft-tissue interventions or passive exercises, the PTA notices signs and symptoms of possible trigger points that have not been previously documented, these findings should be documented and reported to the supervising PT.

Pain: A Final Note

On occasion the PTA may be faced with the circumstance that the patient's complaints of pain do not match observed behaviors of the patient. In this case, it is not the role of the PTA to judge the patient and conclude that the patient is malingering or "faking" the condition. Instead the PTA should objectively document his or her observations and discuss them with the supervising PT.

VITAL SIGNS

An objective measure of physiologic status, particularly as related to cardiopulmonary function, can be obtained quickly through measurement and assessment of vital signs. Body temperature is discussed in the section on inflammation; heart rate, blood pressure, respiration, and pulse oximetry are discussed here. It may be observed that vital signs are not routinely assessed in the outpatient clinic that serves mainly patients with orthopedic diagnoses. However, as the profession of physical therapy strives toward achieving the status of a recognized point of entry for the health care consumer, we must shift our perception of routine procedures to include a more thorough and comprehensive assessment of the patient's overall health status and responses to our treatments.

The student is encouraged to become proficient with effective assessment of vital signs through repeated practice on a variety of subjects and on subjects in different positions (supine versus sitting, versus standing), as well as subjects performing different activities (e.g., activities of daily living [ADL] and exercise).

It is not within the scope of this text to discuss or review detailed physiology related to cardiopulmonary function or pathology. General guidelines for collecting vital sign data and determining when modification to planned interventions is warranted are discussed.

Pulse (Heart Rate)

Heart rate should be measured at the time of evaluation to establish a baseline rate and subsequently when beginning any exercise program or new activity. Accepted values for normal heart rate in adults range from 60 to 100 beats per minute (BPM).[10] Factors that influence heart rate include age, gender, emotional state, medications, exercise or conditioning level, and systemic or local heat.[26]

In addition to the quantitative measure, the quality of the pulse should be noted. Often in a setting where the PTA is working primarily with healthy clients (e.g., trained or conditioned athletes), it may be sufficient to perform a 6-second beat-count and multiply by 10 to quickly determine the cardiovascular response to an activity. However, if the PTA perceives any abnormal quality to the pulse, such as an irregular rhythm or a "thready" pulse (lacking distinct beats), the heart rate should be monitored for a full minute.[26] In such a case, if the abnormality has not previously been noted, this finding should be reported to the supervising PT immediately. Otherwise, as in the case with other assessment procedures, the PTA should employ the same technique as the PT uses during the initial evaluation to enhance consistency and better determine any deviation from the baseline measure.

Textbooks commonly used by PTA educational programs offer specific guidelines for setting exercise intensity using heart rate as a determinant.[10,19,26] An increase in the pulse of more than 20 BPM with activity that lasts for more than 3 minutes after rest should be reported to the supervising PT.[14]

Respiration

As with pulse, respirations should be assessed for both rate and quality. In the healthy adult, normal respiratory rate ranges from 12 to 20 breaths per minute.[26] Variations in the range of normal respiration rate are expected among age groups. Other factors influencing respirations include age, body size, stature, exercise, body position, environment, emotions/stress and pharmacologic agents.[26]

At rest, respiration should be smooth and steady, with uniform chest movement. Observe for excessive use of accessory breathing muscles (anterior upper quarter, anterolateral shoulder, and cervical muscles), which may indicate ventilatory compromise (e.g., chronic obstructive pulmonary disease, asthma, chronic bronchitis caused by smoking, or other pathologic conditions). Also observe to ensure that chest expansion is symmetric bilaterally. Because respiration includes voluntary control, it is best to discreetly assess respiration in conjunction with heart rate to avoid the patient inadvertently altering breathing pattern or rate in response to feeling self-conscious if he or she is aware that the PTA is observing the rise and fall of the chest. The rate is counted for 30 seconds and multiplied by 2, or if irregularities are noted, a full 60 second count is preferred. Refer to the section of this chapter on fatigue for information relating specifically to the assessment of pulmonary response to exercise and activity.

Blood Pressure

Assessment of blood pressure provides an objective measurement of vascular resistance to blood flow at a given time. The pressure exerted by blood is influenced by various factors and conditions, including age and cardiac output, both of which are directly proportional to systolic blood pressure.[26] Obviously, age is a nonmodifiable factor, so an increase in systolic blood pressure of elderly patients may not necessarily indicate an active pathologic process. As always, these findings should be noted in relation to the baseline measurement obtained by the supervising PT during the initial examination.

The PTA working with patients who have musculoskeletal dysfunction or impairment is most concerned with noting responses in blood pressure as new therapeutic activities are introduced or advanced during the course of progression through the established plan of care. Most notably, blood pressure is affected by exercise and activity level in the following ways. Cardiac output increases proportionally to increased physical activity.[16] An even greater and potentially dangerous increase in blood pressure also may occur if the patient holds his or her breath during periods of exertion with exercise. Patients may do this subconsciously in an effort to increase the weight-bearing function of the abdominal cavity, which becomes more stable with an attempt at strong exhalation against a closed glottis, nose, and mouth.[26] As noted in the discussion about pain, the PTA must be alert to the patient's total response to interventions and data collection techniques. When the observant PTA notices that the patient is holding his or her breath during exertion, the patient should be educated in techniques to avoid this behavior. The PTA also may want to reassess blood pressure at this time, although the effect on blood pressure from this activity, known as the *Valsalva maneuver*, is transient. It is particularly critical that the Valsalva maneuver be avoided by patients with a known history of hypertension or cardiac disease.[16]

Another important blood pressure response that may occur during a physical therapy session is a sudden drop in blood pressure, called *orthostatic hypotension*. This rapid drop in blood pressure is associated with a sudden change in the patient's position. It is most frequently the result of the patient being immobile or recumbent for prolonged periods of time, and baseline measurements should be determined before the initiation of upright activities. Signs of orthostatic hypotension include lightheadedness, weakness, dizziness, or diaphoresis.[14] If not addressed (by returning the patient to at least a semi-reclined position), the patient may lose consciousness. Because of the rapid change in blood pressure, the PTA must be prepared to assess the blood pressure immediately upon the change in position. The blood pressure response is critical to obtain, record, and report because the symptoms associated with orthostatic hypotension can also be caused by other serious medical conditions.

Three final points should be noted by the student PTA. First, the PTA should check to be sure of any precautions or contraindications for the assessment of blood pressure that may be present. If the patient has a history of circulatory or lymphatic drainage compromise in one upper extremity, blood pressure must be assessed in the contralateral upper extremity.[26] Second, as mentioned in relation to assessment of other vital signs, the PTA student should practice taking and monitoring blood pressure on a variety of healthy individuals to reinforce a sense of values and ranges considered normal. Finally, the psychomotor skill involved with applying and securing the blood pressure cuff and attached sphygmomanometer, applying and holding the stethoscope diaphragm, pumping air into the bulb, releasing pressure from the cuff, and reading the meter while listening for the blood pressure sounds (called *Korotkoff sounds*) does take coordination and skill. Although the process is basic and consistent, practice reinforces efficient application in actual patient care situations.

Pulse Oximetry

In addition to the measurement of vital signs described, pulse oximetry is a tool used to provide instant information about a subject's cardiopulmonary status. Specifically, the pulse oximeter is a noninvasive probe (in the form of a clip-on device placed on the ear, finger, foot, or nose) that provides a digital readout of oxyhemoglobin saturation. Most commonly, this device is used to identify hypoxemia, monitor the patient's tolerance to activity, and to evaluate patient response to treatment.[26] However, for the patient in the hospital setting who has coexisting cardiopulmonary and musculoskeletal involvement, pulse oximetry is a viable tool for establishing goals to address tolerance to progressive activities.

The standard normal value for oxygen saturation ranges from 95% to 100%; this value is not expected to change with activity or exercise in the healthy individual.[14] This level noticeably decreases in patients with chronic respiratory disease; the PTA must be aware of normal ranges for a given individual in this case. Activity should be halted if the value of oxygen saturation drops below 90% in the acutely ill patient or below 86% in the patient with chronic lung disease.[16] If the referring physician has indicated any other specific level of oxygen saturation to use as a guideline for a given patient, the PTA must be sure to be aware of this level, so that exercise tolerance will not be exceeded. PTAs should also assess other vital signs, skin and nail bed color, tissue perfusion, mental status, breath sounds, and respiratory pattern in patients with whom they use pulse oximetry.[14]

Vital Signs and Exercise

As the profession of physical therapy evolves, with the pursuit of uniform direct access throughout the country, PTs will more often be the "point of entry" for the health care consumer. Along with this increased autonomy and recognition also come increased responsibilities of physical therapy providers, including PTAs, to assess and monitor the patient's general health status, making decisions and judgments accordingly. For the PTA working with orthopedically involved patients, this responsibility includes being aware of normal and expected vital signs, values, and responses and monitoring for the unexpected.

Certain responses in vital signs are expected with exercise. In a "Scientific Statement" published by The American Heart Association,[13] detailed guidelines for exercise testing and training are provided, taking into consideration the cardiovascular health status of the patient. Abnormal blood pressure responses include the absence of an increase in systolic pressure or a drop in systolic pressure with exercise; a normal response is an increase that correlates to the rate and intensity of exercise initiation.[19] If the patient's systolic blood pressure elevates to >250 mm Hg or if the diastolic pressure elevates to >110 mm Hg during exercise, the activity should be discontinued.[14] Further, the systolic pressure should not rise >20 mm Hg with minimal to moderate exercise or >40 to 50 mm Hg with intensive exercise.[14] Diastolic blood pressure is not expected to increase or decrease more than 10 mm Hg with exercise in the healthy adult.[14] Refer to Box 2-3 for a summary of abnormal responses of vital signs to exercise.

Fatigue

In general, the PTA is expected to be competent in performing data collection techniques and selected interventions such that they can make appropriate modifications based on patient responses.[2] In relation to fatigue, this may translate as observing and reporting abnormal responses to activity and making modifications to the interventions within the context of the PT's plan of care. Fatigue may be specific to an individual muscle or muscle group, or it may affect the entire body, manifesting as cardiopulmonary (also called

---

BOX 2-3

Abnormal Responses to Exercise

- Heart rate increases more than 20 to 30 BPM above resting heart rate
- Heart rate decreases below resting heart rate
- Systolic blood pressure increases more than 20 to 30 mm Hg above resting level
- Systolic blood pressure decreases more than 10 mm Hg below resting level
- Oxygen saturation drops below prescribed level
- Patient becomes short of breath or respiratory rate increases to a level not tolerated by the patient
- Electrocardiogram changes

From Hillegass EA: *Essentials of cardiopulmonary physical therapy*, ed 3, St Louis, 2011, Saunders.

cardiorespiratory or *general*) fatigue.[19] Frequently, associated symptoms such as dyspnea, chest pain, palpitations or headache are associated with cardiopulmonary fatigue.[14]

A muscle in a state of fatigue is unable to generate a normal contraction, which may manifest by decreased force, ROM, or quality of the contraction. The patient may complain of discomfort or cramping in the muscle being exercised.[19] When a muscle is fatigued, the patient may compensate by consciously or subconsciously substituting with another muscle or muscle group that performs the same or similar action. For this reason, it is very important for the PTA to be particularly familiar with muscle actions and potential substitutions and observe patients during exercise activities. In terms of quality of motion, fatigue may result in tremulous or jerky motions, instead of a smooth contraction through the ROM.[19]

Generalized fatigue is apparent when the patient is experiencing dyspnea or inability to breathe normally with activity, indicating a decreased ability of the body to use oxygen efficiently.[19] One tool that has been determined to be a fairly good indicator of a patient's pulmonary tolerance to exercise is a standardized scale referred to as the *Borg scale,* or the *Rate of Perceived Exertion scale* (RPE).[16] This instrument calls for the patient to place an objective grade on the amount of exertion he or she perceives with exertion, thus making a subjective report more measurable. A similar instrument, the Dyspnea Scale is used for rating the level of shortness of breath, or dyspnea.[16] As with all standardized instruments, the PTA uses the form, instrument, or technique consistent with that of the supervising PT. If the PT chose to use a standardized instrument to document examination data related to the patient's tolerance to activity, it is likely that a goal addressing that impairment is included in the plan of care, with the outcome to be measured using the same instrument.

ASSESSMENT OF MUSCULOSKELETAL STRUCTURES

Detailed reviews of anatomy and function of specific structures are not covered here because the scope of this chapter is limited to the PTA's role in assessment. Rather, this section provides information relating to entry-level data collection techniques and assessment procedures pertaining to structures involved with musculoskeletal diagnoses commonly encountered by the PTA.

End-Feel

End-feel is the term used to describe the barrier encountered that prevents further motion at the end of passive ROM in a joint. Because different types of tissue have different characteristics and qualities to their

constituency, there are associated normal (physiologic) and abnormal (pathologic) end-feels for each tissue. Normal end-feels are described simply as soft, firm, or hard.[25] Other terms used to denote normal end-feels include *soft tissue approximation,* such as occurs with knee flexion; *muscular stretch,* such as occurs with hip flexion with the knee straight; *capsular stretch,* as denoted in extension of metacarpophalangeal joints of the fingers; *ligamentous stretch,* as found in forearm supination; or *bone contacting bone,* such as occurs with elbow extension.[25] Obviously these terms are descriptive of the specific anatomic relationships of structures that normally limit the motion of each joint. The PTA student is encouraged to practice assessing the different normal end-feels on a variety of subjects, because the exact perception varies depending on the structure and build of each individual tested.

When one of the end-feels (described in the preceding) is noted in a joint that normally exhibits a different end-feel, it is considered to be abnormal or pathologic end-feel. Abnormal end-feels may be classified as soft, firm, hard, or empty. A soft end-feel occurs sooner or later in the ROM than is usual for a joint, or in a joint that normally has a firm or hard end-feel, and is described as feeling "boggy." A firm end-feel occurs sooner or later in the ROM than is usual, or it may be noted in a joint that normally would have a soft or hard end-feel. Hard end-feels occur sooner or later in the ROM than is normal for a joint or in a joint that normally has a soft or firm end-feel, and a bony grating or bony block is noted. An empty end-feel is when no real end-feel is noted because pain prevents the examiner from reaching the end of ROM.[25] Resistance is not noted with an empty end-feel other than the patient/client's protective muscle splinting or spasm.[25] As always, when the PTA recognizes these abnormal circumstances, these findings must be documented and reported to the evaluating PT.

Skeletal Muscle Tissue

Skeletal muscle tissue has various characteristics that allows it to function as it does. Three such characteristics are excitability, contractility, and extensibility. Excitability (or irritability) refers to the ability of skeletal muscle tissue to be stimulated; contractility is the ability of skeletal muscle tissue to contract or shorten; and extensibility is the ability of skeletal muscle to extend or stretch, and to return to its resting length after having contracted.[32]

Strength Testing

It is beyond the scope of this text to provide detailed instruction in the performance of techniques used to measure strength of specific muscles. However, because specific strength increases are frequently included as physical therapy goals, the PTA must be competent with measuring strength, by use of both specific and gross testing techniques. Procedures for assessing muscle strength to determine changes or unexpected findings are discussed here.

When the plan of care includes goals related to increase in specific muscle grades, the PTA must use the same technique for assessing the muscle strength as the evaluating PT used at the time of the initial examination and evaluation. In general, specific manual muscle testing takes into account the precise attachments, action, and position of a muscle during movements or isometric contractions against gravity. Scales for specific muscle grades are also precise, based on word/letter or number scales with strict definitions for each. A table is an organized and convenient way to record data relating to muscle strength testing; an example of a table format is provided in Table 2-4.

In contrast to specific manual muscle testing, gross manual muscle testing techniques are used to quickly determine a nonprecise, yet objective measurement of functional strength. This technique might be used as an efficient method to determine a patient's readiness to progress with exercise or gait activities. This method also may be used to gather data about any changes in the patient's status since the initial examination or last therapy session. In general, movements should be resisted bilaterally and, when possible, simultaneously on both sides for easy comparison. Positions or test movements do not necessarily take gravity into account but focus more on functional positions and movements, such as shaking hands, grasping the therapist's fingers, or lowering and rising to and from a squatting position. In addition to gross strength, the PTA should be alert for any signs of pain or discomfort with resisted muscle testing. Again, when conducting gross manual muscle tests, the PTA is not attempting to obtain a precise measurement of strength, but rather is gathering data relevant to the patient's progress toward goals; readiness to progress through the established plan of care; and status, in terms of changes in condition. The PTA must document and report any unexpected changes or previously undocumented data related to muscle strength to the supervising PT.

If the PTA observes signs of pain with resisted movements during strength testing, he or she must make certain that the test is being performed in such a way as to avoid causing active insufficiency of muscles being tested. Kendall and co-workers[18] define active insufficiency as: "The inability of a Class III or IV two-joint (or multijoint) muscle to generate an effective force when placed in a fully shortened position." Thus, active insufficiency can result from improper positioning of a two-joint or multijoint muscle and causes a cramping type of pain. Pain experienced with muscle testing during a properly performed technique could be indicative of an inflammatory state or strain of the tissues being stressed. Because the musculotendinous tissue is responsible for sustaining joint position during resistance, the presence of pain with muscle testing, even if the result indicates intact strength, points to involvement of the muscle or tendon. Once again, if these data represent a change from the initial examination or evaluation data, it should be documented and reported to the evaluating PT.

Another indication of muscle weakness or the possibility of undiagnosed musculoskeletal or neuromuscular pathology is change in muscle mass or tone. Changes in mass may manifest as either atrophy (muscle wasting) or hypertrophy (excessive mass). The PTA should be able to recognize changes in mass as well as make observations about any pattern of these manifestations, such as the involvement of a specific muscle versus a muscle group; the involvement of muscles innervated by common peripheral or spinal nerve segments; and the involvement of unilateral, asymmetric muscles or groups versus bilateral, symmetric involvement.

Tone refers to the resistance of muscle tissue to passive elongation or stretch and is determined through observation of movements for quality of motion and control of motion (including grading and coordination) and through palpation.[26] True changes in muscle tone should also be noted in the context of patterns of involvement such as described in the preceding and should be differentiated from a local muscle guarding or splinting response.

Stretching and Palpation

In general, the stage of inflammation determines when pain is felt with movement. During the acute stage of inflammation, pain is usually encountered before tissue resistance; during the subacute stage, pain is usually synchronous with tissue resistance; and during the chronic stage, pain usually occurs after tissue resistance is encountered.[26] An increase in complaints of pain with stretching is reported in the event that a previous stretching or strengthening exercise program has been performed too vigorously or aggressively.

Table 2-4	Sample Format for Recording Muscle Strength		
Joint/Motion Shoulder	Muscle Test Grade*		Other Response†
	Right	Left	
Flexion	4−/5	2+/5	
Extension	4/5	3/5	
Internal rotation	4/5	3−/5	
External rotation	4+/5	3−/5	

*Measurements represent example of ascending 0 to 5 scale.
†"Other Responses" could include notation regarding the presence of pain, etc.

In addition to pain at end range, muscle and tendon tissue that is in a state of inflammation or injury is tender to palpation over the involved area. Trigger points also may be noted upon palpation (see previous discussion of trigger points).

Muscle tenderness or soreness to palpation is not by itself an accurate indicator of the tissues involved because referred pain can also manifest as tenderness. However, the PTA should note and document the location and degree of tenderness or soreness for purposes of comparison to initial examination findings and possibly as a measure of progress toward goals, if the supervising PT addressed this area in the plan of care. A previously unnoticed pattern of tenderness revealed while the PTA is working with the patient should also be documented and reported to the supervising PT because patterns of the distribution of tender points represent the hallmark characteristic of conditions such as fibromyalgia. It is also important to note that the core features of fibromyalgia syndrome include widespread pain lasting more than 3 months, and widespread local tender points that are described as painful upon palpation.[14]

As with pain on stretching contractile tissue to end range, palpable tightness or spasm also may occur after exercise or other activity that is too vigorous or aggressive. A muscle may respond to overwork by subconscious splinting or guarding, which results in a feeling of tightness or increased tension to palpation. When increased tightness or spasm is noted upon palpation, modifications to the level of activity or exercise could be warranted within the parameters of the established plan of care.

Flexibility

The loss of the muscle or tendon unit's ability to obtain full length results in decreased flexibility. Decreased flexibility may be differentiated from decreased joint ROM or loss of accessory motions, which may result from involvement of intraarticular structures (discussed in the section on joints).

The end-feel associated with a loss of muscle or tendon flexibility secondary to increased tension in a muscle is described as *muscular* end-feel, and *muscle-spasm* end-feel relates to when joint movement is stopped abruptly with some rebound due to muscles contracting reflexively to prevent further joint movement.[15]

In terms of assessment, the PTA should use a technique consistent with that used by the evaluating PT. Because a loss of flexibility is a problem that may have a significant impact on function, it is an area frequently addressed in the physical therapy plan of care. Examination techniques and subsequent goals may be addressed in terms of specific quantitative outcomes or be more functionally based. An example of a quantitative measurement is the use of goniometric measurements. As with manual muscle testing, detailed instruction in goniometry techniques is beyond the scope of this text. The most important elements of goniometric measurement are accuracy and consistency among testers and testing techniques. PTA educational programs are organized to allow the student to establish a solid foundation in human anatomy, typically including specific emphasis on the musculoskeletal system and structures. To be effective with the application of assessment or data collection techniques such as goniometry, the student is strongly encouraged to ensure that he or she possesses this critical knowledge base. In addition to a solid grasp of skeletal and superficial anatomic landmarks, the student must learn other principles associated with goniometric testing, such as the differences among passive, active, and active-assisted ROM. It is common for the novice to document goniometric measurements as an indicator of flexibility, failing to indicate whether the data represent the patient's ability to actively move through the range or whether passive overpressure was applied to obtain the measurement. The functional implications relating to this concept are significant.

Another technique that may be used to obtain and document information related to flexibility is a functional measurement, such as measuring the distance between the patient's fingertips and the floor during forward flexion (e.g., to measure hamstring flexibility). Although this technique may have specific functional implications, many factors may confound the results and make it less specific to the area of focus. For example, forward trunk flexion performed in this manner may be limited by loss of mobility in the lumbar spine, not the hamstring group. Again, for purposes of data collection to accurately assess the patient's progress, the PTA must employ the same technique as the supervising PT for each patient case. Furthermore, there should be consistency among PTs and PTAs within a practice setting to ensure continuity of care for the patient and valid outcome measurements.

Overuse

As in the case with overuse caused by overaggressive or vigorous exercise (active strengthening or passive stretching), the PTA must be alert for signs of overuse or cumulative stress to contractile tissue, particularly tendons. Signs of tendinitis (the inflammatory condition that results from overuse) include painful but strong resisted isometric contraction (e.g., with manual muscle testing techniques), and possibly pain at end range with stretching, as well as tenderness to palpation over the site of irritation, often near or at the tendinous insertion of the involved muscle. The PTA must not dismiss the possibility that a patient progressing through an exercise program may develop signs and symptoms of tendinitis, even if this is not the original reason for referral. As discussed earlier, the long-term effects of inflammation can have serious implications. Therefore it is imperative for the PTA to present this information to the supervising PT so that modifications to the plan of care can be made to avoid further excessive stresses to these tissues.

Bones

Of primary importance to the physical therapy clinician is the need to rule out conditions or disease processes that are beyond the professional scope of physical therapy, warranting medical diagnosis and treatment. Even without the advent of direct access to physical therapy care, it is possible that a patient may be referred to physical therapy in error for treatment of a condition that in fact requires strict medical attention. The main consideration with bone tissue is fracture. The potential exists for the fracture to be missed on initial examination (medical or physical therapy). An existing fracture also may progress, in terms of malalignment, in the case of a hairline or crack fracture, in which case referral for immobilization may be indicated. Therefore it is critical for the PTA to have an understanding of the signs and symptoms of fracture, regardless of the severity. Common signs and symptoms include pain and local tenderness, deformity, edema, ecchymosis, and a loss of overall function and mobility.[8]

If the patient exhibits exquisite point tenderness over a localized site other than a ligament or other supportive structure, a fracture may be indicated versus other musculoskeletal involvement (e.g., a ligamentous sprain).[14] The PTA should also be aware that fractures can occur as a result of relatively minor trauma, such as sneezing or lifting a sack of groceries out of the car. Often times this occurs in patients who have osteoporosis.[8] Because of the high prevalence and risk of osteoporosis, the astute PTA must recognize the possibility of vertebral compression fractures in a patient with complaints of mid or low back pain. Though sudden impact fractures are the most common type of fracture, the PTA must also be aware of the possibility of stress and pathologic fractures. A stress fracture is a microscopic disruption or break in a bone that is not displaced and produces pain that is described as a localized tenderness or deep aching pain that increases with activity and improves with rest.[14] Pathologic fractures occur in bones that are weakened by disease or tumors and frequently occur spontaneously with very little or no stress. They can be local to the cause, such as with infections, cysts, or tumors, or generalized, as in osteoporosis, Paget's disease, or disseminated tumors.[27]

Joints and Ligaments

Accessory Joint Motions

As a component of evaluation, the PT assesses ligamentous integrity and accessory joint motions for the purposes of differential diagnosis and making decisions on which to base the plan of care. It is the position of the American Physical Therapy Association that spinal and peripheral joint mobilization techniques are interventions performed exclusively by the PT.[6] Although the PTA is not responsible for these elements of physical therapy patient care, it is nonetheless important that he or she understands the implications of assessment procedures that may reveal problems with structures that contribute to joint integrity.

The term *accessory joint motions* refers to "motions between adjacent joint surfaces that occur when a bone moves through a range of motion; includes slides (glides), distractions, compressions, rolls, and spins."[26] Accessory joint motions are also described as motions that occur during active motion, but are not under voluntary control.[19] Another term used to describe these motions is arthrokinematics. For the accessory motions of roll, slide, and spin to occur in a joint, there must be adequate capsule laxity.[19] Roll occurs when one bone within a joint rolls on another bone within the joint. It always occurs in the same direction as bone motion, and new points on one bone meet new points on the other bone.[19] The slide accessory motion relates to the concave-convex rule. If the surface of the moving bone segment is convex, sliding is in the direction opposite of the angular movement of the bone; and if the surface of the moving bone is concave, sliding is in the same direction as the angular movement of the bone.[19] Spin takes place when there is rotation about a stationary axis, and a point on the moving surface creates an arc as it spins. Abnormal findings that may be noted in the presence of impaired accessory motions include decreased joint ROM, a capsular end-feel during stretching techniques, and substitution or compensatory attempts by the patient to obtain full motion.

Distraction and Compression

Distraction (a manual separating of adjacent joint surfaces) and *compression* (a manual approximation of joint surfaces) are assessment techniques that can provide information about the involvement of tissues or structures that serve to provide support to the joint (ligaments); that lie between the joint surfaces (cartilage); or that are directly affected by joint mechanics (bursae). In the presence of mechanical or structural problems that result in impingement on structures located within or near a joint, distracting the joint may produce a relief of symptoms such as pain (radiating or local) or dysesthesia. The PTA's role in this case is to report and document any previously undocumented findings that may provide information as to the nature of the patient's problem.

Likewise, if the PTA notices an increase in the patient's symptoms such as pain, or signs such as crepitus (joint noise resulting from changes—usually increased coarseness or roughening—of the joint surfaces) during approximation or weight-bearing activities, he or she should suspect degenerative or inflammatory conditions and should document these findings and report them to the supervising PT.

Bursae are fluid-filled sacs that are located near tendinous insertions to reduce friction with motion. Bursae also may develop as an adaptive mechanism in the presence of excessive friction. An inflamed bursa sometimes is visible near a joint as a small, soft, encapsulated protrusion that is tender to touch. With bursitis, movement of the nearby joint will be painful and/or motion may be restricted in a noncapsular pattern.[15] Any signs of a pathologic or inflamed bursa should be documented and reported to the supervising PT. Changes in exercise programs or functional activities should be incorporated into the plan of care. If a patient presents with a lump under the skin, joint pain and swelling, fever, chills, malaise and redness, the patient may be exhibiting signs of gout and requires referral for further medical workup if this condition has not been diagnosed previously.[14]

Ligamentous Integrity

During the course of administering components of the physical therapy plan of care for the patient with history or diagnosis of ligament sprain, the PTA must be able to assess the patient's readiness to progress with interventions that will increase stresses to the healing tissue. Ligamentous laxity or improper healing results in decreased joint stability, which may manifest as complaints from the patient that the joint or weight-bearing extremity feels as if it may "give." In this case the PTA should consult with the supervising PT before initiating progressive activities; failure to modify interventions in this case may result in impaired healing, regression of healing, or permanent tissue damage.

If the PTA notices the sudden onset of increased edema, heat to touch, and extremely painful and limited mobility during the course of treatment of a patient with a ligament sprain, the supervising PT must be consulted to seek medical referral to rule out hemarthrosis (bleeding inside the joint capsule).[19]

GAIT

For the PTA to be proficient with assessment of gait, he or she must first obtain a solid understanding of the normal mechanics of walking. Once this underlying knowledge is present, the PTA observes the patient walking, compares the pattern against the normal gait pattern, and notes the deviations. As with all assessment procedures, the PTA must ensure that the techniques he or she employs are consistent with those used by the supervising PT. Gait assessment should be performed on flat surfaces, as well as uneven when indicated, and with the patient both wearing and not wearing shoes. The shoes also can be examined for signs of abnormal

wear, such as scuff marks on the toe of one shoe or flattening of one side of the shoe sole.

Deviations in gait primarily occur as a result of pain, weakness, or other imbalance between muscle strength and flexibility. Typically the short-term goals in the plan of care will address the specific cause of the deviation, with the long-term goal or outcome addressing the overall quality or function of gait. The PTA is responsible for assessing those components of gait that have been specifically addressed in the plan of care. For example, a patient exhibiting an uncompensated Trendelenburg gait during the initial evaluation may have a goal addressing increased gluteus medius strength on the involved side. In this case, the PTA observes the patient's gait to assess for changes in the Trendelenburg pattern and measure strength of the gluteus medius for comparison to initial evaluation data.

The PTA also plays a role in determining if a patient is ready to progress to gait training activities with a lesser assistive device. To make appropriate recommendations, the PTA must be familiar with advantages and disadvantages of various assistive devices and must understand purposes and limitations of each. The PTA should keep in mind that ultimately the patient will be best served by the assistive device that allows for maximum safety, independence, and the most normal gait pattern.

BALANCE

According to the Normative Model,[2] the PTA is to be competent in performing balance, coordination, and agility training. Three physiologic systems linked to balance control include somatosensory (musculoskeletal and neuromuscular components), visual, and vestibular. The vestibular system involves the structures and organs of the inner ear, which play a key role in maintaining upright posture, equilibrium, and orientation, all components of balance. Although the application of interventions designed to correct vestibular problems is beyond the skill level of an entry-level PTA, he or she must be aware that patients who report symptoms of vertigo, dizziness, balance problems, coordination problems, trouble focusing or tracking objects, hearing loss, tinnitus, nausea, vomiting, motion sickness, ear pain, headaches, or a sensation of fullness in the ears may need further physical therapy or medical assessment to rule out or confirm involvement of vestibular conditions. (Detailed information about vestibular disorders can be found on the website of the Vestibular Disorders Association at www.vestibular.org.)

A patient who constantly or frequently looks at the floor during ambulation or other activities that challenge balance is likely excessively depending on visual input to compensate for somatosensory impairment (e.g., weakness, loss of sensation, or limited joint mobility). In this case, ongoing assessment should include

---

BOX 2-4

Sample SOAP Documents

S: c/o UEs feeling tired with parallel bars and pregait activities

O: Prior to gait training, GMMT reveals overall strength WFL, with the exception of poor hip clearance with WC push-up. 50% of attempts, pt. requires specific instructions and tactile guidance with proper hand placement with sit-to-stand and stand-to-sit; otherwise carries out this task properly. In parallel bars, pt took 3 steps forward and back + mod assist; stand with trunk and (L) LE flexed and does not push adequately with UEs.

A: Concerns re: difficulty maintaining NWB status (R) LE with pre-amb activities because of insufficient shoulder depression strength; as a result, thus pt. is not ready to begin gait training with walker. Pt. will benefit from ex. to increase shoulder depression strength to enhance use of assistive device for NWB (R) LE.

P: Include push-up blocks with ther ex next visit; progress with gait training with walker, NWB (R) LE as indicated.

Signature, PTA

---

these components or musculoskeletal or neuromuscular integrity according to the plan of care as established by the evaluating PT. Data collection and documentation must relate changes in the patient's musculoskeletal and neuromuscular function (e.g., ROM, loss of sensation, or weakness) to balance.

Likewise, the patient with visual impairment may depend heavily on musculoskeletal and neuromuscular control to compensate for this deficit. In this case the PTA may notice that the patient reaches for props or ambulates with a wide base of support.

DOCUMENTATION

Documentation is a critical element of the patient's physical therapy experience. Unfortunately, all too often in the present health care environment, the focus of documentation emphasizes reimbursement for services at the cost of cutting short other very important purposes of effective record keeping. In addition to serving as a permanent record of the patient's physical therapy episode of care, documentation is used as a communication tool among members of the health care team; it also may be an effective tool for quality assurance or management within a service or department to measure consistency between providers, set standards for assessment and interventions, and measure effectiveness of outcomes.

The *Physical Therapist Assistant Clinical Performance Instrument*[5] lists the following sample entry-level behaviors associated with the criterion, "Produces documentation to support the delivery of physical therapy services":

■ "Documents aspects of physical therapy care, including selected data collection measurements, interventions, response to interventions, and communicates with family and others involved in delivery of patient care.

■ Produces documentation that follows guidelines and format required by the clinical setting and law.

■ Documents patient care consistent with guidelines and requirements of regulatory agencies and third-party payers.

■ Produces documentation that is accurate, concise, timely, and legible.

■ Demonstrates technically correct written communication skills."[5]

This discussion focuses on the PTA's role in documenting assessment. Even early in his or her educational experience, the PTA student learns to recognize the standard elements of the subjective objective assessment plan (SOAP) format of documentation; this format is effective as a tool to organize one's thoughts and the content of a treatment note, even if it is not the standard format used by a given facility.

In the subjective section of the note, the PTA would document any patient reports related to functional status or disability. In the objective section of the SOAP note, the PTA would document treatment performed, including frequency, duration, and intensity; patient education; equipment provided; and changes in patient's status including observed changes during or after treatment.[29] In the plan section of the SOAP note the PTA would indicate the intervention(s) for the next patient visit, what the patient is to be doing between treatments, as well as steps that will be taken to reach the established goals.[21] So how does assessment fit into the PTA's documentation?

The assessment is the key portion of documentation that links subjective and objective data to the physical therapy goals, outcomes, and plan. Thus, in the assessment section of the note, "...the PTA summarizes the information in the S and O sections and reports the progress being made toward accomplishing the goals."[21]

Box 2-4 provides a sample SOAP note, written with the intent of offering an example of an effectively documented assessment by a PTA.

Summary

This chapter began with reference to the rapid changes occurring in the physical therapy profession today. It is imperative for PTAs just entering the profession to possess an awareness and understanding of the issues surrounding the dynamics of this evolution. As PTA students gain an understanding of the foundational principles and core documents that affect their clinical and professional roles and function, they will be better equipped to be active participants in these discussions. This chapter was designed with this outcome in mind and focused on the PTA's role in the performance and documentation of assessment procedures used in the care of patients with musculoskeletal disorders.

❖ GLOSSARY

Assessment: "The measurement or quantification of a variable or the placement of a value on something."[4]

Centralization: The increase of signs and symptoms in the immediate area of the lesion.

Evaluation: The specific process reserved solely for the PT, in which clinical judgments are made from the base of data obtained during the examination.

Examination: The preliminary gathering of data and performing various screens, tests, and measures to obtain a comprehensive base from which to make decisions about physical therapy needs for each individual patient, including the possibility of referral to another health care provider.

Judgment: "Decisions made within the clinical environment that are based on the established physical therapy plan of care. With consideration toward safety, a problem-solving process is applied that includes decision rules (e.g., codes, protocols), thinking, data collection, and interpretation."[5]

Peripheralization: The spread of pain to areas outside of or distant from the immediate area of involvement.

Referred pain: Pain that is "felt in an area far from the site of the lesion, but supplied by the same or adjacent neural segments."[14]

Trigger points: "Small, localized tender areas found within skeletal muscles, fascia, tendons, ligaments, periosteum, and pericapsular areas."[30]

Visceral pain: Pain that originates from a body organ.

REFERENCES

1. Alvarez DJ, Rockwell PG: Trigger points: diagnosis and management, *Am Fam Phys* 65(4):653–660, 2002.
2. American Physical Therapy Association: *A normative model of physical therapist assistant education: version 2007*, Alexandria, Va., 2007, American Physical Therapy Association.
3. American Physical Therapy Association: *Professionalism in physical therapy: core values*, Alexandria, Va., 2003, APTA.
4. American Physical Therapy Association: *Guide to physical therapist practice*, ed 2, Alexandria, Va., 2001, American Physical Therapy Association.
5. American Physical Therapy Association: *Physical therapist assistant clinical performance instrument*, Alexandria, Va, 1998, American Physical Therapy Association.
6. American Physical Therapy Association: Position statement: Procedural interventions exclusively performed by physical therapists. HOD 06-00-30-36, 2000.
7. Standards of Ethical Conduct for the Physical Therapist Assistant, HOD S06-00-13-24. House of Delegates Standards, Policies, Positions, and Guidelines. Alexandria, Va., American Physical Therapy Association, 2005.
8. Boissonnault WG: *Primary care for the physical therapist examination and triage*, St Louis, 2005, Saunders.
9. Crowley L: *An introduction to human disease pathology and pathophysiology correlations*, ed 6, New York, 2004, Jones and Bartlett.
10. Duesterhaus Minor SD, Duesterhaus Minor MA: *Patient care skills*, ed 5, Upper Saddle River, NJ, 2006, Pearson Prentice Hall.
11. Ehrman PM, Gordon P, Visich PS, et al: *Clinical exercise physiology*, Champaign, Ill, 2003, Human Kinetics.
12. Esterson PS: Measurement of ankle joint swelling using a figure of 8, *J Orthop Sports Phys Ther* 1(1):51–52, 1979.
13. Fletcher GF, Balady GJ, Amsterdam EA, et al: Exercise standards for testing and training: A statement for health care professionals from the American Heart Association, *Circulation* 104:1694–1740, 2001.
14. Goodman CC: *Kelly Snyder TE: Differential diagnosis for physical therapists screening for referral* St Louis, 2007, Saunders.
15. Hertling D, Kessler RM: *Management of common musculoskeletal disorders: physical therapy principles and methods*, ed 4, Philadelphia, 2006, Lippincott Williams & Wilkins.
16. Hillegas EA: *Essentials of cardiopulmonary physical therapy*, ed 3, St Louis, 2011, Saunders.
17. Karges JR, Mark BE, Strikeleather SJ, et al: Concurrent validity of upper-extremity volume estimates: Comparison of calculated volume derived from girth measurements and water displacement volume, *Phys Ther* 83(2):134–145, 2003.
18. Kendall FP, McCreary EK, Provance PG: *Muscles: testing and function*, Baltimore, 1993, Williams & Wilkins.
19. Kisner C, Colby LA: *Therapeutic exercise: foundations and techniques*, ed 5, Philadelphia, 2007, FA Davis.
20. Kloth LC, McCulloch JM: *Wound healing: alternatives in management*, ed 3, Philadelphia, 2002, FA Davis.
21. Lukan M: *Documentation for physical therapist assistants*, ed 2, Philadelphia, 2001, FA Davis.
22. Magee DJ: *Orthopedic physical assessment*, ed 5, St Louis, 2008, Saunders.
23. May BJ: *Home health and rehabilitation: concepts of care*, Philadelphia, 1999, FA Davis.
24. Merskey H, Bogduk N: *Classification of chronic pain*, ed 2, Seattle, 1994, International Association for the Study of Pain.
25. Norkin CC, White DJ: *Measurement of joint motion: a guide to goniometry*, ed 4, Philadelphia, 2009, FA Davis.
26. O'Sullivan SB, Schmitz TJ: *Physical rehabilitation: assessment and treatment*, ed 5, Philadelphia, 2007, FA Davis.
27. Porth CM: *Essentials of pathophysiology concepts of altered health states*, ed 2, Philadelphia, 2007, Lippincott Williams & Wilkins.
28. Prentice WE, Voight ML: *Techniques in musculoskeletal rehabilitation*, New York, 2001, McGraw-Hill.
29. Quinn L, Gordon J: *Functional outcomes documentation for rehabilitation*, St Louis, 2003, Saunders.
30. Tan JC: *Practical manual of physical medicine and rehabilitation*, St Louis, 1998, Mosby.
31. Tatro-Adams D, McGann S, Carbone W: Reliability of the figure-of-eight method on subjects with ankle joint swelling, *J Orthop Sports Phys Ther* 22(4):161–163, 1995.
32. Thibodeau GA, Patton KT: *Anatomy & physiology*, ed 2, St Louis, 1993, Mosby.

REVIEW QUESTIONS

Short Answer

1. What is the most basic, effective method of controlling transmission of infectious agents?
2. List typical signs and symptoms of myocardial infarction (heart attack) that may occur concurrently with the pattern of pain identified as early warning signs of a heart attack.
3. What is the term used to describe increasing pain symptoms in the immediate area of the lesion (as opposed to spreading pain)?
4. List five factors that affect respiration rate.
5. What is the term used to describe joint noise that results from degenerative joint changes?
6. What are two potential long-term complications of chronic, unresolved inflammation?

True/False

7. Enlarged and tender lymph nodes are a normal and expected localized response to inflammation.
8. Signs of a deep venous thrombosis include pale skin, increased local temperature, edema, and pain.
9. Assessing patients' vital signs is not necessary on a routine basis in the outpatient, orthopedic clinical setting.
10. The Valsalva maneuver should be taught to patients to use during exercise to increase trunk stability.
11. Fractures can occur as a result of relatively minor trauma, and they can also occur spontaneously with little or no stress.
12. For accurate data collection related to gait, assessment should be performed only on level surfaces and only while the patient ambulates with shoes on.
13. Examination of the patient's shoes may provide information about the mechanism of a gait deviation.
14. Fractures associated with osteoporosis may be asymptomatic, or silent, and diagnosed after healing during medical workup for subsequent fractures.
15. The patient does not play an active role in establishing the severity of general fatigue he or she may experience during activity.

3 Flexibility and Stretching

Harvey W. Wallmann

LEARNING OBJECTIVES

1. Describe viscoelasticity and the properties associated with collagen.
2. Explain the stress-strain curve and factors that influence change.
3. Discuss Golgi tendon organs (GTOs) and muscle spindles.
4. Discuss how temperature affects connective tissue.
5. Define and discuss range of motion, flexibility, and stretching.
6. Outline various methods used to measure flexibility.
7. Identify and describe various stretching techniques.
8. Discuss precautions and essential components of stretching program development.
9. Discuss at least two proposed benefits of stretching.
10. Explain how stretching might negatively impact activity performance.
11. Describe the clinical applications for stretching soft-tissue contractures.
12. Describe and contrast the differences and similarities between scar tissue and adhesions.

KEY TERMS

Adhesion

Collagen

Contracture

Creep phenomenon

Deformation

Golgi tendon organs

Load

Muscle spindles

Remodeling

Strain

Stress

Viscoelasticity

CHAPTER OUTLINE

Enhancing flexibility is an important component of a fitness program[7] and is useful, not only for sport-specific activities, but also for activities of daily living (ADLs). The need for flexibility is particularly necessary if mobility has been impaired, resulting in compromised range of motion (ROM). ROM is the amount of movement available to a joint moving within its anatomic range. Muscular imbalances due to shortened muscles may lead to faulty postural alignment that may lead to injury and joint dysfunction. The ability to restore ROM is crucial when implementing or following a rehabilitation program; consequently, being able to incorporate stretching exercises to restore flexibility as well as normal ROM and function becomes a primary goal for the physical therapist assistant (PTA).

Many clinicians emphasize that having a more flexible body is more efficient, improves muscle balance, and more easily undergoes strength and endurance training. Overall purported benefits of flexibility due to stretching include injury prevention, quicker recovery from workouts, a reduction in post exercise soreness, and facilitation of relaxation.[2,129] However, the effects of stretching on performance is somewhat more controversial. Some literature shows that it may potentially help improve performance,[48] whereas other literature and research reveal potential detrimental effects on maximal performance activities after stretching.[66,113,124,131] Research into flexibility and stretching is ongoing in an attempt to determine the effects of stretching on the body. Consequently, some of the long-held beliefs about stretching, especially regarding performance, are being challenged.

PROPERTIES OF CONNECTIVE TISSUE

Before discussing the concepts of flexibility and stretching, a general review of several biomechanical concepts will be discussed to help form a foundation for later material. Specifically, concepts of **viscoelasticity, stress,** and **strain,** along with associated variables related to tensile load will be discussed in relation to **collagen.**

Just as amino acids are the building blocks of protein, tropocollagen is the building block of collagen (Fig. 3-1). Collagen fibers are made of short subunits (fibrils) and are found in varying amounts within the different connective tissues: bone, tendon, muscle, skin, hyaline cartilage, and joint capsule.[20,41,119] Collagen is a protein building block of connective tissue and it provides the strength needed to withstand high levels of tension and force during movement and exercise. There are more than 20 types of collagen, but the majority of the collagen in the body consists of types I, II, and III.[38] Of these, type I collagen is the most abundant in the body.

Type I collagen fibers are thick fibers gathered into bundles and display very little elongation when placed under tension (they have an ability to resist pulling).

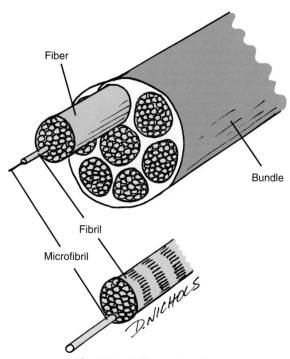

Fig. 3-1 Collagen bundle.

Type II collagen fibers, on the other hand, are thinner and possess slightly less tensile strength. These fibers are observed primarily in tissues such as articular cartilage and the nucleus pulposus. Type III collagen serves mainly in a structural support capacity and is found in expansible organs (e.g., arteries, liver, lungs).[58] It is also common in fast growing or healing tissue and is often seen at the early stages (phase 1) of wound repair. It is later replaced by the tougher type I collagen.[90]

Elastin is a structural protein present in tendons in amounts of less than 1%.[35,136] Tissues with greater amounts of elastin usually demonstrate greater degrees of flexibility. Elastin assists collagen in the recovery of tissues after stress.

Stress and Strain

Stress or **load** is given in units of force/area, where the units may be pounds per square inch or Newtons per square centimeter.[96] Therefore stress is directly related to the magnitude of force and inversely related to the unit area, but is independent of the amount of a material.[97] The complementary measure related to stress is strain or **deformation.** Strain is usually dimensionless, since the units of measure cancel each other out, but units are often provided (e.g., inches/inch) to give a perspective of scale applied to the loads.[96]

The relation of stress and strain is dependent on several factors. These include the material properties used, the magnitude of the stresses, and the rate of stress application. Subsequently, the graphical representation of stress and strain is different for each type of material discussed. This representation is known as the

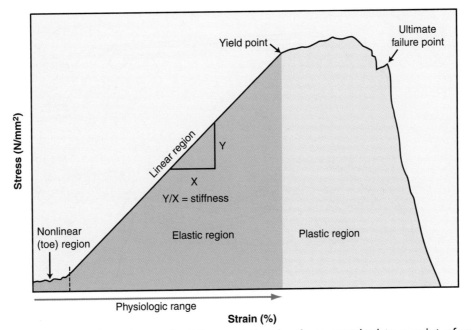

Fig. 3-2 The stress-strain relationship of an excised ligament that has been stretched to a point of mechanical failure (disruption). (From Neumann DA: *Kinesiology of the musculoskeletal system: foundations for rehabilitation*, ed 2, St Louis, 2010, Mosby.)

stress-strain or *load-deformation curve*.[92] Figure 3-2 demonstrates the various regions within the stress-strain curve, with each region demonstrating a biomechanical property of a tissue.

The toe region represents how a slightly pulled tissue (i.e., a ligament) produces only a small amount of tension within the tissue; it indicates that the collagen fibers within the tissue must first be pulled tight before a stretch can be induced. This minimal amount of tension simply results in the slack of the tissue being taken up with no stretch being encountered. The elastic region represents a linear change in strain, which occurs if the tissue continues to be pulled at higher stress levels. A good example of this linear relation is similar to the model of a stretched rubber band. The greater the load on the rubber band, the more the rubber band stretches. So, as the tension on the rubber band is removed, the band shortens, nearing its original length. Given this behavior, it is referred to as the *elastic zone*. The amount of stretch (strain) applied to the tissue in this zone is generally experienced during many body movements. Note that the slope (the angle of the curve) in this zone is indicative of the relative stiffness of the tissue. Stiffness is defined as the change in force per unit change in length.[41] As such, the stiffer the tissue, the steeper the slope. So tissues such as ligaments will only change length at higher levels of stress compared with tissues of less stiffness, such as loose connective tissue.

The upper level of the elastic region marks a transition from the linear slope to one where the slope begins to flatten. This is called the *plastic region* and is a point where an increasing level of stress on the tissue results in proportionately increased changes in tissue length,

probably due to microscopic failure of the tissue. This is termed the plastic zone because of the tissue damage resulting in permanent deformation (plastic deformation). Unlike the elastic region, the plastic energy is not recoverable in its entirety when the load is removed; additionally, there is a change in its resting length. Continued stretch in the plastic region would result in additional deformation of the tissue and would occur until it reached its initial point of failure. The toe region can include strains up to 3%; the elastic region, from 6% to 10%; and the plastic region, from 10% to 15%.[41,112]

Viscoelasticity

All connective tissue exhibits the property of viscoelasticity, which is simply a combination of the behavior of the properties of elasticity and viscosity.[73,76] Elasticity refers to a material's ability to return to its original state following strain or deformation (i.e., change in length or shape) after a removal of the stress or load. This mutable change is termed elastic deformation and is similar to the changes that occur in a rubber band under high rates of strain. The rubber band rapidly conforms to a new length and is able to return to its original resting length when the stress is removed. However, the rubber band breaks if the degree of stress exceeds the strain capabilities (Fig. 3-3). Viscosity refers to a material's ability to resist a change in form or to dampen shearing forces. Tissues exhibiting viscosity have time-dependent and rate-dependent properties when forces are applied to them.

The rate at which tissues are stretched has a profound effect on the degree or percent of strain. As mentioned, tensile (distractive) or compressive forces will produce

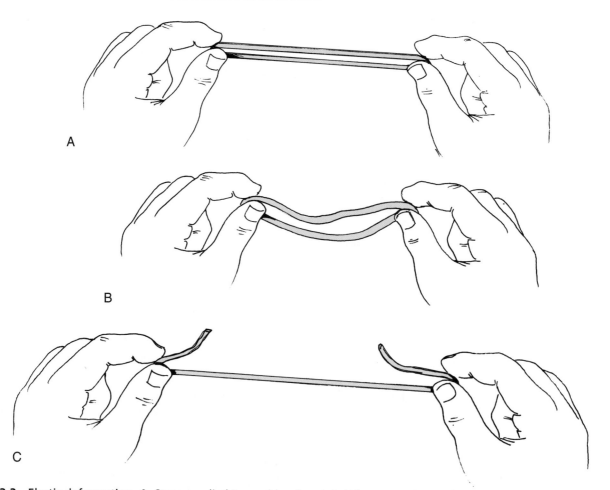

Fig. 3-3 Elastic deformation. **A,** Stress applied to a rubber band. **B,** When stress is removed the rubber band returns to its original length. **C,** If the stress exceeds the strain capabilities of the band, it can break.

deformation on viscoelastic materials, but will allow return to their original state after removal of the force. Given normal conditions, however, viscoelastic materials do not immediately return to their original state. Viscoelastic materials, unlike pure elastic materials, have time-dependent properties. Slower rates of stress produce greater amounts of strain or elongation, whereas faster rates of stretch produce much smaller amounts of elongation.[29,35,119] As such, they are sensitive to the applied force duration. Tissues gradually lengthen when they are subjected to constant or repeated stress of long duration.

So a viscoelastic material subjected to either a constant compressive or tensile load will initially respond by rapidly deforming; it continues to deform over a finite length of time even if the load remains constant. This deformation of the tissue will continue until a state of equilibrium is reached when the load is balanced. This is called the *creep phenomenon* (Fig. 3-4),[76] which simply means the gradual increase in tissue length that occurs when maintaining a constant stress (or force). For example, if one uses a constant force against the muscle with slow and passive stretching, the muscle will

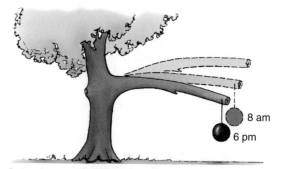

Fig. 3-4 Creep. The branch of the tree is demonstrating a time-dependent property associated with a viscoelastic material. Hanging a load on the branch at 8 AM creates an immediate deformation. By 6 PM, the load has caused additional deformation in the branch. (From Panjabi MM, White AA: *Biomechanics in the musculoskeletal system*, New York, 2001, Churchill Livingstone.)

eventually elongate. However, the tissue does not return to its original length immediately when unloaded because of the collagen's viscous property.[73] Essentially, the longer the duration of the applied force, the greater the deformation or stretching of the tissue.

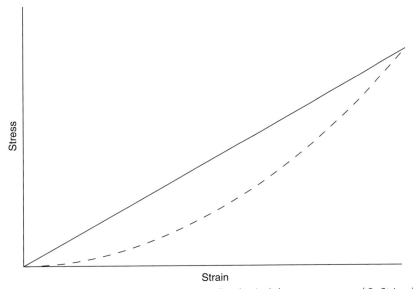

Fig. 3-5 **The hysteresis loop.** (From Placzek JD: *Orthopaedic physical therapy secrets*, ed 2, St Louis, 2006, Mosby.)

Another term frequently used is stress-relaxation, or force-relaxation. Unlike creep, this occurs when a viscoelastic material experiences a constant strain (no deformation occurs). In this case, a high initial stress placed upon a tissue decreases over time until equilibrium is reached and the stress equals zero, resulting in relaxation of the tissue. Consequently, no change in length is produced. For example, if a muscle is held at a certain length over time, a reduction in stress would occur, but there would be no change in length (no stretch occurs).

The loading and unloading of tissue is influenced by its viscoelastic properties. This loading and unloading is quantified by measuring the hysteresis area (Fig. 3-5). The loading (solid line) and unloading (dashed line) phases represent a measurement of the stress and strain that is applied to a tissue and then released. The hysteresis area lies between the two lines and represents the amount of energy dissipated in the loading and unloading process.[41,73]

The ability of tissues to recover after stress is extremely important in relation to flexibility. Woo and colleagues[136] have shown that increasing the levels of stress produces an increase in collagen within ligaments and tendons, whereas reducing the levels of stress causes weakening in connective tissues. Recovery is the ability of tissues to return to their previous resting state. However, it does not imply that permanent elongation or microscopic damage has not occurred. Plastic deformation is force dependent under slow rates of stress and is used to describe permanent change in a tissue. For example, when a low degree of stress is applied to a plastic spoon, the spoon slowly deforms to a new shape. The spoon breaks if the stress is applied too fast (Fig. 3-6). Lehman and colleagues[74] and Warren and co-workers[126]

have demonstrated that recovery of the tissue's resting length had occurred after microscopic failure had begun.

Along with stress and the rate of stress applied to tissues, temperature also affects connective tissue extensibility as well as the rate of creep. High temperatures in the range of 37° C (98.6° F) to 40° C (104° F) affect the viscoelastic properties of connective tissue and increase the rate of creep.[29,73] The higher the temperature (approximately 45° C [113° F] is the therapeutic upper limit), the greater the degree of elongation with stress before tissue failure.[108] Because connective tissue's viscoelastic and plastic changes occur at higher temperatures, there is less microscopic damage under stress at these temperatures. Studies by Warren and colleagues[127] have demonstrated that a temperature of 45° C is needed to reduce tissue damage during strains of 2.6% or less. So to stretch out a connective tissue structure, one should heat it and use a large load over a long period of time to produce creep.[96] Low temperatures decrease the rate of creep.

Muscle or contractile tissue responds to stretch by elastic and plastic deformation properties in ways similar to connective tissue. Obviously the contractile properties of muscle allow for the greatest degree of freedom of movement around a joint. Although connective tissue is considered a passive resistant to joint motion, muscle tissue is considered an active restraint to joint motion by virtue of its elastic and contractile elements. Active exercise (muscular contractions) affects intramuscular temperature. Increases to approximately 39° C are observed in exercised muscle.[6] Commonly used passive thermal agents that increase tissue temperature are moist heat and ultrasound. The judicious use of active exercise and passive thermal agents before and during stretching programs enhances the effectiveness of the prescribed program.

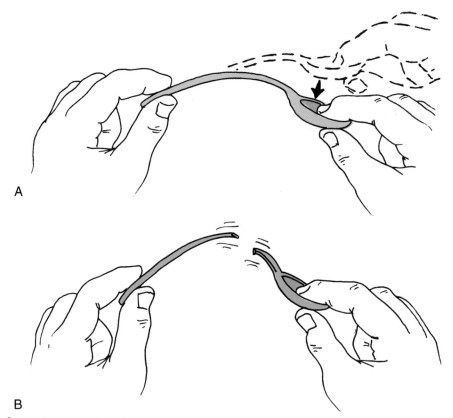

Fig. 3-6 Plastic deformation. **A,** A low degree of stress is applied to a plastic spoon. The spoon will deform slowly and accommodate to a new shape. **B,** If stress is applied suddenly and with great force, the spoon will break.

FLEXIBILITY

Kisner and Colby[64] define flexibility as the ability of a muscle to relax and yield to a stretch force. Others have defined flexibility as the ability to move muscles and joints through a full ROM.[12,102] In essence, flexibility refers to the degree of normal ROM available. Therefore, flexibility can refer to various measurable components of joint motion. Muscles, tendons, ligaments, skin, joint capsule, and bone geometry all influence the degree of movement in joints. For example, a muscle can stretch or elongate, creating a measurable effect on the joint or joints upon which it acts. If a muscle becomes damaged by trauma or disease or becomes shortened because of immobilization, its ability to stretch and allow freedom of joint motion is affected. Flexibility will diminish over time if tissues are not stretched or exercised using regular and proper stretching regimens.[2] As such, the goal of any flexibility program would be to improve or maintain ROM at all joints.

Different classifications of flexibility currently exist, depending on how the tissue is stretched. For example, static flexibility occurs as a result of static stretching, whereas dynamic flexibility relates to moving through a ROM with normal or rapid velocity.[2] However, evidence does not support the existence of flexibility as a single general characteristic of the body. Instead, it is specific to particular joints, joint actions, or movements and is highly variable among different individuals.[53] An understanding of the properties and components of various connective tissues is fundamental in delivering various stretching and flexibility regimens.

Measuring Flexibility

It is important to assess overall flexibility by measuring ROM at specific joints, because no one composite test provides an index of an individual's flexibility characteristics.[53,54] Subsequently, some measurements of overall flexibility are somewhat difficult, since they involve a complexity of movements over several joints (e.g., sit and reach test).

Measuring joint ROM is accomplished by using standard goniometric instruments. The measuring device most commonly used to measure ROM is the universal goniometer (Fig. 3-7), which is a protractor with degree measurements. The goniometer arms are placed along the proximal and distal components of a joint with the axis centered over the joint, which are then moved in accordance with the body part being measured. The goniometer can be used to measure joint position and ROM at almost all joints of the body.[95] Other types of goniometers used less frequently in the clinical setting are the inclinometer, the pendulum goniometer, and the fluid goniometer.

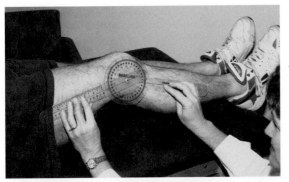

Fig. 3-7 Measuring joint motion with a goniometer.

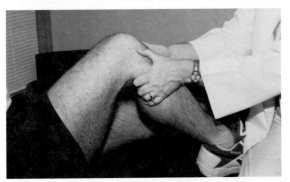

Fig. 3-8 Joint stability is measured by manually applied clinical tests. Anterior drawer test of the knee is shown.

Consistency in measurement is crucial; therefore it is important to use the same type of goniometer for a specific patient each time that patient is measured. Because different goniometers may provide slightly different results, they should not be interchangeable in their use in the clinical setting. For example, when using an inclinometer as the measuring device, it should be used for all future measurements for that patient to ensure consistency.[96] For documentation purposes, most authorities recommend using goniometry rather than visual estimates because of its increased accuracy and reliability of measurement.[128,137]

Joint stability differs from joint ROM in that the ligaments and surface geometry of joint articulations dictate static joint integrity (stability). A patient may demonstrate limited ROM in knee flexion and extension (by goniometry); however, anterior and posterior joint mobility may be excessive and unstable (Fig. 3-8). On the other hand, a patient may demonstrate normal joint ROM, yet when tested statically the joint may be very stable, tight, and unyielding to pressure.

The sit and reach test (Fig. 3-9, *A-B*), standing toe touch for back and hamstring flexibility (Fig. 3-9, *C*), seated hip external rotation test (Fig. 3-9, *D*), and standing knee recurvatum test generally are less specific flexibility tests. These tests and others are used to provide very general assessment of multijoint flexibility. Such tests also can be used as stretching techniques to improve limitations in

movement. However, objective clinical documentation of joint ROM is made by joint goniometry.

Factors Affecting Flexibility

In addition to muscles, tendons, and their surrounding fascia, other structures, such as bone, fat, connective tissue lesions, skin, and postural problems, may all lead to flexibility and joint ROM limitations.[5] Other factors that may affect flexibility are age and gender.[14,25]

STRETCHING

Stretching involves elongating the muscles and tendons to the end of the available ROM. As such, applying a tensile force to a muscle results in a transient deformation, which elongates the musculotendinous unit, resulting in a stretch.[2,40] Given that the mechanical behavior of connective tissue is primarily influenced by the amount of collagen available,[73,119] the amount of stretching that takes place is dependent on the type of connective tissue present (i.e., skin, fascia, ligaments, tendons, joint capsules, and muscle fascia).

Although gradually increasing flexibility to increase ROM is the main goal, other adaptations occur from a regular stretching program. For example, research has shown that as a result of training, the stretch reflex may be reset to a different level.[133,134] Several types of stretching exercises have been detailed in the literature and will be described in this section.

Stretching Principles

Stretching is effective primarily because of its mechanical and neurophysiologic effects.[69,119] As mentioned, the muscle-tendon unit responds viscoelastically during stretching. However, some stretching exercises are based on the neural inhibition of the muscle undergoing stretch as well. In this case, a decreased reflex activity would result in reduced resistance to stretch, resulting in further gains of joint ROM. Most likely, both mechanisms are responsible.

It is important to note that stiffness relates to a tissue's ability to resist stretch and indicates the amount of deformation proportional to the load applied.[81] So, the stiffer the tissue, the less compliance it has and the less likely it is to stretch; conversely, less stiffness means greater compliance. It stands to reason then that flexibility training is designed to decrease the stiffness of the muscle-tendon unit.[69,119] Furthermore, a rapidly applied stretch results in a greater resistance to that stretch.

Both mechanical and neurophysiologic components are inherent within muscular flexibility.[43,50,105,118,119] However, some researchers believe that the ability of stretching to produce greater flexibility is primarily a result of the viscoelastic nature of muscle and connective tissue.[84,119] As such, the most resistance to stretching probably is due to the connective tissue framework and

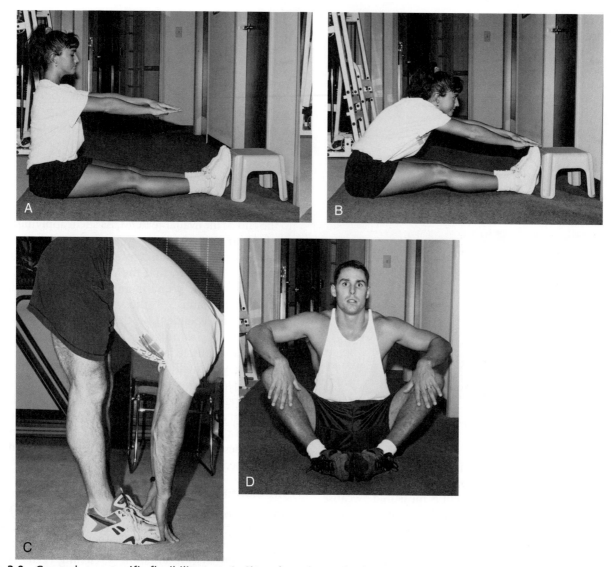

Fig. 3-9   General, nonspecific flexibility test. **A,** Sit and reach test for hamstrings and low-back flexibility, starting position. **B,** End position of sit and reach test. **C,** General, nonspecific standing toe-touch flexibility test for the hamstring and lower back. **D,** Seated hip external rotation butterfly stretch.

sheathing from within and around the muscle and not the muscle itself (since the muscle itself can be stretched to 150% of its resting length); this includes the epimysium, perimysium, and endomysium and may even include the sarcolemma.[107,109,116,117]

On the other hand, many researchers suggest that the immediate result of stretching is attributed to neurophysiologic phenomena.[69] They categorize these phenomena as either a stretch tolerance or active contractile responses and claim that the limiting factor during stretching is the muscular resistance secondary to reflex activity. A stretch tolerance simply means an accommodation to the discomfort of stretching over time. With this philosophy, the aim of stretching is to inhibit the reflex activity, subsequently decreasing the resistance and improving ROM. Several other researchers agree and recommend certain types of stretching for its reduction in reflex activity.[3,43,50] **Muscle**

spindles and **Golgi tendon organs** are the mechanoreceptors responsible for the contractile responses (Fig 3-10).

Warm-up

Warm-up is necessary to help prepare the tissue for activity. Stretching alone before exercise is not recommended by most researchers and health professionals.[65,66,111,124] As such, the purpose of warm-up exercises, including stretching, is to prepare the body for the stresses it will encounter during an activity or sport and is necessary for increasing the core body temperature. Heat is produced with muscle contraction, thereby increasing the intramuscular temperature.[23] ROM increases as a result of warmed tissue.[107] A warmed muscle will be able to contract more forcefully and relax more quickly,[15] thereby enhancing work production for those muscles used.[16] In training, a general body warm-up is needed

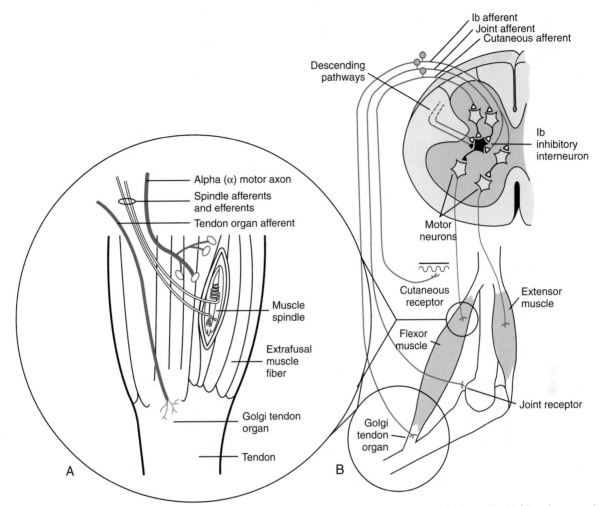

Fig. 3-10 **A,** Muscle spindle and Golgi tendon organ (GTO). Fibers of the muscle spindle (intrafusal fibers) are activated by stretch. Type Ia and II sensory afferents of the spindle send information about stretch and the stretch velocity to the spinal cord. Nerve impulses then return to the muscle (extrafusal fibers) through the efferent alpha motor neurons that cause the muscle to contract and resist the stretch. The Golgi tendon organs exist in series as the junction between extrafusal muscle fibers and tendons. The sensory afferents of the GTO are known as *type Ib* and are sensitive to changes in tendon tension that occur with either muscle stretch or contraction. **B,** Reflex action of Ib afferent fibers from GTO. Ib inhibitory neurons receive input from GTO, spindles, joint cutaneous receptors, and descending pathways. (**A,** Redrawn from Kandel E, Schwartz J, and Jessell T, editors: *Principles of neural sciences,* ed 3, East Norwalk, Conn, 1991, McGraw-Hill. **B,** Modified from Kandel E, Schwartz J, and Jessell T, editors: *Principles of neural sciences,* ed 4, New York, 2000, McGraw-Hill.)

first. The beneficial effects of a warm-up before strenuous activities include the following:

■ Blood flow to working muscles is increased.
■ Temperature in working muscles is increased.
■ Cardiovascular response to sudden, dynamic exercise is improved.
■ Breakdown of oxyhemoglobin for the delivery of oxygen to the working muscles is increased.

With warm-up, the risk of connective tissue and contractile tissue damage is reduced. Warm-up protocols usually last from 10 to 25 minutes or more and may vary somewhat, depending on the nature of the activity or event.[8] The warm-up should be intense enough to cause an increase in body temperature, but not so intense as to cause fatigue. So one should taper the warm-up 5 to 10

minutes before the actual event.[3] It is clinically assumed, of course, that a more compliant muscle can be stretched further and is therefore less susceptible to injury.[48]

However, some think that the warm-up period may not be the best time to stretch for increasing ROM, primarily because of increased tissue stiffness. Since the concept of stretching to prevent injury has come under question, benefits of stretching before activity may be incorrect. Activity of gradually increasing intensity (dynamic stretching) may be more appropriate than static stretching as a warm-up activity.[96] Some researchers have examined the combination of stretching and active warm-up and have shown that the decrease in stiffness mainly results from increased muscle temperature and not stretching.[85,104]

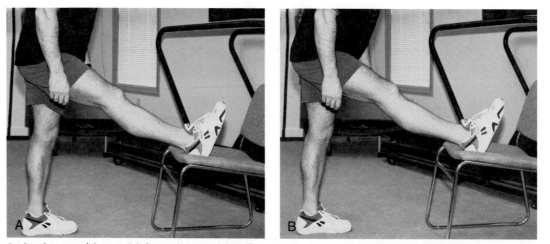

Fig. 3-11 A, Static stretching. Initial starting position for standing hamstring stretch. **B,** Ending position for standing hamstring stretch (note trunk flexion). The muscle will slowly conform to an elongated position by maintaining stress on the tissue for a period of time.

Increasing intramuscular temperature to help increase ROM may also be achieved through external means.[110] Henricson and colleagues[57] reported on results that followed the application of heat to the hip. Although heat alone did not improve hip ROM, stretching without heat did increase hip ROM, and stretching with heat combined gave the greatest increase in ROM, maintaining it for 30 minutes. These results are consistent with others,[62,74,127] who report that collagen extensibility increases and musculotendinous stiffness decreases with heat. Bear in mind, however, that most authors recommend using exercise as the primary way of increasing intramuscular temperature.[96] It has not been definitively shown whether a general warm-up serves to improve sports performance.[17,18,21,46]

Stretching Techniques
In discussion of flexibility and associated stretching programs, the stretching of nonpathologic muscle must be separated from stretching noncontractile connective tissue. Improving muscle extensibility in nonpathologic conditions and in adaptive muscle shortening after injury or immobilization requires a complement of active exercise techniques and thermal agents. Types of stretching exercises are static stretching (active and passive), ballistic stretching, dynamic stretching, and proprioceptive neuromuscular facilitation (PNF) techniques (contract-relax, contract-relax with agonist contraction, and hold-relax). Research has shown that all four techniques have been shown to increase flexibility.[31,56,61,80,82,105] Essential to a successful stretching program for improving flexibility is the proper execution of the exercises.

Static stretching
The most common form of stretching exercise that is used to safely increase the ROM in a joint is static stretching. This form of stretching allows one to sustain

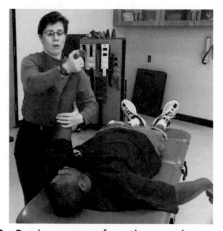

Fig. 3-12 Passive range of motion can be complete in one plane or a combination of planes of motion. (From Huber FE, Wells CL: *Therapeutic exercise: treatment planning for progression*, ed 2, St Louis, 2007, Saunders.)

a controlled stretch by placing a muscle in a fully elongated position and holding that position for a period of time (Fig. 3-11). A passive static stretch implies that the force is applied externally (i.e., with a partner or gravity-assisted) (Fig. 3-12). If an opposing muscle action is used to aid the stretch, then the stretch is called an *active static stretch*. However, to obtain optimal passive stretching, all voluntary and reflex muscular resistance must be eliminated.

Research supports that slow passive stretching through the ROM will not produce muscle activity in normal relaxed subjects.[13,107] As such, the muscle should be slowly and passively stretched to a new length, so that the stretch reflex is not elicited. Additionally, the stretch should not elicit pain.[3,105] As is described later, the stretch is maintained for an extended period of time before being returned to its starting position. Subsequently, a lengthening of the muscle is accomplished.

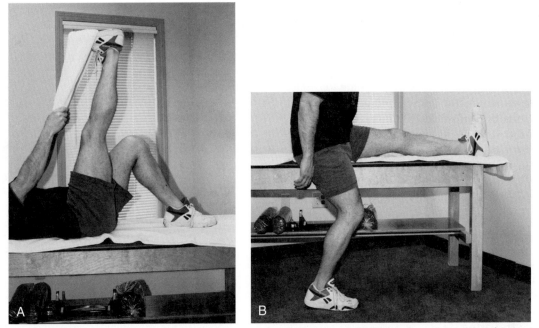

Fig. 3-13 **A,** Supine static hamstring stretch using a towel. **B,** Sitting hamstring stretch.

Athletes use static stretching before sports activities as part of a warm-up before a workout and as part of a cooldown after a workout. Because intramuscular temperature rises to approximately 39° C during exercise,[6] active general body movements can improve muscle temperature before stretching is done. Most warm-up programs use primarily active static stretches, using gravity to assist the stretch.

Studies on rat tail tendons[74] demonstrated that ruptures occurred with 31% of normal loads when temperatures were at 25° C, whereas increasing temperatures to 45° C delayed tendon rupture until 102% of normal load. This demonstrates that stretching at normal body temperatures may damage tissue,[127] but elevating tissue temperature before and during prolonged stretch is less damaging.[126,127]

Static stretching has distinct advantages, such as reduced chance of exceeding strain limits of tissues, reduced energy requirements compared with other forms of stretching, and reduced potential for muscle soreness.[29,108,136] The ease and practicality of teaching patients to perform static stretching is another advantage. For example, hamstring stretches can be taught with the patient in various positions (Fig. 3-13). The general goals of static stretching are to prevent or minimize the risk of soft-tissue injury from participation in sports or physical activities, improve movement and increase flexibility, and prevent contracture.[8,64]

Ballistic stretching

Another technique used quite often by athletes is ballistic stretching (Fig. 3-14). Many believe that this is the least desirable technique, because it potentially places the tissue at risk secondary to the use of jerking or

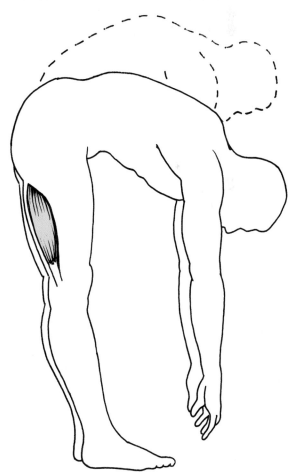

Fig. 3-14 Ballistic stretching requires a relatively high velocity bounce at the end-range of motion. Typically ballistic stretching techniques are reserved for an athletic population in preparation for high-velocity, ballistic, and sometimes violent physical activity.

bouncing movements at the end of the ROM to stretch the muscles.[71] Athletes use dynamic, high-velocity, and even violent motions during sporting events and require extraordinary flexibility to prevent or reduce the risk of potential musculoskeletal injury. Relatively high-velocity or quick bouncing may not be appropriate for many patients. The potential for tissue damage exists in all forms of exercise, but ballistic stretching may increase the risk of connective tissue and contractile tissue trauma, although a narrow segment of patients may benefit.

The reason ballistic stretches are considered undesirable is that they stimulate the muscle spindles during the stretch. This results in a continuous resistance to further stretch, which then causes a high rate of tension strong enough to potentially injure the musculotendinous unit.[65,107,123] Ballistic stretching does not imply aggressive, violent, high-velocity stretches throughout the ROM; instead it involves a slight but progressively greater bounce at the end of the range achieved through static stretching.

Dynamic stretching

A type of stretching technique that has become increasingly popular is dynamic stretching. With dynamic stretching, muscular contraction is used to stretch a muscle; the effect is to increase or decrease the joint angle where the muscle crosses, thereby elongating the musculotendinous unit as the end ROM is obtained.[10] What sets dynamic stretching apart is that it uses activity-specific movements, thereby preparing the muscles by taking them through the movements used in a particular sport. An example of this would be a sprinter who would walk using exaggerated long strides, thus emphasizing hip flexion and extension (Fig. 3-15). This subsequently actively contracts and stretches the muscles used by the sprinter, namely the hip flexors and extensors.[60] Dynamic stretching does not incorporate end range ballistic movements that are bouncy or jerky in nature. Rather, all movements are under control.[96]

Proprioceptive neuromuscular facilitation

Another technique used to facilitate ROM increases via stretching is called *proprioceptive neuromuscular facilitation* (PNF). PNF is a system of therapy that uses different techniques designed to promote neuromuscular responses via stimulation of the proprioceptive system.[122] These techniques use volitional contractions to increase ROM by decreasing the resistance caused by the spinal reflex pathways.[24] PNF stretching uses movements in diagonal patterns along with an isometric contraction before the stretch; this allows greater gains in ROM than stretching alone. However, depending on the clinical setting, many clinicians have modified the various PNF patterns, deviating from the proposed diagonal patterns originally described by Knott and Voss[64a] to straight plane patterns. As a result, it is difficult to determine if the effects of PNF treatment are consistent among practitioners and in the research literature.

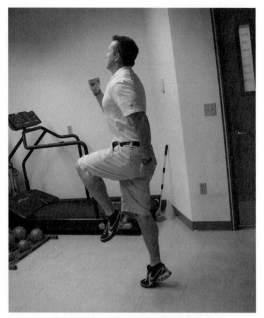

Fig. 3-15   Dynamic stretching.

PNF stretching techniques, which are based on the stretch reflex, appear to increase ROM through the stimulation of the proprioceptors[2] and have been found to produce greater increases in ROM than static stretching.[91,101] Two neurophysiologic sensory receptors involved with the stretch reflex are the Golgi tendon organs (GTOs) and the muscle spindle. The GTOs are inhibitory sensory receptors located within the musculotendinous junction that signal tension in a muscle (see Fig. 3-10, *B*). Stimulation of the GTO results in self-inhibition of that muscle, termed autogenic inhibition. They also signal minute changes in muscle tension, thereby providing information about muscle contraction.[63]

Muscle spindles are excitatory specialized fibers within the muscle (see Fig. 3-10, *A*) that are sensitive to changes in muscle length as well as maintenance of that length. When a muscle is stretched, the spindles send messages to the spinal cord, which in turn signals the muscle to contract. The classic clinical demonstration of the stretch reflex is produced by tapping the relaxed patellar tendon, which causes the reflexive contraction of the quadriceps. The muscle spindles within the quadriceps are activated by the quick stretch of the patellar tendon, causing the quadriceps to contract reflexively (Fig. 3-16).[63]

Despite the advantages, PNF stretching has some disadvantages as well. For example, it is more time consuming than other methods, requires skillful application by trained professionals to be effective, and may lead to mild complaints of patient discomfort.[108] Some of the more commonly used techniques are contract-relax, contract-relax with agonist contraction, and hold-relax.

The contract-relax technique involves instructing the patient to relax the affected muscle while the therapist

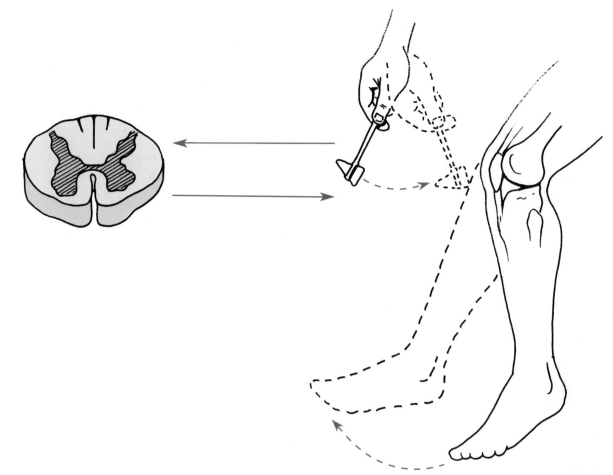

Fig. 3-16 Muscle spindle activation by quick stretch-reflex between the spinal cord and quadriceps.

passively moves the limb to the limit of motion (until the person feels a stretch). The patient is instructed to actively contract the restricted muscle (antagonist) against the manually applied resistance of the therapist for 5 to 8 seconds.[1] The patient is then instructed to relax while the therapist passively moves the limb to the new limits of motion, at which point the clinician holds the stretch for 10 seconds (Fig. 3-17). This relaxation of the antagonist muscle during contraction is an example of autogenic inhibition. The process is repeated by continuing from the new limit of pain-free motion until the required number of repetitions is performed or until no more range is gained.[1]

In the contract-relax with agonist contraction technique, there is a contraction of the opposite (agonist) muscles instead of the shortened or restricted muscles.[1] In this case, the limb is taken to the point of stretch while the clinician applies manual resistance against the muscle being stretched for 5 to 8 seconds (as in the contract-relax method). The muscle is then relaxed while the agonist muscle concentrically contracts; this facilitates the stretch using the principle of reciprocal inhibition (Fig. 3-18). In reciprocal inhibition, voluntary isometric contraction of the agonist

muscle group results in a subsequent reflex inhibition on the muscle groups being stretched (reciprocal inhibition). The clinician again takes up any slack and holds the new position for 10 seconds before continuing.

The hold-relax technique is similar to contract-relax. However, with this technique, the patient actively moves the limb to the end of pain-free motion. The patient isometrically contracts against the force applied by the therapist at the end of the ROM for 5 to 8 seconds as resistance is slowly increased. After holding the contraction for the requisite amount of time, the patient is instructed to relax. The patient then actively stretches the limb to the new limits of motion (Fig. 3-19).[1]

Duration, Frequency, and Intensity of Stretching

The specific duration, frequency, intensity, and number of stretching repetitions varies in the literature. Stretch duration depends upon the joint targeted, the flexibility goal, and the type of stretching technique used. Generally, static stretches may be held in a fully elongated position for anywhere from 10 to 60 seconds, with most research recommending that stretches

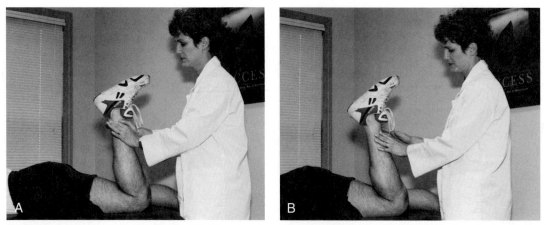

Fig. 3-17 Proprioceptive neuromuscular facilitation, contract-relax technique. **A,** The patient actively contracts against manually applied resistance for 5 to 8 seconds. **B,** The patient then relaxes while the therapist passively moves the limb to the new limits of motion.

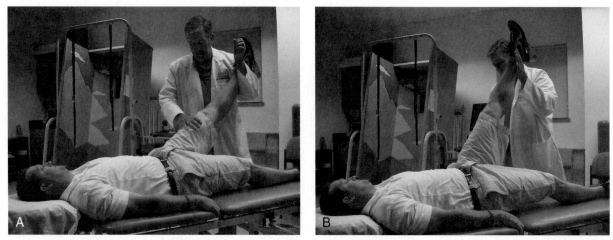

Fig. 3-18 Proprioceptive neuromuscular facilitation, contract-relax with agonist contract technique. **A,** The limb is taken to the point of stretch while the clinician applies manual resistance against the muscle being stretched for 5 to 8 seconds. **B,** The muscle is then relaxed while the agonist muscle concentrically contracts.

be held between 15 and 30 seconds.[8-10,81,103,122] An attempt is then made to extend the stretched position farther within tolerable limits (Fig. 3-20). However, because of the structural diversity of tissue, predicting the duration of stretch for each tissue becomes very difficult.[73] Current American College of Sports Medicine (ACSM) guidelines recommend 3 to 5 repetitions for each stretching exercise.[98]

The limits of motion achieved during a stretching program depend on the patient's tolerance, age, pathologic condition (if any), motivation, and commitment. The muscle's ability to adapt is a prolonged process. Patients must be cautioned not to exceed their pain limits and must receive counseling about the fact that many sessions of stretching are needed to produce change and lasting improvement. Approximately 6 weeks of stretching are necessary to demonstrate significant increases in muscular flexibility.[37] An individual must stretch at least three times per week to

improve flexibility. An individual must stretch at least 1 day per week to maintain the flexibility gained during the program.[108]

Intensity

Increases in ROM can be significantly affected by the intensity of the stretch.[107,125] Structural damage subsequent to stretching could result with increased levels of force and may result in structural weakening of the muscle-tendon unit, thereby increasing the risk of injury.[94,120] The appropriate intensity for static stretching is to stretch slowly and hold the position at low force levels. This is most often communicated to the individual as pain-free or mild discomfort.

How long does it last?

There is little reported on the long-lasting effects of stretching. Some researchers have reported that stretching techniques using cyclic and sustained stretching

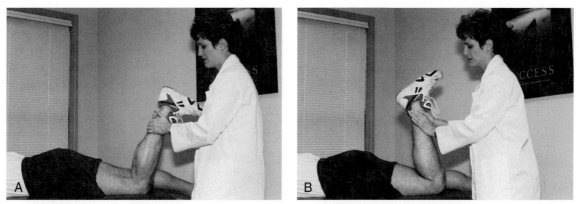

Fig. 3-19 Proprioceptive neuromuscular facilitation hold-relax technique. **A,** The patient isometrically contracts against the force applied by the therapist for 5 to 8 seconds. **B,** The patient relaxes and the therapist passively moves the limb to new limits of motion.

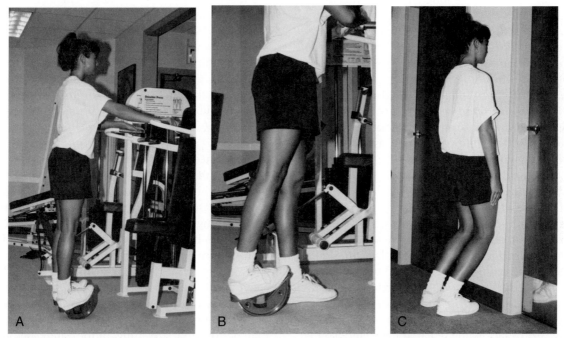

Fig. 3-20 Examples of static stretching positions and techniques for the gastrocnemius-soleus complex. **A,** Standing bilateral calf stretch. **B,** Single limb static calf stretch. **C,** Gastrocnemius-soleus stretch.

for 15 minutes on 5 consecutive days increased hamstring muscle length with a significant percentage of the increased length being retained 1 week posttreatment.[115] Others reported that the knee ROM was able to be maintained for 3 minutes, but had returned to prestretched levels in 6 minutes[36]; whereas other researchers have reported that increased ROM from stretching remained for up to 90 minutes.[45,89] These differences have been explained by variations in warm-up, stretching position, stretching force, and stretching duration.[138] Some research has shown that stretching at least once a week after a 30-day training program will maintain the gained flexibility.[123]

Comparisons of Different Stretching Techniques

All stretching techniques previously discussed have been shown to increase flexibility and ROM.[47,49,79] However, it has not been adequately defined in the literature as to the appropriate stretching frequency and duration for long-lasting changes in flexibility.[100] It is also not completely evident which stretching technique increases flexibility most effectively. Ballistic stretching and static stretching appear to be similar in their effects on flexibility,[56,61,105] yet existing research indicates that dynamic stretching may produce about the same flexibility gains as static and ballistic stretching.[10]

Although many studies have revealed that PNF may be the preferred method for increasing flexibility over static and ballistic stretching,[27,42,52,101,118] direct comparison between methods is very difficult to determine because of the differences in methodology, experimental design, procedures, and measurement instruments and the use of inadequate control groups.[96] Additionally, some studies found no significant differences between techniques.[56,79,86,91] Some authors have reviewed stretching studies and reported conflicting evidence as to the efficacy of these methods[44,52]; they reported that most of the differences between studies were probably due to variations in training methods, measuring instruments, and confounding variables.

Proposed Stretching Benefits

Enhanced Flexibility

Research has shown that a long-term, routine stretching program can result in increased long-term flexibility, whereas an acute stretching program does not.[10,66] Wiktorsson-Moller and colleagues[130] reported that stretching significantly increased hip ROM for flexion/extension, hip abduction, knee flexion, and ankle dorsiflexion. The effect was significantly greater than that obtained by massage and warming up separately or combined. Similarly, Williford and associates[132] showed that increases in flexibility could occur as a result of a static stretching training program.

Relief of Muscular Soreness

Previous research has indicated that slow stretching exercises were able to reduce postexercise muscular soreness,[30,32] but other research, examining the effect of static stretching on soreness, revealed no significant effect on perceived pain compared with a control group.[83] Later research showed that stretching had no effects on decreasing exercise soreness over the postexercise period or immediately after an acute bout of stretching.[22,51] In fact, some research has demonstrated that stretching may actually cause muscle soreness. In a study investigating the effects of static and ballistic stretching on delayed onset muscle soreness (DOMS), researchers found that similar bouts of static and ballistic stretching induced significant increases in DOMS in subjects unaccustomed to such exercise.[114]

Muscle Relaxation

The literature has shown that chronic increased muscular tension can result in negative side effects, such as high blood pressure, headaches, ulcers, and muscle and joint pain.[72] Subsequently, many individuals use certain types of stretching as a way to facilitate muscle relaxation. An example of this type of flexibility training is used in yoga.[2] The belief here is that chronic tension affects muscles so that they become less strong, less supple, and not as capable of absorbing the shock and stress of various types of movements. As such, stretching may be implemented to facilitate muscular relaxation, thereby decreasing stress and muscular tension.[33,34] A possible explanation may be that, with stretching, the muscle spindles may adapt to the stretch, or while held at a constant length, force relaxation may occur, which would decrease the tension on the muscle. In examining electromyograms (EMGs) before and after warm-up, Mohr and colleagues[88] found that muscle activity during static stretching of the gastrocnemius muscle for about 30 seconds was significantly lower and therefore sufficient to attain muscle relaxation.

Injury Prevention

Evidence is not clear as to whether stretching before or after exercise actually decreases the chance of injury. Some research has shown that stretching may decrease the rate of injury.[28,55,87,106] Researchers also stated that stretching, as part of a warm-up or a rehabilitation program, decreased the percentage or recurrence of injuries.[39] On the other hand, research has also shown that stretching is not effective in preventing injury.[121] A 12-week training study of 1538 male army recruits revealed that stretching had little influence on injuries associated with weight-bearing physical training such as running, marching, and walking.[99]

Performance Enhancement

Many assume that performance is enhanced by preactivity stretching and usually point to sports that require extreme ROM at particular joints (e.g., gymnastics and pitching). However, no conclusive data support a correlation between flexibility and/or stretching and performance. It is generally agreed that a warm-up is necessary before exercising in order to perform an activity safely and successfully.[65] Of course, stretching is widely accepted as an important part of the warm-up. Furthermore, many have traditionally believed that performing stretching immediately before physical activity will improve performance.[48] Though it is plausible that increased flexibility may potentially improve performance in many activities where ROM is necessary to perform certain skills, whether preperformance stretching can actually improve performance is questionable.[66,113,131] Some studies have reported that preperformance stretching neither helps nor inhibits performance,[49,67] whereas other studies have revealed negative performance effects.[45,68,124]

The reason for these negative effects, according to some researchers, is probably that the muscle-tendon unit becomes weaker after acute stretching and is thereby less able to produce high intensity force. Consequently, there is a period of time during which the muscle-tendon unit stays stretched (lag period), in which it may need to "take up the slack" before peak tension is reached. Therefore stretching immediately before a performance task may cause a strength deficit, resulting in impeded performance.[124] Because of this, it has been suggested that low intensity muscle contractions should be performed immediately before sport performance (i.e., dynamic stretching).[19]

When to Stretch

Very little literature is available to determine when stretching should take place in an exercise program. Some believe that stretching should be part of the warm-up to enhance musculotendinous extensibility, but should not constitute the entire warm-up.[70] Wiktorsson-Moller and associates[130] showed that warm-up before stretching resulted in significant changes in joint ROM. Some think that stretching should not be performed at the beginning of a warm-up routine.[70,107] They believe that the tissue temperatures may be too low for optimal muscle-tendon function, subsequently leading to a less compliant tissue, which may not adequately prepare the tissue for activity. As such, many authors recommend at least 5 minutes of light progressive exercise before stretching.[107] Conversely, some discourage exercise before stretching, stating that warmed up muscle tissue does not necessarily stretch better nor is it less likely to be injured.[93]

Some researchers found that stretching should be performed after an exercise session because of the improved joint ROM.[85] However, Cornelius and colleagues[26] revealed that performing static stretching before, after, and both before and after each workout in a 6-week program did not make a difference in increasing ROM. All produced significant increases in ROM.

Stretching of Soft-Tissue Contractures

The stretching of soft-tissue contractures involves muscle, capsule, tendon, ligament, bursa, and skin. Many options exist for the therapist when prescribing stretching exercises for patients after immobilization or injury, which differ from static, ballistic, or PNF stretching. Long-duration, low-load static stretching has been an effective technique that produces long-lasting connective tissue changes.[29,74,126,127] The PTA must recognize adaptive changes that occur in various soft tissues after injury or immobility.

Initially, scar tissue is formed, which may result in the development of a scar contracture if the tissue is not adequately mobilized. A **contracture,** in this case, is defined as a permanent or transient limitation of movement or shortening of muscle or other soft tissues; in other words, a contracture is the result of healed tissue that forms a fixed, rigid scar and causes cosmetic deformity or functional deficits.[58] Scar tissue formation may be the result of **adhesions** and other tissue damage (Fig. 3-21, *A*). An adhesion involves a limitation of function resulting from scar tissue that forms between structures.

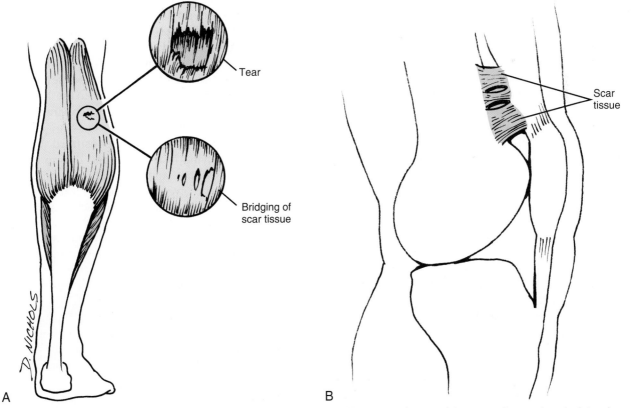

Fig. 3-21 Scar tissue. **A,** Scar tissue formation. **B,** Adhesions formed between the quadriceps tendon and underlying bone results in a limitation of function.

For example, when scar tissue forms after knee surgery, it can bind down and cross-link collagen tissue, resulting in adhesions around the patella, suprapatellar pouch, and quadriceps tendon (Fig. 3-21, *B*).

Generally, immature scar is defined as adaptable for up to 8 weeks and becomes progressively less changeable for up to 14 weeks. Scar becomes quite inextensible at 14 weeks and is termed inadaptable, or mature scar.[4] Adaptable scar is highly vascular, with many cells (including myofibrocytes) that give the scar the ability to contract. Immature scar tissue also has a high rate of **remodeling**,[4] which is the process of tissue restructuring in response to stress or immobilization.[29]

As new scar tissue is formed, the collagen fibers become highly unorganized and arranged randomly, creating an immobile structure.[78] Adaptable or immature scar tissue becomes increasingly organized and oriented, with specific directional lines of stress. The formation of collagen fibers are in response to stress imposed from mechanical loads.[58] Where stretching is concerned, the PTA must be attentive to the following critical components:

■ The nature of scar tissue is time dependent and stress reactive.
■ Immature, adaptable scar tissue is fragile.
  ■ At 5 days, new scar is only 10% of its maximum potential strength.
  ■ At 40 days, new scar is 40% of its maximum strength.
  ■ At 60 days, new scar is 70% of its maximum strength.
  ■ At 12 months, new scar is approximately 100% of its maximum strength.
■ New scar tissue organizes and aligns itself along lines of stress; therefore appropriately applied stress helps to remodel unorganized scar.
■ Low-load, long-duration stretching of joint contractures in combination with thermal agents to preheat extensible connective tissue has proved effective in the treatment of soft-tissue contracture.[59,75,77] Long-duration stretching means stretching over a period of 20 to 60 minutes.

Clinically, the following areas are involved in a low-load, prolonged stretch technique:
1. Preheat the involved structures with moist heat or ultrasound.[29]
2. Place the involved structures in a position of comfort, not maximum stretch. This is an extremely important point. To elicit relaxation, the involved structures must be placed in a supported and comfortable gravity-assisted position.
3. Maintain moist heat application during the entire course of treatment (20 to 60 min).
4. Apply stress or load gradually and minimally. With new immature scar, gravity alone may be enough to clinically effect change. With mature scar, only slightly greater loads should be used. This is a critical point. Lentell and colleagues[75] found that the magnitude of force used in their study (0.5% of body weight) to create a significant long-lasting change in motion fostered such relaxation that many subjects were not even aware of stretching taking place during the procedure. In an effort to gain knee extension after surgery, for example, it would behoove one to use this technique to avoid reflexive splinting or muscle guarding (Fig. 3-22).
5. Allow the patient to rest or recover for a few minutes during the course of treatment if the sensation of stretch becomes too uncomfortable.
6. Maintain heat application for 5 to 10 minutes after removal of the loads. Some researchers[107] have advocated the use of ice packs after stretch in this protocol. Lentell and colleagues[75] did not find cooling to be effective in their study. However, cooling the involved structures after stress may be effective in selected cases where pain and an inflammatory response are present.
7. Initiate isometric contractions after the application of heat and passive stretching to enhance strength gains at the new end of ROM.

Lentell and colleagues[75] demonstrated the effectiveness of applying heat before and during low-load, prolonged stretching and external rotation of non-pathologically involved shoulders. Heat application before and during such stretching was clinically superior

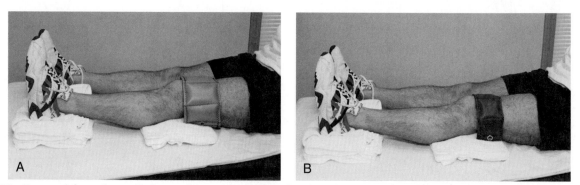

Fig. 3-22 External force is applied to enhance passive low-load prolonged stretch. **A,** Excessive weight causes reflexive muscle splinting and guarding. **B,** Only very light resistance is necessary to elicit appropriate relaxation.

to bouts of stretching alone, stretching plus ice, and a heat-stretch-ice protocol. Clinically, few contraindications exist when attempting to gain motion after specific surgical procedures.

Adhesions are desirable and, in fact, are a surgical goal in selected cases. Desirable permanent shortening of connective tissue is needed to prevent a functional loss of movement in some knee surgeries and surgical correction of some shoulder instabilities. If an attempt is made to fully regain external shoulder rotation after surgery to correct recurrent dislocation, the intent to scar down and protect the joint from further dislocation may be derailed. In this case, it is wise to gain functional motion very slowly to allow enough time for a mature scar to form (14 weeks).

The clinical application of low-load, prolonged stretch can be modified to varying degrees depending on the surgical procedure, time constraints of healing, and goals of the rehabilitation program. For example, supine wall slides are a modified technique that uses some of the points of low-load, prolonged stretch (Fig. 3-23). When attempting to gain knee flexion range, it is wise to preheat the quadriceps muscles and suprapatellar pouch before stretching. Next, the patient is placed in a supine position and the foot of the involved limb put on a towel against a wall. To reduce friction against the wall, the contact surface of the towel is lightly coated with baby powder so it will slide more easily against the wall. As the patient relaxes, gravity assists in knee flexion and the foot slides down the wall.

This concept can be modified further. In keeping with the example of gaining knee flexion range, the use of isotonic exercise equipment can be helpful. With the patient in a seated position on a knee extension

machine, moist heat or ultrasound can be used before and during the stretch (Fig. 3-24). Many knee extension machines are manufactured with an adjustable range-limiting device that allows the patient to adjust the starting and stopping angle of the exercise. Before the stretch is begun, the patient's hips are secured with straps to keep them from rising during the treatment. An angle is selected that is comfortable to the patient. As the tissues are continually heated, a very gradual increase in the flexion angle is initiated. The angle does not have to be excessive to be effective. Thus the protocol remains essentially the same, but the equipment and the position of the patient are changed.

The knee serves as an excellent example to further describe and clarify methods to improve ROM by prolonged static stretching. To gain knee extension range, the patient can be supine with moist heat applied behind the knee (popliteal fossa) and on the hamstring and quadriceps. The heel of the involved limb is placed on a small folded towel (Fig. 3-25, *A*). If the knee is contracted to −20°, for example, towels are added under the hot packs under the knee to ensure a very comfortable starting position. During the course of treatment, small layers of towel can be removed gradually to allow for improved range of knee extension. As a progression to this technique, a small vertical force can be applied on the knee. Care should be taken to ensure that this force is sufficiently small (1 to 2 lb or lighter) and that it is applied superior to the patella to avoid compressive forces between the patella and femur (Fig. 3-25, *B-C*).

The patient is brought to a sitting position to enhance this stretch further. A towel is used to dorsiflex the involved foot, and the patient is instructed to slowly lean forward to stretch the hamstrings (Fig. 3-26, *A*). Simultaneous isometric quadriceps sets also are used to improve strength at the new limits of knee extension.

Gaining knee extension can be achieved in a prone position as well (Fig. 3-26, *B*). However, care must be

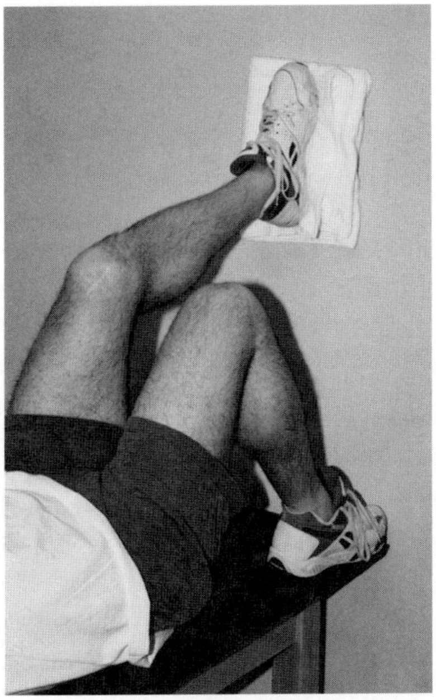

Fig. 3-23 Supine wall slides to gain knee flexion motion.

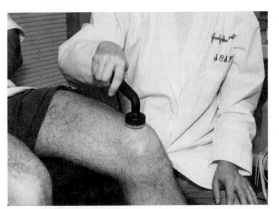

Fig. 3-24 Thermal agents of moist heat and ultrasound applied before passive stretching techniques help elevate tissue temperature and aid in soft-tissue extensibility and patient relaxation.

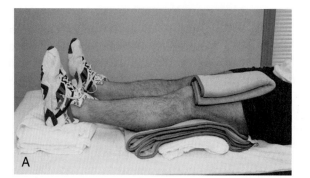

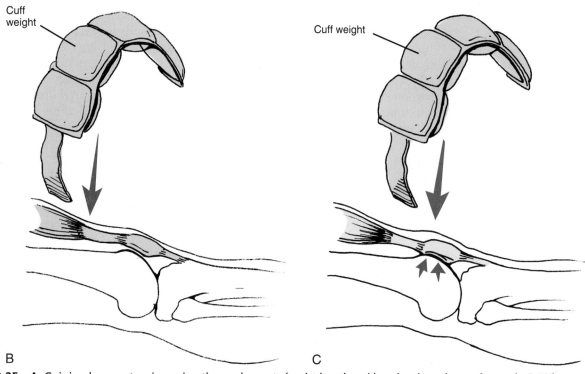

Fig. 3-25   A, Gaining knee extension using thermal agents (moist heat) and low-load, prolonged stretch. **B,** When applying resistance on the knee to gain extension, it is essential that the resistance be placed superior to the patella. **C,** If resistance is placed directly on the patella, there is a sharp concentration of force, which increases patellofemoral compression.

taken to elevate the patella off the table and thereby prevent excessive patellofemoral compression. This is done by placing a small folded towel superior to the patella. This position works well when only slight degrees of motion are needed (5° to 10° of knee extension). This procedure also can be done on an isotonic exercise apparatus following the same process as described with gaining knee flexion on an isotonic exercise machine. Knee extension range also can be improved in a sitting position, with or without the aid of isotonic exercise equipment (Fig. 3-26, *C*).

There are many commercially available tools that use the concept of low-load, prolonged stretch. Dynasplint (Dynasplint Systems, Inc.) and Pro-glide (LMB) are two examples of dynamic splints used to progressively load selected joints to gain motion (Fig. 3-27). An arrangement of pivot points and incrementally

adjustable degrees of tension provides the levels of stress needed to effect change in joint motion. The selection of patients for use of one of these splints must be made carefully. Skin integrity is an issue that must be addressed in the elderly population. Metal hinges and spring-loaded tension flanges may not be appropriate for this population because of the weight of the devices and the patient's potential for skin breakdown.

Simple tools for dynamic stretching can be used at home. A wand, cane, or shortened broomstick can be used for general shoulder flexibility (Fig. 3-28, *A*). Increased mobility can be gained by using the unaffected arm to assist the affected extremity (Fig. 3-28, *B*).

Codman's pendulum exercises are effective for gaining relaxation and small degrees of motion in the shoulder. Relaxation is paramount to the effectiveness of this exercise. In one exercise technique, the patient

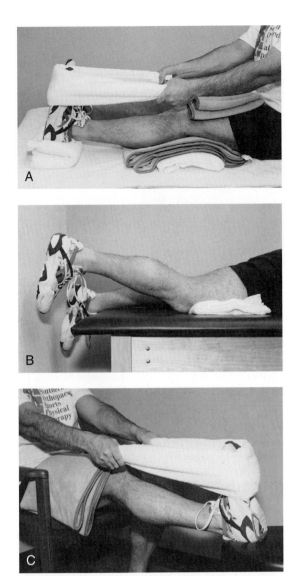

Fig. 3-26 **A,** Seated passive towel stretch. **B,** Passive prone knee extension stretch. Note the use of towels placed under the quadriceps to elevate the patella off the table to reduce patellofemoral compression. **C,** Stretch is enhanced by using a towel to dorsiflex the foot of the involved limbs. Instruct the patient to flex the trunk forward.

is placed prone on a treatment table and a very light weight is held in the hand of the affected extremity. This light distraction force is used in conjunction with gradual, light oscillations in various directions (Fig. 3-29). Relaxation is enhanced by applying moist heat followed by ultrasound to the affected joint before pendulum exercise. When one is teaching the oscillation component of this exercise, it must be made clear that muscular contractions must not be used to initiate and maintain the prescribed motions. The oscillation movements can be initiated by gently swinging the upper body or torso.

Summary

It is necessary to have knowledge of the basic biomechanical and physiologic properties of tissues supporting human movement. Understanding these properties and the effects of exercise and activity on the tissue allows the clinician to modulate appropriate variables in order to recommend patient-specific therapeutic exercise programs that impact strength, coordination, endurance, and flexibility.

❖ GLOSSARY

Adhesion: A limitation of function resulting from scar tissue that forms between individual structures.

Collagen: A fibrous building block of connective tissue that provides strength during movement and exercise.

Contracture: A permanent or transient limitation of movement or shortening of muscle or other soft tissues.

Creep: A viscoelastic property in which there is a change in the shape (deformation) of tissue without actual loss of continuity.

Deformation: Temporary deformations display transient elastic properties. Permanent deformations display plastic properties. Change in loads results in change in deformations.

Golgi tendon organs: A proprioceptive sensory receptor organ that is located at the insertion of skeletal muscle fibers into the tendons of skeletal muscle.

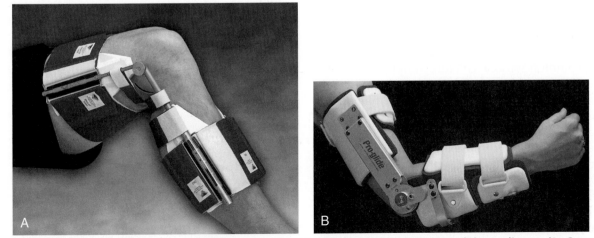

Fig. 3-27 **A,** Dynasplint commercial appliance for low-load prolonged stretch. **B,** Pro-glide appliance. (**A,** Courtesy of Dynasplint Systems, Inc., Severna Park, Md. **B,** Courtesy DeRoyal Medical Products, Powell, Tenn.)

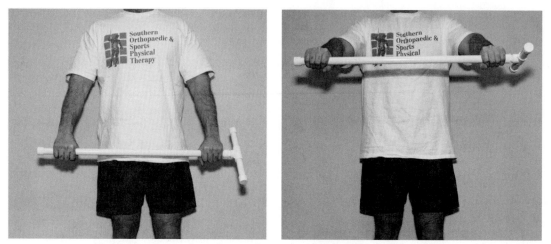

Fig. 3-28   A wand can be used to enhance motion of the shoulder.

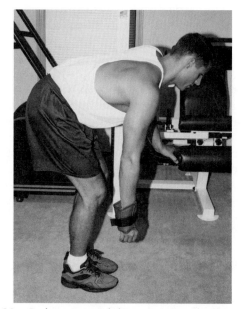

Fig. 3-29   Codman's pendulum exercise. For the exercise to be effective, the patient must relax completely and allow the affected arm to hang and gently oscillate in various directions.

Load: The force sustained by the body. Types of loads include compression, tension, shear, and torsion.

Muscle spindles: Sensory receptors within the belly of a muscle, which primarily detect changes in the length of the muscle.

Remodeling: A process that alters the structure of connective tissue in response to stress.

Strain: The relative measure of the deformation of a body as a result of loading. Strain equals the change in length or original length of a tissue.

Stress: Intensity of internal force. Stress equals force divided by area. It can be compressive, tensile, or shear.

Viscoelasticity: Stress or strain behavior that is time rate dependent.

REFERENCES

1. Adler SS, Beckers D, Buck M: *PNF in practice: an illustrated guide,* ed 2, Berlin, 2000, Springer.
2. Alter MJ: *Science of flexibility,* ed 2, Champaign, Ill, 1996, Human Kinetics.
3. Anderson B, Burke ER: Scientific, medical, and practical aspects of stretching, *Clin Sports Med* 10:63–86, 1991.
4. Arem AJ, Madden JW: Effects of stress on healing wounds: I. Intermittent noncyclical tension, *J Surg Res* 20:93–102, 1976.
5. Arnheim DD, Prentice WE: *Principles of athletic training,* Madison, 1997, Brown & Benchmark.
6. Asmussen E, Boje O: Body temperature and capacity to work, *Acta Physiol Scand* 10:1–21, 1945.
7. Aten D, Knight K: Therapeutic exercise in athletic training: principles and overview, *Athl Train* 13:123–126, 1978.
8. Baechle TR, Earle RW, National Strength, & Conditioning Association (U.S.): *Essentials of strength training and conditioning,* ed 2, Champaign, Ill, 2000, Human Kinetics.
9. Bandy WD, Irion JM: The effect of time on static stretch on the flexibility of the hamstring muscles, *Phys Ther* 74:845–850, 1994.
10. Bandy WD, Irion JM, Briggler M: The effect of static stretch and dynamic range of motion training on the flexibility of the hamstring muscles, *J Orthop Sports Phys Ther* 27:295–300, 1998.
11. Bandy WD, Irion JM, Briggler M: The effect of time and frequency of static stretching on flexibility of the hamstring muscles, *Phys Ther* 77:1090–1096, 1997.
12. Bandy WD, Sanders B: *Therapeutic exercise: techniques for intervention,* Baltimore, 2001, Lippincott Williams & Wilkins.
13. Becker RO: The electrical response of human skeletal muscle to passive stretch, *Surg Forum* 10:828–831, 1960.
14. Bell RD, Hoshizaki TB: Relationships of age and sex with range of motion of seventeen joint actions in humans, *Can J Appl Sport Sci* 6:202–206, 1981.
15. Bergh U: Human power at subnormal body temperatures, *Acta Physiol Scand Suppl* 478:1–39, 1980.
16. Bergh U, Ekblom B: Influence of muscle temperature on maximal muscle strength and power output in human skeletal muscles, *Acta Physiol Scand* 107:33–37, 1979.
17. Bishop D: Warm up I: potential mechanisms and the effects of passive warm up on exercise performance, *Sports Med* 33:439–454, 2003.
18. Bishop D: Warm up II: performance changes following active warm up and how to structure the warm up, *Sports Med* 33:483–498, 2003.

19. Bracko MR: Can stretching prior to exercise and sports improve performance and prevent injury? *ACSM's Health & Fit J* 6:17–22, 2002.

20. Burgeson RE, Nimni ME: Collagen types. Molecular structure and tissue distribution, *Clin Orthop Relat Res* 282:250–272, 1992.

21. Burnley M, Doust JH, Jones AM: Effects of prior warm-up regime on severe-intensity cycling performance, *Med Sci Sports Exerc* 37:838–845, 2005.

22. Buroker K, Schwane J: Does postexercise static stretching alleviate delayed muscle soreness? *Phys Sports Med* 17:65–83, 1989.

23. Ciullo JV, Zarins B: Biomechanics of the musculotendinous unit: relation to athletic performance and injury, *Clin Sports Med* 2: 71–86, 1983.

24. Condon SM, Hutton RS: Soleus muscle electromyographic activity and ankle dorsiflexion range of motion during four stretching procedures, *Phys Ther* 67:24–30, 1987.

25. Corbin CB, Noble L: Flexibility: A major component of physical fitness, *J Phys Educ Rec* 1980 51:23–24, 1980.

26. Cornelius WL, Hagemann RW Jr, Jackson AW: A study on placement of stretching within a workout, *J Sports Med Phys Fitness* 28:234–236, 1988.

27. Cornelius WL, Hinson MM: The relationship between isometric contractions of hip extensors and subsequent flexibility in males, *J Sports Med Phys Fitness* 20:75–80, 1980.

28. Cross KM, Worrell TW: Effects of a static stretching program on the incidence of lower extremity musculotendinous strains, *J Athl Train* 34:11–14, 1999.

29. Currier DP, Nelson RM: *Dynamics of human biologic tissues*, Philadelphia, 1992, FA Davis.

30. de Vries HA: Electromyographic observations of the effects of static stretching upon muscular distress, *Res Q* 32:468–479, 1961.

31. de Vries HA: Evaluation of static stretching procedures for improvement of flexibility, *Res Q* 33:222–229, 1962.

32. de Vries HA: Quantitative electromyographic investigation of the spasm theory of muscle pain, *Am J Phys Med* 45:119–134, 1966.

33. de Vries HA: Physical fitness programs: does physical activity promote relaxation, *J Phys Educ Rec* 46:52–53, 1975.

34. de Vries HA, Wiswell RA, Bulbulian R, et al: Tranquilizer effect of exercise. Acute effects of moderate aerobic exercise on spinal reflex activation level, *Am J Phys Med* 60:57–66, 1981.

35. DeLee J, Drez D, Stanitski CL: *Orthopaedic sports medicine: principles and practice*, Philadelphia, 1994, Saunders.

36. DePino G, Webright W, Arnold B: Duration of maintained hamstring flexibility after cessation of an acute static stretching protocol, *J Athlet Train* 35:56–59, 2000.

37. Dotson CO, Humphrey JH: *Exercise physiology: current selected research*, New York, 1985, AMS Press.

38. Dutton M: *Orthopaedic examination, evaluation, and intervention*, New York, 2004, McGraw-Hill.

39. Ekstrand J, Gillquist J: The avoidability of soccer injuries, *Int J Sports Med* 4:124–128, 1983.

40. Enoka R: *Neuromechanical basis of kinesiology*, ed 2, Champaign, Ill, 1994, Human Kinetics.

41. Enoka RM: *Neuromechanics of human movement*, Champaign, Ill, 2002, Human Kinetics.

42. Etnyre BR, Abraham LD: Antagonist muscle activity during stretching: a paradox re-assessed, *Med Sci Sports Exerc* 20: 285–289, 1988.

43. Etnyre BR, Abraham LD: H-reflex changes during static stretching and two variations of proprioceptive neuromuscular facilitation techniques, *Electroencephalogr Clin Neurophysiol* 63:174–179, 1986.

44. Etnyre BR, Lee EJ: Comments on proprioceptive neuromuscular facilitation techniques, *Res Q Exerc Sport* 58:184–188, 1987.

45. Fowles JR, Sale DG, MacDougall JD: Reduced strength after passive stretch of the human plantarflexors, *J Appl Physiol* 89: 1179–1188, 2000.

46. Genovely H, Stamford BA: Effects of prolonged warm-up exercise above and below anaerobic threshold on maximal performance, *Eur J Appl Physiol Occup Physiol* 48:323–330, 1982.

47. Gibble P, Guskiewicz K, Prentice W, et al: Effects of static and hold-relax stretching on hamstring range of motion using the flexibility LE1000, *J Sport Rehabil* 8:195–208, 1999.

48. Gleim GW, McHugh MP: Flexibility and its effects on sports injury and performance, *Sports Med* 24:289–299, 1997.

49. Godges JJ, MacRae H, Longdon C, et al: The effects of two stretching procedures on hip range of motion and gait economy, *J Orthop Sports Phys Ther* 7:350–357, 1989.

50. Guissard N, Duchateau J, Hainaut K: Muscle stretching and motoneuron excitability, *Eur J Appl Physiol Occup Physiol* 58: 47–52, 1988.

51. Gulick DT, Kimura IF, Sitler M, et al: Various treatment techniques on signs and symptoms of delayed onset muscle soreness, *J Athlet Train* 31:145–152, 1996.

52. Hardy L: Improving active range of hip flexion, *Res Q Exerc Sport* 56:111–114, 1985.

53. Harris M: A factor analytic study of flexibility, *Res Q Exerc Sport* 40:62–70, 1969.

54. Harris ML: Flexibility, *Phys Ther* 49:591–601, 1969.

55. Hartig DE, Henderson JM: Increasing hamstring flexibility decreases lower extremity overuse injuries in military basic trainees, *Am J Sports Med* 27:173–176, 1999.

56. Hartley-O'Brien SJ: Six mobilization exercises for active range of hip flexion, *Res Q Exerc Sport* 51:625–635, 1980.

57. Henricson A, Fredriksson K, Persson I, et al: The effect of heat and stretching on range of hip motion, *J Orthop Sports Phys Ther* 6:110–115, 1984.

58. Hertling D, Kessler RM: *Management of common musculoskeletal disorders: physical therapy principles and methods*, ed 4, Philadelphia, 2006, Lippincott Williams & Wilkins.

59. Hettinga DL: II. Normal joint structures and their reaction to injury, *J Orthop Sports Phys Ther* 1:83–88, 1979.

60. Holcomb W: Stretching and warm-up. In Baechle T, Earle R, editors: *Essentials of strength training and conditioning*, ed 2, Champaign, Ill, 2000, Human Kinetics.

61. Holt LE, Travis TM, Okita T: Comparative study of three stretching techniques, *Percept Mot Skills* 31:611–616, 1970.

62. Hunter SK, Enoka RM: Sex differences in the fatigability of arm muscles depends on absolute force during isometric contractions, *J Appl Physiol* 91:2686–2694, 2001.

63. Kandel ER, Schwartz JH, Jessell TM: *Principles of neural science*, ed 4, New York, 2000, McGraw-Hill.

64. Kisner C, Colby LA: *Therapeutic exercise: foundations and techniques*, ed 5, Philadelphia, 2007, FA Davis.

64a. Knott M, Voss P: *Proprioceptive neuromuscular facilitation*, ed 3, New York, 1985, Harper and Row.

65. Knudson D: Stretching during warm-up: do we have enough evidence? *J Phys Educ Rec Dance* 70:24–32, 1999.

66. Knudson D: Stretching: from science to practice, *J Phys Ed Rec Dance* 69:38–45, 1998.

67. Knudson D, Bennett K, Corn R, et al: Acute effects of stretching are not evident in the kinematics of the vertical jump, *J Strength Cond Res* 15:98–101, 2001.

68. Kokkonen J, Nelson AG, Cornwell A: Acute muscle stretching inhibits maximal strength performance, *Res Q Exerc Sport* 69: 411–415, 1998.

69. Komi PV, IOC Medical Commission, International Federation of Sports Medicine: *Strength and power in sport*, Oxford, UK, 1992, Blackwell Scientific.

70. Kulund DN, Tottossy M: Warm-up, strength, and power, *Orthop Clin North Am* 14:427–448, 1983.

71. Lamontagne A, Malouin F, Richards CL: Viscoelastic behavior of plantar flexor muscle-tendon unit at rest, *J Orthop Sports Phys Ther* 26:244–252, 1997.

72. Larson LA, Michelman H: *International guide to fitness and health*, New York, 1973, Crown.

73. Lederman E: *Fundamentals of manual therapy: physiology, neurology, and psychology*, New York, 1997, Churchill Livingstone.

74. Lehmann JF, Masock AJ, Warren CG, et al: Effect of therapeutic temperatures on tendon extensibility, *Arch Phys Med Rehabil* 51:481–487, 1970.

75. Lentell G, Hetherington T, Eagan J, et al: The use of thermal agents to influence the effectiveness of a low-load prolonged stretch, *J Orthop Sports Phys Ther* 16:200–207, 1992.

76. Levangie PK, Norkin CC: *Joint structure and function: a comprehensive analysis*, ed 3, Philadelphia, 2001, FA Davis.

77. Light KE, Nuzik S, Personius W, et al: Low-load prolonged stretch vs. high-load brief stretch in treating knee contractures, *Phys Ther* 64:330–333, 1984.

78. Longacre JJ, Children's Hospital (Cincinnati Ohio). Research Institute, Research Group for the Facially Crippled: The ultrastructure of collagen: its relation to the healing of wounds and to the management of hypertrophic scar; [proceedings, May 30-31, 1973, Research Institute of Children's Hospital]. Springfield, Ill, 1976, Thomas.

79. Lucas RC, Koslow R: Comparative study of static, dynamic, and proprioceptive neuromuscular facilitation stretching techniques on flexibility, *Percept Mot Skills* 58:615–618, 1984.

80. Madding S, Wong J, Medeiros J: Effect of duration of passive stretch on hip abduction range of motion, *J Orthop Sports Phys Ther* 8:409–416, 1987.

81. Magnusson SP, Simonsen EB, Aagaard P, et al: Mechanical and physical responses to stretching with and without preisometric contraction in human skeletal muscle, *Arch Phys Med Rehabil* 77:373–378, 1996.

82. Markos PD: Ipsilateral and contralateral effects of proprioceptive neuromuscular facilitation techniques on hip motion and electromyographic activity, *Phys Ther* 59:1366–1373, 1979.

83. McGlynn GH, Laughlin NT, Rowe V: Effect of electromyographic feedback and static stretching on artificially induced muscle soreness, *Am J Phys Med* 58:139–148, 1979.

84. McHugh MP, Magnusson SP, Gleim GW, et al: Viscoelastic stress relaxation in human skeletal muscle, *Med Sci Sports Exerc* 24:1375–1382, 1992.

85. McNair PJ, Stanley SN: Effect of passive stretching and jogging on the series elastic muscle stiffness and range of motion of the ankle joint, *Br J Sports Med* 30:313–317, 1996.

86. Medeiros JM, Smidt GL, Burmeister LF, et al: The influence of isometric exercise and passive stretch on hip joint motion, *Phys Ther* 57:518–523, 1977.

87. Millar AP: An early stretching routine for calf muscle strains, *Med Sci Sports* 8:39–42, 1976.

88. Mohr KJ, Pink MM, Elsner C, et al: Electromyographic investigation of stretching: the effect of warm-up, *Clin J Sport Med* 8: 215–220, 1998.

89. Moller M, Ekstrand J, Oberg B, et al: Duration of stretching effect on range of motion in lower extremities, *Arch Phys Med Rehabil* 66:171–173, 1985.

90. Monaco JL, Lawrence WT: Acute wound healing an overview, *Clin Plast Surg* 30:1–12, 2003.

91. Moore MA, Hutton RS: Electromyographic investigation of muscle stretching techniques, *Med Sci Sports Exerc* 12:322–329, 1980.

92. Neumann DA: *Kinesiology of the musculoskeletal system: foundations for physical rehabilitation*, ed 1, St Louis, 2002, Mosby.

93. Noakes T: *Lore of running*, ed 3, Champaign, Ill, 1991, Leisure Press.

94. Noonan TJ, Best TM, Seaber AV, et al: Identification of a threshold for skeletal muscle injury, *Am J Sports Med* 22:257–261, 1994.

95. Norkin CC, White DJ: *Measurement of joint motion: a guide to goniometry*, ed 2, Philadelphia, 1995, FA Davis.

96. Nyland J: *Clinical decisions in therapeutic exercise: planning and implementation*, Upper Saddle River, NJ, 2006, Pearson Prentice Hall.

97. Oatis CA: *Kinesiology: the mechanics and pathomechanics of human movement*, ed 1, Philadelphia, 2004, Lippincott Williams & Wilkins.

98. Pollock ML, Gaesser GA, Butcher JD, et al: American College of Sports Medicine Position Stand. The recommended quantity and quality of exercise for developing and maintaining cardiorespiratory and muscular fitness, and flexibility in healthy adults, *Med Sci Sports Exerc* 30:975–991, 1998.

99. Pope RP, Herbert RD, Kirwan JD, et al: A randomized trial of pre-exercise stretching for prevention of lower-limb injury, *Med Sci Sports Exerc* 32:271–277, 2000.

100. Pratt K, Bohannon R: Effects of a 3-minute standing stretch on ankle-dorsiflexion range of motion, *J Sport Rehabil* 12:162–173, 2003.

101. Prentice WE: A comparison of static stretching and PNF stretching for improving hip joint flexibility, *Athl Train* 18:56–59, 1983.

102. Prentice WE, Voight ML: *Techniques in musculoskeletal rehabilitation*, New York, 2001, McGraw-Hill.

103. Roberts JM, Wilson K: Effect of stretching duration on active and passive range of motion in the lower extremity, *Br J Sports Med* 33:259–263, 1999.

104. Rosenbaum D, Hennig EM: The influence of stretching and warm-up exercises on Achilles tendon reflex activity, *J Sports Sci* 13:481–490, 1995.

105. Sady SP, Wortman M, Blanke D: Flexibility training: ballistic, static or proprioceptive neuromuscular facilitation? *Arch Phys Med Rehabil* 63:261–263, 1982.

106. Safran MR, Garrett WE Jr, Seaber AV, et al: The role of warmup in muscular injury prevention, *Am J Sports Med* 16:123–129, 1988.

107. Sapega AA, Quedenfeld RA, Moyer RA, et al: Biophysical factors in range of motion exercise, *Phys Sports Med* 9:57–65, 1981.

108. Scully RM, Barnes MR: *Physical therapy*, Philadelphia, 1989, Lippincott.

109. Shear CR, Bloch RJ: Vinculin in subsarcolemmal densities in chicken skeletal muscle: localization and relationship to intracellular and extracellular structures, *J Cell Biol* 101:240–256, 1985.

110. Shellock FG, Prentice WE: Warming-up and stretching for improved physical performance and prevention of sports-related injuries, *Sports Med* 2:267–278, 1985.

111. Shrier I: Stretching before exercise does not reduce the risk of local muscle injury: a critical review of the clinical and basic science literature, *Clin J Sport Med* 9:221–227, 1999.

112. Simon SR: *American Academy of Orthopaedic Surgeons: Orthopaedic basic science*, Rosemont, Ill, 1994, American Academy of Orthopaedic Surgeons.

113. Smith CA: The warm-up procedure: to stretch or not to stretch. A brief review, *J Orthop Sports Phys Ther* 19:12–17, 1994.

114. Smith LL, Brunetz MH, Chenier TC, et al: The effects of static and ballistic stretching on delayed onset muscle soreness and creatine kinase, *Res Q Exerc Sport* 64:103–107, 1993.

115. Starring DT, Gossman MR, Nicholson GG Jr, et al: Comparison of cyclic and sustained passive stretching using a mechanical device to increase resting length of hamstring muscles, *Phys Ther* 68:314–320, 1988.

116. Stolov WC, Weilepp TG Jr: Passive length-tension relationship of intact muscle, epimysium, and tendon in normal and denervated gastrocnemius of the rat, *Arch Phys Med Rehabil* 47:612–620, 1966.

117. Street SF: Lateral transmission of tension in frog myofibers: a myofibrillar network and transverse cytoskeletal connections are possible transmitters, *J Cell Physiol* 114:346–364, 1983.

118. Tanigawa MC: Comparison of the hold-relax procedure and passive mobilization on increasing muscle length, *Phys Ther* 52: 725–735, 1972.

119. Taylor DC, Dalton JD Jr, Seaber AV, et al: Experimental muscle strain injury. Early functional and structural deficits and the increased risk for reinjury, *Am J Sports Med* 21:190–194, 1993.

120. Taylor DC, Dalton JD, Seaber AV, et al: Viscoelastic properties of muscle-tendon units. The biomechanical effects of stretching, *Am J Sports Med* 18:300–309, 1990.

121. van Mechelen W, Hlobil H, Kemper HC, et al: Prevention of running injuries by warm-up, cool-down, and stretching exercises, *Am J Sports Med* 21:711–719, 1993.

122. Voss DE, Ionta MK, Myers BJ, et al: *Proprioceptive neuromuscular facilitation: patterns and techniques*, ed 3, Philadelphia, 1985, Harper & Row.

123. Wallin D, Ekblom B, Grahn R, et al: Improvement of muscle flexibility. A comparison between two techniques, *Am J Sports Med* 13:263–268, 1985.

124. Wallmann HW, Mercer JA, McWhorter JW: Surface electromyographic assessment of the effect of static stretching of the gastrocnemius on vertical jump performance, *J Strength Cond Res* 19:684–688, 2005.

125. Walter J, Figoni SF, Andres FF, et al: Training intensity and duration in flexibility, *Clin Kinesiol* 50:40–45, 1996.

126. Warren CG, Lehmann JF, Koblanski JN: Elongation of rat tail tendon: effect of load and temperature, *Arch Phys Med Rehabil* 52:465–474, 1971.

127. Warren CG, Lehmann JF, Koblanski JN: Heat and stretch procedures: an evaluation using rat tail tendon, *Arch Phys Med Rehabil* 57:122–126, 1976.

128. Watkins MA, Riddle DL, Lamb RL, et al: Reliability of goniometric measurements and visual estimates of knee range of motion obtained in a clinical setting, *Phys Ther* 71:90–96, 1991.

129. Wharton J, Wharton P: *The Wharton's stretch book*, New York, 1996, Three Rivers Press.

130. Wiktorsson-Moller M, Oberg B, Ekstrand J, et al: Effects of warming up, massage, and stretching on range of motion and muscle strength in the lower extremity, *Am J Sports Med* 11:249–252, 1983.

131. Wilkinson A: Stretching the truth. A review of the literature on muscle stretching, *Aust J Physiother* 38:283–287, 1992.

132. Williford HN, East JB, Smith FH, et al: Evaluation of warm-up for improvement in flexibility, *Am J Sports Med* 14:316–319, 1986.

133. Wolpaw JR: Acquisition and maintenance of the simplest motor skill: investigation of CNS mechanisms, *Med Sci Sports Exerc* 26:1475–1479, 1994.

134. Wolpaw JR, Carp JS: Memory traces in spinal cord, *Trends Neurosci* 13:137–142, 1990.

135. Woo SL, Buckwalter JA, American Academy of Orthopaedic Surgeons, et al: Injury and repair of the musculoskeletal soft tissues: workshop, Savannah, Ga, June 1987, Park Ridge, Ill, 1988, American Academy of Orthopaedic Surgeons.

136. Woo SL, Matthews JV, Akeson WH, et al: Connective tissue response to immobility. Correlative study of biomechanical and biochemical measurements of normal and immobilized rabbit knees, *Arthritis Rheum* 18:257–264, 1975.

137. Youdas JW, Carey JR, Garrett TR: Reliability of measurements of cervical spine range of motion–comparison of three methods, *Phys Ther* 71:98–104, 1991.

138. Zito M, Driver D, Parker C, et al: Lasting effects of one bout of two 15-second passive stretches on ankle dorsiflexion range of motion, *J Orthop Sports Phys Ther* 26:214–221, 1997.

REVIEW QUESTIONS

Short Answer

1. Is muscle tissue considered to be an active or passive restraint to joint motion?
2. Name three types of stretching techniques.
3. A(n) _____ is an inhibitory neurophysiologic sensory receptor involved with the stretch reflex.
4. The _____ is an excitatory specialized fiber found in muscle.

True/False

5. Stress is the amount of tension or load placed on tissues.
6. Tissue temperature does not affect connective tissue extensibility.
7. Active exercise has an effect on intramuscular temperature and tissue extensibility.
8. Ballistic stretching is superior to other forms of active stretching.
9. Low-load, long-duration static stretching is a technique used to stretch soft-tissue contractures.
10. Research has shown that performing static stretching before or after a workout does not make a difference in increasing ROM.
11. Research has shown that an acute stretching program can result in increased long-term flexibility.

4 Strength

Marc Campolo

LEARNING OBJECTIVES

1. Name the noncontractile and contractile elements of muscle tissue.
2. Give examples of concentric and eccentric contractions.
3. State two definitions of strength.
4. List methods used to measure strength.
5. Compare muscle contraction types related to tension produced and energy liberated.
6. Identify clinical features of delayed onset muscle soreness (DOMS).
7. List three clinically relevant exercise programs to enhance strength.
8. Explain opened and closed kinetic chain exercise.
9. Identify goals and applications of strength training programs for the elderly.

KEY TERMS

Actin
Atrophy
Closed kinetic chain (CKC) exercise
Concentric
Delayed onset muscle soreness (DOMS)
Eccentric
Endomysium
Epimysium
Fasciculi

Fast twitch (FT) (type II, white glycolytic) muscle fiber
Hypertrophy
Isometric
Myofibrils
Myosin
Open kinetic chain (OKC) exercise
Perimysium
Plyometrics
Power

Progressive resistance exercise (PRE)
SAID principle
Slow twitch (ST) (type I, red oxidative) muscle fiber
Strength
Tension
Work

CHAPTER OUTLINE

Strength training is physical activity intended to increase muscle strength and mass.[46] Adults who engage in strength training are less likely to experience loss of muscle mass and functional decline.[63]

Maintaining, enhancing, and regaining strength are critical for improving body function during all phases of recovery after surgery, injury, or disease affecting the musculoskeletal system. Strength training, resistance training, and weight training are synonymous and refer to physical conditioning that uses isometric, isotonic, or isokinetic exercise to develop muscle.[28] Resistance exercise is any form of active exercise in which a dynamic or static muscle contraction is resisted by an outside force, applied either manually or mechanically. Therapeutic exercise is resistance training that is applied in a systematic and individualized manner designed to improve, restore, or enhance physical function. The physical therapist assistant (PTA) must understand the basic foundations of strength development and, more importantly, how to apply principles of strength gaining during recovery after immobilization, surgery, or musculoskeletal injury. In this chapter the PTA is introduced to basic concepts and universally accepted principles that can be applied in numerous clinical situations with various orthopedic pathologies.

A muscle's strength or **tension**-generating capacity is determined by a number of diverse but interrelated factors, including neural control (motor unit recruitment and rate coding; the number and rate at which the motor units are fired), cross-sectional area (muscle fiber number and size), muscle fiber arrangement (angle of pennation or how fibers are aligned in relation to a imaginary line between the muscle's origin and insertion), muscle length (length tension ratio; muscle produces the greatest tension when it is near or at the physiologic resting position at the time of contraction), angle of pull (muscle's tension generating capacity is increased when the tendon is perpendicular to the bone), and fiber type distribution (high percent of type I: low force production, fatigue resistant; or type IIA and IIB: high force production, rapid fatigue).[6,41] One also has to consider other factors, such as energy stores of the muscle, recovery from exercise, fatigue, age, gender, and state of health of the muscle; they may effect tension generation.

A basic understanding of muscular composition and gross structure helps clarify concepts of therapeutic exercise and provides a foundation for developing advanced principles and applications of strength.

GENERAL MUSCLE BIOLOGY

The body of an individual muscle is surrounded by noncontractile connective tissue called the *epimysium.* Within the muscle are bundles of fibers called *fasciculi,* which are surrounded by another noncontractile connective tissue called the *perimysium*. The **endomysium** is a noncontractile connective tissue that surrounds each individual muscle fiber. The individual muscle fibers are composed of **myofibrils** that lie parallel to each other and the muscle fiber itself (Fig. 4-1, *A*). The structural components of the myofibrils are called *myofilaments*, and they comprise two predominant proteins, actin and myosin. The functional, or contractile, unit of a muscle fiber cell is called the *sarcomere* (Fig. 4-1, *B*). **Myosin** (a thick protein) and **actin** (a thin protein) are actively involved with the mechanics of muscular contraction, which involves a complex and highly structured series of chemical and mechanical events.

The extraordinarily complex biochemical excitation–contraction coupling and mechanical actions of muscular contraction are described in physiology textbooks. In simple terms, the neurologic stimulus to contract a muscle causes the release of acetylcholine, which initiates the release of calcium. The calcium ions bond with troponin and tropomyosin, two proteins within the actin filaments. This allows actin–adenosine triphosphate (ATP) to react with myosin–adenosine triphosphatase (ATPase), producing energy so the thick myosin and thin actin filaments can "slide" past each other, generating tension and producing contraction of the muscle.

Muscle Fiber Types

Generally two distinct types of muscle fibers have been identified in humans. These fibers are classified by their contractile and metabolic characteristics (Fig. 4-2).

Slow twitch (ST) (type I, red oxidative) muscle fibers possess relatively large and numerous mitochondria, triglycerides, and oxidative enzymes (succinic dehydrogenase [SDH]), which allow for aerobic work. They also have relatively low myosin-ATPase and glycolytic activity, as well as slower calcium handling ability and shortening speed. This type of fiber is specialized for muscular endurance activities. These fatigue-resistant fibers contract slowly but are highly efficient for prolonged aerobic events.

Fast twitch (FT) (type II, white glycolytic) muscle fibers, by contrast, are anaerobic. These fibers are not as vascular as type I fibers, but they fire, or contract, at a higher speed than type I fibers and with more force. These fibers have a very high level of myosin-ATPase, which provides energy for speed of contraction and tension; they also have low myoglobin content and very few mitochondria. However, they are larger in diameter than red fibers. These fibers are used mainly in activities that require speed, strength, and power.

Type II fibers can be further broken down into three distinct subclassifications: type IIA; type IIAB; and type IIB.[49,73] These fiber types differ mainly in terms of

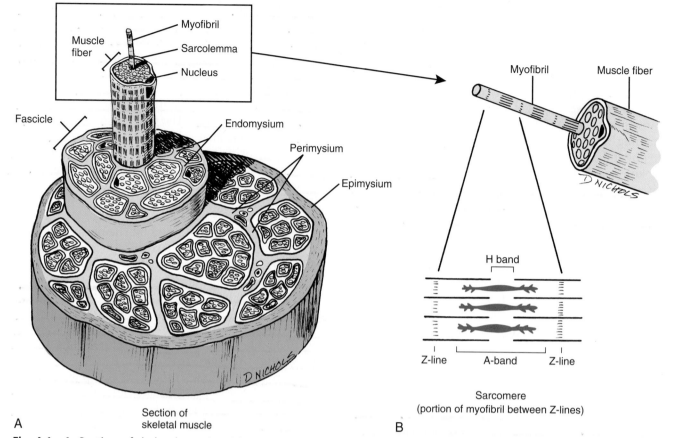

Fig. 4-1 **A,** Section of skeletal muscle with contractile and noncontractile connective tissue. **B,** Functional or contractile unit of skeletal muscle fiber cell.

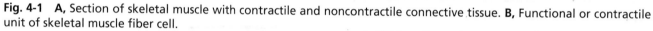

contraction velocity and endurance and are classified as intermediate fiber types with both aerobic and anaerobic capacities.

- The type IIA (fast-oxidative-glycolytic [FOG]) fiber has a fast contraction speed and a moderate capacity for energy transfer from both aerobic and anaerobic sources.
- The type IIB (fast-glycolytic [FG]) fiber possesses the greatest anaerobic capacity and the fastest shortening speed.
- The type IIAB fiber is rare and undifferentiated and may contribute to reinnervation and motor unit transformation.

The motor unit is the basic unit of movement. It consists of the anterior motor neuron and all the muscle fibers it innervates. A motor unit contains only one specific muscle fiber type. Motor unit recruitment is the adding of motor units to increase force. The Henneman size principle proposes an orderly recruitment of motor units within a motor neuron pool during a defined movement task.[36a] When a low force is needed, only the slow twitch motor units (type I) are activated; and with increasing force requirements, larger and faster motor units (type IIA, type IIB) are recruited. Therefore the orderly recruitment of muscle fibers during contraction proceeds according to increased force requirements, as shown in Fig. 4-3.

TYPES OF MUSCLE CONTRACTIONS

The three true types of muscle contractions are **concentric, eccentric,** and **isometric.** Two other terms have been used to describe muscle contractions: isotonic and isokinetic. These are not types of contractions but rather terms used to describe events.

Concentric

In a concentric contraction, tension is produced and shortening of the muscle takes place (Fig. 4-4, *A*). The action produced by a concentric contraction brings together or approximates the origin and insertion of the contracting muscle. In a concentric exercise, tension is developed and shortening of the muscle occurs to overcome an external force, such as a weight.

Eccentric

An eccentric muscle contraction is sometimes referred to as a *lengthening contraction.* In an eccentric contraction, tension is produced; however, lengthening of the muscle occurs so that the net action is opposite that produced

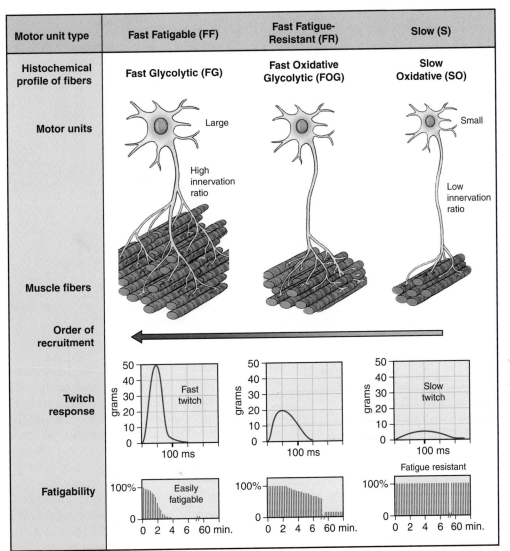

Motor unit type	Fast Fatigable (FF)	Fast Fatigue-Resistant (FR)	Slow (S)
Histochemical profile of fibers	Fast Glycolytic (FG)	Fast Oxidative Glycolytic (FOG)	Slow Oxidative (SO)
Motor units	Large / High innervation ratio		Small / Low innervation ratio
Muscle fibers			
Order of recruitment			
Twitch response	Fast twitch		Slow twitch
Fatigability	Easily fatigable		Fatigue resistant

Fig. 4-2 Classification of motor unit types from muscle fibers based on histochemical profile, size, and twitch (contractile) characteristics. A theoretical continuum of differing contractile and morphologic characteristics is shown for each of the three motor unit types. It is important to note that the range of any single characteristic may vary considerably within any given motor unit (either within or between whole muscles). (From Neumann DA: *Kinesiology of the musculoskeletal system: foundations for rehabilitation*, ed 2, St Louis, 2010, Mosby.)

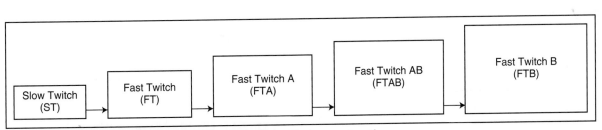

Fig. 4-3 Progressive orderly recruitment of muscle fibers during contraction.

by a concentric contraction (Fig. 4-4, *B*). The origin and insertion of the contracting muscle move farther apart during the contraction. Eccentric exercise involves loading of a muscle, causing a physical lengthening of the muscle as it attempts to control the load when lowering the weight. For example, as one slowly descends to sit in a chair and moves from a standing to a sitting position, the quadriceps muscles must eccentrically contract to control the rate of descent or one would suddenly fall into the chair.

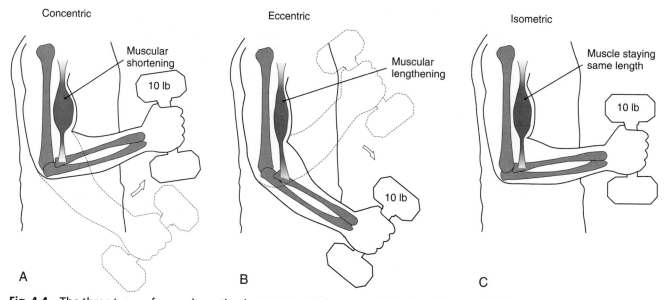

Fig. 4-4 The three types of muscular activation: concentric (**A**), eccentric (**B**), and isometric (**C**). (From Mansfield PJ, Neumann DA: *Essentials of kinesiology for the physical therapist assistant*, St Louis, 2009, Mosby.)

Isometric

In an isometric contraction, tension is produced but no joint movement or action takes place (Fig. 4-4, C). Isometric exercise involves a muscle contraction against a force with no significant movement occurring. Examples include pushing or pulling against an immovable object or holding a weight in a particular position. Isometric exercises are used when joint movement is restricted or not possible. A form of isometric exercise is a muscle-setting exercise. Setting exercises are muscle contractions performed without movement or resistance. An example is a quadriceps set, or quad set. (The word "set" is used to describe an isometric contraction.) If the quadriceps contracts as a knee is held straight, tension is produced within the muscle but no change in joint angle takes place. Clinically, setting exercises are used to decrease pain, facilitate muscle contraction, increase circulation, and retard muscle atrophy.

Isotonic

An isotonic muscle contraction is not an accurate name for what happens physiologically. The name implies that the resistance, force, load, or tension remains constant, but actually the tension or force created in a muscle during this type of action must change as the joint angle changes. For example, when one lifts a barbell (constant resistance), the amount of force generated by the contracting muscle varies at different angles during the movement, even though the weight itself remains constant. This occurs because changes in the muscle length as well as the muscle tendon's angle of pull alter the mechanical advantage of the muscle throughout the movement, resulting in variations of force developing capacity. Therefore a more precise and descriptive term,

isoinertial,[55] can be used in place of isotonic. The term isotonic is used in this book to describe the action of variable velocities of movement with a constant load. Examples of isotonic resistance equipment are barbells, dumbbells, and ankle weights, which are collectively referred to as *free weights*.

Isokinetic

In an isokinetic contraction, the speed or velocity of movement is held constant regardless of the magnitude of force applied to the resistance. Any force applied results in an equal reaction force supplied by the machine throughout a given range of motion (ROM). This is accomplished by a rate-limiting computerized dynamometer. Examples of isokinetic equipment are Cybex, Biodex, Lido, and Kin-Com. Isokinetic exercise is called *accommodating resistance*. The theoretical construct is that if a patient provides maximal effort during a repetition, the machine will provide variable resistance, stressing the muscle maximally throughout the full ROM, unlike the resistance provided with isotonic exercise. This equipment also provides an object force measurement throughout the ROM of a joint and can be a valuable tool for strength assessment.

DEFINITIONS OF STRENGTH AND POWER

Strength is a broad term. Generally strength is the ability of a muscle to generate force, or more specifically the maximum force generated by a single muscle or related muscle group.[50] Other definitions of strength include "The ability to exert force under a given set of conditions defined by body position, the body movement by which force is applied, movement type, and movement speed"[36] and "The maximal force a muscle or muscle group can generate at a specified velocity."[45] The American Physical Therapy Association defines muscle strength as "the muscle force exerted by a muscle or group of muscles to overcome resistance under specific set of circumstances"; muscle performance as "the capacity of a muscle or group of muscles to generate forces"; muscle power as "the work produced per unit time or the product of strength and speed"; and muscle endurance as "the ability to sustain forces repeatedly or to generate forces over a period of time."[5] Functional strength has been described as the ability of the neuromuscular system to produce, reduce, or control forces, contemplated or imposed, during functional activities, in a smooth, coordinated manner.[41]

To help clarify strength clinically, it is perhaps most useful to consider strength in terms that describe performance.

- **Work** is used to describe the result or product of a force exerted on an object and the distance the object moves.[36]
  - This term is expressed as Work = Force × Distance.
- Force can be described as either linear or rotary.[66]
  - Linear force is described as Force = Mass × Acceleration.
  - Rotary force is expressed as Force = Mass × Angular acceleration.
- Torque is the ability to cause rotational movement.
  - Torque is expressed as Torque = Force × Perpendicular distance from the axis of rotation.
- **Power** is defined as the time rate of doing work, which can be expressed in several ways.[55]
  - Power = Work/Time = Force × [Distance/Time]
  - Power = Force × [Distance/Time]
  - Power = Force × Velocity
- Velocity is defined as a vector that describes displacement.

Overall, these terms help describe resultant muscular performance as they relate to the development of strength.

MEASURING STRENGTH

Strength can be measured by six methods:
1. Manual muscle testing
2. Cable tensiometry
3. Dynamometry
4. Isotonic one-repetition maximum lift
5. Isokinetics
6. Functional strength assessment

Manual muscle testing (MMT) is a isometric method of muscle testing that is designed to measure muscle strength requiring no equipment other than the examiner's hands. This technique was introduced in the early 1900s and its use is widely accepted in the health care professions.[61] It is used to generally grade a muscle's isometric contraction capacity at a specific joint angle against a manually applied force or gravity. Performing a MMT requires extensive time, effort, and attention to detail while performing the correct technique to ensure that the results obtained are as accurate as possible.[61] The tester must have a comprehensive and detailed understanding of kinesiology to accurately and consistently reproduce manual grading of muscle strength (performance). The grading scale for this test is clinically easy to use and is outlined in Table 4-1. The disadvantage of isometric strength testing is that because muscle length is held constant, isometric strength testing provides muscle strength data at only one point in the range.[59] MMT is valid from grades 0 to 5; however, when MMT scores exceed grade 4, the MMT loses it ability to discriminate between gradations of strength. In cases where measurement and documentation of

Table 4-1	*Manual Muscle Test Scale*
Score	**Description**
Grade 5/Normal	Patient can hold the position against maximum resistance, has complete range of motion. There is a wide range of normal.
Grade 4/Good	Patient can hold the position against strong to moderate resistance, and has full range of motion. Grade 4/good and below represents true clinical weakness.
Grade 3+/Fair +	Patient can complete a full range of motion against gravity and hold end position against mild resistance.
Grade 3/Fair	Patient can tolerate no resistance but can perform the movement through the full range of motion.
Grade 2+/Poor +	Patient has full range of motion in the gravity eliminated position and can take some resistance.
Grade 2/Poor	Patient has full range of motion in the gravity eliminated position.
Grade 2–/Poor –	Patient can complete partial range of motion in the gravity eliminated position.
Grade 1/Trace	The examiner can detect visually or by palpation some contractile activity.
Grade 0/Zero	The muscle is completely quiescent on palpation or visual inspection.

From Hislop HJ, Montgomery J: *Daniels and Worthingham's muscle testing: techniques of manual examination*, ed 7, St Louis, 2002, Saunders.

strength level is critical above a MMT grade 4, an alternative form of measuring strength should be used.[59]

Cable tensiometry is used to isometrically measure a muscle's strength (Fig. 4-5). Essentially this tool is a mechanical form of manual muscle testing. The tensiometer provides the advantage of versatility for recording force measurements at virtually all angles of a joint's ROM and may be more sensitive for grading muscle strength above grade 4. This method is used primarily to measure strength in normal subjects in research projects. Many tests were developed in the 1950s to describe static force or isometric strength by use of the cable tension method.[15,16]

Dynamometry is used extensively in physical therapy. Hand-held dynamometers (Fig. 4-6) are used to quantify grip strength, and the standing-back dynamometer is used to evaluate back extension strength. In this latter example, many factors contribute to the subject's ability to generate tension or force during the back pull, including the patient's motivation, degree of pain (if any), arm length, leg length, height, weight, and the obvious contribution from other muscle groups. These variables make dynamometry an unreliable, nonspecific testing tool.

An isotonic one-repetition maximum lift is used to test strength using commercially available exercise equipment or barbells and dumbbells. In this method the patient performs a single, full ROM lift, such as a bench press (Fig. 4-7), shoulder press, or arm curl, for a particular muscle group. Applying this method is difficult because the tester and patient must first establish a reasonable starting weight through trial and error, fatigue becomes a factor if many trials are needed, and precise performance or execution of the proper lift is determined subjectively by the tester. This method is best used for normal subjects, in a sports medicine environment, or with uninvolved body parts not necessary for stabilization of a disabled joint.

Perhaps the most widely used and clinically relevant method of objective, reproducible strength testing is through isokinetics. The data collected with isokinetic testing document strength (force production), torque, power, and work.[60] As stated, isokinetics employs a fixed speed, or velocity, of movement that allows for maximum loading throughout the full ROM. If a patient experiences pain during any part of the test, or does not apply a maximum force throughout the entire ROM, the velocity remains constant with a variable resistance that is totally accommodating to the individual.[19] To test for strength, slow speeds (30° to 60° per second) are generally used.[48] Because isokinetic equipment can be interfaced with computers, a hard-copy graph of the data can be used for evaluation and exercise prescription. In addition to being a valid and reliable tool for strength testing, isokinetics also can evaluate neuromuscular endurance, speed of muscle contraction, and muscular power.[40]

The determination of an individual's readiness to return to normal levels of activity is a common issue in rehabilitation. To resolve this issue, clinicians have incorporated functional testing following rehabilitation. Functional testing involves the evaluation of broad skills necessary to perform complex movements versus traditional methods that focus on isolated joint testing. This is particularly important when dealing with athletes who may be returned to activity too soon after rehabilitation because of inaccuracies in the assessment of their functional ability resulting from more traditional assessment methods.[18]

Examples include the following:

■ One-leg hop for distance: The patient performs a single-leg hop for distance with each lower extremity.
■ Single-leg triple hop for distance: The patient performs a single-leg triple hop for distance with each lower extremity.

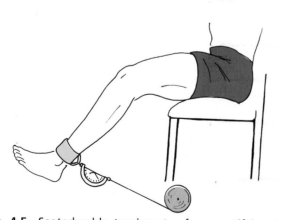

Fig. 4-5 Seated cable tensiometer for quantifying isometric quadriceps strength.

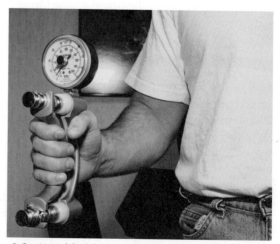

Fig. 4-6 Hand-held grip dynamometer for measuring grip strength.

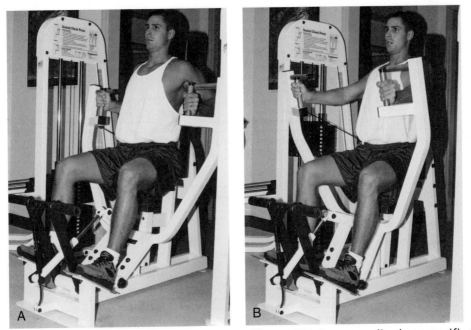

Figure 4-7   Concentric and eccentric one-repetition maximum lift test. This is a generalized nonspecific method to determine strength with commercial isotonic equipment. **A,** Starting position. **B,** End position.

- Timed single-leg hop (minitrampoline): The patient hops on the trampoline a maximum number of times in 30 seconds.
- Vertical jump: The patient performs a two-legged vertical jump for height.

COMPARISON OF MUSCLE CONTRACTION TYPES

Generally, muscle contractions are characterized by the amount of tension the contraction produces and the amount of energy liberated (ATP use) by the contraction. The most common clinically applicable way to strengthen muscle is with concentric and eccentric contractions using isotonic (isoinertial)[55] progressive resistive exercise (PRE). Ankle or cuff weights, hand-held weights (dumbbells), and weight machines are examples of isotonic equipment used in physical therapy practice.* Elftman[23] has demonstrated that the production of maximal force of contraction by various methods occurs in a predictable fashion, as seen in Fig. 4-8.

The force of contraction is expressed as the amount of tension developed per unit of contractile tissue. In terms of energy liberated (ATP use), eccentric muscle contractions use the least ATP, and concentric contractions use the most (Fig. 4-9).[3]

Based on this information, it appears that eccentric muscle contractions are more energy efficient and produce greater tension per contractile unit than both concentric and isometric contractions. However, Davies[19] points out that much of the tension produced by eccentric muscle contraction results from stress imposed on the noncontractile serial elastic components (perimysium, epimysium, and endomysium) of the muscle. Therefore eccentric muscle contractions stimulate both contractile and noncontractile elements, whereas concentric contractions and isometrics focus on the contractile elements.[60]

The PTA must consider the context in which each muscle contraction type is used clinically. Fundamentally implementing multiple muscle contraction types during all phases of rehabilitation is well supported.[8,35,69] In comparing muscle contraction types, it is best to view the decision concerning which type to use, when to use it, and in what pathologic conditions it should be used as a progression or continuum rather than a choice of one type over another. Davies[19] has described a classic model of exercise progression (Box 4-1) that can be used as a general guide. Certain criteria must be established for the progression from one type of contraction to another.

First, exercise variables and parameters must be understood so that necessary adjustments can be made in a patient's exercise prescription (Box 4-2).The criteria established for progressing from one exercise mode to another is based on many factors and is patient specific. In general, pain usually dictates the time frame for progression, although swelling also does to a lesser degree. The sequence proceeds from the least intense to more challenging exercises with increased joint forces and metabolic demands.

---

*Cybex, Nautilus, Rehab Systems, Body Masters, Universal, and Paramount are all examples of companies that produce lines of exercise equipment for strength training used in both fitness and physical therapy facilities. This equipment is typically available in single- and multi-station units.

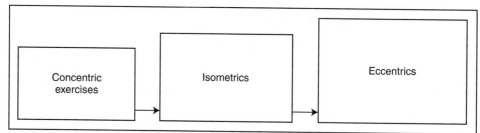

Fig. 4-8   Progression of maximal force production from least to most.

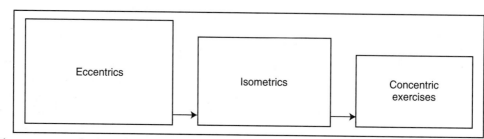

Fig. 4-9   Relative amounts of adenosine triphosphate used in muscle contraction.

BOX 4-1
Davies Model of Exercise Progression (1985)
■ Isometric/eccentric contractions, multiple angle ■ Isometrics (submax effort) ■ Multiple angle isometrics (max effort) ■ Short arc concentric-isokinetics (submax effort) ■ Short arc isotonics-concentric/eccentric ■ Short arc concentric isokinetics (max effort) ■ Full ROM concentric isokinetics (submax effort) ■ Full ROM isotonics-concentric/eccentric ■ Full ROM concentric isokinetics (max effort) ■ Full ROM eccentric isokinetics (submax effort) ■ Full ROM eccentric isokinetics (max effort)

From Davies G: *A compendium of isokinetics in clinical usage and rehabilitation techniques*, Onalaska, Wis, 1987, S & S Publishers.

Some of the advantages and disadvantages of concentric and eccentric isotonic exercise and isokinetic exercise equipment are outlined for general comparison in Table 4-2.

MUSCLE RESPONSE TO EXERCISE

Strength training must be individually tailored to meet the goals of recovery. As stated by DeLee and colleagues,[21] "Function increases with use; functions we do not use, we lose. The intensity, duration, and frequency of activity are all related to the functional capacity that is developed."

Muscle tissue morphology is mutable; that is, it has the ability to change. Muscle mutability has two distinct categories, **hypertrophy** and **atrophy**.

BOX 4-2	
Therapeutic Exercise Parameters	
Frequency	Daily, 3 days a wk, 2 days a wk (QD = once daily, bid = twice daily)
Intensity	Amount of resistance, full range of motion, short arc of motion, velocity of contraction (slow, moderate, fast)
Duration	6 weeks, 8 weeks, 10 weeks
Type of resistance	Isotonic, isokinetic
Muscle contraction type	Concentric, eccentric, isometric
Degree of resistance	Total amount of weight or force applied
Number of repetitions	1 to 15
Number of sets	1 to 5
Length of rest between sets	Short rest for aerobic-metabolic pathway, long rest (2 to 3 min) for anaerobic pathways
Order of exercise	Exercise large muscle groups first, progress to smaller muscle groups
Degrees of effort	Low intensity (submax effort), high intensity (max effort)

The stimuli for adaptive changes in skeletal muscle are described as frequency, intensity, and duration.[12] Human skeletal muscle responds and adapts to these stimuli and is characterized by the nature, rate, magnitude, and duration of the stimulus.[8] In a clinical

Table 4-2	Comparison of Isotonics versus Isokinetics

Commercially Available Machines and Free Weights	Isokinetics
ADVANTAGES	
• Low cost (relative)	• Can exercise over a wide velocity (0° to 300° or more)
• Has both concentric and eccentric components	• Accommodates to pain and fatigue
• Easy to instruct patients	• Low compressive forces at high speeds
• Objective increase in muscle performance by increasing weight	• Provides objective permanent record of data
• Can perform static or isometric contractions	• Valid and reliable
DISADVANTAGES	
• Momentum is involved	• Very expensive
• Not safe if patient has pain during the motion of lifting	• Some models do not provide eccentrics
	• Takes time to switch machine for other body parts (time consuming)

situation, the stimulus provided to human muscle is the conditioning or training program. These programs are based on certain principles that lead to the necessary adaptive changes, which in turn affect function. The principles of overload, specificity, and reversibility[25] as well as progression and transfer of training[6] provide the foundation for the strength training programs used in physical therapy and are as follows.

The overload principle[6] is the guiding principle of exercise prescription. If muscle performance is to improve, a load that exceeds the metabolic capacity of the muscle must be applied. A muscle must be challenged to perform at a level greater than that to which it is accustomed.

The **specific adaptations to imposed demands**[25] **(SAID) principle** in part defines specific adaptations and alterations in response to highly specific demands. After injury, muscle reeducation helps the patient adapt and prepare for return to function.

Specificity[6] is the training of a patient in a specific manner to produce a specific adaptation or training outcome.

The progression principle[6] dictates that the intensity of program must become progressively greater in order to continue to make gains.

The transfer of training[6] principle describes the carryover of training effects from one variation of exercise or task to another.

The reversibility principle[25] indicates that changes in a body's systems are transient unless training induced improvements are regularly used for functional activities or a person participates in a maintenance program. This can begin within 1 to 2 weeks after cessation of exercises.

In general, type I muscle fibers (red [high myoglobin content] and oxidative) respond more favorably to low-intensity (low tension), high-volume (sets and repetitions) exercise than type II (white [low myoglobin content] and glycolytic) muscle fibers. High-volume, low-intensity exercise is repetitive, and gross muscle movements occur (e.g., bicycling, running, swimming, and rowing). In this type of training, oxidative capabilities increase and relative percent of oxygen increases in type I muscle fibers in the specific muscle or muscle groups used.

In strength training programs, a desirable and predictable morphologic adaptive change is hypertrophy, which is the compensatory increase in individual muscle fiber size as a result of increases in and synthesis of the contractile proteins actin and myosin.[32] Type II muscle fibers increase more than type I fibers do. This can be observed in comparing the body types of long-distance runners with the larger, more muscular physiques of sprinters. The physiques of long-distance runners and most aerobic athletes are thinner, possess less body fat, and have smaller muscles that are more adapted to endurance activities. Highly specific, or absolute strength, programs use a high-tension (heavy loads) and low-volume protocol. This type of training program requires relatively short bouts of progressive overload to stimulate the type II muscle fibers.

Biochemical adaptations of muscle occur in specifically applied strength training programs. After intense strength training, significant increases appear in glycogen, ATP, and creatine phosphate; increased activity and quantity of enzymes involved with anaerobic glycolysis, creatine kinase, and myokinase also are seen.[17]

Hyperplasia (the development of new muscle fibers) or longitudinal fiber splitting may occur in response to high-intensity strength training programs. Gonyea and colleagues[33] reported in animal studies that an increase of 19% of the total number of muscle fibers occurred in cat forelimb muscles after weight lifting. This phenomenon has not been proven in humans. The predominant change in response to high-intensity strength training programs is hypertrophy of existing skeletal muscle fibers. The relative contribution (if any) of hyperplasia or muscle fiber splitting has not been determined.[12] Induced hypertrophy in injured or postoperative muscle tissue is important because hypertrophy relates to a potential to generate greater tension.

It is interesting to note that passive stretching of innervated muscle tissue creates tension and also results in fiber hypertrophy. The change in fiber size associated with this stretch-induced hypertrophy results from increased protein turnover.[12] This feature has clinical relevance in muscle recovery during immobilization.

DELAYED ONSET MUSCLE SORENESS

The clinical features of exercise-induced muscle soreness are diffuse and general, occurring in the absence of specific, intense injury.[57] Acute muscle strain can be differentiated from exercise-induced soreness primarily by the history leading to the injury. With an acute strain, the patient is able to relate a specific event or episode that caused the injury.[57]

Based on this distinction, the PTA can identify complaints of diffuse muscle soreness resulting from new or unaccustomed exercise.[57] However, if the patient can describe a history of local, intense pain after a specific episode, an acute muscle strain must be considered.[57]

Although the PTA does not interpret and define complaints of pain without consulting with the physical therapist (PT), the assistant must be able to accurately identify and describe the nature and disposition of any pain, based on the patient's complaints and relevant history, and be able to communicate this information to the PT.

After a specific exercise program, muscle soreness is an anticipated by-product of intense eccentric exercise.[29,30,40,52,65,68] The degree and presence of after-exercise muscle soreness appear to be greater with these eccentric programs than with concentric exercise programs.[11,40,52,54,65,72]

Symptoms of **delayed onset muscle soreness (DOMS)** include pain, swelling, tenderness, reduced ROM, and stiffness.[3,40,52,65] Albert[3] reports five general theories concerning the process of DOMS:

1. Lactic acid theory
2. Torn tissue theory
3. Tonic muscle spasms theory
4. Connective tissue damage theory
5. Tissue fluid theory

The lactic acid and tonic muscle spasms theories do not appear to be related to DOMS.[1,2,62,75] Studies[49,51] show evidence that the primary cause of muscle soreness after exercise is skeletal muscle damage. Greater tensions produced by eccentric exercise contribute to the initial muscle damage, although isometric and concentric contractions are not absolved of producing latent muscle soreness. In fact, isometric exercise and concentric exercise can produce DOMS even in well-trained athletes.

Conventional methods of treating DOMS are listed in Table 4-3.

Treatment of DOMS remains controversial. One recent study[64] found ice, a traditional treatment method, to be ineffectual, whereas other studies[7,26] found vibration and compression, nontraditional treatment methods, to be effective.

A recent review[67] of the current strategies for treating DOMS revealed the following:

■ Pharmacologic aids, nonsteroidal antiinflammatory drugs (NSAIDs): Although there are some inconsistency

Table 4-3	Suggested Treatment Techniques for Delayed Onset Muscle Soreness
Type	**Efficacy**
Rest	None
Nonsteroidal antiinflammatory drugs	Highly successful
Steroidal antiinflammatory drugs	Moderately successful
Electrical stimulation	Proposed only
Exercise	Highly successful
Transcutaneous electrical nerve stimulation	Highly successful
Stretching	Mixed success
Iontophoresis	Not successful
Cryotherapy	Not successful
Calcium antagonists	Proposed only

From Albert M: *Eccentric muscle training in sports and orthopaedics*, New York, 1991, Churchill Livingstone.

in findings, NSAIDs such as ibuprofen have the potential to alleviate some of the symptoms of DOMS.

■ Therapeutic treatments using physical modalities: Treatment using conventional therapies, such as icing, massage, or stretching, also proved inconsistent. Nonconventional treatments such as acupuncture, herbal remedies, and hyperbaric oxygen therapy were found to have limited use. However, the review did indicate that of all the therapies examined, icing the affected area appeared to be the most effective.

■ Dietary methods using nutritional supplements: Additional supplementation with antioxidants (vitamins C and E) and supplements such as arnica, coenzyme Q and L-carnitine appears to be of little use.

The authors concluded that "It would appear that we are still no closer to establishing a conclusive approach to the treatment of the symptoms of DOMS. In the interim, several possible treatments, such as the use of NSAIDs and cryotherapy (icing), have the potential to help alleviate the pain associated with DOMS."

It appears the most prudent approach is to ease into any unfamiliar exercises (especially eccentrics), and if patients do end up with DOMS they should be educated that with appropriate rest and recovery, DOMS should run its course in 2 to 3 days and they'll be able to get back to their training relatively pain free.

VELOCITY OF MUSCLE CONTRACTIONS

Muscle contraction velocity and speed of limb movement are not the same. If two arms are bending at the same speed but one arm is holding a weight, the muscle bending the arm with more weight must produce a greater speed of contraction to overcome the resistance. Therefore more tension is developed in the muscle lifting the heavier arm, even though the speed of limb movement is the same.

Slower speeds of muscle contraction can produce greater force and tension than the same muscle moving at a higher rate of speed. A slower contracting muscle moving a heavy resistance can produce greater tension than a faster contracting muscle lifting a lighter resistance.[54] When slow speeds of full arc resistance exercise are used to generate greater tension and strength, joint compression forces and torque are increased as well. Therefore to minimize the negative or unwanted effects of joint compression (Fig. 4-10), a program of isometric exercise may be more appropriate in some instances.

Initially strength programs focus on using slow-speed tension to produce isometric contractions and spare the negative effects of excessive joint motion, torque, and compressive forces found in full ROM slow-speed isotonic (concentric and eccentric) exercises. Fast and slow contraction speeds can be distinguished with isokinetic exercise. By controlling the speed of limb movement with an isokinetic apparatus, better control of joint compression forces can be achieved. (Speed is defined isokinetically as control of limb movement, not necessarily the actual speed of muscle contraction.) A slow speed of limb movement using an isokinetic apparatus may be 60° per second, and a fast speed may be 300° per second.

Higher speeds of limb movement require the resistance to be lighter than in a slower moving limb with greater resistance. Isokinetic testing and exercise use the concept of velocity spectrum training, which is the ability to control limb speeds within a range of slow to fast speeds. Higher speeds of limb movement produce less joint compression and lower forces relative to slow-speed, high-resistance training.

Functionally, human limbs move at various speeds and with various degrees of motion. Velocity spectrum training allows a patient to train at speeds of motion that more closely approximate normal human limb speeds.[10,58,77] For example, a training program using the velocity spectrum concept may include submaximal contractions at slow speeds (60° to 90°/s) for two sets of 8 to 12 repetitions, then contractions at incrementally increasing speeds up to 240° per second or higher for two or three sets of 15 repetitions. This may not be appropriate for athletes, because the functional speeds of movements in athletics far exceed the capability of the isokinetic dynamometer.

In a comparison of isokinetic and isotonic exercise, most isotonic exercise is performed at approximately 60° per second,[19] whereas isokinetic exercise can be adjusted specifically to train the affected area at speeds

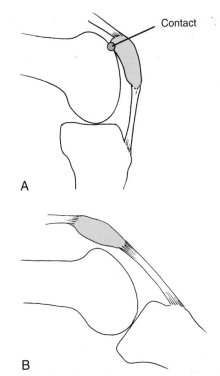

Fig. 4-10 **A,** With the knee flexed to 90° there are resultant increases in patellofemoral compression with excursion of the knee (leg) into extension. **B,** With the knee in extension there is less patellofemoral compression.

more closely duplicating normal functional speeds of movement. The higher velocity contractions used with isokinetic exercise allow for the following:

■ Improved functional speeds of contraction
■ Reduced joint compression forces
■ Accommodation of patient's pain (the patient will not undergo more force than he or she can safely produce)

Using velocity spectrum training with isokinetics allows the progression from multiangle isometrics (0 deg/s) to slow speeds (60 deg/s) for greater tension and torque, to higher speeds (240 deg/s and faster) for functional activities and lower compressive forces.

CLINICALLY RELEVANT EXERCISE PROGRAMS

Although there are many strength training protocols, three broad fundamental strength protocols are used extensively in physical therapy. The DeLorme[22] **progressive resistance exercise (PRE)** protocol is still used widely for strength training programs after injury to the musculoskeletal system. This program uses the classic and well-recognized exercise of three sets of 10 repetitions of resistance. Its protocol states that the patient must establish a maximum weight that can be lifted for 10 repetitions. This is termed the 10 RM (repetitions maximum). To initiate the program the patient performs 10 repetitions at half (50%) of the predetermined 10 RM. The next set of exercise is performed at three fourths (75%) of the 10 RM. Finally, the third set is performed for 10 repetitions at the established 10 RM (100%).

The DeLorme protocol calls for an arbitrary increase in resistance each week. It allows for a systematic and gradual progression during each exercise session by providing a warm-up period using submaximal contractions before the 10 RM.

The following is an example of a Delorme protocol that provides progressive loading with a warm-up built in:

- Set 1 = 10 reps at 50% of 10 RM
- Set 2 = 10 reps at 75% of 10 RM
- Set 3 = 10 reps at 100% of 10 RM

Performing three sets of 10 repetitions at the same resistance is a common clinical practice, however, it is not the DeLorme protocol and is less efficient because it does not overload the muscle in the same manner, nor does it involve built-in warm-up.

The Oxford program[78] is the opposite of the DeLorme protocol. Although it begins by establishing the individual's 10 RM, the second set is performed at three fourths (75%) of the 10 RM and the following set at half (50%) of the established 10 RM. Each set involves 10 repetitions. The method reportedly takes advantage of the muscle's fatigue during exercise.

There are fundamental differences in philosophy between the DeLorme PRE protocol and the Oxford technique. The DeLorme program calls for a progressive overload during each session by adding resistance while the muscle fatigues. The Oxford technique calls for reducing resistance as the muscle fatigues. Both programs were developed in the 1950s, and since then many variations and combinations have been used to discover the most effective and efficient means to regain strength after an injury.

The Oxford regimen provides regressive loading and takes into consideration muscle fatigue:

- Set 1 = 10 reps at 100% of 10 RM
- Set 2 = 10 reps at 75% of 10 RM
- Set 3 = 10 reps at 50% of 10 RM

To objectively control the progression or resistance with exercise programs, Knight[44] established the daily adjustable progressive resistance exercise technique (DAPRE). Instead of using three sets of 10 repetitions as DeLorme and Oxford did, Knight's program calls for four sets with variable repetitions. The protocol calls for establishing the patient's 6 RM instead of 10 RM, with the number 6 based on research by Berger[9] as the optimum number of repetitions for developing strength.

The first set is performed at half (50%) of the established working weight for 10 repetitions. The second set is performed at three fourths (75%) of the 6 RM for six repetitions. The third set is performed at the full previously established maximum weight, but the patient is asked to perform as many repetitions as possible with this weight. The number of repetitions performed in this set is used to determine the weight used in the fourth set. The goal of this technique is to establish a maximum resistance that can be performed for six repetitions.

As the individual's strength increases, the number of repetitions in the third set increases, which increases the weight in the fourth set. The hallmark of this program is understanding the guidelines used to adjust the working weight of the third and fourth sets.[21] The DAPRE adjusted working weight guide is as follows:

Set 1	10 reps	50% of 6 RM
Set 2	6 reps	75% of 6 RM
Set 3	max reps	100% of 6 RM
Set 4	max reps	Adjust weight based on # reps performed in set 3

Third Set Number of Repetitions	Fourth Set Change
0 to 2	Reduce weight 5 to 10 lb
3 to 4	Reduce weight 5 to 10 lb
5 to 7	Keep weight the same
8 to 12	Increase weight 5 to 10 lb
13 or more	Increase weight 10 to 15 lb

The rationale for the weight adjustments described in the preceding list is to modify resistance during the fourth set to maintain the goal of keeping repetitions between five and seven, whereas encouraging maximum resistance to influence strength increases and morphologic changes, such as hypertrophy.

In this protocol, the exact weight used by the patient is highly specific and tailored to the individual and goals of recovery. Adjustments in weight are made to accommodate the specific healing constraints of the injury and the individual tolerance level of the patient. Thus extremely close communication and supervision of the patient are necessary. With the DeLorme PRE program and Oxford program, the patient works with a percentage of an established weight each session and advances in resistance once each week. The DAPRE protocol requires daily adjustments; it takes advantage of the fact that submaximal work does not provide the necessary stimulus for maximal gains in strength. By reducing the volume of repetitions to six and adjusting the weight so that a maximal load is used for six repetitions, the intensity of work is increased.

The National Strength and Conditioning Association[6] makes the following recommendations:

Training Goal	Load (%1 RM)	Goal Repetitions	Goal Sets
Strength	≥85	≤6	2-6
Power	80-90	1-2	3-5
Hypertrophy	67-85	6-12	3-6
Muscle Endurance	≤67	≥12	2-3

Other protocols have suggested[70] that by initially focusing on muscular hypertrophy, a greater potential for strength would exist. Because the cross-sectional area of muscle would be increased by a program of higher volume, the potential to develop greater amounts of tension is increased by reducing the volume of exercise and increasing the loads used.

The rule of tens is followed in isometric exercise protocols that are commonly used in rehabilitation.[60] This rule states that the patient must perform 10-second contractions for 10 repetitions with a 10-second rest between each repetition.[19] The patient is taught to perform isometric contractions by gradually developing tension for 2 seconds, maintaining a maximal contraction for 6 seconds, then gradually decreasing tension for 2 seconds (Fig. 4-11).

While one is performing isometric exercise, an overflow of strength occurs approximately 10° above and below the angle (Fig. 4-12) at which the exercise is occurring.[43] Multiple-angle isometrics are taught at 10° increments to achieve strength gains throughout a described ROM.

A circuit training program is a predetermined, organized sequence of exercise. Traditionally, this type of program is used for general body conditioning and total fitness. A general circuit program calls for the performance of one or two exercises for each body part in sequence (Table 4-4). Usually a rest period of 30 seconds to 1 minute is allowed between sets. If resistance exercise equipment is used, circuit weight-training programs also tax the aerobic metabolic pathway to a degree. The movement from one station to another does not allow for maximum recovery and high-intensity loads, but it does provide an adequate stimulus for both aerobic and anaerobic work.

The clinical delivery of specific exercise protocols depends on many factors. The patient's pathologic condition; time constraints for healing of specific tissues; and degree of swelling, pain, function, and motivation all play a role in determining the most appropriate program to use and when to use it. In making an organized, systematic progression from one program to another, following specific guidelines is a responsible and appropriate plan for strength training programs for a wide variety of musculoskeletal system injuries.

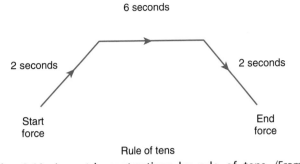

Fig. 4-11 Isometric contractions by rule of tens. (From Davies G: *A compendium of isokinetics in clinical usage and rehabilitation techniques*, Onalaska, Wis., 1987, S & S Publishers.)

Plyometrics

Plyometric exercises are intense power-generating exercises that are traditionally confined to sport-specific functional training near the end of a rehabilitation program. *Plyo* comes from the Greek word *plythein*, meaning to increase, and *metric* refers to measure. Plyometrics is a system of exercising that uses the stretch reflex to develop muscle contraction speed.[76]

Plyometric exercises are also highly adaptable for use with the general orthopedic patient population. However, the inherent nature of plyometrics requires the patient to be prepared for high-intensity, task-specific, dynamic exercise.

The principles behind plyometrics are based on the neurophysiologic responses from the Golgi tendon organs (GTOs) and muscle spindles.[76] The most rudimentary example of plyometrics is the depth jump (Fig. 4-13). As the foot of the patient contacts the ground (amortization phase), the muscle spindles respond by causing a reflex muscular contraction. Albert[3] states, "The greater and more quickly a load is applied to a muscle, the greater the firing frequency of the muscle spindle with a corresponding stronger muscle contraction." The fundamental goal of plyometric exercise is to minimize the amortization phase of the exercise, which, in this example, is contact with the ground.

All forms of jumping, skipping, and hopping can be used in a plyometric exercise program.[76] Upper body exercises, such as throwing and catching a weighted object, are examples of plyometrics. An isotonic supine leg press hop is an example of plyometrics used to develop rapid, eccentric loading with a corresponding rapid, concentric contraction.

Plyometrics must be used judiciously and principally as an end component in a phase progression program. The fundamental concept of plyometrics involves ballistic, high-velocity movement patterns, which cannot be used during early rehabilitation when tissues are still healing. Plyometrics can be added to increase function as the patient progresses from one program or phase to another.

Many isotonic strength training programs involve lifting a load from a seated, supine, or standing position. These exercises are meant to isolate and strengthen specific

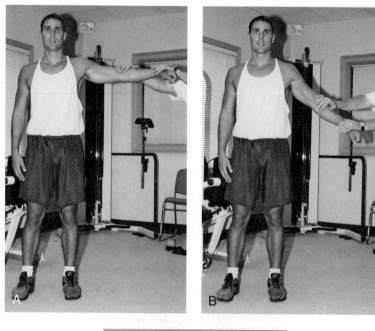

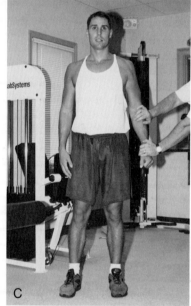

Fig. 4-12 Multiangle isometric shoulder abduction. **A,** Isometric hold in approximately 90° of abduction. **B,** Midrange isometric shoulder abduction. **C,** Isometric set in 0° of abduction.

muscle groups throughout a single plane of motion. Plyometrics, on the other hand, focus on weight-bearing functional activities that duplicate high-velocity, multiplane, normal human movement.[76] Therefore the PTA must recognize that the value of plyometrics is primarily to prepare the patient to return to function. Naturally not all patients recovering from an orthopedic injury require an intense plyometric exercise program. If, however, the patient desires to return to dynamic sporting activities, or his or her job requires dynamic or ballistic physical labor, then plyometrics are appropriate conditioning to enable one to withstand high levels of both eccentric and concentric loads.

Closed Kinetic Chain Exercise

During any exercise, if the distal portion of the exercising segment is weight bearing or fixed, it is called a *closed kinetic chain (CKC) exercise.* An **open kinetic chain (OKC) exercise** involves the distal segment moving freely in space, such as a seated knee extension. A CKC is best described as a system of interdependent articulated links. For example, in a weight-bearing leg (Fig. 4-14), as the knee is flexed, the entire chain or link system joining the ankle to the knee and to the hip is affected. In an OKC system, such as the arm (Fig. 4-15), the shoulder and elbow are fixed, whereas the distal

Table 4-4	Sample Circuit Weight Training Program		
Exercise	Repetitions	Sets	Rest
Leg press	10	2	30 s between each set
Leg extension	10	2	30 s between each set
Leg curl	10	2	30 s between each set
Bench press	10	2	30 s between each set
Supine fly	10	2	30 s between each set
Shoulder press	10	2	30 s between each set
Lateral pull-down	10	2	30 s between each set
Bent over row	10	2	30 s between each set
Bicep curl	10	2	30 s between each set
Triceps press-down	10	2	30 s between each set

wrist segment moves freely in space. Davies[20] states, "In a closed kinetic chain, motion at one joint will produce motion at all of the other joints in the system in a predictable manner."

The human body functions as a combination of both open- and closed-chain activities such as walking and stair climbing. The primary advantage of CKC exercises is the highly functional nature of the exercises, which use concentric and eccentric muscle contractions synchronously to produce functional movement. In a strength training program, combinations of OKC and CKC exercises should be used to condition the patient to perform purposeful, functional activities.

In knee rehabilitation programs,[14,56] for example, quadriceps strengthening can be achieved through knee extension exercises (which are open chain), or leg press exercises or squats (which are closed chain). In many cases, patients are introduced to therapeutic exercises by way of submaximal isometric muscle contractions. More intense and demanding exercises are added as pain, strength, and function allow. OKC resistance exercises can be employed to further stimulate growth in strength. In some cases, the PT institutes CKC exercises early in the recovery phase of rehabilitation. For example, CKC exercises are frequently used within the first few weeks after anterior cruciate ligament reconstructive surgery. In addition, select open-chain exercises (those that do not place unwanted forces on the newly repaired tissues) are used. CKC exercises may not be appropriate for some patients with osteoarthritis or other conditions where vertical, compressive loads would exacerbate the condition.

The general rationales for using closed-chain exercises in rehabilitation programs are as follows:

■ In theory, CKC exercises are more functional than OKC exercises (this can be refuted)
■ Loading of the affected joint(s) produces an increase in kinesthetic awareness
■ Improved neuromuscular coordination is achieved

■ CKC exercises are nonisolation exercises that produce muscular co-contractions

Caution must be used when prescribing CKC activities during rehabilitation when pain, swelling, dysfunction, or muscle weakness is present.[20] Because an articulated joint system is being exercised under these conditions (limited ROM, pain, swelling, etc.), unpredictable compensation may occur in the joint(s) superior and inferior to the affected joint.[20] Therefore OKC exercise must be used to isolate and strengthen the weakened area before progressing to CKC exercises.

Periodization of Strength Training Programs

Periodization involves a predictable pattern of exercise volume, intensity, and rest periods that enhance strength-developing capabilities.[71] Its main components are cycles, or periods, of strength training. Many fundamental strength programs call for a progressive resistance exercise system without consideration for variations in frequency, intensity, duration, and recovery. The periodization model takes into consideration progressive cycles of various training loads and degrees of intensity during strength programs.[71]

Periodization can involve any of three cycles: microcycle, mesocycle, or macrocycle. The microcycle is the smallest unit of time (usually weeks), and accumulated microcycles form a mesocycle. The mesocycle is traditionally a few months long and consists of multiple microcycles that vary in volume, frequency, and intensity. The macrocycle is the largest segment of time (it can be a year long) and involves a collection of mesocycles.

Periodization of strength training programs in the clinical rehabilitation setting was originally designed for and used extensively in athletics and is justified by following a series of defined protocols directed specifically at developing strength while minimizing fatigue and overtraining of the recovering orthopedic patient.

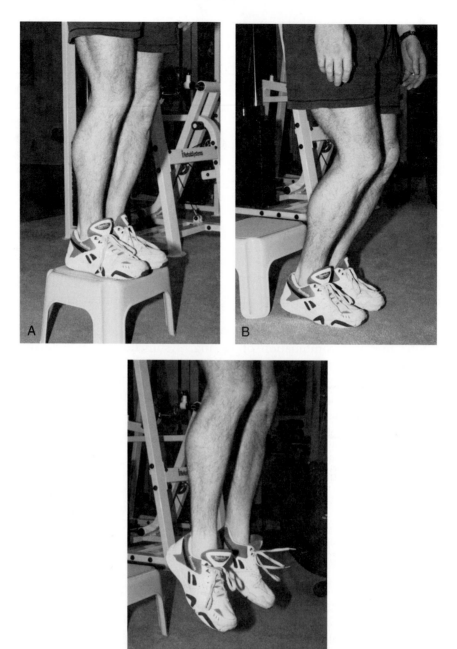

Fig. 4-13 Plyometric depth jump. **A,** Starting position on a short stool. **B,** Without jumping up, the patient steps off the stool down to the ground with both feet simultaneously. The time spent on the ground is called the *amortization phase.* **C,** Rapid concentric contraction follows the amortization phase, which results in a powerful leap.

The fundamental goals and objectives of a classic periodization program are outlined in Figure 4-16. This is only a basic example, which must be modified to meet the specific rehabilitation goals for recovering patients. It can be adapted for many patients who require strength as part of their rehabilitation program.

In a periodization program, instead of constantly striving to increase resistance during each treatment or each week by use of the same system of sets and repetitions for a recovering patient, an attempt should be

made to cycle the program into specific phases. In general the first phase (microcycle) strives to develop basic strength and muscular hypertrophy. There are small alterations in sets (between three and six sets) and repetitions (between 8 and 12) in each week of rehabilitation, and a high volume of exercise is used, dictating a lower intensity level (~65% to 70% of the 1 RM). This phase can be called the *preparatory phase,* or *initial rehabilitation protocol.* The second phase (mesocycle) is designed to enhance strength by increasing the loads

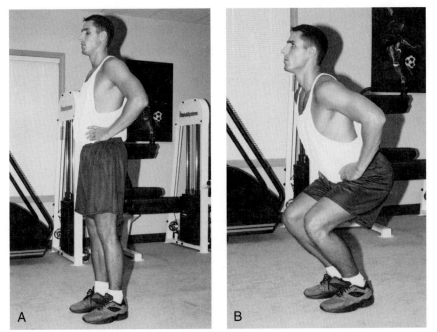

Fig. 4-14 A closed kinetic chain. **A,** Starting position of a standing squat or leg bend maneuver. **B,** Motion of the knee produces predictable motion in all joints within the kinetic chain. With knee flexion the resultant change in joint position of the ankle, hip, and spine is noticeable.

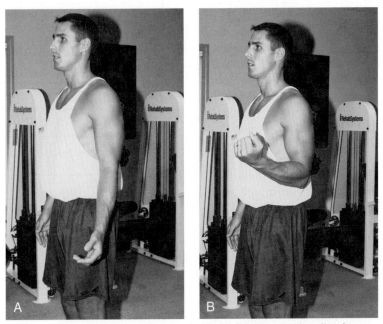

Fig. 4-15 An open kinetic chain. **A,** Beginning position of elbow flexion. **B,** The distal arm and wrist segments move freely in space.

used (85% of 1 RM) and decreasing the volume of exercise to three to five sets of four to six repetitions. This mesocycle, as well as the first, may last for 2 or 3 months. Remember that during each mesocycle there are numerous microcycles (weeks) where various changes are made to reduce chronic overwork. The second phase of this basic example is called the *first transition phase* or *active rehabilitation phase.*

The traditional athletic model for this modified periodization program is described in Figure 4-17. The strength protocol should be modified to fit the specific needs of each individual.

Strength Training for Older Populations
Strength training programs for the geriatric population include special considerations. In an elderly population,

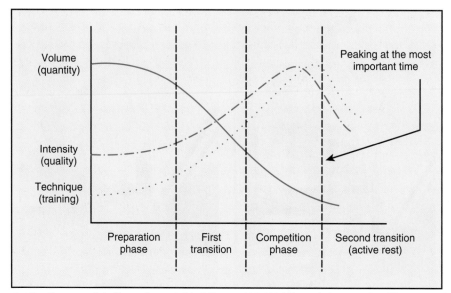

Fig. 4-16 Classic periodization model. (From Stone MH, O'Bryant HS: *Weight training: a scientific approach*, Minneapolis, 1987, Burgess Internationals.)

declines in muscle performance, force-generating capabilities, and concomitant muscle mass are well documented.[39,47] Therefore strength training programs for the elderly are focused on delaying muscle atrophy, improving function, and increasing force-generating capabilities by stimulating muscle hypertrophy. Note that resistance exercise programs for healthy, older populations show significant improvements in muscle strength, muscle volume (hypertrophy), and other parameters of muscle structure and function.[74] Thompson[74] reports that studies show that "Given an adequate training stimulus, older men and women show similar gains compared to young individuals after resistive training." In addition, McCartney and colleagues[51] report that "Long term resistance training in older people is feasible and results in increases in dynamic muscle strength, muscle size, and functional capacity."

A study by Evans[24] concludes that "exercise may minimize or reverse the syndrome of physical frailty, which is so prevalent among the most elderly. Because of their low functional status and high incidence of chronic disease, there is no segment of the population that can benefit more from exercise than the elderly."

Another study by Henwood and Taaffe[37] found that cessation of training resulted in only a modest loss of muscle power and strength which was recouped with retraining. This is important, considering that the elderly tend to take extended vacations and have family commitments that require breaks from training.

One must consider multiple morbidities and degenerative joint disease when developing strength training programs for the elderly. Unstable, chronic, and complex medical problems may preclude certain types of strength training programs. For example, in cardiovascular disease, chronic obstructive pulmonary disease,

Preparation → Transition 1 → Competition → Transition 2 (active rest)				
Phase	Hypertrophy	Basic strength	Strength & power	Peaking or maintaining
Sets	3 - 10	3 - 5	3 - 5	1 - 3
Reps	8 - 12	4 - 6	2 - 3	1 - 3
Days/wk	3 - 4	3 - 5	3 - 5	1 - 5
Times/day	1 - 3	1 - 3	1 - 2	1
Intensity cycle (weeks)	2 - 3/1	2 - 4/1	2 - 3/1	—
Intensity	low	high	high	very high to low
Volume	high	moderate to high	low	very low

Fig. 4-17 Traditional athletic model of a modified periodization program. (From Stone MH, O'Bryant HS: *Weight training: a scientific approach*, Minneapolis, 1987, Burgess Internationals.)

and other conditions, a protocol of general, very low-intensity gross body movement may be more beneficial and safer than isometric or isotonic resistance exercise. In advanced cases of osteoarthritis of the knee and hip, it is prudent to avoid vertical compression loads and full ROM-heavy isotonic exercise. Pain and swelling from osteoarthritic lesions, bone spurs, and osteophytes (Fig. 4-18) can be exacerbated by the tibiofemoral vertical compressive loads involved in leg press or squatting exercises.

In general, studies support the fact that high-intensity resistance training promotes force-generating capabilities in aged muscle[42] and that resistance training enhances muscle hypertrophy in elderly people.[13,31] In one study,[27] a very small population of very old (89- to 90-year-old) men and women showed the beneficial effects of isotonic resistance exercise for this age group. When they trained for 8 weeks, three times per week, the force-generating capacity of the trained muscles increased 174% ± 31%. The muscle mass of this group increased 9% ± 4.5%. In addition, two subjects improved in ambulation, no longer requiring the use of a cane. A hypothesis drawn from these findings suggests that increased force-generating capacity can be correlated with increased function.[38]

The previously outlined resistance exercise protocols (DeLorme, Oxford, and Knights DAPRE protocols) may be inappropriate for disabled elderly persons. However, modifications of these programs have provided some guidance in developing strength programs for elderly persons.[38] Frontera[31] states, "The isotonic resistance protocol that produced the greatest increases in force-generation capacity and attenuated atrophy to the greatest extent in older human muscle was three sets of eight repetitions of exercise performed at an intensity of 80% of a muscle's 1 RM, 3 days a week for 12 weeks." Studies also support the need to closely monitor heart rate, blood pressure, respirations, and subtle signs of distress during any exercise program for elderly persons.[38]

As with any resistance program to elicit strength, intensity of effort is the key element in the magnitude of functional or morphologic change in muscle tissue.[13,31] In the elderly population, intensity of effort must take into account age, history of cardiovascular or pulmonary disease, history of orthopedic pathologic conditions, present disease states, osteoarthritis, and multiple medical conditions present.

General recommendations for strength training in the older adult are as follows[4,50]:

- Get physician approval
- Initially, supervise closely
- Monitor vital signs
- Start with low resistance and low number of repetitions
- Progress by increasing repetitions, then by small amounts of resistance
- Avoid high resistance to decrease stress on joints
- Train two to three times per week with 48-hour rest intervals

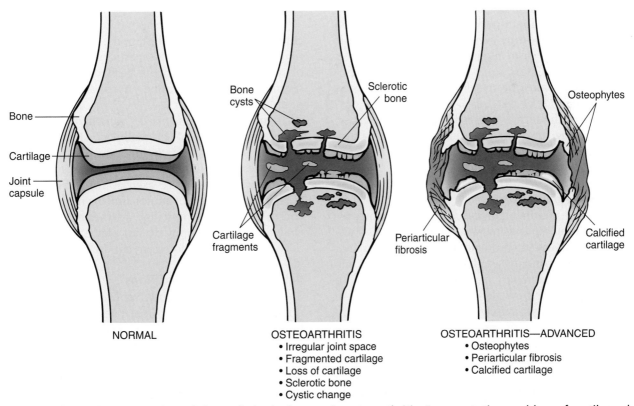

Fig. 4-18 Schematic presentation of the pathologic changes in osteoarthritis. Fragmentation and loss of cartilage denude the subchondral bone, which undergoes sclerosis and cystic change. Osteophytes form on the lateral sides and protrude into the adjacent soft tissues, causing irritation, inflammation, and fibrosis. (From Damjanov I: *Pathology for the health professions*, ed 3, St Louis, 2006, Saunders.)

- Use a balance of flexion and extension exercises
- Use supported positions if a decrease in balance is noted

Strength Training for Younger Populations

A clear definition of the age range of this special population must be made at the outset to clarify and define the application of resistance exercise and the physiologic adaptation to the precise mode of training. *Prepubescent* and *child* are synonymous terms used to describe both boys and girls before the onset of secondary sex characteristics.[34] The general range of prepubescence is 11 years for girls and 13 years for boys.[34] The terms pubescent and adolescent are synonymous descriptive terms related to girls 12 to 18 years old and for boys 14 to 18 years old.[34]

In general, these definitions correspond to the classic Tanner stage classification system. Tanner stage I represents preadolescence or ages before the onset of secondary sex characteristics. Tanner stages II through IV describe various levels of development of secondary sex characteristics within adolescence. Tanner stage V is defined as adulthood.[34] Other definitions that must be clarified are strength, weight training, resistance training, and weight lifting. The use of the terms strength training, weight training, and resistance training are used to describe submaximal progressive resistance exercise to improve strength, whereas weight lifting describes an attempt to lift maximum weight for a single repetition as a competitive sporting event. Examples are Olympic weight lifting (e.g., clean and jerk, snatch lift) and power lifting (e.g., bench press, squat, dead lift). The appropriate terminology must be specific to denote the precise intent of the mode of exercise.

The use of the terms progressive resistance exercise, weight training, resistance training, or strength training are both appropriate and practical in the context of orthopedic rehabilitation.

Physiologic Adaptations

Preadolescent children (Tanner stage I) do not possess circulating androgenic-anabolic hormones (testosterone) that act to stimulate hypertrophy, muscular strength, and secondary sex characteristics. Historically this single irrefutable fact has led many researchers to state, "prepubertal boys do not significantly improve strength or increase muscle mass in a weight training program because of insufficient circulating androgens."[34] However, the complexity of strength acquisition is dependent on many factors, including hypertrophy, increases in muscle cross-sectional area, motor activation, central nervous system stimulation, genetic control, and psychological drive, as well as circulation levels of endogenous hormones.[34]

Several leading researchers and scientists have identified that preadolescent children can significantly increase strength with appropriately applied resistance exercise protocols.[34] However, current evidence strongly suggests that neuromuscular activation, motor coordination, and intrinsic muscular adaptations contribute to preadolescent strength gains.[34] In fact, when investigating the effectiveness of nine studies supporting strength gains in children younger than 13 years, researchers found a 71.6% increase in strength versus control group.[35]

Injury Risk

In nonpathologic conditions, PRE for preadolescent and adolescent children is both safe and effective, providing a few conditions are strictly followed. Also the nature of the specific type of training is directly related to the risk of injury. Namely, unsupervised weight training poses no greater risk for injury when compared with other sports or recreational activities common to this age group.[34]

Injuries specific to this age group include disruption of the primary growth centers of ossification, the physeal plates. The secondary growth centers, the apophyses, are at risk of injury from traumatic and chronic traction at these sites.

Specific sites of injury occurring from nonsupervised weight lifting include the wrist, shoulder, elbows, lumbar spine, and knee. Estimates are more than 17,000 injuries occur annually to adolescents participating in nonsupervised weight lifting or power lifting.[34]

Other researchers have found no evidence of subclinical or clinical manifestations of musculoskeletal injury in prepubertal boys participating in 20 weeks of resistance training on the basis of bone scans and serum extraction of creatine phosphokinase (a marker of muscle damage).[34]

Therefore well-supervised, submaximal resistance exercise with use of nonballistic, slow, controlled motions is both effective and safe for preadolescent and adolescent children. The mechanism of physiologic adaptations of resistance exercise for this population is primarily a result of motor unit recruitment, motor control, and neuromuscular activation. Morphologic changes via hypertrophy do not play a role in strength development in preadolescent children.[34]

Relevant Clinical Applications

The specific therapeutic intervention of strength development in children follows a parallel progression of bone and soft-tissue healing. Each contraction type (isometric, concentric, eccentric) is appropriately used during the defined stages of tissue healing (acute inflammatory, stage I; fibroplasia, stage II; and maturation, stage III), depending on radiographic confirmation of osseous union and stability, as well as soft-tissue healing constraints. In concert with specifically applied flexibility techniques (autogenic and reciprocal inhibition, covered in Chapter 3), strength acquisition in children using the foundation of therapeutic exercise parameters—frequency, intensity, duration, muscle contraction type, degree of resistance, number of repetitions, number sets, length of rest between sets, speed of contraction, and order of exercise—as well as a clearly defined model of exercise progression (see Davies model of exercise progression), the preadolescent can be expected to develop strength primarily by neurogenic activation.

Though the American Academy of Pediatrics (AAP) is against weight lifting, power lifting, and body building, it does approve of strength training programs for children and teens. The training may use free weights, the individual's own body weight, machines, and/or other resistance devices to attain this goal (Box 4-3).

THERAPEUTIC EXERCISE EQUIPMENT USED IN STRENGTH TRAINING

The most commonly used strength training tools are ankle or cuff weights. These extremely versatile pieces of equipment are easily adapted to many programs, body parts, and age groups. Thera-Band, surgical tubing, or latex rubber bands are popular, inexpensive, highly adaptable, very portable (for home use), and effective tools. They allow for diagonal patterns of resistance, as well as those involving a single plane. Some manufacturers have added handles to ends of thick rubber cords to enhance the versatility of this equipment.

Dumbbells also are used extensively in physical therapy. Inexpensive, portable, and versatile, dumbbells also can be used to develop excellent ROM and unilateral or bilateral motions. Barbells also can be used but are cumbersome; barbells are effective in sports medicine practices where young athletes should develop overall strength and fitness, not usually in acute rehabilitation environments or hospital physical therapy departments.

Wall pulleys or cable column systems are used in most rehabilitation departments. The amount of resistance used with pulleys can vary from a few to more than 100 pounds. Cable columns are extremely useful for both upper extremity and lower extremity strength training and can be used for many age groups and conditions. They also allow for use of diagonal movements such as those used in proprioceptive neuromuscular facilitation.

There are many commercially available isotonic exercise systems.* Generally, isotonic exercise machines are fairly adaptable, provide a wide range of resistance (5 to 500 lb for some leg machines), and are mechanically adjustable to accommodate different body types.

> ### BOX 4-3
> #### AAP Recommendations for Strength Training
>
> - Have a medical evaluation by your pediatrician before starting a strength training program.
> - Kids should be able to complete 8 to 15 repetitions in a set: The greatest benefits and smallest risks occur when 8 to 15 repetitions can be performed with a given weight before adding weight in small increments.
> - The goal is not lifting as much as you can. Instead, kids can slowly begin adding weight in small increments as they are able to easily finish their sets.
> - Be sure to include a warm-up and cooldown routine to all workouts.
> - Aerobic conditioning and all major muscle groups should be included in the strength training program.
> - Workouts should be about 20 to 30 minutes long, 2 to 4 times a week.
> - Make sure child is well supervised as he starts lifting weights, especially if he is doing it at home and won't be supervised by a trainer at school or a gym.

Individual pieces can be expensive ($3000 or more for a single leg press machine), and a full system may cost $30,000 or more. Various types of muscle contractions can be used with isotonic exercise machines, including concentric and eccentric contractions, isometric static holds, and unilateral or bilateral movements; these exercises can be done using a wide degree of contraction velocities. As discussed, 1 RM testing can be performed on isotonic systems.

Space availability also is a consideration when one acquires exercise equipment. Whereas the footprint of many of these machines is small, a space of several hundred square feet to a few thousand feet may be needed for complete systems. Most of these systems use weight stacks, cables, straps, cams, and chains, but some use pneumatic (air), hydraulic, or electromagnetic resistance.

Isokinetic exercise systems are used extensively in physical therapy practices for testing, documentation, medicolegal presentations, rehabilitation, and velocity spectrum training. These systems generally are very expensive, with a single multi-joint system costing $40,000 or more.[†]

These systems are extremely adaptable to most major body parts (knee, ankle, hip, wrist, elbow, shoulder, and back attachments are available with most systems), and therapeutically these systems are perhaps the most versatile of all strength training tools. Protocols and training

---

*Some of the more common systems are the Universal, Paramount, Nautilus, Body Masters, and Cybex systems.

[†]Some common multi-joint systems are the Cybex, Lido, Kin-Com, Biodex, Isotechnologies, and Ariel systems.

BOX 4-4

Example of Knee Rehabilitation

PROTOCOL VERSATILITY USING ISOKINETIC TECHNOLOGY

To Gain Knee Motion
■ Continuous passive motion

To Initiate Muscle Contractions
■ Use isometric mode. Progress to multiangle isometric, from 0° to 120° of knee motion at 20° increments.

To Progress Strength
■ Use isotonic modes. For example, knee extension (concentric)
■ Quads followed by knee flexion (eccentric)
■ Quads from 60°/s to 180°/s (five sets: 60°, 90°, 120°, 150°, and 180°).

Progress to Isokinetics
■ Knee extension (concentric).
■ Quads followed by concentric hamstrings velocity spectrum training: (eight sets: 30°, 60°, 90°, 120°, 150°, 180°, 210°, and 240°).

BOX 4-5

Application for Inertial Training

CONDITIONS	INDICATIONS
Submaximal plyometrics	Painful arc remediation
Neuromuscular training	Mechanical, reproducible joint pain
Training of tendon tissue	Capsular afferents and coordination
Alteration of electro-mechanical delay	Proposed prevention of bone loss
Physiologic crossover effects	

From Albert M: *Eccentric muscle training in sports and orthopaedics,* New York, 1991, Churchill Livingstone.

---

modes that are generally available with most isokinetic systems are as follows:
■ Passive
  ■ Continuous passive motion
  ■ Active assistive range of motion
■ Isometric
  ■ Multiangle isometrics
■ Isotonic
  ■ Types of contraction modes:
    ■ Concentric/eccentric
    ■ Concentric/concentric
    ■ Eccentric/concentric
    ■ Eccentric/eccentric
■ Isokinetic
  ■ Types of contraction modes:
    ■ Concentric/eccentric
    ■ Concentric/concentric
    ■ Eccentric/concentric
    ■ Eccentric/eccentric

Isokinetic systems typically function from 0 degrees per second to 350 to 400 degrees per second. These systems are designed to isolate, test, and rehabilitate single joints. Unfortunately, it is very time consuming to change from one leg to another or from one joint (knee) to another (ankle). The versatility of these systems is presented in Box 4-4.

The impulse inertial exercise apparatus is a system used for submaximal plyometric training. The impulse system provides limited ROM (by design), high-velocity, low-intensity, concentric, and eccentric loading. The application of inertial exercise involves rapid, coordinated, cyclic, and dynamic motions with reduced loads or resistance. The impulse system can be used for upper and lower extremity exercise. Extremely adaptive components with various handles allow for the duplication of sports such as tennis, racquetball, and golf. Clinically, this system is used mainly for neuromuscular coordination and strength in limited degrees of motion. The clinical delivery of inertial exercise is shown in Box 4-5.[3]

❖ GLOSSARY

ATP use in muscle contractions: Concentric contractions use more ATP than isometric contractions. Eccentric contractions use the least.

Closed kinetic chain (CKC) exercise: Resistance exercise—a system of predictably interdependent articulated biomechanical links, a system that stimulates joint afferent neuromechanoreceptor input, highly functional, proprioception, and kinesthetic awareness—nonisolation exercise.

Components of muscle contraction and strength development: Calcium, potassium, and sodium ions; axoplasmic transport; efficient neuromuscular activation; muscle contraction types; activation of motor units; modes of exercise frequency—intensity and duration of contraction types, rest recovery, adaptation.

Contractile tissue: Myofibril—two basic proteins, myosin and actin.

Contraction types: Concentric, eccentric, and isometric.

Exercise and program design variables: Choice of exercise, metabolic demands, order of sequence of exercises, sets and repetitions (consider Delorme protocol, Oxford protocol, or DAPRE), loads used, ratio of rest to exercise, frequency of exercise, and progression.

Exercise modifications: Precise identification of anatomic pathology; limit ROM to accommodate pain and biomechanical limitations; adjust resistance; use slow, controlled precision movements; control velocity.

Force production: Eccentric contractions create more force than isometric contractions. Concentric contractions produce the least force.

General adaptation syndrome: Alarm stage, resistance stage, exhaustion stage, and adaptation.

Increase in blood flow to exercising muscle: Immediate blood flow response may increase vascular supply tenfold.

Muscle fiber types: Fast twitch (type II)—white, glycolytic, speed, strength, and power; slow twitch (type I)—red, oxidative, fatigue resistant.

Noncontractile tissue: Epimysium, perimysium, and endomysium.

Periodization: Microcycle—daily or weekly changes in intensity, frequency, duration of exercise; mesocycle—monthly changes; macrocycle—annual adaptations.

SAID principle: Specific adaptation to imposed demands.

Specific proprioceptive closed-chain neuromuscular training: Multiangle, closed-chain functions; reciprocal, coordinated, balanced, full body, or joint-specific dexterity, considering joint position, movement, direction, speed, amplitude, and deceleration.

Strength adaptations: Early increases in strength do not parallel increases in hypertrophy. Early increases in strength are caused by increased neuromuscular activation and efficiency. Evoked hypertrophy is a time-dependent adaptive response to increased loads.

Vascular response to exercise: At rest, blood flow is estimated at 2 to 3 mL per 100 mL of muscle per minute.

REFERENCES

1. Abraham WM: Exercise induced muscle soreness, *Phys Sports Med* 7:57, 1979.
2. Abraham WM: Factors in delayed muscle soreness, *Med Sci Sports Exer* 9:11, 1977.
3. Albert M: *Eccentric muscle training in sports and orthopaedics,* New York, 1991, Churchill Livingstone.
4. American College of Sports Medicine: *ACSM's guidelines for exercise testing and prescription/American College of Sports Medicine,* ed 8, Baltimore, 2009, Lippincott Williams & Wilkins.
5. American Physical Therapy Association: *Guide to physical therapy practice,* ed 2, Alexandria, Va, 2003, American Physical Therapy Association.
6. Baechle TR, Earle RW: *Essentials of strength training and conditioning,* ed 2, Champaign, Ill, 2000, Human Kinetics.
7. Bakhtiary AH, Safavi-Farokhi Z, Aminian-Far A: Influence of vibration on delayed onset of muscle soreness following eccentric exercise, *Br J Sports Med* 41(3):145, 2007.
8. Belka D: Comparison of dynamic, static, and combination training on dominant wrist flexor muscles, *Res Q* 39:244, 1968.
9. Berger RA: Optimum repetitions for the development of strength, *Res Q Exerc Sport* 33:334–338, 1962.
10. Brinkman JR, et al: Rate and range of knee motion in ambulation, *Phys Ther* 62(5):632, 1982.
11. Byrnes WC, et al: Delayed onset muscle soreness following repeated bouts of downhill running, *J Appl Physiol* 59:7109, 1985.
12. Caplan A, et al: Skeletal muscle. In Woo SL-Y, Buckwalter J, editors: *Injury and repair of the musculoskeletal soft tissues,* Rosemont, Ill, 1988, American Academy of Orthopaedic Surgeons.
13. Charette SL, et al: Muscle hypertrophy response to resistance training in older women, *J Appl Physiol* 70:1912–1916, 1991.
14. Chu DA: Rehabilitation of the lower extremity, *Clin Sports Med* 14(1):205–222, 1995.
15. Clarke HH: Improvements of objective strength tests of muscle groups by cable tension methods, *Res Q* 21:399, 1950.
16. Clarke HH, et al: New objective strength tests of muscle groups by cable tension methods, *Res Q* 23:136, 1952.
17. Conroy BP, Earle RW: Bone, muscle and connective tissue adaptations to physical activity. In Baechle TR, editor: *Essentials of strength training and conditioning,* Champaign, Ill, 1994, Human Kinetics.
18. Cordova M, Armstrong C: Reliability of ground reaction forces during a vertical jump: implications for functional strength assessment, *J Athl Train* 31(4):342–345, 1996.
19. Davies GJ: *A compendium of isokinetics in clinical usage and rehabilitation techniques,* ed 3, Onalaska, Wis, 1987, S & S Publishers.
20. Davies GJ: *Course notes. Open and closed kinetic chain exercises and their application to testing and rehabilitation: advances on the knee and shoulder,* Cincinnati, 1993, Cincinnati Sports Medicine and Orthopaedic Center.
21. DeLee J: Therapeutic exercise modalities. In DeLee JC, Drez Jr D, Miller MD: *Orthopaedic sports medicine,* Philadelphia, 1989, Mosby.
22. DeLorme TL, Watkins A: *Progressive resistance exercise,* New York, 1951, Appleton-Century.
23. Elftman H: Biomechanics of muscle, *J Bone Joint Surg* 48:363, 1966.
24. Evans WJ: Exercise training guidelines for the elderly, *Med Sci Sports Exerc* 31(1):12–17, 1999.
25. Faulkner JA: New perspectives in training for maximum performance, *JAMA* 205:741–746, 1986.
26. Fedorko BF: *The effects of continuous compression as a therapeutic intervention on delayed onset muscle soreness following eccentric exercise,* 2007, University of Pittsburgh, PhD (dissertation).
27. Fiatarone MA, et al: High intensity strength training in nonagenarians: effects on skeletal muscle, *JAMA* 263:3029–3034, 1990.
28. Fraleigh J: Strength training: not just for the young, *Montvale* 71(11):41, 2008.
29. Francis KT: Delayed muscle soreness: a review, *J Orthop Sports Phys Ther* 5:10, 1983.
30. Friden J, Sjostrom M, Ekblom B: Myofibrillar damage following intensive eccentric exercise in man, *Int J Sport Med* 4:170–176, 1983.
31. Frontera WR, et al: Strength conditioning in older men: skeletal muscle hypertrophy and improved function, *J Appl Physiol* 64:1038–1044, 1988.
32. Gollnick PD: Fiber number and size in overloaded chicken anterior latissimus dorsi muscle, *J Appl Physiol* 54:1292, 1983.
33. Gonyea W, Ericson GC, Bonde-Peterson F: Skeletal muscle fiber splitting induced by weight-lifting exercise in cats, *Acta Physiol Scand* 99:105–109, 1977.
34. Guy JA, Michel LJ: Strength training for children and adolescents, *J Am Acad Orthop Surg* 9:26–31, 2001.
35. Hakkinen K, Komi PV: Effect of different combined concentric and eccentric muscle work regimes on maximal strength development, *J Hum Mov Stud* 7:33, 1981.
36. Harman E: Strength and power: a definition of terms, *J Strength Cond Res* 15(6):18–20, 1993.
36a. Henneman E, Somjen G, Carpenter DO: Excitability and inhibitability of motoneurons of different sizes, *J Neurophysiol* 28(3): 599–620, 1965.
37. Henwood TR, Taaffee DR: Detraining and retraining on older adults following long-term muscle power or muscle strength specific training, *J Gerontol* 63A(7):751–758, 2008.
38. Hopp JF: Effects of age and resistance training on skeletal muscle: a review, *Phys Ther* 73(6):361–373, 1993.
39. Jzankoff SP, Norris AH: Effect of muscle mass decreases on age-related BMR changes, *J Appl Physiol* 43:1001–1006, 1977.
40. Kellis E, Baltzopoulos V: Isokinetic eccentric exercise, *Sports Med* 19(3):202–222, 1995.
41. Kisner C, Colby LA: *Therapeutic exercise: foundations and techniques,* ed 5, Philadelphia, 2002, FA Davis.

42. Klitgaard H, et al: Function, morphology and protein expression of aging skeletal muscle: a cross-sectional study of elderly men with different training backgrounds, *Acta Physiol Scand Suppl* 140:41–54, 1990.

43. Knapik JJ, et al: Angular specificity and test mode specificity of isometric and isokinetic strength training, *J Orthop Sports Phys Ther* 5(2):58–65, 1983.

44. Knight KL: Quadriceps strengthening with the DAPRE technique: case studies with neurological implications, *Med Sci Sport Exerc* 17(6):646–650, 1985.

45. Knuttgen H, Kramer W: Terminology and measurement in exercise performance, *J Appl Sports Sci Res* 1:1–10, 1987.

46. Kruger J, Carlson S, Kohl H III: Trends in Strength Training: United States, 1998-2004, *Morb Mortal Wkly Rep* 55:769–772, 2006.

47. Kuta I, Parizkova J, Dycka J: Muscle strength and lean body mass in old men of different physical activity, *J Appl Physiol* 29:168–171, 1970.

48. Mangine R, Heckman TP, Eldridge VL: Improving strength, endurance and power. In Scully RM, Barnes MR, editors: *Physical therapy*, Philadelphia, 1989, JB Lippincott.

49. McAllister RM, Amann JF, Laughlin MH: Skeletal muscle fiber types and their vascular support, *J Reconstr Microsurg* 9(4):313–317, 1993.

50. McArdle WD, Katch VL: *Exercise physiology: energy, nutrition, and human performance*, ed 5, Baltimore, 2002, Lippincott Williams & Wilkins.

51. McCartney N, et al: Long-term resistance training in the elderly: effects on dynamic strength, exercise capacity, muscle, and bone, *J Gerontol Appl Biol Sci Med Sci* 50(2):97–104, 1995.

52. Miles MP, Clarkson PM: Exercise-induced muscle pain, soreness, and cramps, *J Sports Med Phys Fitness* 34(3):203–216, 1994.

53. Newham DJ, et al: Pain and fatigue after concentric and eccentric muscle contractions, *Clin Sci* 64:55, 1983.

54. Newham DJ, et al: Ultrastructural changes after concentric and eccentric contractions of human muscle, *J Neurol Sci* 61:109–122, 1983.

55. Norkin CC, Levangie PK: *Joint structure and function: a comprehensive analysis*, ed 2, Philadelphia, 1992, FA Davis.

56. Nyland J, et al: Review of the afferent neural system of the knee and its contribution to motor learning, *J Orthop Sports Phys Ther* 19(1):2–11, 1994.

57. Page P: Pathophysiology of acute exercise induced muscular injury: clinical implications, *J Athl Train* 30(1):29–34, 1995.

58. Palmieri G: Weight training and repetition speed, *J Appl Sport Sci Res* 1(2):36–38, 1987.

59. Reese NB: *Muscle and Sensory Testing*, ed 2, St Louis 2005, Saunders.

60. Rothstein JM, Lamb RL, Mayhew TP: Clinical uses of isokinetic measurements: critical issues, *Phys Ther* 67:1840, 1988.

61. Schmitt WH, Cuthbert SC: Common errors and clinical guidelines for manual muscle testing: "the arm test" and other inaccurate procedures, *Chiropr Osteopat* 16(16):1746–1340, 2008.

62. Schwane J, et al: Blood markers of delayed onset muscle soreness with downhill treadmill running, *Med Sci Sports Exerc* 13:80, 1981.

63. Seguin R, Nelson ME: The benefits of strength training for older adults, *Am J Prev Med* 25(Suppl 2):141–149, 2003.

64. Sellwood KL, Brukner P, Williams D, et al: Ice-water immersion and delayed-onset muscle soreness: a randomised controlled trial, *Br J Sports Med* 41(6):392, 2007.

65. Smith LL, et al: Impact of a repeated bout of eccentric exercise on muscular strength, muscle soreness and creatine kinase, *Br J Sports Med* 28(4):267–271, 1994.

66. Soderberg G: *Kinesiology: application to pathological motion*, Baltimore, 1986, Williams & Wilkins.

67. DOMS treatment: a review of the current strategies for treating DOMS, *Sports Injury Bulletin* , 2009.

68. Stauber WT: Eccentric action of muscles: physiology, injury and adaptation, *Exerc Sport Sci Rev* 19:157, 1989.

69. Steadman JR: Rehabilitation of athletic injury, *Am J Sports Med* 7:147, 1979.

70. Stone M: Literature review: explosive exercise and training, *J Strength Cond Res* 15(3):6–19, 1993.

71. Stone MH, et al: Periodization, *NSCA J Part I reprinted* 15(1):29, 1993.

72. Talag TS: Residual muscular soreness as influenced by concentric, eccentric and static contractions, *Res Q Exerc Sport* 44:458, 1973.

73. Talmadge RJ, Roy RR, Edgerton VR: Muscle fiber types and function, *Curr Opin Rheumatol* 5(6):695–705, 1993.

74. Thompson LV: Aging muscle: characteristics and strength training, *Issues Aging* 18(1):25–30, 1995.

75. Waltrous B, Armstrong R, Schwane J: The role of lactic acid in delayed onset muscular distress, *Med Sci Sports Exerc* 13:80, 1981.

76. Wilk KE, et al: Stretch-shortening drills for the upper extremities: theory and clinical application, *J Orthop Sports Phys Ther* 17(5):225–239, 1993.

77. Wyatt MP, Edwards AM: Comparison of quadriceps and hamstring torque values during isokinetic exercise, *J Orthop Sports Phys Ther* 3(2):48–56, 1981.

78. Zinowieff AN: Heavy resistance exercise: the Oxford technique, *Br J Phys Med* 14:129, 1951.

REVIEW QUESTIONS

Short Answer

1. How many muscle fiber types have been identified in humans?
2. Aerobic exercises require muscle fibers that are primarily _____ . (oxidative or glycolytic)
3. Organize the following five muscle fiber types into a numeric sequence of recruitment, proceeding from the lowest force requirements (1) to the greatest (5): _____ Fast twitch (type II) _____ Fast twitch (type IIAB) _____ Slow twitch (type I) _____ Fast twitch (type IIA) _____ Fast twitch (type IIB)
4. List the five ways muscular strength is measured.
5. Organize the following muscle contraction types in orderly sequence from greatest (3) to least (1) use of ATP: _____ Eccentrics _____ Concentrics _____ Isometrics
6. Organize the following muscle contraction types in orderly sequence from greatest (3) to least (1) force production: _____ Concentrics _____ Isometrics _____ Eccentrics
7. Name the two categories of muscle mutability.
8. What does SAID stand for?
9. Name the three stimuli for adaptive changes in skeletal muscles.
10. A patient returns to the outpatient physical therapy department and reports localized, specific muscle pain and describes an isolated event of lifting a box, which immediately increased pain. Describe the appropriate course of action the PTA will take to manage this patient's complaints of increased pain.

True/False

11. Isokinetic and isotonic do not describe muscle contractions but rather are terms used to define and describe events using true muscle contractions.
12 Manual muscle testing can be used to determine a muscle's power, work capacity, and force production.
13. Clinically it is important to choose one contraction type throughout the course of recovery from injury.
14. In terms of muscle hypertrophy, type I fibers hypertrophy more than type II fibers.

15. Stretching an innervated muscle creates tension, which results in muscle hypertrophy.
16. Muscle soreness is never an anticipated byproduct of new or more intense exercise.
17. Plyometric exercises are functionally appropriate exercises to use for all orthopedic patients.
18. Closed kinetic-chain exercises always must be deferred until the final phase of recovery.

19. High intensity strength training for the elderly is not safe or effective and does not lead to improved function.
20. Studies demonstrate that muscle size (hypertrophy), strength (force generation), and function (gait and balance) can be improved in elderly people with appropriately applied high-intensity resistance exercise.

5 Endurance Training

Jason Brumitt

LEARNING OBJECTIVES

1. Recognize the differences between muscular and cardiovascular endurance.
2. Define activities/exercises that are aerobic or anaerobic.
3. Describe benefits associated with cardiovascular fitness training.
4. Compare moderate- and vigorous-intensity exercises.
5. Describe methods to measure exercise intensity.
6. Describe the role of aerobic exercise for patients with an orthopedic injury.
7. Define the training parameters to improve muscular endurance.

KEY TERMS

Borg rating of perceived exertion

Cardiovascular endurance

Catabolism

Karvonen method

Maximal heart rate (MHR)

Maximal oxygen uptake (VO$_2$ MAX)

Muscular endurance

Oxidative system

Target heart rate (THR)

CHAPTER OUTLINE

Cardiovascular Training
    Energy Metabolism for Aerobic Training
    Benefits of Cardiovascular Fitness Training
Minimum Aerobic Exercise Guidelines for Americans
    Exercise Guidelines for Adults
    Exercise Guidelines for Children
Additional Methods to Measure Exercise Intensity
    Target Heart Rate and Estimated Maximum Heart Rate

Borg Rating of Perceived Exertion
Methods of Aerobic Training
Aerobic Exercise for Patients with an Orthopedic Injury
Muscular Endurance Training
Glossary
References
Review Questions
    Short Answer
    True/False

The ability to perform repetitive activities, participate in recreational pursuits, or to compete in sports requires adequate endurance capacity. The performance of an endurance activity (or exercise) may require involvement from one's muscular system, cardiovascular system, or both. **Muscular endurance** describes the ability of a muscle, or muscles, to perform at a particular level for prolonged period of time. **Cardiovascular endurance** describes the ability of one's cardiovascular system to allow the performance of prolonged aerobic activities. Both the muscular and cardiovascular systems require training to improve and/or maintain endurance capacity. In addition, training both systems will help to improve one's fitness level, reduce the risk of developing certain acute or chronic conditions, and help restore function after injury.

The purpose of this chapter is to define muscular and cardiovascular conditioning, review the metabolic pathways associated with each form of endurance training, discuss the physical and physiologic changes that occur when performing an endurance fitness program, present the recommended minimum training requirements, and address the functional role of endurance training for the rehabilitation client.

CARDIOVASCULAR TRAINING

Energy Metabolism for Aerobic Training

The **catabolism** of macronutrients (carbohydrates, proteins, and fats) creates energy for the human body. These fuel sources are ultimately converted into adenosine triphosphate (ATP), the main energy source for muscular function. Three metabolic pathways (Box 5-1) in the human body are responsible for the production of ATP. Energy metabolism may occur either with (aerobic metabolism) or without (anaerobic metabolism) the presence of oxygen.

When an endurance-based activity is initiated, the initial production of ATP is supplied by the ATP-creatine phosphate (ATP-CP) and the glycolysis systems. The ATP-CP system can only provide enough ATP for approximately 15 seconds of activity and the glycolysis system can only supply up to an additional 2 minutes worth of ATP. Continuation of an endurance-based activity requires the constant supply of oxygen for the

body to continue to produce ATP.[2,11,25] The **oxidative system** produces approximately 19 times the ATP (38 to 39 ATP, dependent upon the fuel substrate) as produced by the phosphagen energy system (2 ATP).[11,25]

Benefits of Cardiovascular Fitness Training

More than 60% of adults in the United States are considered either overweight or obese.[16,21] Obesity is a leading risk factor for developing heart disease, diabetes, hypertension, and some cancers. Obesity may also contribute to the development of certain musculoskeletal injuries.[15] An individual with a chronic disease who initiates an aerobic exercise program may experience a decrease in the severity of symptoms associated with their disease. Likewise, participating in a regular aerobic fitness program may help to reduce the risk of developing a chronic disease.

There are many positive physical and physiologic changes that occur when one participates in a cardiovascular fitness program. Individuals who perform a cardiovascular fitness program have a lower risk of developing many chronic diseases including cardiovascular disease, type 2 diabetes, and some cancers.[3,5,12,17-19,26,29,32,33] Additional training benefits associated with regular participation in an aerobic exercise program include reduction/control of one's weight, an increase in muscular strength, a reduction in the risk of falls, and a reduced mortality.[9,13]

The most notable physical and physiologic changes associated with regular participation in an aerobic exercise training are[4,23,25]:

- Increased size and number of mitochondria
- Increased myoglobin content
- Increased heart weight and size
- Increased cardiac output and stroke volume
- Improved mobilization and use of fat and carbohydrates
- Selective hypertrophy of type I slow twitch oxidative muscle fibers
- Decreased resting heart rate and submaximal heart rate
- Decrease in adipose tissue
- Increased blood volume and hemoglobin
- Reduced systolic and diastolic blood pressure
- Significantly improved oxygen extraction rates from the blood

MINIMUM AEROBIC EXERCISE GUIDELINES FOR AMERICANS

The Centers for Disease Control and Prevention (CDC) has provided physical activity guidelines for children, adults, healthy pregnant or postpartum women, and older adults.[1,9] Table 5-1 presents the minimum aerobic exercise guidelines suggested to improve one's aerobic fitness.[1,9]

BOX 5-1

Metabolic Pathways in the Human Body Responsible for the Production of ATP

- The ATP-CP system
- Glycolysis
- The oxidative system

Table 5-1	*Minimum Weekly Aerobic Exercise Guidelines for Adults*		
Intensity Level	Adults	Older Adults (65 years of age or older)	Healthy Pregnant or Postpartum Women
Moderate intensity aerobic activity	2 hours and 30 minutes weekly	2 hours and 30 minutes weekly	2 hours and 30 minutes weekly
Vigorous intensity aerobic activity	1 hour and 15 minutes weekly	1 hour and 15 minutes weekly	May continue vigorous intensity activities, such as running, if performing these exercises before her pregnancy.
Combination	Equal amount of moderate and vigorous intensity aerobic activity	Equal amount of moderate and vigorous intensity aerobic activity	N/A

From Centers for Disease Control and Prevention: Physical activity for everyone (website): www.cdc.gov/physicalactivity/everyone/guidelines/index.html. Accessed March 15, 2010.

Exercise Guidelines for Adults

The minimum exercises guidelines for adults, older adults, and healthy pregnant or postpartum women are based on the volume of moderate or vigorous intensity aerobic activity one performs.[9] The CDC has provided both relative and absolute guidelines to help one appreciate the intensity of his or her exercise session.[9] The talk test may be used to determine the relative intensity of an exercise session.[9] If one is able to talk during exercise, that exercise is of moderate-intensity. If one is unable to speak more than a few words before needing to pause for a breath, then they are likely performing a vigorous intensity exercise. The absolute intensity guidelines are based on the amount of energy one typically uses during 1 minute of exercise.[9] Examples of moderate intensity exercises include walking briskly, water aerobics, doubles tennis, and cycling at a pace less than 10 miles per hour.[9] Running, swimming laps, singles tennis, cycling faster than 10 miles per hour, and hiking are all examples of vigorous intensity exercises.[9]

The CDC recommends that as adults' fitness level improves, they should increase their level of either moderate intensity aerobic activity to 5 hours a week, or to 2½ hours of vigorous intensity aerobic activity each week, or to an equal mix of both types.[9]

Exercise Guidelines for Children

The number of children and adolescents who are considered overweight or obese has at least doubled during the past twenty years.[21] Recent studies have demonstrated that the likelihood that one will be obese as an adult increases if he or she was obese as a child.[31] To combat pediatric obesity, children and adolescents need to participate in daily physical activity. A lack of physical education in many school districts limits the opportunities during the day for a child to exercise.[20]

The CDC recommends that children perform at least 60 minutes of moderate intensity exercises each day.[9,30] In addition, children should perform vigorous intensity exercises at least 3 times a week.[9] The physical therapy team may play a crucial role in educating a family as to the importance of daily physical activity for a child as well as developing and implementing a fitness program for the child.[8]

ADDITIONAL METHODS TO MEASURE EXERCISE INTENSITY

In a clinical exercise physiology setting the efficiency of one's aerobic fitness may be determined by measuring the maximum volume of oxygen consumed during exercise. This measure has been termed the **maximal oxygen uptake** or the Vo_2 MAX.[2,11,25] Using this number, a clinician can prescribe a particular exercise intensity based on a percentage of one's Vo_2 MAX.

Most physical therapy clinics do not possess the necessary equipment required to record a patient's maximal oxygen uptake. Several methods have been developed that allow clinicians to measure and prescribe a particular exercise intensity without needing high-tech equipment.

The aforementioned talk test (previous section) is one manner to determine a client's aerobic exercise intensity. Two other methods used to measure aerobic intensity are the target heart rate/estimated maximum heart rate method and the perceived exertion method.[9]

Target Heart Rate and Estimated Maximum Heart Rate

The CDC recommends that an individual who is performing moderate intensity exercise should do so at a target heart rate range of 50% to 70% of one's maximum heart rate (beats per minute).[9] When an individual performs vigorous intensity exercise, their **target heart rate (THR)** should be 70% to 85% of their **maximal heart**

Table 5-2	*Target Heart Rate Calculations for a 30-Year-Old Individual*	
	Moderate Intensity Exercise	**Vigorous Intensity Exercise**
Formula	MHR × (0.50) or (0.70)	MHR × (0.70) or (0.85)
Lower limit	(220 − 30) × 0.50 = 95 beats per minute	(220 − 30) × 0.70 = 113 beats per minute
Upper limit	(220 − 30) × 0.70 = 113 beats per minute	(220 − 30) × 0.85 = 162 beats per minute

Maximum heart rate (MHR) = 220 − age.

Table 5-3	*Target Heart Rate Calculations Using the Karvonen Method*
	Moderate Intensity Exercise
Formula	MHR (or HR_{max}) = 220 − 30 = 190
50% MHR	[(190 − 70) × 0.50] + 70 = 130
70% MHR	[(190 − 70) × 0.70] + 70 = 154

Target heart rate (THR) = [(HR_{max} − HR_{rest}) × % Intensity] + HR_{rest}; *MHR*, maximum heart rate.

rate (MHR).[9] How is the MHR measured? To calculate a client's/patient's MHR, the individual's age is subtracted from 220 (e.g., 220 − 30). To establish the THR, the MHR is multiplied by the desired intensities. These two calculations (Table 5-2) will provide the lower and upper limit target heart rates for someone who is performing moderate or vigorous intensity exercises.[9]

The **Karvonen method** has been suggested as an alternative method of calculating THR.[25] The Karvonen method differs from the aforementioned technique in that it accounts for one's resting heart rate. In the previous example (see Table 5-2), the THR for a 30-year-old individual performing moderate intensity exercise is 95 to 113 beats per minute. If this individual has a resting heart rate of 70 beats per minute, the THR range would be 130 to 154 beats per minute (Table 5-3).

Borg Rating of Perceived Exertion

The **Borg Rating of Perceived Exertion** scale may be used to assess exercise intensity based on an individual's perception of exertion. While the client is exercising, ask him or her to rate how hard he or she is exercising based on the Borg scale. The Borg scale ranges from 6 to 20 points, with a 6 corresponding to "no exertion at all" and a 20 corresponding to "maximal exertion."[6] The client/patient should be asked to view the scale each time when measuring perceived exertion. The Borg scale has also been found to correlate with one's heart rate.[6,7] This is a helpful feature allowing the clinician to monitor exercise intensity level based on an estimate of heart rate. To determine heart rate from the Borg scale, multiply the perceived rating (e.g., 13) by a factor of 10 (e.g., 130 beats per minute).

METHODS OF AEROBIC TRAINING

Aerobic conditioning programs are either continuous or discontinuous. Continuous aerobic activities provide no rest interval during the entire bout of exercise. Examples of continuous activities are jogging, walking, running, cycling, and stair climbing.

Discontinuous aerobic activities are also known as *interval training activities*. A discontinuous aerobic exercise routine may include similar exercises used during continuous aerobic programs; however, during interval training, repeated exercise bouts are interspersed with rest intervals. Discontinuous training routines may be beneficial for patients who have limited exercise tolerance.

AEROBIC EXERCISE FOR PATIENTS WITH AN ORTHOPEDIC INJURY

Patients who have been diagnosed with an orthopedic injury will benefit from the inclusion of aerobic exercise as part of their rehabilitation program. The physical therapy team must consider tissue healing parameters when implementing an exercise. An acute injury or surgery may require a period of rest (or activity avoidance) in order to avoid additional injury or protect the surgical repair.

Evidence suggests that aerobic fitness activities should be included in a rehabilitation program for a patient recovering from a back injury.[27] Riding a stationary bicycle or walking on a treadmill (Fig. 5-1, *A-B*) may help to facilitate initial aerobic training. However, sitting on the saddle seat of a stationary ergometer may be uncomfortable or provoke symptoms for many patients with back problems. A recumbent cycle, with its large bucket seat (Fig. 5-1, *C*) to provide lumbar support, may be preferred by many clients. Patients who are unable to tolerate land based aerobic exercises may benefit from walking on an underwater treadmill. Immersion in the water can provide enough buoyancy during walking, unloading the spine, allowing the patient to exercise without exacerbating symptoms (Fig. 5-1, *D*).

Patients who have sustained a lower extremity injury or are recovering after a lower extremity surgery can maintain or improve cardiorespiratory fitness using an upper body ergometer (UBE) (Fig. 5-2, *A*). The UBE is ideal for individuals who are contraindicated from either bearing weight or performing range of motion activities with their involved lower extremity. The single-leg stationary bicycle ergometer exercise (Fig. 5-2, *B*)

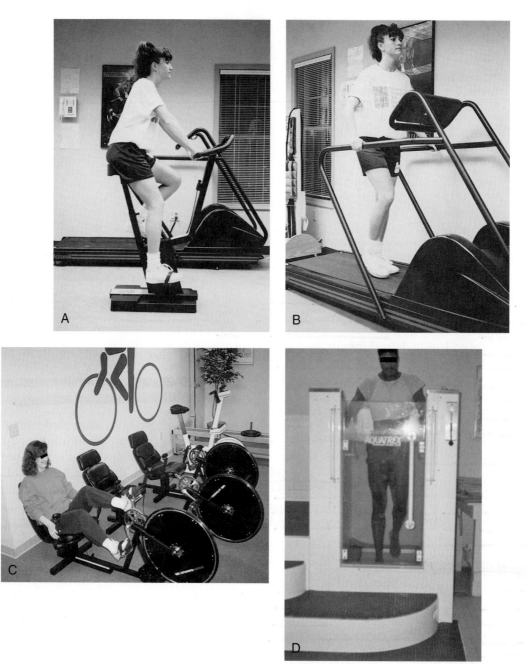

Fig. 5-1 A, Seated stationary bicycle ergometer. **B,** Standard treadmill. **C,** Recumbent bicycle ergometer. Large bucket seat used in a recumbent position may allow some patients to tolerate seated aerobic activities. **D,** Underwater treadmill. The buoyancy of the water may allow early vertical loading and the initiation of normalized gait mechanics.

may also be safely initiated by a patient before beginning double-leg cycling.

Older patients with hip, knee, or ankle osteoarthritis (degenerative joint disease) may also benefit from a UBE training program. The vertical compressive loads experienced during treadmill walking, stair climbing, or even stationary cycling may cause or increase one's symptoms.

Patients with upper extremity conditions can use a stationary cycle or treadmill for endurance training. Patients also can be instructed to use one-arm cycling

on a UBE (Fig. 5-3) to maintain upper body aerobic fitness.

Modifications can be made on stationary cycles to allow for continued aerobic conditioning after an ankle injury or surgery. Typically the seat height should allow for slight knee flexion (~10°) at the end of the pedal stroke. With the seat in normal position, the foot generally plantar flexes toward the end of the pedal stroke, causing stress to the anterior talofibular ligament. Therefore the seat height is lowered for a patient with a severe ankle sprain to allow for

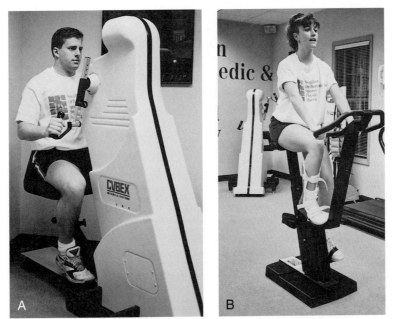

Fig. 5-2 **A,** For patients with lower extremity injuries, an upper body ergometer allows continued aerobic activities during periods of immobilization. **B,** In some cases, a single-leg stationary cycle ergometer can be used for cardiovascular fitness during periods of immobilization.

a complete pedal stroke and keep the ankle joint in neutral (Fig. 5-4).

Stair climbing, seated rowing, and cross-country ski machines are popular aerobic tools but must be used judiciously. Stair climbers require the patient to be correctly positioned vertically and maintain balance (holding the hand rails) to perform the exercise correctly. Therefore stair climbers are inappropriate or unsafe for many patients during the acute stage or immediate postorthopedic surgery period. Rowing machines require both a pulling motion with the arms and hip and knee flexion and extension. These simultaneous motions make modifications for use with specific orthopedic problems quite difficult. Cross-country ski machines require bilateral, reciprocal leg and arm motions and are also difficult to modify for orthopedic patients with acute disorders. However, stair climbers, rowing machines, and cross-country ski machines can be effective tools in aerobic conditioning programs after the acute phase of recovery from injury or surgery.

MUSCULAR ENDURANCE TRAINING

Even though they share the term *endurance*, muscular endurance and cardiovascular endurance are not one and the same. One can demonstrate functional muscular endurance but not possess functional cardiovascular endurance. What is the difference? As mentioned earlier in the chapter, cardiovascular endurance involves one's cardiovascular system to perform an aerobic activity. For an activity to be considered aerobic, the oxidative energy system is used.

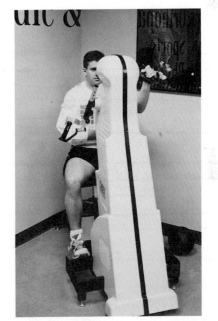

Fig. 5-3 A one-arm, upper body cycling activity with an upper body ergometer is also an effective aerobic exercise activity.

On the other hand, muscular endurance exercises typically only use the ATP-CP and glycolysis energy systems.

The key variables that define how a muscle(s) is(are) being trained are: the number of repetitions performed during a set, the amount of weight lifted during the set, and the period of rest between sets.

To increase muscular endurance, sets of high repetitions should be performed. At least 15 repetitions

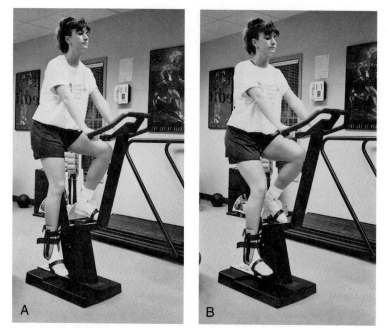

Fig. 5-4 **A,** Normal seat elevation for the performance of a seated bicycle ergometer allows for greater plantar flexion motion. Plantar flexion may be contraindicated with acute and subacute sprains of the lateral ligament complex of the ankle. **B,** With the saddle seat lowered, the affected ankle can be maintained in a more appropriate neutral position during periods of aerobic activity on the cycle ergometer.

should be performed per set.[2,10] Each repetition should be performed at or below 67% of one's 1 RM (repetition maximum). A period of 1 to 2 minutes should be allowed for rest in between each set. Table 5-4 compares variables associated with the four main types of muscular training: power, strength, hypertrophy, and endurance.

Muscular endurance training plays a key role when rehabilitating patients with an orthopedic injury.[14,22,24,27,28] Using the muscular endurance training principles allows the physical therapy team to prescribe strengthening exercises during the subacute phase of healing (see Chapter 11) while reducing the risk of overstressing the healing tissue.

Table 5-4	Training Variables Associated with Training Goals		
Training Goal	Repetitions Goal	Load (%of 1 RM)	Rest Interval Between Sets (min)
Power	1-2	80-90	2-3
Strength	≤6	≥85	2-3
Hypertrophy	6-12	67-85	2-3
Endurance	15+	≤67	1-2

❖ GLOSSARY

Borg rating of perceived exertion: A scale used to assess exercise intensity based on an individual's perception of exertion.

Cardiovascular endurance: The ability of one's cardiovascular system to allow the performance of prolonged aerobic activities.

Catabolism: A metabolic process that breaks down compounds, such as degradation of glucose to CO_2 and H_2O, causing the release of energy.

Karvonen method: An alternative (to the Borg) method of calculating target heart rate.

Maximal heart rate (MHR): The maximum number of beats per minute that the heart is able to pump. MHR is measured by subtracting the patient's age from 220.

Maximal oxygen uptake (VO$_2$ MAX): The maximum volume of oxygen consumed during exercise. This measurement shows the patient's level of aerobic fitness.

Muscular endurance: The ability of muscle(s) to perform at a particular level for prolonged period of time.

Oxidative system: An energy system known as the *aerobic system* because its operation requires a constant supply of O_2.

Target heart rate (THR): The optimum number of beats per minute that the heart should pump during moderate or vigorous intensity exercise. THR is calculated by multiplying the patient's MHR by either 0.70 (for moderate intensity) or 0.85 (for vigorous intensity).

REFERENCES

1. American College of Sports Medicine Position Stand: The recommended quantity and quality of exercise for developing and maintaining cardiorespiratory and muscular fitness, and flexibility in healthy adults, *Med Sci Sports Exerc* 30(6):975–991, 1998.
2. Baechle TR, Earle RW, Wathen D: Resistance training. In Baechle TR, Earle RW, editors: *Essentials of strength training and conditioning*, ed 3, Champaign, Ill, 2008, Human Kinetics.
3. Ballard-Barbash R, Hunsberger S, Alciati MH, et al: Physical activity, weight control, and breast cancer risk and survival: clinical trial rationale and design considerations, *J Natl Cancer Inst* 101(9):630–643, 2009.
4. Barnard RJ, Edgerton VR, Peter JB: Effects of exercise of skeletal muscle. I. Biochemical and histochemical properties, *J Appl Physiol* 28(6):762–766, 1970.
5. Blair SN, Morris JN: Healthy hearts—and the universal benefits of being physically active: physical activity and health, *Ann Epidemiol* 19(4):253–256, 2009.
6. Borg G: *Borg's perceived exertion and pain scales*, Champaign, Ill, 1998, Human Kinetics.
7. Borg G: Psychophysical bases of perceived exertion, *Med Sci Sports Exerc* 14(5):377–381, 1982.
8. Brumitt J: The role of the certified strength and conditioning specialist in preventing childhood obesity, *Strength Condition J* 28(4):54–56, 2006.
9. Centers for Disease Control and Prevention: *Physical activity for everyone* (website). www.cdc.gov/physicalactivity/everyone/guidelines/index.html. Accessed March 15, 2010.
10. Cooper LW, Powell AP, Rasch J: Master's swimming: an example of successful aging in competitive sport, *Curr Sports Med Rep* 6(6):392–396, 2007.
11. Cramer JT: Bioenergetics of exercise and training. In Baechle TR, Earl RW, editors: *Essentials of strength training and conditioning*, ed 3, Champaign, Ill, 2008, Human Kinetics.
12. Dalleck LC, Allen BA, Hanson BA, et al: Dose-response relationship between moderate-intensity exercise duration and coronary heart disease risk factors in postmenopausal women, *J Womens Health (Larchmt)* 18(1):105–113, 2009.
13. Donnelly JE, Blair SN, Jakicic JM, et al: American college of sports medicine position stand. Appropriate physical activity intervention strategies for weight loss and prevention of weight regain for adults, *Med Sci Sports Exerc* 41(2):459–471, 2009.
14. Durall CJ, Udermann BE, Johansen DR, et al: The effects of preseason trunk muscle training on low-back pain occurrence in women collegiate gymnasts, *J Strength Cond Res* 23(1):86–92, 2009.
15. Durstine JL, Moore GE: *ACSM's exercise management for persons with chronic diseases and disabilities*, ed 2, Champaign, Ill, 2003, Human Kinetics.
16. Flegal KM, Carroll MD, Ogden CL, et al: Prevalence and trends in obesity among US adults, 1999-2000, *JAMA* 288(14):1723–1727, 2002.
17. Firestone B, Mold JW: Type 2 diabetes: which interventions best reduce absolute risks of adverse events? *J Fam Pract* 58(6):E1, 2009.
18. Giada F, Biffi A, Agostoni P, et al: Exercise prescription for the prevention and treatment of cardiovascular diseases: part II, *J Cardiovasc Med (Hagerstown)* 9(6):641–652, 2008.
19. Giada F, Biffi A, Agostoni P, et al: Joint Italian Societies' Task Force on Sports Cardiology. Exercise prescription for the prevention and treatment of cardiovascular diseases: part I, *J Cardiovasc Med (Hagerstown)* 9(5):529–544, 2008.
20. Grunbaum JA, Kann L, Kinchen S, et al: Youth risk behavior surveillance – United States, 2003 *Morb Mortal Wkly Rep* 53(SS-2):1–95, 2004.
21. Hedley AA, Ogden CL, Johnson CL, et al: Prevalence of overweight and obesity among U.S. children, adolescents, and adults, *JAMA* 291(23):2847–2850, 2004.
22. Kell RT, Asmundson GJ: A comparison of two forms of periodized exercise rehabilitation programs in the management of chronic nonspecific low-back pain, *J Strength Cond Res* 23(2):513–523, 2009.
23. Kiessling K: Effects of physical training on ultrastructural features in human skeletal muscle. In Pernow B, Saltin B, editors: *Muscle metabolism during exercise*, New York, 1971, Plenum Press.
24. Lorig KR, Sobel DS, Stewart AL, et al: Evidence suggesting that a chronic disease self-management program can improve health status while reducing hospitalization: a randomized trial, *Med Care* 37(1):5–14, 1999.
25. McArdle WD, Katch FI, Katch VL: *Exercise physiology. energy, nutrition, and human performance*, ed 4, Baltimore, 1996, Williams & Wilkins.
26. McGavock JM, Eves ND, Mandic S, et al: The role of exercise in the treatment of cardiovascular disease associated with type II diabetes mellitus, *Sports Med* 34(1):27–48, 2004.
27. McGill SM: *Low back disorders. Evidence-based prevention and rehabilitation*, ed 2, Champaign, Ill, 2007, Human Kinetics.
28. Nikander R, Mälkiä E, Parkkari J, et al: Dose-response relationship of specific training to reduce chronic neck pain and disability, *Med Sci Sports Exerc* 38(12):2068–2074, 2006.
29. Sandrock M, Schulze C, Schmitz D, et al: Physical activity throughout life reduces the atherosclerotic wall process in the carotid artery, *Br J Sports Med* 42(10):539–544, 2008.
30. Strong WB, Malina RM, Blimkie JR, et al: Physical activity recommendations for school-age youth, *J Pediatr* 146:732–737, 2005.
31. Styne DM: Childhood and adolescent obesity, *Pediatr Clin North Am* 48:823–854, 2001.
32. Taylor RS, Brown A, Ebrahim S, et al: Exercise-based rehabilitation for patients with coronary heart disease: systematic review and meta-analysis of randomized controlled trials, *Am J Med* 116(10):682–692, 2004.
33. Thompson PD, Buchner D, Piña IL, et al: Exercise and physical activity in the prevention and treatment of atherosclerotic cardiovascular disease: a statement from the Council on Clinical Cardiology (Subcommittee on exercise, Rehabilitation, and Prevention) and the Council on Nutrition, Physical Activity, and Metabolism (Subcommittee on Physical Activity), *Arterioscler Thromb Vasc Biol* 23: e42-e49, 2003.

REVIEW QUESTIONS

Short Answer

1. According to the CDC what is the minimum number of hours a week that an adult should perform moderate intensity aerobic exercises?
2. Calculate the MHR for a 40-year-old male.
3. The Borg scale has a range of numbers starting at _____ and ending at _____.
4. A 25-year-old football player has fractured his right fibula. The orthopedic surgeon believes that he can return to competition in 3 to 4 weeks. At this moment, the football player is not allowed to bear weight on his right lower extremity. Which exercises would be most appropriate for him to maintain cardiovascular fitness?

True/False

5. Cardiovascular endurance and muscular endurance are one and the same.
6. A distance runner primarily uses the glycolytic pathway to produce ATP.

6 Balance and Coordination

Bryan Riemann

LEARNING OBJECTIVES

1. Define and contrast balance and coordination.
2. Discuss the mechanoreceptor system and define four mechanoreceptors.
3. List static and dynamic balance and coordination tests and activities.
4. Define proprioception and kinesthetic awareness.
5. Discuss several factors that contribute to balance dysfunction.
6. Identify functional closed kinetic chain proprioceptive exercises.
7. Discuss the rationale for proprioceptive training for the upper extremity.

KEY TERMS

Balance

Base of support

Coordination

Golgi tendon organs

Mechanoreceptors

Muscle spindles

Neuromuscular control

Postural equilibrium

Proprioception

CHAPTER OUTLINE

EXERCISE IN ORTHOPEDIC DISORDERS

Rehabilitation after an acute injury, surgery, immobilization, or chronic orthopedic condition must address all the components of normal function. Regaining lost strength, reducing pain and swelling, improving flexibility, enhancing local muscular endurance, and building cardiovascular fitness are obvious and vital areas requiring specific therapeutic interventions. Sometimes less apparent, but equally important, is the need to address the motor control and neuromuscular elements to promote synchronous, fluid, and stable motor function of the injured part within the context of the distal and proximal body parts. Furthermore, secondary to the interdependence of coordination, posture, and **balance** to gait and functional movements, attention must also be placed on these elements for complete recovery from injury. Long-term convalescence reduces strength, flexibility, and cardiorespiratory fitness, as well as the use of vestibular and afferent neural input needed for balance and coordination.

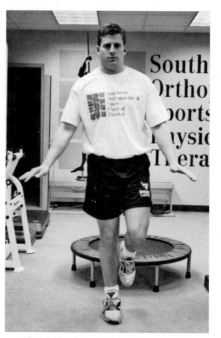

Fig. 6-1 Single-leg stance test.

DEFINITIONS OF BALANCE, PROPRIOCEPTION, NEUROMUSCULAR CONTROL, AND COORDINATION

Balance is often considered as the ability to maintain the center of mass (COM) over the **base of support.**[12] This definition is only appropriate, however, when the base of support is fixed, such as standing in a constant location on two feet. The base of support is defined as the area contained within the parts of the body making physical contact with the external environment (Fig. 6-1).[9] During dynamic situations, such as gait and functional activity, the base of support does not remain fixed to a constant location. Rather, as part of locomotion, the base of support moves, increasing the challenge to the elements responsible for maintaining balance. For this reason, the concept of balance also needs to include consideration to these circumstances. **Postural equilibrium** is a broader term that refers to balancing all forces acting on the body's COM to maintain COM within the limits of stability with optimal joint segment alignment.[1] Forces that challenge postural equilibrium arise from gravity, unexpected perturbations (i.e., stumbling over an unforeseen obstacle), or performance of voluntary motor activities (i.e., picking up a bag of groceries). Maintaining postural equilibrium is accomplished by the postural control system, the collection of sensory sources (somatosensory, vision, and vestibular), central nervous system, and the musculoskeletal system, all serving to maintain postural equilibrium. The somatosensory sources relevant to postural equilibrium are the mechanoreceptor populations residing in joint, muscle, connective, and ligamentous tissues. Because these tissues are often damaged during orthopedic injury, postural equilibrium may be disturbed following injury because of sensory disruptions, musculoskeletal disruptions, or both.[9]

Performing motor tasks effectively and efficiently requires not only postural equilibrium, but also effective coordination of the many muscles serving to move and stabilize the joints upon which they cross. **Coordination** has been defined as the ability to produce patterns of body and limb motions in the context of environmental objects and events.[13] For example, picking up an object from a table requires coordinating the shoulder, elbow, and wrists joints to put the hand and fingers into position so the object can be grasped. Essential to coordinating joint positions is sufficient sensory (afferent) information regarding joint position, movement (kinesthesia), and movement resistance/tension. The afferent information contributing to these three elements, joint position, movement (kinesthesia), and movement resistance/tension, is referred to as *proprioception.*[12] When the proprioception elements are consciously perceived, they are referred to as the *conscious perceptions of proprioception.*[12] Proprioception is vital for neuromuscular control. From a joint stability perspective, **neuromuscular control** refers to the subconscious activation of muscles occurring in preparation for and in response to joint motion and loading.[12]

Mechanoreceptors

Mechanoreceptors are the sensory receptors that are responsible for converting mechanical events (e.g., movement, tension) into neural signals that can be conveyed to the central nervous system.[7] As mentioned previously, mechanoreceptors are located in muscle, tendon, ligament, joint capsules, and in skin and connective (fascial) tissues. Each mechanoreceptor has specific stimuli (e.g., light touch versus tissue lengthening) and thresholds (e.g., magnitude of stimuli required) to which it will respond.[6] Mechanoreceptors most susceptible to disruption during orthopedic injury include the receptors located in the musculotendinous, ligaments, and joint capsules. Mechanoreceptors located in the musculotendinous tissues include the muscle spindles and Golgi tendon organs. **Muscle spindles** are responsible for conveying information regarding muscle length and rate of length change. Unique to muscle spindles is their adjustable sensitivity via the gamma motor neurons. **Golgi tendon organs,** located across a musculotendinous junction are responsible for conveying information regarding muscle tension. Located in the ligaments and joint capsules are Ruffini receptors, Pacinian corpuscles, Golgi tendon-like endings and free nerve endings. Collectively, based on their threshold and adaptation characteristics, these four mechanoreceptors provide the central nervous system with information regarding speed of joint position and movement and host tissue load levels.

BALANCE AND COORDINATION TESTS

To prescribe appropriate balance and coordination exercises, it is essential to have data related to present balance and coordination status. Most often, coordination is evaluated by using the simple tests such as those outlined in Box 6-1. Although quantifying a patient's coordination abilities can be easily accomplished by counting the number of repetitions completed in a given time frame or the number or percentage of successes per number of attempts, qualitatively examining and describing the patient's abilities and difficulties (e.g., steadiness, control, speed) can also be useful.

Interestingly, balance tests and specific balance treatment activities are rarely separated, and the same movements are used for fundamental balance exercises and clinically relevant balance tests. Recall that three sensory sources, somatosensory, visual, and vestibular, contribute afferent information to the central nervous system so that appropriate muscle actions can be selected. By manipulating the conditions in which balance tasks are conducted, different aspects of the postural control system may be more selectively challenged.[9] For example, having a patient stand with eyes closed heightens their reliance on somatosensory and vestibular information. In addition, manipulating the base of support and support surface characteristics can also change the challenge imposed upon the postural control system. For example, compared to double-leg stance, single-leg stance requires that the postural control system reorganize itself over a narrow and short base of support, with the additional advantage that bilateral comparisons can be made.

BOX 6-1

Coordination Tests

Finger to nose: A reciprocal motion test in which the patient touches the tip of the index finger to the tip of the nose.

Finger opposition: A reciprocal motion test in which the patient alternately touches the tip of each finger with the tip of the thumb.

Fixation-position hold: A static position test in which the arms are held horizontally or the knees extended.

Heel on shin: A reciprocal motion and accuracy test in which the patient is supine and is asked to slide the heel of one leg from the ankle to the knee of the opposite leg.

Pronation-supination: A reciprocal motion test in which the palms are rotated up and down.

Tapping foot or hand: A reciprocal motion test in which the patient is asked to repeatedly tap the ball of one foot while keeping the heel in contact with the floor. With the hand, the patient is asked to tap hand on knee.

Throwing and catching a ball: A reciprocal motion test in which the patient is asked to receive and deliver a ball.

Functionally, periods of single-leg stance are often interspersed in many activities of daily living, such as walking, turning, climbing stairs, and putting on a pair of pants. Further, during activities of daily living, one does not usually solely concentrate on maintaining balance, but rather on the details of the task (e.g., reaching up to remove the correct book from a shelf). Additionally, during activities of daily living, situations arise where unexpected challenges (perturbations) to postural equilibrium occur. Thus comprehensive balance assessment and training frequently call for a progressive battery of specific tasks of incremental difficulty and should include not only static stances with varying bases of support and support surface characteristics, but also tasks that involve voluntary movement and task completion and unexpected perturbations.[9] Close observation of the patient's protective reactions during loss of balance is a critical component of all balance tests and training activities. Immediate corrective action by the patient to maintain balance is necessary to move the patient from low-level balance activities to more challenging, complex maneuvers.

Box 6-2 summarizes common progressions used with respect to stances, support surfaces, and vision. For example, the static double-leg stance test with the eyes open is often the first test performed. This very simple test is made more challenging by having the patient maintain balance on both legs with his or her eyes closed. Next, the patient can then stand on a high-density foam

BOX 6-2

Progressive Balancing Exercises

Seated: Eyes open, eyes closed, manually applied postural stress. Throwing and catching a ball.

Seated: Uneven surface, physioball (Swiss ball). Eyes open, eyes closed.

Standing: Double-leg standing—eyes open, eyes closed, manually applied postural stress, weight shifting
Single-leg standing—eyes open, eyes closed, postural stress

Surface changes: All standing drills can be advanced by changing the inclination and type of surface:
■ Concrete
■ Carpet (short, dense, thick)
■ Asphalt
■ Tile (slick), linoleum
■ Grass, loose gravel, dirt

Minitrampoline: Double-leg standing—eyes open, eyes closed, hopping
Single-leg standing—eyes open, eyes closed, hopping

Foam padding: Double- and single-leg standing, ambulation, eyes open, eyes closed

Balancing devices: Biomechanical ankle platform system (BAPS) board, kinesthetic ability training (KAT) device, balance board, seated position, standing position, double-leg and single-leg standing-eyes open, eyes closed

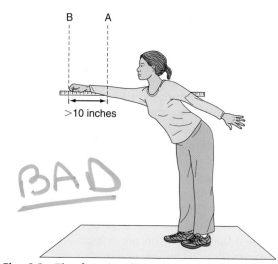

Fig. 6-2 The functional reach test. *A,* Starting position. *B,* Normal functional reach of more than 10 inches. (From Cameron MH, Monroe LG: *Physical rehabilitation: evidence-based examination, evaluation, and intervention,* St Louis, 2008, Saunders.)

surface with eyes open and closed, followed by standing on low-density foam with eyes open and closed. After that, the patient can stand on inclined or declined surfaces and unstable surfaces such as minitrampolines, rocker boards, and wobble boards, again using the eyes open to eyes closed progression. Similar eyes open to eyes closed and support surface progressions can be used with the patient using single-leg and tandem stances.

After a patient has mastered static stances under a variety of visual and support surface conditions, balance tasks can be progressed to include concurrent voluntary movements and tasks. Reaching tasks are very practical and functional test that determine a patient's ability to perform simple daily tasks. Tests can be performed with the patient seated or standing using the upper or lower extremity (Fig. 6-2). Patients are offered a target that is slightly out of reach to test their ability to shift their center of mass to their limits of stability. Automatic activities, such as catching a ball, can also be performed in sequence from a seated to a standing position. The velocity, angle, and direction of throwing the ball to the patient challenges the patient's ability to rapidly move arms and trunk out of static balance state, and back to equilibrium.

More dynamic balance tests requiring the patient to maintain a base of support, negotiate a single plane or multidirectional movement, and keep the body in motion are also useful. Walking in a straight line for a prescribed functional distance (e.g., from a chair to the bathroom) is a simple test to administer. Adding directional changes, such as turning a corner or negotiating a random series of obstacles provides information concerning the patient's dynamic balance.

Quantifying performance during many of the previously mentioned tasks can be done using noninstrumented or instrumented measures. Noninstrumented measures include variables such as length of time in equilibrium,[5,9] error scoring systems,[10,11] and distances reached with arms or legs.[1,8] During the dynamic tests, such as tandem walking (straight line, heel-to-toe sequencing), the distance traveled during a specified time period can be recorded. Instrumented measures often involve technology that record the forces exerted on a support surface (force platforms) or sensors that detect movement and position of the support surface. In addition to providing objective measures of balance performance, some also provide real time biofeedback to facilitate weight transfer within base of support boundaries.

As an additional objective measurement of static balancing abilities, Wolfson and associates[14] designed the postural stress test (PST) to help quantify static balance. This test measures a patient's ability to maintain balance during a series of progressive graded destabilizing forces. It is clinically cumbersome in that it involves applying a belt to the patient's waist and attaching a weight-pulley system behind the patient. Without the patient's knowledge, a weight is applied to the pulley system, which provides a sudden posterior force necessitating rapid correction of the postural interference. The test is graded on a scale from 0 to 9, with 0 representing a total inability to correct balance, and 9 representing no loss of balance. In addition to assessing a patient's ability to withstand destabilizing perturbations, the PST may also serve as a training task.

BALANCE TRAINING IN ORTHOPEDICS

In concert with regaining strength and motion, specific functional tasks must be incorporated into the rehabilitation plan to accentuate muscular coordination, neuromuscular control, and postural equilibrium during dynamic activities. Duncan[4] has identified several factors that may significantly contribute to balance dysfunction:

- Perception
- Behavior
- Range of motion
- Biomechanical alignment
- Weakness
- Sensory
- Synergistic organization strategy
- Coordination
- Adaptability

Many studies have demonstrated how injury, surgery, immobilization, and rehabilitation programs without specific balance and proprioceptive training can have a profound negative effect on balance and neuromuscular control. It can be concluded from these studies that the physical therapist assistant must (PTA) clearly recognize that injury, surgery, and non–weight-bearing immobilization negatively affect the proprioceptive pathways, as well as use of proprioceptive information by the central nervous system for neuromuscular control and balance. Functional balance and coordination training combined with closed kinetic chain (CKC) resistive exercises allows for afferent neural input from peripheral joint mechanoreceptors, which in turn may promote restoration proprioception, neuromuscular control, and balance.

Specific Balance Tasks in Orthopedics

As described in the testing section, many of the tasks used as balance tests are also used for balance training, using the same progression principles. This section will describe some additional balance tasks that are used for training. It is important to recognize that a rehabilitation protocol rarely suggests a comprehensive, specific sequence using the balance activities described in this chapter. Generally, tasks and drills are initiated and progressed according to the abilities and desired goals of the patient.

In cases of lower extremity injury with long-term, bedbound convalescence, manual resistive hip and knee extension with varying joint positions may be appropriate to initiate restoration of normal proprioceptive pathways. Once a patient may assume an upright position, progressive balance training may begin in a seated position. Similar progressive sequencing as with the standing tasks can be used, with the patient first attempting to maintain balance with the eyes open, then with the eyes closed. Progressions can include movements such as reaching tasks and the lifting of objects. Manually applied external forces (perturbations) can be applied while the patient's eyes are closed to initiate reflexive balance training. Comparable to using foam and unstable surface for standing progressions, a large physioball or Swiss ball can be used as part of a seated static and dynamic balancing program to increase the challenge to the postural control system (Fig. 6-3, *A*). The physioball, which is a rather demanding exercise apparatus, has many applicable and creative uses in balancing and strengthening programs for various orthopedic patients. One very challenging exercise is the performance of support sit-ups on the physioball (Fig. 6-3, *B*). Obviously this particular exercise is for a rather active population, and not for all patients.

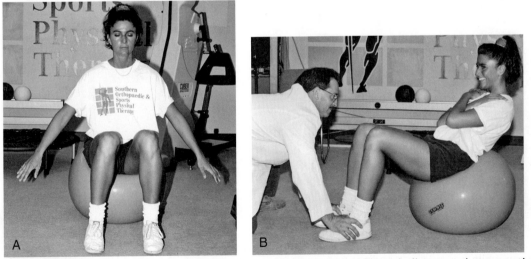

Fig. 6-3 A, Sitting trunk balance can be progressed using a physioball (Plyoball) to challenge and test a patient's ability to demonstrate protective reactions and appropriate muscular corrective action while seated. **B,** Supported partial direct sit-ups for improving trunk balance and strength on a large diameter physioball (Plyoball).

Once a patient is weight bearing, progressive balance training can begin with vertical weight bearing (double-leg standing). For proper gait mechanics, weight shifting (changing base of support from one leg to another) is critical. Thus, after the patient masters double-leg standing static balance, the physical therapist assistant should begin training the patient to shift balance from one leg to the other. The next progressions can include the aforementioned visual, support surface, and base of support progressions. For teaching and safety purposes, all single-leg balance drills should be initiated on the uninvolved limb. As confidence and motor learning progress, the patient then performs the balance activity on the involved limb. In all cases of balance training, manual support and spotting is provided as required. As a means to document progress, the length of time the patient can maintain equilibrium can be recorded.

Other functional CKC exercises that replicate the specific demands of daily activities or athletic skills serve to restore coordination and balance, as well as the factors contributing to balance dysfunction listed in the previous section. Unfortunately, progressively demanding tasks are sometimes omitted from rehabilitation programs, with reliance put on increased clinical strength tests, greater range-of-motion grades, and reduced pain and swelling, as objective data leading to discharge from formal therapy. Examples of functional CKC exercises include double- and single-leg squats on stable and unstable surfaces, forward and backward gait, sidestepping (lateral steps), heel-to-toe walking, and braiding steps (carioca). Progressively challenging tasks that stimulate the patient's ability to safely and accurately negotiate obstacles and make multidirectional changes while in motion are important.

It is important that advanced functional balance drills, such as hopping, be included in the programs of patients returning to high levels of physical activity. Hopping drills can range from simple vertical leaps to quite challenging combinations of vertical and horizontal patterns. Hopping is useful with an athletic population and can be done on a flat, hard surface or on a minitrampoline (Fig. 6-4, *A*). The forgiving, uneven rebound surface of the minitrampoline adds an appropriate challenge for progressive balance training. Additionally, a wobble board (Fig. 6-4, *B*) or the kinesthetic ability trainer (Fig. 6-5) can be used to challenge single- or double-leg proprioception. Using the minitrampoline after hip, knee, or ankle injury for static standing balance and for single-leg or double-leg hopping is unique and challenging for many patients. As with other balance drills, single-leg or double-leg standing or hopping can progress from eyes open to eyes closed.

Inclusions of tasks in which sudden perturbations challenge balance are also important components of a balance training program. For example the clinician can apply sudden force to the patient while the patient is standing on one leg with the eyes closed (Fig. 6-6). Applying the manual postural stresses in different directions and with varying degrees of force can further challenge the ability to "right" or correct balance. Another method of perturbing balance is to use elastic tubing secured to a patient. The clinician begins the task

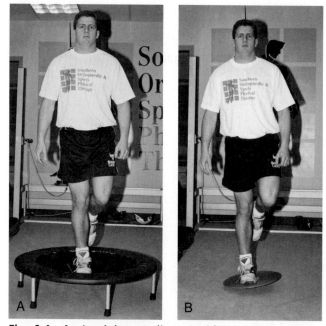

Fig. 6-4 **A,** A minitrampoline provides a unique, challenging, and forgiving surface to encourage balance and proprioception while hopping or standing. **B,** A wobble board or BAPS board can be used to challenge single- or double-leg proprioception and balance.

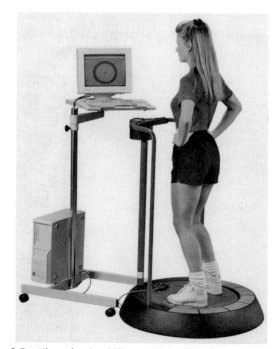

Fig. 6-5 **Kinesthetic ability trainer.** (Courtesy of Breg, Inc., Vista, Calif.)

by applying tension through the tubing. By suddenly releasing the tubing, the patient is suddenly presented with an immediate challenge to postural equilibrium.

Many commercial training devices have been developed to assist with balance training. Most commonly used is the biomechanical ankle platform system (BAPS). The name is misleading because this unit can be used for a wide variety of lower extremity conditions. The generic names for this tool are wobble board and balance board (Fig. 6-7). This device is very adaptable, portable, and affordable for many physical therapy environments. Initially, double-leg support progresses to single-leg standing. One of the most challenging balance drills is performing single-leg standing on a balance board with the eyes closed.

Balance and Proprioceptive Training for the Upper Extremity

Many household chores involve the repetitive use of the arms and shoulders to lift, pull, and carry. Industrial workers, manual laborers, and assembly line workers all use their arms and shoulders in vigorous weight-bearing positions (weight bearing in these instances refers to overhead lifting, pulling, and climbing maneuvers.). Athletes in particular use their arms and shoulders to perform sports skills. Gymnasts require extraordinary flexibility, strength, and glenohumeral stability during demanding upper-body, weight-bearing activities. With the upper extremity in contact with a secure surface, it is incorporated into defining the base of support.

As mentioned, injury, surgery, and immobilization lead to significant alterations in proprioception. Specific proprioceptive exercises have been proposed that, when used in conjunction with proprioceptive neuromuscular facilitation exercises, rhythmic stabilization strengthening exercises, and general range of motion, may contribute to improved proprioception in the upper extremity.

The upper extremities can be progressed in much the same way as the lower extremities. Although many of these exercises are often considered to be specific for an athletic population, they can be adapted to the general orthopedic population who must rely on dynamic vigorous weight-bearing shoulder and arm activities to accomplish tasks of daily living. With both arms in contact with the ground, weight shifting between the arms can be conducted on firm and unstable surfaces. In addition, while in a similar position, eyes open and eyes closed, balancing can be conducted on the same support surfaces used for standing balance (Figs. 6-7, 6-8, A1-A2). Beginning with two arms, this exercise can be intensified by having the patient use one arm with the eyes open and closed. Global stability of the glenohumeral joint can be enhanced effectively with the use of medicine balls and physioballs (Fig. 6-8, B1-B2). The patient begins the progression of this exercise by kneeling in front of the ball and placing both hands on the ball. As the exercise progresses, extraordinary joint stability, strength, and balance are required to maintain equilibrium.

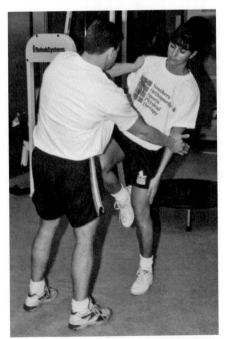

Fig. 6-6 To test and challenge a patient's protective reactions, the clinician can apply a sudden external force while the patient's eyes are closed. Close protection and support must be provided by the clinician during this activity.

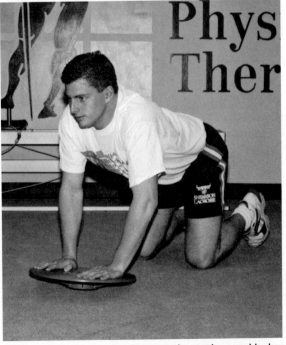

Fig. 6-7 For upper extremity proprioception and balance training, a wobble board can be used; initially, both arms are involved. As the patient gains strength, balance, and confidence, one arm can be used.

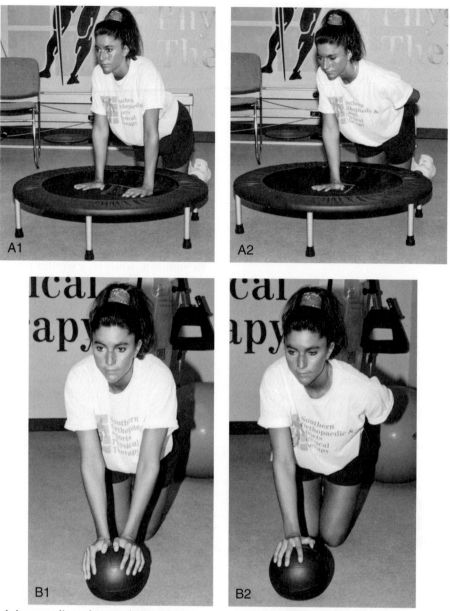

Fig. 6-8 **A1,** The minitrampoline also can be used to encourage closed chain proprioception for the upper extremities. **A2,** Progressing this activity will have the patient perform one-arm balancing, push-ups, and hopping maneuvers on the forgiving surface of the minitrampoline. **B1,** A small physioball (Plyoball) also can be used to encourage dynamic closed-chain proprioception for the upper extremities. **B2,** Closed-chain, weight-bearing activities can be progressed by having the patient balance and support on one arm on a Plyoball.

Summary

Underlying all motor activities are specific processes to ensure that postural equilibrium is maintained. Disruptions to balance, postural equilibrium and coordination often accompany orthopedic pathology. Additionally, orthopedic conditions often produce alterations in proprioception, motor control, coordination and neuromuscular control thereby requiring specific elements to be incorporated into rehabilitation programs to promote their restoration. Often the same tasks used for balance assessments can be used for training. Progressions can be made by changing stances, support surfaces, visual conditions and tasks. Similar progressions can also be incorporated into upper extremity rehabilitation programs.

❖ GLOSSARY

Balance: The ability to maintain the center of mass (COM) over the base of support.[12]

Base of support: The area contained within the parts of the body making physical contact with the external environment.[9]

Coordination: The ability to produce patterns of body and limb motions in the context of environmental objects and events.[13]

Golgi tendon organs: Fibers responsible for conveying information regarding muscle tension.

Mechanoreceptors: Sensory receptors responsible for converting mechanical events into neural signals that can be conveyed to the central nervous system.[7]

Muscle spindles: Fibers responsible for conveying information regarding muscle length and rate of length change.

Neuromuscular control: Subconscious activation of muscles occurring in preparation for and in response to joint motion and loading.[12]

Postural equilibrium: The balance of all forces acting on the body's COM to maintain it within the limits of stability with optimal joint segment alignment.[1]

Proprioception: The afferent information contributing to joint position, joint movement (kinesthesia), and movement resistance/tension.

REFERENCES

1. Bellew J, Fenter P: Control of balance differs after knee or ankle fatigue in older women, *Arch Phys Med Rehabil* 87:1486–1489, 2006.
2. Crotts D, Thompson B, Nahom M, et al: Balance abilities of professional dancers on select balance tests, *J Orthop Sports Phys Ther* 23:12–17, 1996.
3. Crutchfield CA, Shumway-Cook A, Horak FB: Balance and coordination training. In Scully RM, Barnes MR, editors: *Physical therapy*, Philadelphia, 1989, JB Lippincott.
4. Duncan PW: *Balance dysfunction: implications for geriatric and neurological rehabilitation. Course Notes*, Nov. 1994, Advanced Educational Seminars, Inc.
5. Ekdahl C, Jarnlo G, Andersson S: Standing balance in healthy subjects, Evaluation of a quantitative test battery on a force platform, *Scan J Rehabil Med* 21:187–195, 1989.
6. Erikson R: Stimulus coding in topographic and nontopographic afferent modalities: on the significance of the activity of individual sensory neurons, *Psychol Rev* 75:447–465, 1968.
7. Grigg P: Peripheral neural mechanisms in proprioception, *J Sport Rehabil* 3:2–17, 1994.
8. Hertel J, Braham R, Hale S, Olmsted-Kramer L: Simplifying the star excursion balance test: analyses of subjects with and without chronic ankle instability, *J Orthop Sports Phys Ther* 36(3):131–137, 2006.
9. Riemann B: Is there a link between chronic ankle instability and postural instability? *J Athl Train* 37(4):386–393, 2002.
10. Riemann B, Caggiano N, Lephart S: Examination of a clinical method of assessing postural control during a functional performance task, *J Sport Rehab* 8:171–183, 1999.
11. Riemann B, Guskiewicz K, Shields E: Relationship between clinical and forceplate measures of postural stability, *J Sport Rehabil* 8:71–82, 1999.
12. Riemann B, Lephart S: The sensorimotor system, part I: the physiologic basis of functional joint stability, *J Athl Train* 37(1):71–79, 2002.
13. Turvey M: Coordination, *Am Psychol* 45(8):938–953, 1990.
14. Wolfson LI, Whipple R, Amerman P, Kleinberg A: Stressing the postural response: quantitative method for testing balance, *J Am Geriatr Soc* 34:845–850, 1986.

REVIEW QUESTIONS

Short Answer

1. Name two ways to increase the intensity of the double-leg stance test (DLST).
2. Studies have demonstrated that many elderly people fall during walking, ascending and descending stairs, and turning. Which activity or test is most appropriate for developing single-leg stance equilibrium?
3. List three Plyoball exercises that can be used to increase dynamic trunk balance, proprioception, and strength.

True/False

4. The joint mechanoreceptor system (afferent neural input system) is important in regulating changes related to joint movement and body position.
5. Single-leg stance test (SLST) and DLST are examples of balance tests and are never used as treatment activities.
6. High-density foam padding is used for patients to stand and walk on during the final phase of balance training.
7. A high degree of balance is necessary to maintain equilibrium while standing and walking on low-density foam.
8. The reach test shows the patient's ability to reach and challenge the limits or borders of the base of support.
9. Injury, surgery, immobilization, and non–weight-bearing convalescence have a profoundly negative effect on the afferent neural input system.
10. Rehabilitation programs that do not address balance, coordination, and proprioception can result in poor restoration of function and increase the risk of reinjury.
11. Postoperative shoulder patients do not require proprioception exercises because the shoulder is a non–weight-bearing structure.

PART II

REVIEW OF TISSUE HEALING

The physical therapist assistant (PTA) must understand the general healing mechanisms of specific tissues to make sound clinical recommendations, develop a progression of rehabilitation exercises, and readily identify problems associated with immobilization, surgery, or injury. Trauma surgery and immobilization (usually longer than 4 weeks) profoundly affect bone and soft tissues. To understand the events and factors that negatively influence healing, the PTA must be aware of the tissue response to injury, surgery, and immobilization. Different tissues (ligament, tendon, bone, muscle, and cartilage) heal or remodel at different rates.[2]

When beginning therapeutic exercises after ligament surgery, cast removal, or an acute traumatic injury, initial clinical information must include which specific tissues are involved, length of time immobilized, weight-bearing status during immobilization, and which surgical procedure, if any, was performed. These points help the clinician recognize healing constraints of specific tissues, as well as indications and contraindications for modifying therapeutic interventions and functional activities. This section provides information concerning immobilization, stress, exercise, joint protection, inflammation, repair, and remodeling, and it outlines the clinical foundations for specific exercises and progressions.

Three overlapping, interrelated series of events initiate healing: phase I, inflammatory response; phase II, proliferation; and phase III, remodeling and tissue maturation (Fig. II-1).[3]

The five cardinal signs of an acute inflammatory reaction are redness, swelling, pain, heat, and loss of function. The acute phase of inflammation lasts 24 to 48 hours, with the entire inflammatory response generally complete after 2 weeks.[3]

Immediately after injury, vasoconstriction, stimulated by serotonin,[1,5] limits blood and fluid loss for a few minutes. A platelet plug occludes small vessels surrounding the injury site, blocking the flow of blood and fluids away from the site. Other strong chemical mediators responsible for vascular constriction and later tissue permeability are histamine (permeability), serotonin (vasoconstriction), bradykinin (permeability), and prostaglandins (inflammatory regulation, permeability, and pain) (Fig. II-2).[2]

A principal feature of the inflammatory response to injury is the process of ridding the injured area of tissue debris (autolytic wound débridement). This occurs via neutrophils that migrate to the injury site.[3] Other phagocytic cells, macrophages, and lymphocytes help produce enzymes that foster this process.[4]

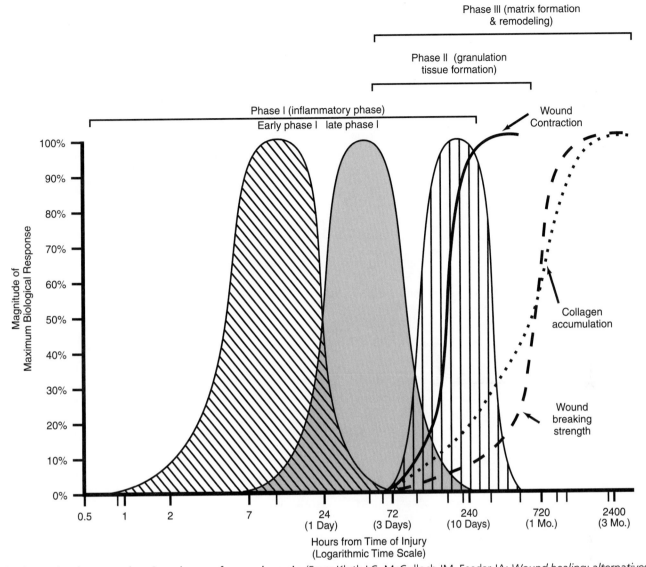

Fig. II-1 The three overlapping phases of wound repair. (From Kloth LC, McCulloch JM, Feedar JA: *Wound healing: alternatives in management*, Philadelphia, 1990, FA Davis.)

The proliferation phase is characterized by fibroplasia, myofibroblast activity, and the organization and production of collagen (Fig. II-3).[3] Collagen formation begins about 5 days after injury.[3] Type III immature collagen predominates, providing very limited structural strength to the injury site. The synthesis, orientation, and deposition of new collagen are random, which reduces scar formation strength.

Phase III, the remodeling phase, begins about 2 weeks after injury and can last from a few months to as long as a year or more.[1] In remodeling, as the name implies, new collagen and connective tissue gradually reorient along the lines of physical stress imposed on the injured site.[1] If tissues are immobilized for prolonged periods, new collagen is laid down highly disorganized and randomly. Active stress or muscular contractions with progressive joint motion promotes longitudinally organized, stronger, more functional collagen arrangements.[1]

Box II-1 outlines basic healing mechanisms.

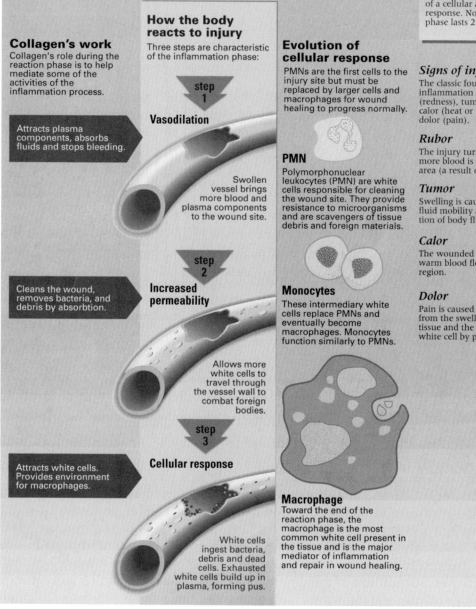

Wounds

REACTION: INFLAMMATION

The inflammatory process

After bleeding is stopped, cellular and vascular responses to the injury are initiated. This is the body's natural damage-control mechanism: it protects the body from foriegn objects at the wound site, cleans the site and brings cells necessary for directing healing in the next stage to the site.

Definition:

Inflammation is part of the reaction phase and consists of a cellular and vascular response. Normally, this phase lasts 2-5 days.

Collagen's work

Collagen's role during the reaction phase is to help mediate some of the activities of the inflammation process.

Attracts plasma components, absorbs fluids and stops bleeding.

Cleans the wound, removes bacteria, and debris by absorbtion.

Attracts white cells. Provides environment for macrophages.

How the body reacts to injury

Three steps are characteristic of the inflammation phase:

step 1

Vasodilation

Swollen vessel brings more blood and plasma components to the wound site.

step 2

Increased permeability

Allows more white cells to travel through the vessel wall to combat foreign bodies.

step 3

Cellular response

White cells ingest bacteria, debris and dead cells. Exhausted white cells build up in plasma, forming pus.

Evolution of cellular response

PMNs are the first cells to the injury site but must be replaced by larger cells and macrophages for wound healing to progress normally.

PMN

Polymorphonuclear leukocytes (PMN) are white cells responsible for cleaning the wound site. They provide resistance to microorganisms and are scavengers of tissue debris and foreign materials.

Monocytes

These intermediary white cells replace PMNs and eventually become macrophages. Monocytes function similarly to PMNs.

Macrophage

Toward the end of the reaction phase, the macrophage is the most common white cell present in the tissue and is the major mediator of inflammation and repair in wound healing.

Signs of inflammation

The classic four clinical signs of inflammation are: rubor (redness), tumor (swelling), calor (heat or warmth) and dolor (pain).

Rubor

The injury turns red because more blood is present in the area (a result of vasodilation).

Tumor

Swelling is caused by increased fluid mobility and accumulation of body fluids in the tissue.

Calor

The wounded area is heated by warm blood flowing into the region.

Dolor

Pain is caused by the pressure from the swelling of nearby tissue and the accumulation of white cell by products.

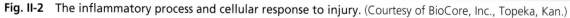

Fig. II-2 The inflammatory process and cellular response to injury. (Courtesy of BioCore, Inc., Topeka, Kan.)

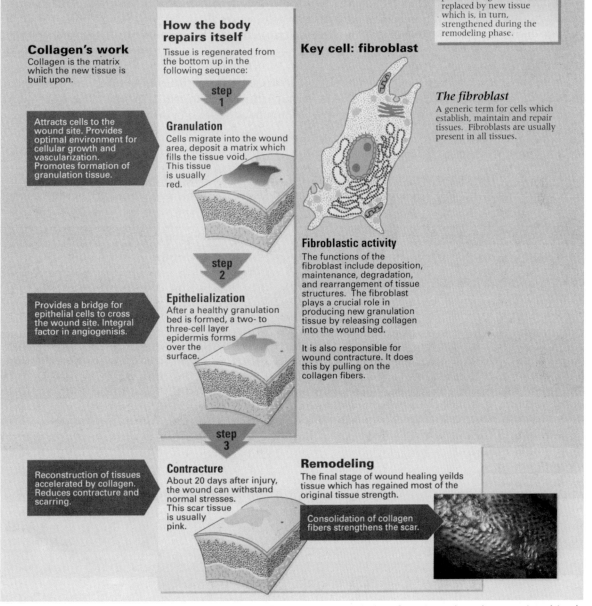

Fig. II-3 Remodeling and regeneration. Collagen and fibroplasia provide key functions that characterize this phase of tissue healing. (Courtesy of BioCore, Inc., Topeka, Kan.)

BOX II-1

Review of Basic Healing Mechanisms

DAYS 2–4

Scar tissue composition: A clot forms in the wound. Connective tissue cells infiltrate the area, with macrophages attracting fibroblasts. In this initial stage of scarring, the tissue is very fragile and easily disrupted because of the predominance of weak and unstable type III collagen. Adhesion is by cellular attachments, and stretching of the scar causes tearing of the cells.

DAYS 5–21

Fibroplasia and contraction: This stage is very cellular. The scar increases in bulk because of fibroplasia, with an increase in the quantity of collagen fibers. This is a highly active stage of collagen synthesis and degradation. Treatment to increase range of motion and function of a joint can be very effective during this stage because of the collagen remodeling process.

DAYS 21–60

Consolidation: The scar contains well-organized collagen. The tissue gradually changes from predominantly cellular to fibrous, with a large amount of collagen fibers. There is a gradual increase in strength of the scar because of an increased stable covalent bonding. During this time, there will be a continuous decrease in the ability of the scar to respond to treatment.

DAYS 60–360

Maturation: Type I collagen fibers are compact and large. The fully mature scar is only 3% cellular and almost totally collagenous. Response to treatment is poor, and hypertrophic and keloid scar tissue increases when stretched in multiple directions.

From Currier D, Nelson R: Mechanisms of connective tissue, In Currier D, Nelson R, editors: *Dynamics of human biologic tissues*, Philadelphia, 1992, FA Davis.

REFERENCES

1. Bushbacher R: Tissue injury and healing. In *Practical guide to musculoskeletal disorders: diagnosis and rehabilitation*, Boston, 1994, Andover Medical Publishers.
2. Cummings GS, Tillman LJ: Remodelling of dense connective tissue in normal adult tissues. In Currier DP, Nelson RM, editors: *Dynamics of human biologic tissues*, Philadelphia, 1992, FA Davis.
3. Kloth LC, Miller KH: The inflammatory response to wound healing. In Kloth LC, McCulloch JM, Feedar JA, editors: *Wound healing: alternatives in management, contemporary perspectives in rehabilitation*, Philadelphia, 1990, FA Davis.
4. Laub R, Huybrechts-Godin G, Peeters-Joris C, et al: Degradation of collagen and proteoglycan by macrophages and fibroblasts, *Biochim Biophys Acta* 721:425–433, 1982.
5. Vander AJ, Sherman JH, Luciano DS: *Human physiology: the mechanisms of body function*, ed 3, Minneapolis, 1980, McGraw-Hill.

7 Composition and Function of Connective Tissue

Erik P. Meira

LEARNING OBJECTIVES

1. Outline components of connective tissue.
2. Discuss the sequence of overlapping events of inflammation.
3. Define fibroplasia.
4. Identify the sources of coagulation.
5. Describe and discuss the various cells of inflammation and their function.
6. Discuss the molecular cascade of arachidonic acid metabolic pathways of lipoxygenase and cyclooxygenase.
7. Define cytokines and growth factors, and discuss their various functions.

KEY TERMS

Apoptosis

Cellular necrosis

Glycosaminoglycans (GAGs)

Ground substance

Maturation

Regeneration

Remodeling

Repair

CHAPTER OUTLINE

CONNECTIVE TISSUE PROPERTIES

The functions of various connective tissues are to bind cells together to form and organize tissues, organs, and systems and to provide a mechanical link between musculoskeletal junctions and the articulations of joints. Generally, connective tissues are made up of cells and the extracellular matrix that they produce. Extracellular matrix is defined as the noncellular components of connective tissue.[4]

Two classic functions of connective tissues are mechanical support for bone and soft tissues and intercellular exchange of oxygen, blood, water, gases, cells, and wastes. Basic mechanical support functions of connective tissues, such as bone, ligament, tendon, muscle, and cartilage,[1,3] are to provide stability and shock absorption in joints,[2] provide a mechanical link system between bones, and transmit muscle forces.[4]

Intracellular exchange relies on the circulation of blood to supply tissues with nutrients and oxygen, and to provide removal of extracellular waste and gases. The basic aggregate components of the extracellular matrix of connective tissues are I-elastin, II-collagen, III-ground substance, IV-proteoglycans and **glycosaminoglycans (GAGs).** V-lipids, phospholipids, proteins, and glycoproteins.

Elastin is a noncollagenous glycoprotein in which molecules are arranged randomly as a constituent of extracellular connective tissue matrix. Elastin is found in varying amounts in tissues requiring high levels of physiologic motion (elasticity). Two special amino acids, desmosine and isodesmosine, are found in elastin. They are directly responsible for the cross-linking arrangement of elastin fiber and its unique ability to deform under stress then return to its original orientation and shape. Primarily, elastin fibers contain the amino acids glycine, proline, alanine, and valine. Characteristically, elastin fibers can elongate about 70% without undergoing fiber disruption.[4]

In contrast to elastin, collagen is the most abundant component of the connective tissue matrix, and 12 to 19 distinct types of collagen exist.[4] Types of collagen are classified according to their structure and tissue distribution. Biochemical properties of connective tissues such as ligament, cartilage, tendon, bone, and muscle are dependent on the specific predominant types of collagen found in the extracellular matrix. The characteristic extensive network of cross-links in collagen significantly contributes to the stability and strength of the extracellular matrix. The basic histochemical profile of collagen includes the amino acids glycine, hydroxyproline, proline, and hydroxylysine. Of these amino acids, proline generally is responsible for resisting tensile forces in collagen.[4] Fibroblasts stimulate collagen synthesis through assembly of polypeptide chains of proline and lysine, which aggregate into a triple helix monomer.[4] **Ground substance** is an amorphous nonfibrous aqueous–gel component of the connective tissue matrix. Generally this substance is responsible for facilitating intercellular exchange of water, oxygen, cells, and gases, as well as providing mechanical support between various tissues.

Proteoglycans are protein and mucopolysaccharide macromolecules subclassified as glycosaminoglycans. Generally, GAGs are responsible for the compressive strength of the cartilage matrix. Proteoglycans are extremely hydrophilic, so they attract and bind water. The major and distinct types of GAGs found in cartilage are chondroitin sulfate, keratan sulfate, and dermatan sulfate, with chondroitin sulfate representing almost 90% of all GAGs in cartilage. These large proteoglycans, specifically chondroitin and keratan, bind together to form a distinct type of GAG referred to as *aggrecan*. Various types of connective tissues, such as ligament, cartilage, tendon, and muscle, contain varying amounts of these large proteoglycans that relate directly to the specific biomechanical and biochemical nature of all connective tissues. The networking capacity of proteoglycans and collagen within all forms and types of connective tissue contributes to the classically distinct nature of strength, stiffness, rigidity, and flexibility of connective tissues.[4]

Noncollagenous proteins and glycoproteins are relatively minor constituents in terms of volume in the extracellular matrix of connective tissues. Generally, these molecules function in matrix organization and cell matrix interactions. They also help with orientation and maintenance of matrix structure. Two important glycoproteins found in the extracellular matrix are fibronectin and laminin. Fibronectin regulates the spread of cells and has strong chemotactic properties that attract and bind various connective tissue cells. Fibronectin is synthesized by many connective tissue cells, including osteoblasts, and may play a role in cell matrix interactions during osteoblast **maturation.** Laminin is a multifunctional glycoprotein found in the extracellular matrix that is important in establishing epithelial tissue and basement membranes during wound healing.

Lipids represent less than 1% of human articular cartilage matrix. The specific function of lipids and phospholipids is not clearly known. However, the presence of lipids in extracellular connective tissue matrix varies with the onset of osteoarthritis (OA).[4]

Specific connective tissue organization of muscle fibers is systematically arranged by endomysium connective tissue. Muscle fibers collectively are bound together to form fascicles. These fascicles are supported by perimysium connective tissue. The connective tissue membrane surrounding the entire muscle is called *epimysium*. Muscle tissue is unique in that it consists of contractile elements that respond to stimuli, as well as passive or elastic elements that resist stretching. Muscle tissue and noncontractile connective tissues such as endomysium, perimysium, and epimysium demonstrate characteristic load deformation viscoelastic properties in response to specific stimuli. Human skeletal muscle exhibits the same viscoelastic properties as other dense connective tissues. In fetal development, these noncontractile connective tissues act as tissue scaffolds to hold, support, and provide continuity of gross form and structure of the muscle's belly. In addition, loose connective tissue of the perimysium serves as a channel for nutrient arteries and vessels, as well as nerves that supply the muscle fibers.[4]

REVIEW OF TISSUE HEALING

Healing of biological tissue is characterized by predictable, orderly, and sequential phases of **repair.** In essence, healing can be broadly classified in a series of three overlapping events: (1) inflammatory response, (2) proliferation, and (3) **remodeling** and tissue maturation. All musculoskeletal tissue proceeds to heal and repair by these individually unique processes.

Inflammatory Response

Acute inflammation is a transient initial phase of injury repair that lasts approximately 5 to 7 days. Directly after trauma, platelets migrate to the injury site and release specific growth factors and chemical mediators, which stimulate homeostasis and initiate the repair process. A fibrin scaffold structure is formed within the trauma bed, creating a matrix that allows for platelet aggregation and adherence to the injury site. This process of platelet activation stimulates synthesis of thrombin, fibrin, and the random organization of clot formation. Platelet plug formation is essentially a four-step process: (1) adhesion, (2) aggregation, (3) secretion, and (4) procoagulant activity (Fig. 7-1).

Adhesion of platelets is the deposition of these cells on the subendothelial matrix. Platelets have a surface receptor glycoprotein that binds to a sticky protein substance referred to as *von Willebrand factor* (vWF) found in the subendothelial matrix. Endothelial cells synthesize vWF, which is released into the circulating plasma, then deposited in the subendothelial matrix in response to exposure from injury.[1,3] Aggregation is simply platelet-to-platelet cohesion via the surface fibrinogen receptor complex of the platelets. Secretion is the release of a number of platelet-derived growth factors (PDGFs) by stimulated platelets. The aggregating stimulators of serotonin, thrombospondin, and thromboxane also are secreted. Procoagulant activity refers to the process of thrombin formation and ensures that coagulation occurs at the site of the platelet plug.

Inflammation

Initially triggered by the release of histamine from mast cells in the surrounding tissue, the inflammatory response is amplified by cytokines (signaling molecules) such as interleukin-1 (IL-1) and tumor necrosis factors (TNFs) that are activated by leukocytes (white blood cells). These leukocytes are involved with phagocytosis, or the engulfment, of cellular debris. Cytokines stimulate vascular permeability allowing mononuclear cells to mobilize, proliferate, and differentiate into monocytes at the injury site. Other cytokines such as platelet-derived growth factor (PDGF), insulin-like growth factor (IGF), and transforming growth factor-β (TGF-β) help organize the specific sequence of migration of neutrophils, macrophages, and then fibroblasts to the injury site.

Fibroplasia

Several days (5 to 7) after the injury, the relative population of fibroblasts increases, whereas inflammatory cells and proinflammatory factors decrease. At this stage there is a proliferation of reparative cells. Fibroblasts stimulate PDGF and TGF-β among others to synthesize and deposit extracellular matrix constituents of fibronectin, laminin, collagen, and glycosaminoglycans.[1,3,4]

This phase also includes angiogenesis, the neovascular budding that helps reestablish oxygen-rich and growth factor–rich blood to new, fragile healing tissue. Angiogenic growth factors involved with the stimulation of this neovascularization are fibroblast growth factor (FGF), tumor necrosis factor-β (TNF-β), and wound angiogenesis factor (WAF). Endothelial cells from intact vascular membranes are mobilized to form new tissue from the secretion of specific enzymes and collagens. The end stages of angiogenesis signal vascular capillary and network tube formation, creating new vascular basement membranes that directly communicate with the injury site.[1,3,4]

Remodeling and Tissue Maturation

The remodeling phase of injury repair is essentially a balance between enzymatic (proteolytic) degradation of excess collagen and the deposition, organization, modification, and maturation of collagen, as well as a systematic regression of inflammatory cells (Fig. 7-2).

Collagenases are enzymes of the metalloproteinase family that act to fragment collagen. The regulation of the rate of collagen synthesis and degradation (turnover) is mediated by specific growth factors such as PDGF, IL, TGF-β, and TNF-β.[4]

Cummings and Reynolds[2] describe remodeling as "the process by which the architecture of connective tissue alters in response to stress." Collagen fibers align parallel to the direction of applied stress, which increases the strength of the scar tissue union. Remodeling also includes absorption of collagen fibers that lie in opposing directions. If controlled properly, the effect of the remodeling phase is that the fibrous union becomes stronger and more supple with fewer adhesions.

Because of the vascularity, dense cell population of myofibroblasts, and nature of its small, fragile collagen fibers, new scar tissue is able to remodel quickly.

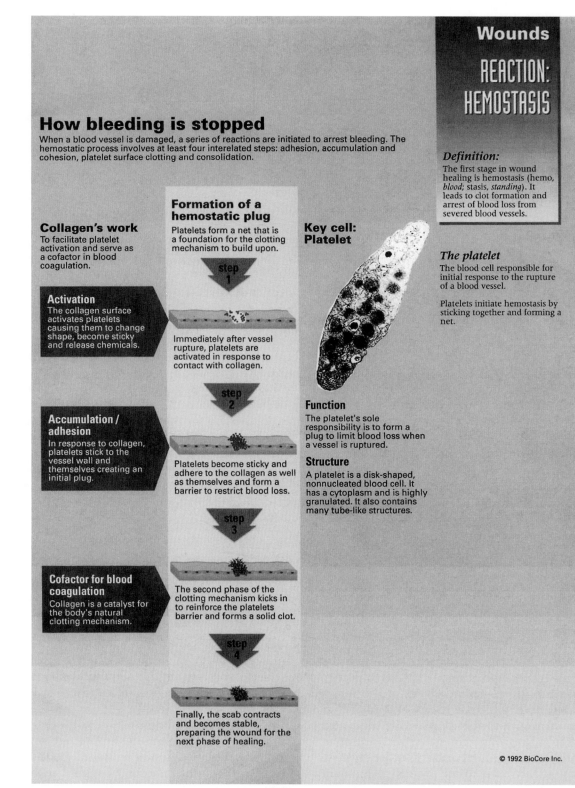

Fig. 7-1 Wound hemostasis. (Courtesy of BioCore, Inc., Topeka, Kan.)

Collagen fibers are initially small and disorganized, and they form a spongy randomly oriented tissue. As remodeling continues, larger, more parallel fibers replace the smaller fibers and orient across the wound, which forms a stronger yet supple repair (Fig. 7-3).[2]

GENERAL CELL TYPES INVOLVED IN INJURY REPAIR

Various cells with complex interactions are involved with tissue homeostasis, injury, and the repair processes. Generally, cell membranes are plasma-based with a

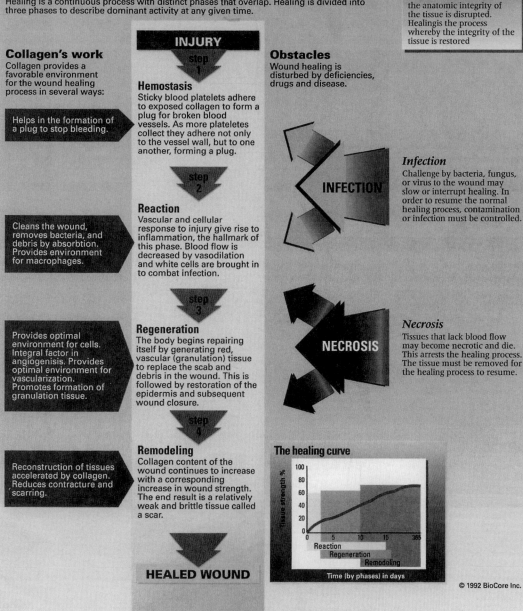

Fig. 7-2 Remodeling and tissue maturation. (Courtesy of BioCore, Inc., Topeka, Kan.)

relatively selective permeable barrier, which promotes bidirectional flow of molecules. The major components of cellular plasma membranes are proteins and lipids. The major relevant class of cell membrane lipids is phospholipids.

Cellular Structure

Organelles define various component structures within cells. Smooth endoplasmic reticulum as a cell organ is involved with the synthesis of steroid hormones, particularly cholesterol. Rough endoplasmic reticulum

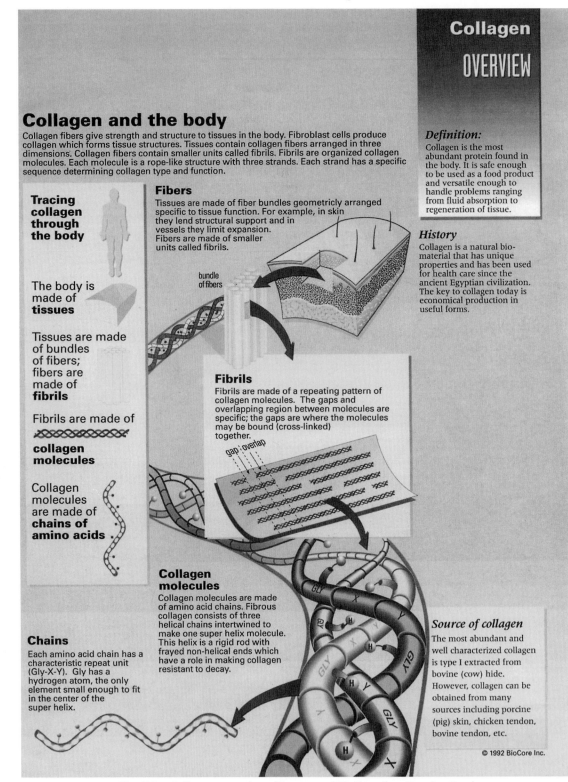

Collagen and the body

Collagen fibers give strength and structure to tissues in the body. Fibroblast cells produce collagen which forms tissue structures. Tissues contain collagen fibers arranged in three dimensions. Collagen fibers contain smaller units called fibrils. Fibrils are organized collagen molecules. Each molecule is a rope-like structure with three strands. Each strand has a specific sequence determining collagen type and function.

Tracing collagen through the body

The body is made of **tissues**

Tissues are made of bundles of fibers; fibers are made of **fibrils**

Fibrils are made of **collagen molecules**

Collagen molecules are made of **chains of amino acids**

Chains

Each amino acid chain has a characteristic repeat unit (Gly-X-Y). Gly has a hydrogen atom, the only element small enough to fit in the center of the super helix.

Fibers

Tissues are made of fiber bundles geometricly arranged specific to tissue function. For example, in skin they lend structural support and in vessels they limit expansion. Fibers are made of smaller units called fibrils.

bundle of fibers

Fibrils

Fibrils are made of a repeating pattern of collagen molecules. The gaps and overlapping region between molecules are specific; the gaps are where the molecules may be bound (cross-linked) together.

gap overlap

Collagen molecules

Collagen molecules are made of amino acid chains. Fibrous collagen consists of three helical chains intertwined to make one super helix molecule. This helix is a rigid rod with frayed non-helical ends which have a role in making collagen resistant to decay.

Collagen OVERVIEW

Definition:
Collagen is the most abundant protein found in the body. It is safe enough to be used as a food product and versatile enough to handle problems ranging from fluid absorption to regeneration of tissue.

History
Collagen is a natural bio-material that has unique properties and has been used for health care since the ancient Egyptian civilization. The key to collagen today is economical production in useful forms.

Source of collagen
The most abundant and well characterized collagen is type I extracted from bovine (cow) hide. However, collagen can be obtained from many sources including porcine (pig) skin, chicken tendon, bovine tendon, etc.

© 1992 BioCore Inc.

Fig. 7-3 Collagen overview. (Courtesy of BioCore, Inc., Topeka, Kan.)

organelles are actively involved with protein synthesis and secretion. Within cells the Golgi apparatus functions primarily as a storage and modification organ for various proteins that have been synthesized in the rough endoplasmic reticulum. Lysosomes and peroxisomes are cellular compartment structures that are involved with enzymatic degradation and oxidation of protein and fatty acids. Mitochondria, the powerhouses of the cell, are actively involved with adenosine triphosphate (ATP) production and protein synthesis.[1,3]

Proteoglycans and Glycoproteins

Proteoglycans are macromolecules consisting of a protein core and bound polysaccharide units referred to as *glycosaminoglycans* (GAGs). GAGs are major components of ground substance within the extracellular matrix of various connective tissues, such as ligament, capsule, muscle, tendon, cartilage, nerve, vessel, and bone. GAGs are synthesized within the endoplasmic reticulum and Golgi apparatus of the fibroblast cells in connective tissues. Several GAGs are identified in musculoskeletal tissues, which significantly contribute to structure, composition, and function of the extracellular matrix of tissues: (1) chondroitin sulfate, (2) dermatan sulfate, (3) keratan sulfate, (4) hyaluronate, (5) aggregen, (6) decorin, and (7) biglycan.[1,3]

Generally, GAGs carry a high negative charge that renders GAGs hydrophilic. Within articular cartilage, GAGs are continuously synthesized, assembled, degraded, and secreted by the extracellular matrix to establish a relative homeostatic environment. Enzymatic degradation of GAGs occurs within lysosome organelles of the chondrocytes.[1,3,4]

Glycoproteins are molecules that organize and maintain the structure of the extracellular matrix. In articular cartilage these are fibronectin, laminin, anchorin, and tenascin.

CELLS OF INFLAMMATION AND REPAIR

The complex cascade of molecular events during the inflammatory phase are mediated by cytokines acting through endocrine (distant cells), paracrine (adjacent cells), or autocrine (same cells) stimulation.

Polymorphonuclear Leukocytes

Granulocytes, or polymorphonuclear leukocytes, differentiate into neutrophils, basophils, and eosinophils when stimulated by cytokine growth factors and colony-stimulating factors. Neutrophils, the most abundant granulocytes, are leukocytes that migrate to damaged tissue after mediation and activation of cytokines, platelet factor 4 (PF4), and TGF-β that are released by platelets. Primary function of neutrophils includes initial phagocytosis of foreign matter, bacteria, and cellular debris from the damaged tissue site. Neutrophils also contribute to the immune system inflammation process by stimulation, vasodilation, and vascular permeability assisting with transportation and migration of molecules and cytokine growth factor–PDGF propagating events to further minimize intense inflammatory reactions.

Mononuclear Leukocytes

Mononuclear leukocytes are single-nucleus cells that are derived from pluripotent hematopoietic stem cells, which differentiate into monocytes and lymphocytes.

Circulating monocytes are mobilized to damaged tissue, where they are activated and become macrophages. Noted as *scavenger cells*, macrophages are leukocytes that display three essential functions during the inflammatory process: (1) phagocytosis, (2) antigen presentation, and (3) production of cytokine growth factors.[1,3,4]

Macrophages synthesize and secrete numerous cytokines, such as TGF-β, PDGF, transforming growth factor-α (TGF-α), and IL-1. The release of these cytokines stimulates proliferation of fibroblasts and collagen deposition and degradation of collagen by secreting enzymes (collagenases) also, which denatures collagen during the inflammatory and remodeling phases.[1,3,4]

Fibroblasts

Fibroblasts, important and highly specialized cells, are actively involved with collagen production of various stages of injury repair. Fibroblastic cell proliferation is activated by cytokines released by platelets and leukocytes. PDGF is responsible for the stimulation of fibroblast proliferation. Fibroblasts serve a critical function in wound healing mechanics. Fibronectin is a glycoprotein produced by fibroblasts, which acts to bind collagen within the extracellular matrix of healing tissue. Myofibroblasts are specialized contractile cell types that are important during the later stages of wound repair, contracting the edges of the wound.

Prostaglandins, Thromboxanes, and Leukotrienes

Prostaglandins and thromboxanes are lipid-derived powerful and important mediators of inflammatory reactions (Fig. 7-4), which are metabolized from arachidonic acids within the cells. Arachidonic acid metabolism is initiated by the degradation of cell membrane phospholipids by phospholipase enzymes. This cell membrane degradation releases arachidonic acid–synthesized cyclooxygenase enzymes, such as COX-1 and COX-2, which results in metabolic conversion to prostaglandins and thromboxanes.

Prostaglandins are generally of three forms[1,3]: (1) prostaglandin E_2 (PGE$_2$), which stimulates smooth muscle relaxation and vasodilation; (2) prostaglandin I_2 (PGI$_2$), which is synthesized in endothelial cells and incites vascular dilation and inhibition of platelet adhesion; and (3) prostaglandin F_2 (PGF$_2$), which is a potent vasoconstrictor and stimulates smooth muscle contractions. These molecules are capable of producing pain and stimulating synthesis of pain-producing chemicals.[1,3] Thromboxanes are synthesized by platelets and are products of the COX pathway along with prostaglandins. These cell-signaling molecules are potent vasoconstrictors and smooth muscle contractors. Leukotrienes are products of an alternate arachidonic acid metabolic pathway. In this pathway, lipoxygenase is converted to leukotrienes, which act as smooth muscle contractors;

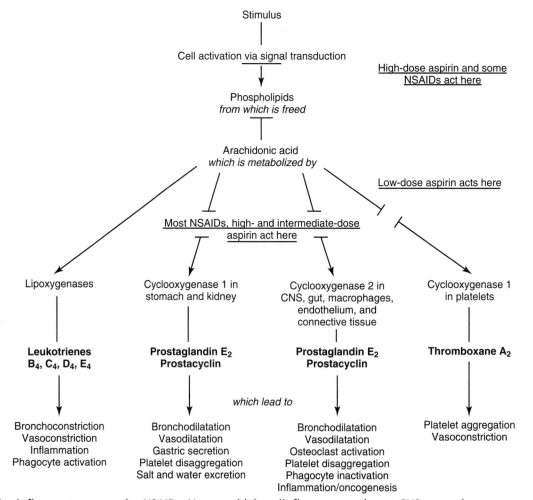

Fig. 7-4 The inflammatory cascade. *NSAIDs,* Nonsteroidal antiinflammatory drugs; *CNS,* central nervous system. (From Goldman L, Bennett JC: *Cecil textbook of medicine,* ed 21, Philadelphia, 2000, Saunders, p. 115.)

lipoxygenase also stimulates bronchoconstriction and is a strong mediator of other various inflammatory chemicals (chemotactic).[1,3]

Various pharmacologic agents involved with antiinflammatory action, namely corticosteroids and nonsteroidal antiinflammatory drugs (NSAIDs), target arachidonic acid for the inhibition of prostaglandins, thromboxanes, and leukotrienes. Specifically, corticosteroids inhibit production of arachidonic acid metabolites (cyclooxygenase and lipoxygenase) by inhibiting the conversion of cell membrane phospholipids to arachidonic acid. Conversely, NSAIDs are post–arachidonic acid inhibitors of the specific cyclooxygenase (COX-1, COX-2) metabolic pathway.

Cytokines

Cytokines, including many growth factors, are a large and complex group (more than 100 identified) of protein-soluble peptide signaling molecules that are synthesized and secreted by all musculoskeletal tissues. They are used for cellular communication and stimulate cell proliferation, differentiation, and regulation of normal growth, homeostasis, injury, disease, and repair (Table 7-1). Generally referred to as *mitogenic,* cytokines are powerful and important immunologic mediators that coordinate and amplify various repair processes of injured musculoskeletal tissues.[1,3]

Cytokines are named for either the biological effects they perform or the tissue on which they exert action. Tumor necrosis factor-α (TNF-α) is a proinflammatory cytokine synthesized and secreted by macrophages, lymphocytes, and monocytes. The biological effects and anatomic target tissues are varied and diverse. General target tissues include stimulation of leukocytes, mononuclear phagocytes, vascular endothelial cells, fibroblasts, chondrocytes, and synovial macrophages. TNF-α activates granulocytes and stimulates other proinflammatory cytokines, which are also important regulators of bone resorption. IL-1 is also a proinflammatory cytokine that is synthesized by various cells. Tissue targets include monocytes, synovial macrophages, fibroblasts, chondrocytes, and endothelial cells. Biologically mediated

Table 7-1	*Types and Functions of Cytokines*	
Type		**Primary Functions**
Interleukins (ILs)	IL-1	Augments the immune response; inflammatory mediator; promotes maturation and clonal expansion of B cells; enhances activity of NK cells; activates T cells, activates macrophages
	IL-2	Induces proliferation and differentiation of T cells; activation of T cells, NK cells, and macrophages; stimulates release of other cytokines (α-IFN, TNF, IL-1, IL-6)
	IL-3 (multicolony colony-stimulating factor)	Hematopoietic growth factor for hematopoietic precursor cells
	IL-4	B-cell growth factor; stimulates proliferation and differentiation of B cells; induces differentiation into TH2 cells; stimulates growth of mast cells
	IL-5	B cell growth and differentiation; promotes growth and differentiation of eosinophils
	IL-6	T- and B-cell growth factor; enhances the inflammatory response; promotes differentiation of B cells into plasma cells; stimulates antibody secretion; induces fever; synergistic effects with IL-1 and TNF
	IL-7	Promotes growth of T and B cells
	IL-8	Chemotaxis of neutrophils and T cells; stimulates superoxide and granule release
	IL-9	Enhances T-cell survival; mast cell activation
	IL-10	Inhibits cytokine production by T and NK cells; promotes B-cell proliferation and antibody responses; potent suppressor of macrophage function
	IL-11	Synergistic action with IL-3 and IL-4 in hematopoiesis; is a multifunctional regulator of hematopoiesis and lymphopoiesis; osteoclast formation; elevates platelet count; inhibits proinflammatory cytokine production
	IL-12	Promotes α-IFN production; induction of T helper cells; activates NK cells; stimulates proliferation of activated T and NK cells
	IL-13	B cell growth and differentiation; inhibits proinflammatory cytokine production
	IL-14	Stimulates proliferation of activated B cells
	IL-15	Mimics IL-2 effects; stimulates proliferation of T cells and NK cells
	IL-16	Proinflammatory cytokine; chemoattractant of T cells, eosinophils, and monocytes
	IL-17	Promotes release of IL-6, IL-8, and G-CSF; enhances expression of adhesion molecules
	IL-18	Induces α-IFN, IL-2, and GM-CSF production; important role in development of T helper cells; enhances NK activity; inhibits production of IL-10
	IL-19	Similar to IL-10
	IL-20	Similar to IL-10
	IL-21	Similar to IL-2, IL-4, and IL-5
	IL-22	Similar to IL-10
	IL-23	Similar to IL-12; promotes memory T cell proliferation

Continued

Table 7-1	*Types and Functions of Cytokines—cont'd*	
Type		**Primary Functions**
	IL-24	Similar to IL-10
	IL-25	Promotes TH2 cytokine production
	IL-26	Similar to IL-10
	IL-27	Similar to IL-12
Interferons (IFNs)	α-Interferon (α-IFN)	Inhibit viral replication; activate NK cells and macrophages; antiproliferative effects on tumor cells
	β-Interferon (β-IFN)	
	γ-Interferon (γ-IFN)	Activates macrophages, neutrophils, and NK cells; promotes B cell differentiation; inhibits viral replication
Tumor necrosis factor (TNF)		Activates macrophages and granulocytes; promotes the immune and inflammatory responses; kills tumor cells; is responsible for extensive weight loss associated with chronic inflammation and cancer
Colony-stimulating factors (CSFs)	Granulocyte colony-stimulating factor (G-CSF)	Stimulates proliferation and differentiation of neutrophils; enhances functional activity of mature PMNs
	Granulocyte-macrophage colonystimulating factor (GM-CSF)	Stimulates proliferation and differentiation of PMNs and monocytes
	Macrophage colony-stimulating factor (M-CSF)	Promotes proliferation, differentiation, and activation of monocytes and macrophages
Erythropoietin		Stimulates erythroid progenitor cells in bone marrow to produce red blood cells

NK, Natural killer; *PMN,* polymorphonuclear neutrophil.

From Lewis SM. *Medical-surgical nursing: assessment and management of clinical problems,* ed 7, St Louis, 2008, Mosby.

effects include inhibition of extracellular matrix synthesis within chondrocytes, stimulation of fibroblast proliferation, proliferation of T cells, and stimulation of other proinflammatory cytokine synthesis. Interleukin-7 is also a proinflammatory growth factor responsible for additional cytokine secretion and stimulation of prostaglandins in epithelial, endothelial, and fibroblastic cells.

Transforming growth factor-β is a potent immunosuppressive cytokine with strong anabolic activity in cartilage. TGF-β also reduces enzymatic degradation activity specifically within cartilage. In addition, TGF-β promotes wound healing, bone formation, and neovascular activity.[1,3,4]

Insulin-like growth factor (IGF) regulates many musculoskeletal functions. Generally, IGF stimulates proteoglycan synthesis, chondrocyte proliferation, and osteoblast matrix synthesis. Target cells for neovascularization include platelets and endothelial cells.

Platelet-derived growth factor contributes significant stimulation toward the repair process of musculoskeletal and vascular tissue. Cell types activated by PDGF include platelets, neutrophils, macrophages, fibroblasts, and endothelial cells. Biological activity activated by PDGF includes homeostasis, initiation of wound repair cascade phagocytic activity, synthesis, and deposition of extracellular matrix constituents and angiogenesis activity.

Vascular endothelial growth factor (VEGF) is an important angiogenic cytokine that stimulates endothelial cell proliferation. VEGF significantly contributes to neovascularization. In addition, VEGF has been identified in the hypertrophic zone of calcified cartilage in the epiphyseal plate. VEGF stimulates endothelial cell ingrowth in this area, possibly enhancing cartilage conversion to bone. VEGF also is responsible for the release of degradative enzymes in the extracellular matrix.

Fibroblast growth factor (FGF) stimulates cell proliferation of cartilage matrix and bone tissue. FGF is also an effective angiogenic stimulant for revascularization after injury. FGF promotes epithelial cell activity during remodeling and neovascular growth.

Overall, tissue disruption and subsequent repair processes initiate and propagate complex cellular events mediated by cytokines. Cytokines regulate, stimulate,

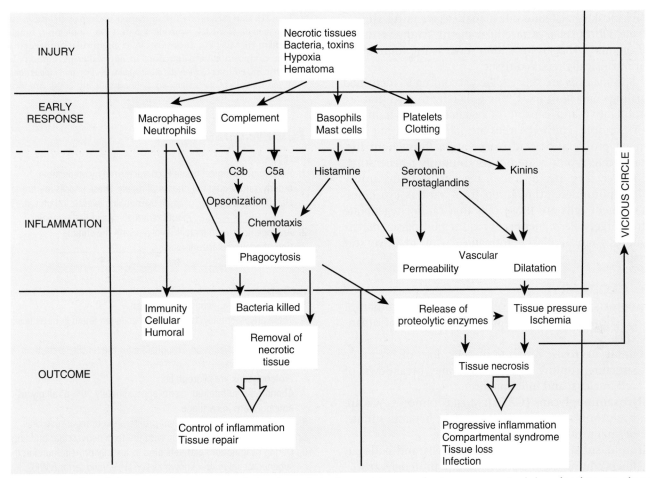

Fig. 7-5 Results of the necrotic process: cellular, hematologic, and immunologic responses to injury lead to repair or further destruction. (From Browner BD, Jupiter J, Levine A, et al: *Skeletal trauma,* ed 2, Philadelphia, 1998, Saunders.)

and express other growth factors to synthesize, proliferate, excrete, and mobilize numerous molecules involved with extracellular matrix deposition, cartilage synthesis, vascular growth, enzymatic degradation, and modulation of inflammatory immune reactions during injury and repair of musculoskeletal and neurovascular repair (Fig. 7-5).[1,3]

GENERAL CELL INJURY AND REPAIR

Cellular hypertrophy is an adaptive response to a specific applied stimulus when cells and tissues are able to physiologically cope with unusual or stressful demands that do not rupture the cell's phospholipid membrane or damage the mitochondria. This situation is essentially a reversible cell injury.[1,3]

However, cells also can become irreversibly damaged. Hypoxia, caused by ischemia, is the most common cause of irreversible cell injury. Tissue or **cellular necrosis** refers to the aggregate morphologic changes after irreversible cell injury. When cells are damaged, specific organelles (lysosomes) are involved with autolysis, or self-killing, leading to tissue necrosis. Cells of

the immune system are involved with the process of heterolysis through phagocytosis and degranulation from active circulating T cells. **Apoptosis** refers to programmed cellular, organelle, and nuclear disassembly and death. Contrasted with necrosis, in which organelles rupture, cell phospholipid membranes tear from intracellular swelling and inflammatory reactions occur from cell debris. Apoptosis is somewhat more organized and systematic without inducing an inflammatory response. Apoptosis is an efficient, controlled process of orderly cellular, organelle, and nuclear shrinkage and disassembly of intracellular structures.[1,3]

GENERAL REPAIR AND REGENERATION PROCESS

The term **regeneration** specifically refers to injured tissue being replaced with identical or similar tissue. The process occurs from the activation of various cytokine growth factors that stimulate the synthesis, differentiation, and proliferation of specialized cells that regenerate the damaged tissue. Repair processes involve adaptive scar tissue replacement within the damaged musculoskeletal tissue rather than regenerative similar tissue. Fibroplasia, extracellular matrix synthesis, deposition, and collagen formation serve as the foundation for intrinsically repaired tissue.

Specific cells are subclassified according to identified healing characteristics. Labile cells refer to cells that are proliferative and capable of regeneration after injury. For example, epithelial cells are labile, requiring continued proliferation and regeneration throughout life. Stable cells typically are not continuously regenerating. However, they are capable of regeneration after injury with appropriate stimulation from various cytokines. Permanent cells are those cells that cannot regenerate after surgery. Permanent cells require fibroplasia, matrix synthesis, and collagen formation with adaptive scar tissue.

✤ GLOSSARY

Apoptosis: Programmed cell death; no inflammation reaction; cell shrinkage with maintenance of organelles.

Cellular necrosis: Swelling of cells, loss of organelle structure, rupture of cell membrane, breakdown of cell nucleus, and inflammation.

Glycosaminoglycans (GAGs): Most common GAGs are hyaluronic acid, chondroitin sulfate, heparan sulfate, dermatan sulfate, and keratan sulfate.

Ground substance: Space between cells and collagen fibers composed of water, salts, and proteoglycans.

Maturation: Process of maturing of granulation tissue to relative avascular fibrous tissue.

Regeneration: Traumatized tissue is replaced by biochemically similar tissues resulting from stimulation and proliferation of local specialized cells.

Remodeling: Collagen and fibrous tissue organization and orientation to a stable scar.

Repair: Traumatized tissue is replaced with scar.

REFERENCES

1. Cell Biology: In *United States medical licensing examination, step I. The Princeton review*, ed 3, New York, 2000, Random House.
2. Cummings GS, Reynolds CA: Principles of soft tissue extensibility of joint contracture management. In Wadsworth C, editor: *Strength conditioning. Applications in orthopaedics*, LaCrosse, Wis, 1998, APTA, Inc.
3. Kent TH, Hart MN: Injury, inflammation, and repair. In *Introduction to human disease*, ed 3, Norwalk, Conn, 1993, Appleton & Lange.
4. Mankin HJ, Mow VC, Buckwalter JA, et al: Articular cartilage structure, composition, and function. In Buckwalter JA, Einhorn TA, Simon SR, editors: *Orthopedic basic science, biology, and biomechanics of the musculoskeletal system*, ed 2, Rosemont, Ill, 2000, American Academy of Orthopedic Surgeons.

REVIEW QUESTIONS

Short Answer

1. Healing of biological tissue is characterized by predictable, orderly, and sequential phases of repair. These phases are broadly classified into a series of three overlapping events: inflammatory, _____ , and remodeling and tissue repair.
2. Angiogenic growth factors involved with the stimulation of neovascularization are _____ , _____ , and _____ .

True/False

3. Elastin is a collagenous proteoglycan.
4. There are essentially three types of collagen found in musculoskeletal tissue.
5. Glycosaminoglycans are responsible for the tensile strength of cartilage matrix.
6. Proteoglycans are hydrophilic.
7. Chondroitin sulfate represents approximately 90% of all glycosaminoglycans in cartilage.
8. Fibroplasia does not represent proliferation of reparative cells.
9. Angiogenesis is synonymous with the term neovascular budding.
10. During coagulation, platelets bind to a sticky protein found in the subendothelial matrix known as *von Willebrand factor* (vWF).
11. Tissue remodeling is a balance between degradation of excess collagen and the deposition, organization, modification, and maturation of collagen, as well as the systematic regression of inflammatory cells.
12. New collagen fibers are organized and firmly and rigidly attached to damaged and healing tissue.
13. Chondroitin sulfate, dermatan sulfate, keratan sulfate, and hyaluronic acid are examples of GAGs found in musculoskeletal tissues.
14. Prostaglandins and thromboxanes are products of the lipoxygenase metabolic pathway of arachidonic acid metabolism.
15. Nonsteroidal antiinflammatory drugs (NSAIDs) are used to affect the cyclooxygenase pathway of arachidonic acid.

8 Ligament Healing

John DeWitt

LEARNING OBJECTIVES

1. Define and discuss the inflammatory response to injury.
2. Describe the phases of healing and sequence of events characteristic of each phase.
3. Identify the five cardinal signs of inflammation.
4. Describe the effects of immobilization on ligaments.
5. Discuss the effects of stress and exercise on ligaments.
6. Identify and discuss practical clinical applications of stress deprivation and protected motion during phases of ligament healing.

KEY TERMS

Collagen
Continuous passive motion (CPM)

Immobilization
Inflammatory reaction

Ligament
Sprain

CHAPTER OUTLINE

LIGAMENT ANATOMY

Ligaments are uniformly classified as dense connective tissue. Macroscopic gross examination reveals ligaments to be opaque, white band or cordlike tissue. Ligaments contain primarily type I **collagen**, fibroblasts, extracellular matrix, and varying amounts of elastin. Type I collagen, the predominant structural collagen in the body, is structurally very strong in mature scars. Conversely, type III collagen is assembled in thin filaments and is more elastic in nature. This type of collagen is usually seen in immature scars and more prevalent in newborns and young children.

Interestingly, certain ligaments (e.g., ligamentum nuchae) contain greater amounts of elastin, which in turn contributes to different mechanical properties than those of ligaments with less elastin. Although considered hypovascular, ligaments demonstrate relative uniform microvascularity that originates from their origin and insertion sites.[24]

Ligaments have a rich sensory innervation of specialized mechanoreceptors and free nerve endings that contribute to proprioception and pain, respectively. Ligament attachment to bone is by direct or indirect transition. Direct ligament insertion into bone represents a gradual change from specific ligament fiber to fibrocartilage to calcified fibrocartilage to bone. With indirect insertion, the superficial layers of ligament fibers attach directly in the periosteum, whereas the deep fibers transition to bone by way of Sharpey's perforating fibers.[24]

MECHANICAL PROPERTIES

Characteristic behavior of ligament substance (e.g., stress–strain, tensile loading) is directly influenced by collagen composition, proteoglycans, glycosaminoglycans (GAGs), orientation of fibers, and actions between extracellular matrix and ground substance. It should be recognized that anatomic location of various ligaments (extraarticular versus intraarticular), as well as cellular, histologic, ultrastructural, and biochemical differences strongly influence ligament mechanical and viscoelastic behavior. These unique differences between various ligaments influence intrinsic healing abilities, physical therapy procedures, and surgical intervention.

INJURY AND REPAIR

As with other vascular tissues, extraarticular ligaments heal in a highly structured, organized, and predictable fashion. Generally, the sequential cascade of events overlaps four stages of repair: Phase I, hemostasis and degeneration; Phase II, inflammation; Phase III, proliferation and migration; and Phase IV, remodeling and degeneration.[11]

In contrast, intraarticular ligaments, although demonstrating an intense vascular response to injury, do not heal spontaneously. The environment of intraarticular synovial fluid tends to dilute hematoma formation between the ends of the injured ligaments while preventing fibrin clot organization and ultimately limiting the intrinsic healing mechanism.[24]

The **inflammatory reaction** to trauma represents Phase I of the injury and repair cascade. Initially the injured ends of **ligament** retract and usually demonstrate a highly disorganized appearance. As the ligamentous microvascularity is disrupted, a hematoma forms between the damaged ends of tissue.

Phase II is marked by a release of extremely potent chemical mediators of vasodilation, cell wall permeability, and pain in response to fibrin clot formation. Prostaglandins, histamine, bradykinins, and serotonin are mobilized to the trauma site to increase capillary permeability and profuse dilation of blood vessels. This action allows migration of specific inflammatory polymorphonuclear cells and lymphocytes to the injured tissue to initiate the action of ingestion (phagocytosis) to remove bacteria and dead tissue. The predominant cell types present during the acute inflammatory phase are neutrophils and lymphocytes. Monocytes are referred to as *macrophages* as they become phagocytes.[24]

The production of type III collagen, extracellular matrix, and, within 2 days, proteoglycans by fibroblasts initiate the beginning of Phase III matrix and cellular proliferation. Fibroblasts rapidly synthesize new extracellular matrix containing high concentrations of water; GAGs; and relatively weak, fragile, and immature type III collagen. Neovascularization (angiogenesis) begins as granulation tissue tenuously attaches to the damaged gap. Gradually the concentration of water, GAGs, and type III collagen decreases over several weeks. Inflammatory cytokines are slowly removed from the injured site. Fibroblastic activity synthesizes type I collagen during this highly cellular phase of repair. There is a marked decrease in vascularity within the repair tissue as the collagen concentration increases. Matrix organization continues as the fibrils of type I collagen slowly arrange and align in response to appropriately applied stress. As the density of collagen, elastin, and proteoglycans increase, the tensile properties of repaired tissue also increase.[23]

Remodeling and maturation of intrinsically repaired ligament tissue is a slow process that characteristically lasts a year or more. This Phase IV tissue repair process is an overlapping transition from the matrix and cellular proliferation phase of tissue healing. During this final phase, active matrix synthesis decreases while type III collagen transitions to type I, improving stiffness. The hallmark of Phase IV remodeling is collagen organization and increases in tensile strength of the repair tissue.

Important consideration must be given to the fact that intrinsically repaired extraarticular ligament does not return to normal, biochemically or biomechanically. Even after considerable time and remodeling of dense connective tissue, ultimate tensile strength may approach only 50% to 70% of normal ligaments up to 1 year after injury.[16,24]

The most common injury of joints are ligament **sprains.** The knee and ankle joints are common areas of sprains, with the incidence of knee ligament sprains, particularly those of the medial collateral ligament (MCL), occurring in as many as 25% to 40% of all knee injuries.[7,19]

Not all ligaments heal at the same rate or to the same degree.[2] For example, the anterior cruciate ligament (ACL) does not appear to heal as well as the MCL of the knee.[25] Factors affecting ligament healing include blood supply and function.[12,25]

Three key conditions must be present for ligaments to properly remodel or heal:[2]
1. Torn ligament ends must be in contact with each other.
2. Progressive, controlled stress must be applied to the healing tissues to orient scar tissue formation.
3. The ligament must be protected against excessive forces during the remodeling process.

The continuum of the healing process outlined here is ligament specific, and healing is related to blood supply, degree of injury, and mechanical stresses applied to the ligament.[2]

Nonsurgical Repair versus Surgical Repair

Ligaments can be repaired surgically or allowed to heal conservatively without surgery, depending on the degree of injury and involvement of supporting tissues. Investigators have shown that untreated ligaments heal by way of scar tissue proliferation rather than true ligament regeneration.[8] Untreated ligament tears are biochemically inferior, possessing a large portion of type III immature collagen, and generally are not healed even at 40 weeks after injury.[8]

The following is a list of grades of injury occurring to ligament tissue. They are graded by severity:

Grade I: Microscopic tearing of the ligament without producing joint laxity

Grade II: Tearing of some ligament fibers with moderate laxity

Grade III: Complete rupture of the ligament with profound instability and laxity

Grade I and II ligament sprains are most common, with only 15% of all knee sprains classified as grade III.[3] Generally, grade I and II ligament sprains can be treated with protective bracing and comprehensive and progressive rehabilitation with appropriate strengthening to provide dynamic muscular support. With grade I and II ligament sprains of the knee (ACL, MCL, posterior cruciate ligament [PCL], and lateral collateral ligament [LCL]), good to excellent results can be anticipated in 90% of those cases treated nonsurgically.[2]

Surgical repair of a grade III sprain frequently involves repair of associated tissues. Cartilage (menisci) and MCL-, LCL-, or PCL-related injury often is seen with primary ACL grade III injury.

Repair versus Nonrepair

The decision to surgically repair a torn ligament is based on several intrinsic and extrinsic factors. The most clinically relevant example is to contrast the differences between tears of extraarticular MCLs with those of intraarticular ACL tears. Not only must the severity of injury (grade) be considered, but also the anatomic location (biomechanical influences) and vascular supply.

By virtue of its extracapsular anatomy, the MCL provides for a greater periarticular vascular response and the ability to protect the ligament from unwanted forces (e.g., varus, valgus, and internal and external rotation), and allows for an appropriate environment to stimulate healing and propagation of motion, collagen synthesis organization and orientation, proteoglycan concentration, and joint function. Therefore all three distinct grades (grades I, II, and III) of isolated MCL tears appear to heal uneventfully without surgical repair. Even though a fibrous repair gap may exist between torn ends of the ligament, resulting in inferior mechanical resistance to tensile loads, the greater cross-sectional area of the healed ligament provides for biochemical properties (e.g., ultimate tensile load to failure) that more closely resemble an uninjured ligament.[24]

Conversely, the relative pristine environment of the ACL is not conducive to intrinsic repair. In addition, the difficulty of protecting the injured ACL from unwanted deforming forces by using commercial or custom braces contributes to and maintains a high-stress force environment of the ACL that limits healing.

Effects of Immobilization

Immobilization, surgery, injury, and rehabilitation of ligaments must take into consideration not only the healing response of the ligament itself, but also that of the ligament–bone interface. Stress deprivation of the ligament and ligament–bone complexes resulting from prolonged immobilization after injury or surgery can have significant and profound negative effects. Joint stiffness after immobilization is related to adhesion formation, active shortening of dense connective tissue (ligament), and decreases in water content.[2] Studies show a gradual deterioration in ligament strength, loss of bone, weakening of cartilage and tendons, significant muscle atrophy, and negative effects on joint mechanics after periods of immobilization (Box 8-1).[1] Immobilization also affects ligament–bone complexes. Studies report that loss of bone directly beneath the junction of ligament and bone reduces the strength of both the insertion site and entire ligament–bone complex.[15]

Rigidly immobilized joints produce chemical and morphologic changes in ligaments 2 and 4 weeks following

BOX 8-1

Effects of Immobilization on Ligament Tissue and Associated Structures

- Reduced physiologic motion
- Decreased afferent neural input
- Muscular atrophy
- Ligament shortening
- Reduction of water content, proteoglycans and glycosaminoglycans
- Bone loss, periosteal bone reabsorption
- Articular (hyaline cartilage) erosion
- Reduced ligament weight
- Reduced ligament size
- Reduced ligament strength
- Adhesion formation
- Increased ligament laxity
- Joint stiffness related to synovial membrane adherence

From Kloth LC, McCulloch JM, Feedar JA: Wound Healing: *Alternatives in management*, Philadelphia, 1990, FA Davis.

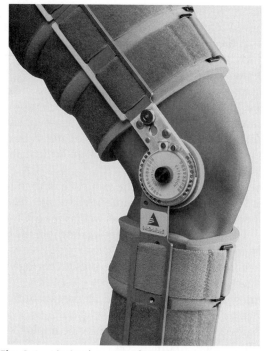

Fig. 8-1 Limited range of motion long leg brace.

injury, respectively.[9] After 8 weeks of immobilization, ligaments lose 20% of their weight; significant atrophy results, and marked infiltration of periarticular connective tissue is observed surrounding the ligament.[9] Although immobilization may be needed to promote healing of damaged tissues, the extended use of rigid immobilization should be limited. As an alternative, limited range of motion braces (Fig. 8-1) can be used to protect healing structures and decrease unwanted external forces, as well as allow for progressive motion of involved joints to minimize the negative effects of immobilization.

The biochemical, histochemical, and morphologic changes that occur in ligament and dense connective tissue in response to immobilization are related to the length of time tissues are immobilized. In addition, both structure and mechanical function of ligament substance, as well as ligament–bone insertion complexes (direct insertion and indirect periosteal insertion with Sharpey's perforating fibers), are significantly affected in response to the quality and duration of immobilization.

The effects of immobilization on dense connective tissue have been described by Cummings and Reynolds[5] as follows: Following only 2 weeks of immobilization, animal studies revealed increased GAG synthesis and concentration, decreased water content, thickening of the joint capsule and ligaments, adaptive muscle shortening and adhesion formation of unopposed articular surfaces. After 4 weeks of immobilization, the biochemical and morphologic changes become more pronounced, with a reduction of GAGs, fissures in articular cartilage, increased ligament stiffness, and decreased capsular remodeling. After 6 weeks of immobilization, joint mobility becomes significantly limited, with thickening noted in the joint capsule, ligaments, and cartilage and

decreased ligamentous compliance. In summary, joint immobilization causes a progression of dense connective tissue remodeling, resulting in joint stiffness.

During the first 2 weeks, adaptive muscle shortening appears to be the primary limiting factor in joint mobility. As immobilization extends to 4 weeks, changes in GAG synthesis and water concentration become more pronounced, resulting in a loss of normal fiber lubrication, spacing, and connective tissue disorganization. As the immobilization period approaches 6 weeks, morphologic and biochemical changes become more evident as the dense connective tissue remodels in a shortened position.[24]

Specifically, immobilization causes more pronounced mechanical and biochemical changes in ligament–bone complex insertion sites compared with ligament substance alone. Generally the area of bone directly beneath the ligament–bone insertion site becomes osteoporotic with osteoclastic activity, resulting in pronounced bone resorption, loss of cortex, and reduced strength of the entire ligament–bone insertion complex.[24]

Exercise

As stated, stress deprivation of ligaments, because of immobilization, results in atrophy.[8,9,16,18,25] Conversely, motion, stress, and general physical activity prescribed for healing ligaments produce hypertrophy and increased tensile strength.[2,9] Research shows that ligament and ligament–bone complex strength is related to the mode and duration of exercise used during rehabilitation.[2] Tipton[23] has shown that endurance types of exercise are more effective in producing larger diameter collagen than nonendurance types of exercise. In addition, the long-term detrimental effects of prolonged immobilization on ligament–bone insertion sites are reversible.[2] In fact, the effects of mobilization and exercise are seen 4 months to 1 year after immobilization.[2]

EFFECTS OF REMOBILIZATION AND EXERCISE

The negative biomechanical, biochemical, and morphologic changes incurred with immobilization generally are reversible. However, there are therapeutically relevant differences between ligament substance and ligament–bone insertion complexes after immobilization.

As stated, ligament substance once injured may regain only 50% to 70% of normal tensile strength after 1 year or more of remodeling.[24] Ligament–bone insertion complexes tend to remodel and regain tensile strength more slowly than ligament tissue after immobilization and therapeutically directed reconditioning. The clinical significance of delayed ligament–bone insertion healing compared with midsubstance tissue repairs is manifested by the relative increase in avulsion injury during this protracted healing interval.[24]

Generally, ligament substance and ligament–bone complexes are sensitive to exercise. These tissues become stronger depending on the type and duration of exercise prescribed. The orientation, composition, synthesis, and concentration of type I collagen and ultimate load to failure, increase in tensile strength, and stiffness of ligament and ligament–bone complexes are observed with appropriately directed exercise.[24]

It is interesting to note that dense fibrous tissue (e.g., tendon or ligament) not only responds to frequency, intensity, and duration of exercise, but also to the specific type of load applied to the tissue. The structural and biochemical adaptation of dense, fibrous tissue varies according to compressive or tensile loads. Tissues subjected to repeated compressions respond by synthesizing larger and greater amounts of proteoglycans than those tissues exposed to tension loads.

Generally, after injury to ligaments, appropriate controlled motion and exercise stimulates ligament repair by improving matrix organization and composition, increasing the weight of injured ligaments, and promoting normalized collagen synthesis and strength.[24]

Continuous Passive Motion

Motion, exercise, and protected progressive stress can influence and determine the degree and type of healing that occur after trauma and subsequent immobilization.[17] Studies have demonstrated that healing is dramatically different in immobilized joints compared with those moved passively through limited motion.[10] Gelberman and colleagues[10] have shown that joints moved passively have well-organized, longitudinally oriented collagen fibers in

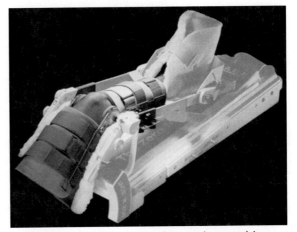

Fig. 8-2 Continuous passive motion machine.

which no adhesions are present. Conversely, joints that were immobilized demonstrated scar tissue and adhesions.

The concept of early protected motion applied to healing soft tissues has resulted in the development of a technique termed **continuous passive motion** (CPM) (Fig. 8-2). CPM is used in the treatment of the following: knee joint contractures; postoperative ACL reconstructions; joint effusions; knee, elbow, and ankle fractures (after immobilization); joint arthrosis; and total knee arthroplasty.[14] Early motion after surgery or immobilization acts to enhance and facilitate connective tissue strength, size, and shape; evacuate joint hemarthrosis (bloody effusion within the joint space); improve joint nutrition; inhibit adhesions; initiate normal joint kinematics; reduce articular surface changes; and minimize other deleterious effects of prolonged immobilization.[14] With postoperative ACL reconstruction, no stretching out of the graft occurs when CPM is used.[4,6,17,20] CPM can be used postoperatively; applied in the operating room; or be done a few days after surgery, immediately upon cast removal, or during the early phases of rehabilitation.

CPM devices have been designed for use on many body parts.[14] The knee is the most common, with the ankle, shoulder, elbow, wrist, hand, and hip joints also benefiting from CPM. The CPM machine is calibrated in cycles per minute and degrees of motion. Progressive increases in the cycle mode and degrees of motion are made gradually so as not to initiate pain or increase the time necessary for healing.

CPM usually is used in conjunction with other agents to reduce swelling and pain. Among these are ice packs, oral or intravenous analgesics, antiinflammatory medications, transcutaneous electrical nerve stimulation (TENS), and joint compression bandages.

Although CPM may be helpful to decrease postoperative pain following ACL reconstruction, systematic reviews suggest that there is no substantial advantage to using CPM, and no difference in long-term outcomes. It is recommend as an adjunct rather than a replacement for a postoperative exercise program.[21,27]

Practical Considerations

The time constraints and healing mechanics of ligaments are well documented.[2,3,8,13,15,16,22,25,28] Careful consideration must be given to the progression of therapeutic exercises and functional activities for patients with ligament injuries. Usually the absence of pain and swelling is an exceedingly poor indicator of healing tissue. With an ACL reconstruction, pain and swelling normally subside within a few weeks, but return of functional joint motion requires a couple of months. Strength values gradually increase, with muscle hypertrophy following slowly.

As the outward clinical signs point to healing, the ligament, being a dynamic tissue, continues to remodel and mature for up to 1 year. Protection of the joint is critical during healing. Functional knee braces with range-limiting devices can have a protective effect for MCL injuries, however no evidence exists that supports the routine use of functional bracing following ACL reconstruction.[26,27] Initiating progressive resistance exercises after knee ligament injury or surgery, while maintaining joint protection, can be challenging. Placing the resistance (weight) above the joint line during straight leg raises (Fig. 8-3) after ACL surgery can be the first phase of progressive resistance while protecting the healing ligament and retraining quadriceps activation.

To strengthen hip adduction with an MCL sprain, resistance initially is applied above the knee joint line so as not to overstress the healing MCL (Fig. 8-4). As the time constraints of healing allow, progressive strengthening of the adductors can involve loading the joint more distally, if joint protection is applied. Awareness of the time necessary for healing and duration of immobilization after trauma, weight bearing status, and degree of injury guide the physical therapist assistant (PTA) in making clinical recommendations about the progression of exercise and the placement of force during rehabilitation.

Developing a progressive therapeutic exercise and functional activities program with ankle sprains is similarly challenging. Generally, a grade II anterior talofibular (ATF) ligament sprain does not produce significant pain or functional limitations after a few weeks of conservative treatment involving splinting, crutch walking (non–weight bearing progressing to full weight bearing), ice, compression, and elevation. The PTA should protect the ligament for many weeks after injury because the process of ligament healing occurs slowly (Fig. 8-5).

Encouraging weight bearing as soon as tolerated, while protecting the joint, helps to establish normal joint kinematics and gait. Protecting the ligaments from further stress not only involves external bracing, but more importantly, includes avoidance of motions that place unwanted force on the healing ligaments. For example, the ATF ligament of the ankle is stressed with plantar flexion and inversion. To protect the ligaments, these two motions should be avoided during the early (postacute) and middle phases of rehabilitation.

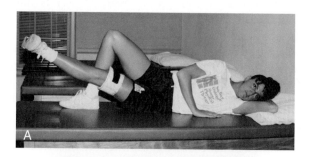

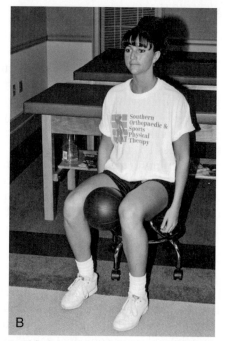

Fig. 8-4   **A,** Side-lying hip adduction exercise with the resistance placed proximal to the knee joint to protect the healing medial collateral ligament. **B,** Isometric hip adduction with the use of a ball placed proximal to the joint line.

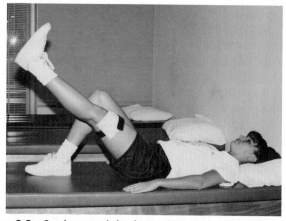

Fig. 8-3   Supine straight leg raises with the resistance placed proximal to the knee joint to reduce anterior translatory forces after anterior cruciate ligament reconstructive surgery.

Early protected motion is encouraged after ligament injury, repair, or immobilization, but caution should be taken to avoid overstressing the ligament or duplicating motions that place unwanted strain too soon after injury. The acute and postacute phases of rehabilitation after ligament injury or repair usually involve pain management techniques, swelling reduction, muscle reeducation (isometric muscle contraction and functional muscle stimulation), CPM, active range of motion, ligament protection devices via range-adjustable bracing, and weight bearing gait maneuvers with crutches as needed. During this early phase of recovery, it is particularly important to avoid excessive motions that may disrupt the intentional scar formation needed for joint stability. The degree of motion, direction of forces, and velocity of joint movement applied during this early postacute phase must be joint specific, functional, and protected. For example, with a cruciate ligament sprain, movements that are allowed include knee flexion and extension but no rotary or torque-producing motions. After an MCL sprain, knee flexion and extension motion can be initiated in the postacute phase (within limits); however, no valgus stress should be applied. As stated, the reason for ligament protection, maintenance of joint stability, and improved motion is that collagen fiber growth and parallel alignment are stimulated by early tensile loading within the normal physiologic range of the healing ligament.

Table 8-1 outlines the stages of ligament healing and subsequent therapeutic interventions that enhance the healing of ligament tissues.

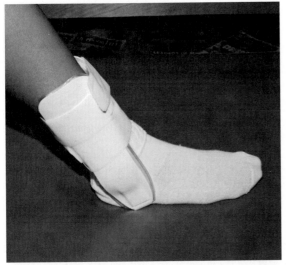

Fig. 8-5 Joint protection from unwanted forces must be considered essential for many weeks after ligament injuries. Shown here is an air–stirrup brace for lateral ligament complex sprain of the ankle.

Table 8-1	*Therapeutic Considerations During Stages of Ligament Healing*			
Timeline	**Immediate**	**Day 3-14**	**Day 14-60**	**Day 60-360**
Description	Hemostasis and degeneration. Weak, fragile tissue.[11,22]	Inflammation. Vasodilation and scar formation. Break down and remove dead cells. Unstable type III collagen.[11]	Proliferation and migration. Angiogenesis. Very gradual changes in collagen strength. Tissue changes from cellular to fibrous.[11,22]	Remodeling and maturation
Treatment	RICE, pain management techniques (TENS, oral IV analgesics). Non–weight bearing or weight bearing as tolerated. Can initiate CPM (within limited range of motion) Protection of ligaments from unwanted stress—usually adjustable range braces or hinged casts. Strict, rigid, long term cast immobilization should be minimized. Isometric muscle contractions. Contralateral limb exercise as tolerated.	Continue RICE. Active progressive motion. Continued ligament protection. Progressive weight bearing. Protected, controlled, active resisted exercise. Cycling (for motion). Isometric exercise progression. Electrical muscle stimulation. Initiate gentle multiangle static holds (isometrics). Avoid excessive motion.	Continue RICE as needed. Begin low-load static stretch if needed. Preheating tissues if needed. Full weight bearing. Isokinetic exercise with continued ligament protection with bracing. Eccentric isotonic exercise. Progressive concentric isotonic exercise. Hydrotherapy—swimming. Progressive cycling. Initiate closed kinetic chain exercise.	Prolonged low-load static stretching. Progressive advanced isokinetic and isotonic exercise. Cycling—stair climbs. Proprioception—balance—coordination exercise. Advanced CKC exercise, progressing to plyometric exercise. Jogging, running, jumping, maintain joint protection with functional bracing as needed.

CKC, Closed kinetic chain; *CPM,* continuous passive motion; *RICE,* rest, ice, compression, elevation; *TENS,* transcutaneous electrical nerve stimulation.

✤ GLOSSARY

Collagen: The primary protein of connective tissue in the human body that comes in 25 different forms and types.

Continuous passive motion (CPM): A form of rehabilitation that is typically done immediately after surgery when there is anticipation that a joint restriction may occur. This form of treatment uses a device known as a *continuous passive motion machine*, which gently moves the joint through a controlled range of motion decided upon by the physician in charge of the patient's care.

Immobilization: An attempt to render a joint in a fixed position. Immobilization in rehabilitation is done to decrease stressful activity to a joint that is inherently unstable. Typically immobilization is done for as short a duration as possible because complications can result from extended immobility.

Inflammatory reaction: A physiologic reaction to injury and tissue damage whose main function is to defend the body against harmful destruction, dispose of dead tissues, and promote healing of injured tissue.

Ligaments: Dense connective tissue.

Sprain: An injury to a ligament or capsular structure. Sprains are graded by their severity. A grade I sprain would indicate minimal damage to tissue, whereas a grade III would indicate complete rupture of the ligament or capsule.

REFERENCES

1. Akeson WH: An experimental study of joint stiffness, *J Bone Joint Surg* 43A:1022–1034, 1961.
2. Andriacchi TP, DeHaven KE, Dahners LE, et al: Ligament: injury and repair. In Woo SL-Y, Buckwalter J, editors: *Injury and repair of the musculoskeletal soft tissues*, Rosemont, Ill, 1988, American Academy of Orthopaedic Surgeons.
3. Buschbacher R: Tissue injury and healing. In *Musculoskeletal disorders: a practical guide for diagnosis and rehabilitation*, Boston, 1994, Andover Medical Publishers.
4. Coutts RD, Toth C, Kaita JH: The role of continuous passive motion in the rehabilitation of the total knee patient. In Hungerford DS, Krackow KA, Kenna RV, editors: *Total knee arthroplasty: a comprehensive approach*, Baltimore, 1984, Williams & Wilkins.
5. Cummings GS, Reynolds CA: Principles of soft tissue extensibility and joint contracture management. In Wadsworth C, editor: *strength and conditioning applications in orthopedics. Orthopedic section*, LaCrosse, Wis, 1998, APTA.
6. Davis D: Continuous passive motion for total knee arthroplasty, *Phys Ther* 64:709, 1984.
7. DeHaven KE, Lintner DM: Athletic injuries: comparison by age, sport and gender, *Am J Sports Med* 14:218–224, 1986.
8. Frank C, Woo SL, Amiel D, et al: Medial collateral ligament healing: a multidisciplinary assessment in rabbits, *Am J Sports Med* 11:379–389, 1983.
9. Gamble JG, Edwards CC, Max SR: Enzymatic adaptation in ligaments during immobilization, *Am J Sports Med* 12:221–228, 1984.
10. Gelberman RH, Van de Berg JS, Lundborg GN, et al: Flexor tendon healing and restoration of the gliding surface: an ultrastructural study in dogs, *J Bone Joint Surg* 65:70–80, 1983.
11. Goodman CC, Tepper SH, McKeough DM: Injury, inflammation, and healing. In Goodman CC, Fuller KS, editors: *Pathology: implications for the physical therapist*, St. Louis, 2009, Saunders.
12. Inoue M, McGurk-Burleson E, Hollis JM, et al: Treatment of the medial collateral ligament I: the importance of anterior cruciate ligament on the varus-valgus knee laxity, *Am J Sports Med* 15:15–21, 1987.
13. Kloth LC, Miller KH: The inflammatory response to wound healing. In Kloth LC, McCulloch JM, Feedar JA, editors: *Wound healing: alternatives in management, contemporary perspectives in rehabilitation*, Philadelphia, 1990, FA Davis.
14. McCarthy MR, O'Donoghue PC, Yates CK, et al: The clinical use of continuous passive motion in physical therapy, *J Orthop Sports Phys Ther* 15:132–140, 1992.
15. Noyes FR, DeLucas JL, Torvik PJ: Biomechanics of anterior cruciate ligament failure: an analysis of strain-rate sensitivity and mechanisms of failure in primates, *J Bone Joint Surg* 56A:236–253, 1974.
16. Noyes FR, Keller CS, Grood ES, et al: Advances in the understanding of knee ligament injury, repair and rehabilitation, *Med Sci Sports Exerc* 16:427–443, 1984.
17. Noyes FR, Mangine RE: Early motion after open arthroscopic anterior cruciate ligament reconstruction, *Am J Sports Med* 1: 149–160, 1987.
18. O'Donoghue DH, Frank GR, Jeter WJ: Repair and reconstruction of the anterior cruciate ligament in dogs: factors influencing long-term results, *J Bone Joint Surg* 53A:710–718, 1971.
19. Powell J: 636,000 injuries annually in high school football, *Athl Train* 22:19–22, 1987.
20. Salter RB, Simmonds DF, Malcolm HW: The effects of continuous passive motion on the healing of articular cartilage defects: an experimental investigation in rabbits, *J Bone Joint Surg* 57A:570–571, 1975.
21. Smith TO, Davies L: The efficacy of continuous passive motion after anterior cruciate ligament reconstruction: a systematic review, *Phys Ther Sport* 8:141–152, 2007.
22. Tillman LJ, Cummings GS: Biologic mechanisms of connective tissue mutability. In Currier DP, Nelson RM, editors: *Dynamics of human biologic tissues*, Philadelphia, 1992, FA Davis.
23. Tipton CM, James SL, Mergner W, et al: Influence of exercise on strength of medial collateral knee ligaments of dogs, *Am J Physiol* 218:894–902, 1970.
24. Woo SL, An K-N, Frank CB: Anatomy, biology, and biomechanics of tendon and ligament. In Buckwalter JA, Einhorn TA, Simon SR, editors: *Orthopedic basic science, biology, and biomechanics of the musculoskeletal system*, ed 2, Rosemont, Ill, 2000, Amercian Academy of Orthopedic Surgeons.
25. Woo SL, Gomez MA, Inoue M, et al: New experimental procedures to evaluate the biomechanical properties of healing canine medial collateral ligaments, *J Orthop Res* 5:425–432, 1987.
26. Wright RW, Fetzer GB: Bracing after ACL reconstruction: a systematic review, *Clin Orthop Relat Res* 455:162–168, 2007.
27. Wright RW, Preston E, Fleming BC, et al: A systematic review of anterior cruciate ligament reconstruction rehabilitation: part I: continuous passive motion, early weight bearing, postoperative bracing, and home-based rehabilitation, *J Knee Surg* 21:217–224, 2001.
28. Zarro V: Mechanisms of inflammation and repair. In Michlovitz S, editor: *Thermal agents in rehabilitation*, Philadelphia, 1986, FA Davis.

REVIEW QUESTIONS

Short Answer

1. Name the four phases of tissue healing.
2. Name the five cardinal signs of inflammation.

3. Organization and production of collagen occur during which phase of healing?

4. For torn ligaments to heal properly, the torn ends must be in _____ to one another. To orient collagen fibers and promote a functional scar, _____ must be applied. In addition, after injury or surgery to a ligament, protection against _____ must be strictly enforced.

5. Discuss the rationale for continuing or discontinuing external support as it relates to the healing constraints of ligament tissue after 2 weeks of progressive rehabilitation for a ligament sprain of the ankle.

True/False

6. Ligaments heal through a process of tissue regeneration.

7. Strict, long-term, rigid cast immobilization is necessary to allow for proper ligament healing.

8. The specific type and duration of exercise used during rehabilitation is not related to ligament and ligament–bone complex strength.

9. The long-term detrimental effects of immobilization on ligament and ligament–bone complex are not reversible.

10. Pain is an excellent guide to judge the degree of healing a ligament has achieved.

11. Ligaments may take 1 year or more to remodel and mature after surgery or injury.

9 Bone Healing

Robert C. Manske
Gary A. Shankman

LEARNING OBJECTIVES

1. Identify and describe the phases of bone healing.
2. Discuss the objectives that serve as the foundation of fracture management and bone healing.
3. Define osteoblasts, osteoclasts, and osteocytes.
4. Define and discuss Wolff's law.
5. Discuss stress deprivation, immobilization, and normal physiologic stress as they apply to fracture healing.
6. Define three complications of bone healing.
7. Outline and describe six areas of descriptive organization of classifying fractures.
8. Describe the five types of pediatric fractures defined by Salter-Harris.
9. Define pathologic fractures and list four types.
10. Discuss how osteoporosis affects fractures.
11. Define osteomalacia.
12. List common methods of fracture fixation, fixation devices, and fracture classifications.
13. Discuss clinical applications of rehabilitation techniques used during bone healing.

KEY TERMS

Bone matrix
Bone types
Cancellous bone
Cortical bone

Osteoblasts
Osteoclasts
Osteocytes
Piezoelectric effect

Remodeling
Repair

CHAPTER OUTLINE

Orthopedic conditions involving bone tissue are extremely common ailments treated in physical therapy. Therefore the physical therapist assistant (PTA) must appreciate the organized, dynamic nature of bone healing and must recognize the various methods of treating injuries to bone. Bone tissue is not a static structure, but a living, dynamic tissue that can actively adapt to its changing needs.

STRUCTURE AND FUNCTION

Bone is an intense metabolically active tissue. Bone has unique mechanical characteristics that are determined primarily by the structural components of bone tissue. Chemically complex, bone tissue is approximately 65% mineral and 35% organic matrix. The major organic constituent of bone is type I collagen, representing about 90% of the dry weight of bone.[35] The remaining 10% is composed of noncollagenous matrix proteins, lipids, phospholipids, proteoglycans, and phosphoproteins. The principal inorganic component of bone is a crystalline calcium phosphate hydroxyapatite.[35] This compound is generally brittle, tolerating only small amounts of deformation before fracture. The remaining tissue volume includes fluid-filled vascular channels and cellular spaces.[12]

Bone Cells

There are three types of bone cells. **Osteoblasts** are functionally distinct cells that form **bone matrix** (osteoid) and synthesize type I collagen,[35] and are commonly found on a bony surface. These cells are unique in that they have a large volume of endoplasmic reticulum, Golgi apparatus, and mitochondria to synthesize collagen and secrete matrix proteins.[35]

Osteoblasts and **osteocytes** are distinguished more by their location than by their structure and function.[15] Osteoblasts are responsible for synthesis, deposition, and mineralization of bone. They are derived from bone marrow and secrete procollagen on all active bone surfaces. Once the osteoblast is done forming bone, it can become an osteocyte.

Osteocytes actually are osteoblasts that are embedded within newly formed mineralized bone matrix.[35] Chemically, osteocytes differ from osteoblasts in that they demonstrate fewer organelles and a greater nucleus to cytoplasmic ratio.[35] These cells represent approximately 90% of mature skeletal tissue and metabolically function to control extracellular concentrations of calcium and phosphorus.[35] Osteoid osteocyte, and osteocytic osteoblasts are cells that are in an intermediate changeover from osteoblast to osteocyte, thus the pure distinction between cells may be more related to developmental stage than differing cell types.[37]

Osteoclasts are giant cell multinucleated bone resorption cells. Osteoclasts synthesize a specific acid phosphatase enzyme and also produce hydrogen ions, which in turn lower the pH environment.[35] The reduced pH increases the solubility of the crystalline phosphate-hydroxyapatite that functions to remove the organic matrix crystals via acid proteolytic degradation.[35] These enzymes remove a thick layer of osteoid covering, allowing osteoclasts to bind to bone and begin resorption if needed.[5]

Types of Bone

The microscopic organization and classification of bone tissue involves two distinct forms that change or adapt as we age: (1) normal, mature lamellar bone; and (2) weak, fragile, immature woven bone (Fig. 9-1).

Woven bone is structurally immature, embryologically (primary) fragile, and weak with a random disorganized collagen arrangement.[3] This random arrangement of collagen fibers allows strength in all directions, while preferring strength in none specifically. Therefore this form of bone is not nearly as strong as mature bone. This specific type of bone is more commonly seen in embryos and newborns, but can also be seen in the adult during fracture **repair** callus, bone tumors, and various bone pathologies.[35]

One of the unique features of woven bone is that it can be deposited without any previous part of a cartilaginous model existing.[23] Woven bone's primary function is to provide temporary, quick acting mechanical support for injured skeletal tissue.

Very early after birth (approximately 2 months to 4 years), woven bone slowly remodels into organized, structurally mature lamellar bone. A clinically relevant feature of woven bone is that its specific mechanical behavior is termed *isotropic*; that is, woven bone does not conform to Wolff's law, so its biomechanical reactions to applied forces and stress is similar in all planes.[3] The disorganized arrangement of collagen fibers in woven bone strongly contributes to this unique characteristic (Fig. 9-2).[3]

Lamellar bone refers to mature remodeled woven bone. Mature bone begins formation at about 1 month after birth[11] and comprises most of the skeleton by age 4 years.[2] The collagen arrangement in lamellar bone is highly structured and organized. This gives normal mature lamellar bone anisotropic mechanical properties that are stress oriented, which characteristically respond to Wolff's law.[3]

Bones are not only classified into various types, but also by their shape. Long bones are considered to have greater length than width. Examples of long bones are the femur and the humerus. These bones are tube shaped with widening at each end. Long bones have a diaphysis, which is the tubular shaped midportion that houses **cancellous bone** and the intermedullary canal where blood cells are formed (Fig. 9-3). The proximal and distal ends of the long bone widen to form a metaphysis, which continues to widen even more into

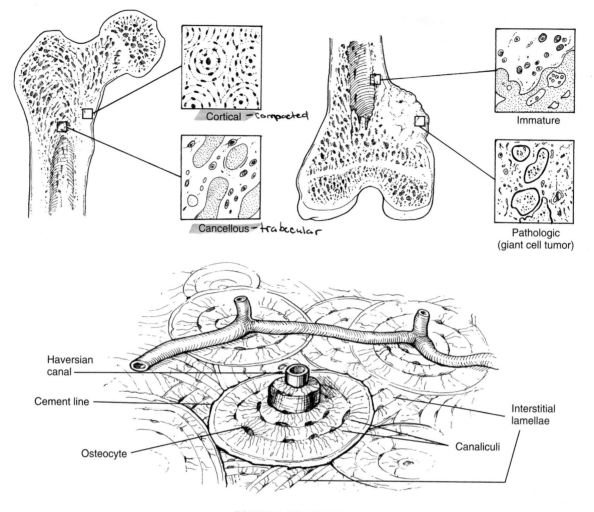

CORTICAL BONE DETAIL

Fig. 9-1 Types of bone. Cortical bone consists of tightly packed osteons. Cancellous bone consists of a meshwork of trabeculae. In immature bone, there is unmineralized osteoid lining the immature trabeculae. Atypical osteoblasts and architectural disorganization are seen in pathologic bone. (From Brinker MR, Miller MD, editors: *Fundamentals of orthopaedics*, Philadelphia, 1999, Saunders.)

the epiphysis or the end of the bone. In growing children, before skeletal maturity, the metaphysis and the epiphysis are separated by an epiphyseal growth plate. This can be a common area of fracture before skeletal maturity, at which time the two ends fuse and demarcation is not detectable.

Short bones are described as such because they are typically equal length in their main dimensions. These bones occur in the hands and feet. Short bones are composed of spongy inner bones that are enclosed by a thick layer of compact bone. Sesamoid and accessory bones are other forms of short bones.

Flat bones are typically larger and appear to serve a purpose in protection of organs. These bones consist of two layers of compact bone with a portion of spongy bone between. Bones like the ribs, sternum, scapula, and skull bones form the majority of flat bones. Many of these flat bones are actually curved and also serve as attachment sites for multiple muscles.

Irregular bones are those that do not seem to fit in the other categories. These include skull, vertebrae, and hip bones. These bones have a thin cortical exterior with a larger spongy interior.

Macroscopic Structure of Bone

Osseous tissue is structurally organized as either cancellous (trabecular bone) or **cortical bone** (compact bone). Cancellous bone is located at the metaphysis of long bones, as well as the vertebrae and other cuboid bones.[3]

Cortical bone, also known as *compact bone,* is located in the diaphyseal portion of long bones. Compact bone is very dense and hard on all surfaces, allowing it to function both structurally and for protection. Approximately 80% to 90% of the volume of cortical bone is calcium.[17] The major structural subunit of cortical-compact bone is the osteon. As described by Bostrom and colleagues,[3] the osteon is a central component of the haversian system.

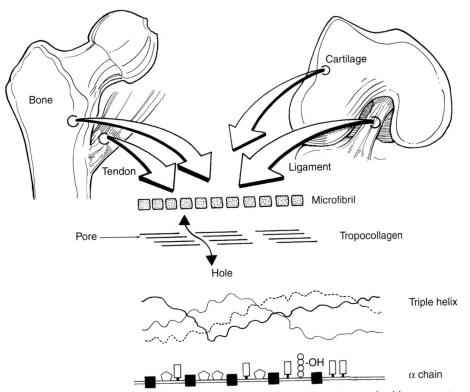

Fig. 9-2 Microstructure of collagen. Collagen is composed of microfibrils that are packed in a quarter-standard fashion to form tropocollagen. Note hole and pore regions for mineral deposition (for calcification). Tropocollagen, in turn, is made up of a triple helix of chains of polypeptides. (From Brinker MR, Miller MD, editors: *Fundamentals of orthopaedics*, Philadelphia, 1999, Saunders.)

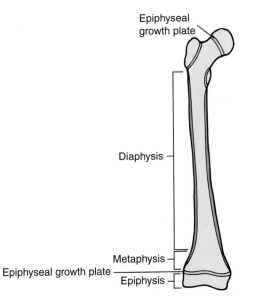

Fig. 9-3 Long bone components. (From Pyrde JA, Iwasaki DH: Fractures. In Cameron MH, Monroe LG, editors: *Physical rehabilitation: evidence-based examination, evaluation, and intervention*, St Louis, 2007, Saunders.)

Haversian bone is the most complex type of cortical bone. It is composed of vascular channels circumferentially surrounded by lamellar bone. This complex arrangement of bone around the vascular channel is called the *osteon*. The osteon is an irregular, branching,

and anastomosing cylinder composed of a more or less centrally placed neurovascular canal surrounded by cell permeated layers of bone matrix.[3] Primary osteons are those that develop into mature bone, while as new haversian canals are constantly formed, secondary osteons form on top of the old. Conversely, trabecular or cancellous bone is uniformly less dense with a large surface area and is significantly metabolically more "active" than cortical bone.[3] In fact, even though cortical bone (compact bone) has four times the mass of trabecular bone, the metabolic activity of trabecular bone is eight times greater than that of cortical bone.[3] Because bone turnover is a surface-oriented event, the profound surface area of trabecular bone explains the greater cellular exchange of cancellous bone.[3]

Bone Architecture

Characteristic differences between cortical bone and trabecular bone are best distinguished by the density and porosity of these two **bone types.**

Visually, cancellous bone, or trabecular bone, appears as a complex lattice of bone matrix fibers or spicules that orient along specific lines of stresses, strains, and compressive forces. Cortical bone, also known as *compact bone*, on the other hand is dense in appearance and is subject to bending, torsion, and compressive forces. Cortical bone also is defined as bone with less than 30%

porosity. Conversely, trabecular bone is generally 50% to 90% porous. Therefore the structure and material characteristics of both cortical and trabecular bone are distinguished by the relative density of each.

Bone Remodeling

The phenomenon of cellular turnover or **remodeling** of bone is a process that occurs on the surface of various portions of bone (periosteal, endosteal, trabecular, and haversian canal).[35] Generally, bone remodeling is a lifelong activity that responds to mechanical stress (torsion bending, compression, tension) according to Wolff's law.[3] In simplified terms, Wolff's law states that intermittent physiologic loads applied to bone stimulate adaptive responses. Removal of mechanical forces on the bone has the opposite effect. That is, when bone does not receive appropriate physiologic stress, osteoclastic activity overwhelms osteoblast production, which in turn reduces bone mass. The Hueter-Volkmann law is the reverse of Wolff's law and is more specifically applied to compression and tensile forces acting on physeal growth plates. Simply stated, this law suggests that compression forces limit bone growth, whereas tensile stress stimulates growth.[3]

Osseous tissue also is responsive to piezoelectric charges. In conjunction with mechanical forces strengthening compression and tensile stress, compression produces an electronegative charge that acts to stimulate osteoblast activity. Tensile stress produces an electropositive charge that stimulates osteoclastic activity. Therefore mechanical laws of stress (Wolff's law) produce electromechanical changes that act to maintain equilibrium between bone formation and bone resorption.

Vascular Supply to Bone

The adult skeletal system receives between 5% and 10% of the body's total cardiac output.[35] Bone receives blood supply from three distinct but interconnected systems: (1) the nutrient artery, (2) metaphyseal–epiphyseal system, and (3) periosteal systems (Fig. 9-4).

The arterial vascular system provides the origin of the nutrient system via a nutrient foramen in the diaphysis of long bones. The total number of nutrient vessels and foramen varies with each bone.[3] The nutrient arteries enter the medullary space, then ascend and descend into the arterioles within the endosteal surface supplying the diaphyseal area of long bones.[3] The metaphyseal-epiphyseal system is supplied by a periarticular complex system of the genicular arteries that penetrates the thin cortices of the metaphysis of long bones.[3] Muscular attachment to the periosteal cortical sites of bone provides nutrition through the periosteal capillary system.[3]

Fractures, internal fixation devices, external fixation, prosthetic joint implants devitalize the microcirculation of the cortical–periosteal and endosteal portion of bone. The resultant ischemia of bone can lead to nonunion and bone infections.[3] These important clinical ramifications of bone circulation disruption are evident when initiating therapeutic interventions of early weight bearing and closed kinetic chain (CKC) resistance exercise after fractures or joint replacement.

OSTEOPOROSIS

Osteoporosis is an age-related heterogeneous bone disease characterized by decreased bone tissue. Osteoporosis occurs when osteoblast (bone formation) activity is surpassed by osteoclast (bone resorption) activity (Fig. 9-5).[21] This creates weaker bones that are subjected to greater rates of fracture. More than 1 million fractures a year can be attributed to osteoporosis[27]; vertebral body compression fractures are the most common.

Causes of osteoporosis may be multifactorial, including hormonal alterations following menopause, prolonged immobilization, diseases, and prolonged steroid administration. Women are at greater risk for developing osteoporosis for several reasons. Age-related cortical bone loss generally begins at about age 40 years,[21] with the rate thereafter being approximately 0.5% annually for both men and women. However, because of lowered

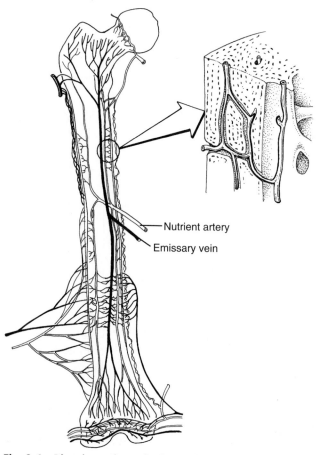

Nutrient artery
Emissary vein

Fig. 9-4 Blood supply to the bone. (From Brinker MR, Miller MD, editors: *Fundamentals of orthopaedics*, Philadelphia, 1999, Saunders.)

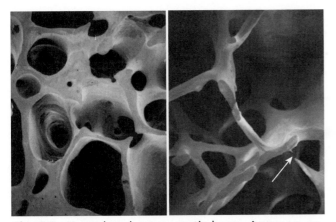

Fig. 9-5 Normal and osteoporotic bone. *Arrow* on osteoporotic bones shows trabecular microfracture. (From Patton KT, Thibodeau GA: *Anatomy and physiology*, ed 7, St Louis, 2010, Mosby.)

estrogen during menopause,[21] women lose bone at a rate of 2% to 8% annually, resulting in a much greater total loss.

Poor absorption of calcium that leads to decreased bone mineralization is called *osteomalacia*.[27] Causes include calcium-deficient diet, accelerated calcium loss, and malabsorption of calcium.[21] Femoral neck fractures are common in patients with osteomalacia.[27]

To appreciate the fragile nature of fractures that occur as a result of osteoporosis or osteomalacia, the following case should be considered:

A frail, elderly woman with osteoporosis suffers resultant multilevel thoracic vertebral body compression fractures. Bed rest with relative immobilization is ordered. She suffers further decrease in bone strength caused by immobilization. Rehabilitation is complicated by osteoporosis and fractures. Combined with the general overall negative effects of immobilization on the body's systems, the effects of immobilization on the remaining skeletal tissue interfere with exercise, sitting, progressive ambulation, and functional activities, forming a vicious cycle that will need to be broken in order for a functional recovery.

CLASSIFICATIONS OF FRACTURES

By definition a fracture is any abnormal disruption in the normal anatomic continuity of bone. Therefore the classification of fractures takes into account the following criteria[32,33]:

■ Site of injury: The area of insult on the bone itself. An epiphyseal fracture describes the site, as does an intraarticular fracture or diaphyseal (shaft) fracture. Generally the site is described as the proximal, middle, or distal portion of a bone (Fig. 9-6).

■ Extent of injury: Complete or incomplete (Fig. 9-7). As the name implies, a complete fracture traverses the bone entirely. Incomplete fractures are commonly described as hairline cracks or greenstick fractures.

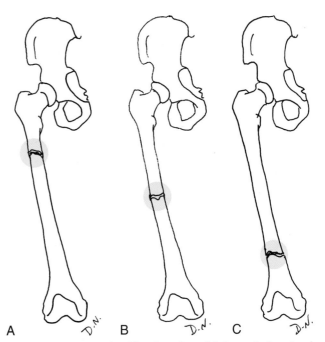

Fig. 9-6 Fracture classification site of injury. **A,** Proximal fracture of the femur. **B,** Middle fracture of the femur. **C,** Distal fracture of femer.

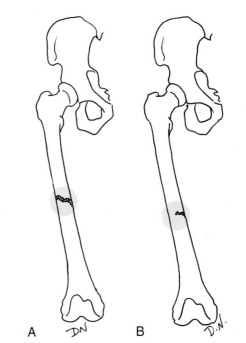

Fig. 9-7 Fracture classification, extent of injury. **A,** Complete fracture of the femur. **B,** Incomplete fracture of femur.

■ Configuration or direction of abnormality: The direction of the fracture. In a transverse fracture, the fracture line goes straight across (horizontally) through the bone; an oblique fracture crosses the bone diagonally. A spiral fracture describes a torsion or rotational injury where the fracture line literally spirals through the bone. An impacted fracture is a long-axis compression injury where the fracture fragments are

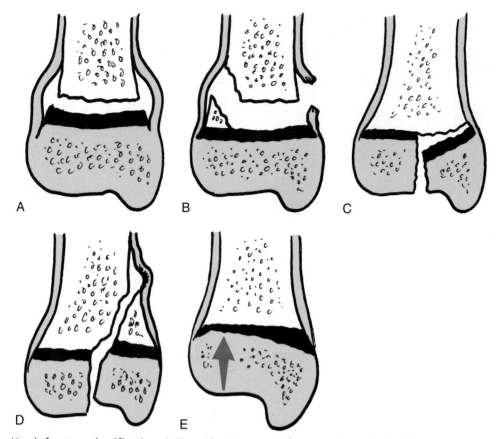

Fig. 9-8 Salter-Harris fracture classification. **A,** Type I is a transverse fracture through the physis. **B,** Type II is same as Type I but also has metaphyseal fragment. **C,** Type III is an intraarticular fracture. Involves both the physis and the epiphysis. **D,** Type IV is the same as Type III, but also involves the metaphysis. **E,** Type V is a crush injury to the physis.

forced together. The fracture is classified as comminuted when more than two fragments are present.

■ Relationship of fracture fragments to each other: Can be displaced, nondisplaced, angulated, twisted, rotated, or overriding. An example is an avulsion fracture where a portion of bone is pulled away as part of a musculotendinous attachment or ligament–bone attachment.

■ Relationship of fracture fragments to the environment: Whether the injury is open (compound fracture) or closed (simple).

■ Complications: Resulting in delayed union, nonunion, or malunion of the fracture fragments. An uncomplicated course of healing is called *uneventful.*

Pediatric fractures have a special classification of injuries involving the epiphysis. Depending on the type of epiphyseal fracture, the eventual growth of the bone can be profoundly affected.

Salter's fracture classification is outlined in Figure 9-8. Type I Salter-Harris fractures, modified by Rang,[27,31-33] are transverse fractures through the physis. Type II fractures are the same as type I, but also have a metaphyseal fragment. Type III fractures involve both the physis and epiphysis. Typically these are intraarticular fractures. Type IV fractures are the same as type III but include the metaphysis. These are significant injuries that can lead to

a reduction in bone growth. Type V fractures are severe injuries classified as crush injuries to the physis. This type of fracture also can lead to the arrest of growth. The PTA should also be aware of the Arbeitsgemeinschaft für Osteosynthesefragen (AO) classification system, which is universally applied to both fracture patterns and the devices used for internal fixation. This system will be discussed later in this chapter.[26]

Other fractures that are commonly seen in children are incomplete fractures. This is typically because a child's bones are more flexible than an adult's. A buckle fracture is one in which a deformation or "bending" of the cortex occurs on one side of the bone. A greenstick fracture is one that involves a linear fracture through one cortical surface and a flexing deformation of the opposite surface. A bowing fracture is one that may be caused by multiple microfractures along the length of a long bone so that the entire bone is bent or curved.

Pathologic fractures are caused by tumors[27] (malignant or primary bone disease), osteoporosis (most common), microtrauma from repetitive overload (stress fractures), or metastatic bone disease (second most common). These usually occur in the elderly person secondary to osteoporosis and can happen spontaneously or with very minor trauma.[27]

COMPONENTS OF BONE HEALING

Most of the adult skeleton (80%) is composed of compact, cortical bone. Approximately 20% of the skeleton is cancellous or spongy bone. Compact bone is extremely dense and unyielding to bending, whereas cancellous bone is more elastic and less dense than cortical bone.[27]

Three types of cells take part in the highly dynamic, reparative process in bone. Osteoblasts help form and synthesize bone. Osteocytes are mature bone cells that account for approximately 90% of all bone tissue. Osteoclasts are active in bone resorption.

The normal dynamic process of bone synthesis and resorption is termed *remodeling.* Remodeling and stress occur together, which profoundly influences bone shape, density, internal architecture, and external configuration.[1,18,22,27] With normal bone remodeling, weight-bearing forces and muscular contractions provide the stress needed for bone formation and adaptation. The absence of physiologic loading, or stress, is detrimental to bone, ligament, cartilage, muscle, and tendons, as well as the cardiorespiratory system. Wolff's law[1] states that intermittently applied stress, as well as changes in function of bone, causes definite changes.[4,22] After a fracture, treatment may involve rigid cast immobilization and non–weight bearing over a period of weeks. This decreased stress on the bone causes rapid osteoclast activity (bone resorption) and decreased osteoblast activity.[28] Therefore although the removal of stress is paramount for healing, the decrease in external force also causes significant bone loss.[27] Bone loss caused by immobilization is reversible after progressive weight bearing, active motion, resistive exercise, and vertical loading (CKC exercise).[27] It is recommended that strict, long-term, rigid cast immobilization be minimized whenever possible.

Although normal stresses promote bone development, excessive stress also can lead to gradual bone resorption.[22] Stress that is unrelenting and does not allow for osteoblastic repair of bone can lead to pathologic accelerated bone resorption and eventual stress fracture.[1,18,22]

Bone remodeling is also influenced by electrical charges when forces are applied to bone. The **piezoelectric effect** describes a negative electric charge toward the concave, or compression, side of a force applied to a bone. An electropositive charge is seen on the tension, or convex, side of the bone. The negative-charge side responds by stimulating osteoblasts, whereas the positive-charge side (tension side) responds by increasing osteoclast activity.[27]

BONE INJURY AND REPAIR

Injury repair and eventual regeneration of osseous tissue is a complex process that involves the bone marrow, bone cortex, periosteum, and external soft tissues.

Trauma to the bone disrupts the biological, mechanical, structural, architectural, and histochemical environment of bone. Classic descriptions of fracture healing are divided into primary (direct) cortical healing and secondary (indirect) fracture healing.

The spontaneous natural course of fracture repair can be described as interfragmentary stabilization by periosteal and endosteal callus formation and by interfragmentary fibrocartilage differentiation, restoration of continuity and bone union by intramembranous and endochondral ossification, substitution of avascular and necrotic areas by haversian remodeling, modeling of the fracture site, and functional adaptation.[1,3,4,8,10,20]

Fracture healing responses differ according to the nature of stabilization provided (direct, internal, compression–appositional, alignment fixation, versus cast immobilization). That is, rigid internal fixation results in primary–direct cortical healing, which is an attempt by the cortex of bone to reestablish mechanical and anatomic continuity. In primary fracture healing the new bone grows directly across the bone ends to unite the fracture site. This form of bone healing is very slow and cannot bridge a fracture gap, thus the two fractured ends are not able to appose each other. This requires rigid fixation with direct contact of cortical bone and an intact intramedullary vasculature. This type of fracture healing response usually is devoid of periosteal soft callus formation. Secondary or indirect fracture repair is noted for external periosteal soft-tissue callus bridging between fracture fragments. In secondary healing, a cartilage matrix is initially formed, which gradually takes on a callus appearance. This method of healing involves adding stability by creating a callus that is actually larger (wider) than the two opposing bones.

Phases of Fracture Repair

In general terms most fractures heal with a combination of primary cortical healing and secondary–indirect healing. The phases of fracture repair are divided into six sequences of events that ultimately lead to functional remodeling of the injured bone.[20] Phase I is inflammation and hematoma formation, Phase II is chondrocyte formation and angiogenesis, Phase III is cartilage and calcification, Phase IV is cartilage removal, Phase V is bone formation, and Phase VI is bone remodeling.[20]

Phase I is characterized by fibrin clot formation. The fracture site creates formation of the inflammatory response. Because of increased vascularity from the injury, a hematoma forms and begins the process of clot formation. The presence of the fibrin clot between fracture fragments acts as a rich source of activating inflammatory molecules essential to the complex cascade of intense cellular activity required for fracture repair. Many cellular processes are involved during this phase that are responsible for attracting, regulating, and differentiating cells that serve to propagate the development of cartilage and revascularization of bone. Animal models demonstrate intramembranous and endochondral bone formation during the first 2 weeks after fracture.[20] This early mass of tissue formed during bone healing is termed a *callus*. The callus is an early precursor to mature calcified bone.

The presence of cartilage within the fracture repair matrix at this point is the hallmark of Phase II repair. Chondrocytes form a V-shaped wedge of tissue between the ends of fractured bone. The matrix formed is type I and II cartilage. Calcification of chondrocytes (cartilage) requires specific enzyme release for phosphate and calcium interactions. During Phase III, there is a gradual decline in proliferative cell activity and an increase in chondrocyte deposition and release of proteolytic enzymes. The calcification process of fibrocartilage is essential before the substitution of woven bone within the fragment gap. Once fibrocartilage is calcified, the ultimate integrity and development of woven bone with resultant remodeling to lamellar bone is dependent on revitalization (vascularity) of injured bone. Eventually, bone reforms into its natural shape.

Angiogenesis (neovascularization) is critical for delivering oxygen, nutrients, inflammatory cells, and fibroblasts to stimulate and support the healing fracture. The vascular response to a healing fracture varies over time. Initially, the three distinct vascular systems of bone are disrupted significantly, reducing blood flow. Over the next several days after fracture, the circulation increases and peaks at approximately 2 weeks.[20] Recognize that although there is a relative increase in vascular budding, the dramatic volume of cellular activity creates a state of hypoxia at the fracture that is highly conducive for cartilage formation.[20]

Process of Bone Healing

Bone healing can be characterized by the following sequence of events:

- Fracture occurs.
- Bleeding occurs, and a hematoma results.
- Granulation tissue is formed by the hematoma (soft callus formation).
- Osteoblasts produce new bone, and a bony or hard callus is formed.
- The callus is gradually reabsorbed, and the anatomic contour of the bone is regained.

As with soft tissue, the immediate inflammatory response lasts 24 to 48 hours and is characterized by the development of granulation tissue, blood clotting, and fibroblast and osteoblast proliferation.[4,27] The repair phase of bone healing signals the development of bone scarring, or callus formation, which is usually detected within the first 2 weeks after injury. The degree of callus formation depends on anatomic alignment of the fragments and the degree and quality of immobilization. If motion occurs through the fracture site during this phase, a soft bone callus (primarily of cartilage) bridges the fragments.[4,27] This type of callus also forms if the union between the fragments is poor, even when immobilization prevents motion.

Primary cortical healing (hard callus) forms with anatomic alignment and fragment apposition, immobilization, and appropriately applied progressive stress. The remodeling phase of bone healing is an extraordinarily long process that can take up to several years to complete and is strongly influenced by Wolff's law.[1]

As with ligament healing, protection of the injury site is vital to a successful outcome. There is an exceedingly narrow line to follow with respect to motion after bone injury. In many cases a reducing plan of immobilization is used to secure the bone fragments, protect the fracture, and provide needed motion for healing. For example, a rigid cast can be applied for a few weeks (2 to 4 weeks), then a limited range hinge brace can be used to protect the healing structures and initiate physiologic motion within set limits. Depending on the severity of the insult, some fractures may require secure immobilization for extended periods to allow for proper healing.

Effects of Immobilization on Bone Tissue

A major goal for bone healing to occur is to immobilize the fracture site. However, when bone tissue does not receive physiologic loads (ambulation, vertical loads, and muscle contractions), the normal remodeling processes are negatively affected. The rate of normal bone remodeling changes when immobilization lasts slightly longer than 1 week.[10] The "turnover" or remodeling of bone during immobilization is characterized by a loss of calcium, resulting in localized bone loss. Immobilization leads to a reduction in the hardness of bone related to the duration of immobilization.[10] By 3 months, bone strength is only 55% to 60% of normal.[36] The relationship between soft tissue structures and bone during periods of immobilization reflects the interdependence of muscular contractions, forces acting on joints, compressive loads, circulation (blood flow affecting nutrition), and motion in maintaining bone remodeling equilibrium.

A definite contrast is seen in the care of healing bone tissue. It is necessary to immobilize the fracture fragments so healing can occur, yet minimize the negative effects of immobilization through the judicious application of progressive motion, exercise, and weight bearing. The length of time needed to regain bone strength after immobilization is considerably longer than the duration of immobilization. Therefore, the length of the immobilization is an important component in the overall process of healing bone tissue.

Complications

Occasionally the process of bone healing leads to three distinct complications:

1. Delayed union
2. Nonunion
3. Malunion

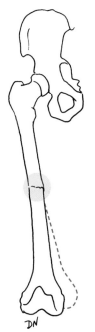

Fig. 9-9 Malunion of the femur. Dotted line indicates normal anatomic alignment.

In delayed union, the dynamic biological repair processes of bone healing occur at a slower rate than anticipated. Brashear and Raney[4] describe delayed union as clinically detectable when firm callus is not present at 20 weeks (for fractures of the tibia and femur) and at 10 weeks (for fractures of the humerus). An important cause of delayed union is "inadequate or interrupted immobilization."[4] Rehabilitation can significantly affect the healing process either positively or negatively. If therapeutic interventions are begun too soon or too vigorously, delayed union may occur because of excessive motion occurring at the fracture site. Unfortunately, the trade-off when caring for delayed bone union cases is the need to provide extended periods of immobilization for healing. However, cast braces and walking casts can be used to provide the weight bearing (Wolff's law) necessary to enhance healing. In nonunion, the healing processes have stopped. Nonunion occurs when there is a significant and severe associated soft-tissue trauma, poor blood supply, and infections.

In malunion, healing results in a nonanatomic position (Fig. 9-9). Malunion is caused by ineffective immobilization and failure to maintain immobilization for an adequate period of time. For appropriate bone healing to occur, anatomic alignment (apposition) of fragments, adequate fixation (external or internal), and length of time of immobilization must occur in concert. If these factors are not balanced, the chance of complications is increased. Regardless of the type of complication, fracture healing fails or is delayed 5% to 10% of the time.[6,9]

Fracture Fixation: Biology and Biomechanics

Rigid anatomic fixation of bone results in primary repair or direct cortical reconstruction. This process generally inhibits periosteal soft tissue bridging callus. The repair process of rigid internal fixation is characterized by haversian remodeling and osteon formation. Creeping substitution is a term used to describe osteoclastic *cutting cones* traversing the cortical fracture fragments, followed by osteoblast formation and revascularization of bone.

The precise application of various internal fixation devices (intermedullary rods, bone plates, and compression screws) to stimulate primary cortical healing are not without inherent risks. The surgical placement of bone plates requires "stripping" the periosteum where the screws and plates are to be fixed. This process obviously devascularizes the periosteal blood supply. In addition, the areas beneath the plate increase the porosity of bone and weaken the mechanical and structural behavior, as well as the architecture of the injured bone. With intramedullary rod application, the medullary canal must be "reamed" to allow for proper anatomic placement of the rod. Again the nutrient arterial system, metaphyseal–diaphyseal system, and medullary circulation are disrupted. During the surgical placement of screws and plates, the surgeon attempts to apply these devices by hand-held screw devices and manual torque wrenches instead of using high-speed drills that might create thermal necrosis of bone and soft tissue, which could contribute to increased bone devitalization.[34,36]

Conversely, nonoperative fracture management involves a complex series of interactions, which stimulate the thermal, chemical, mechanical, and electrical environment of periosteal and cortical bone (Table 9-1).[8,20]

In cases of nonoperative fracture management, the type of repair is referred to as *secondary–periosteal callus*. The natural healing sequence on nonoperative diaphyseal fractures include a period of instability (Phase I) in which there is essentially no true biological support given to the fracture site. The fracture hematoma and proliferative cellular activation provide no mechanical protection of the fragments.

The second phase is the development of the soft callus. Phase II is characterized by the soft-tissue compliance provided the peripheral structures surrounding the fracture fragments. The formation, organization, and gradual maturation of cellular activity in and around the injury site provides for greater stability.[20] As stated by Latta, Sarmiento, and Zych,[20] "peripheral structures supply early vascularization and soft tissue repair. Peripheral soft tissues provide a compliant strength which leads to reduction of acute symptoms long before there is radiographic evidence of healing." Phase III demonstrates a radiographic confirmation of thin "hard callus" (bony ridge).

Table 9-1	Type of Fracture Healing Based on Type of Stabilization	
Type of Immobilization	**Predominant Type of Healing**	**Comments**
Cast (closed treatments)	Periosteal bridging callus	Enchondral ossification
Compression plate	Primary cortical healing (remodeling)	Cutting cone-type remodeling
Intramedullary nail	Early—periosteal bridging callus	Enchondral ossification
	Late—medullary callus	
External fixator	Dependent on extent of rigidity	
	Less rigid—periosteal bridging callus	
	More rigid—primary cortical healing	
Inadequate	Hypertrophic nonunion	Failed endochondral ossification
		Type II collagen predominates

From Brinker MR, Miller MD: *Fundamentals of orthopaedics*, Philadelphia, 1999, Saunders.

Generally, hematoma and cartilage are prevalent along with a gradual revascularization of the interfragmentary gap of soft and hard callus formation. Radiographic confirmation of the disappearance of the fracture line is characteristic of Phase IV, the fracture line consolidation phase.

During this stage of nonoperative diaphyseal fracture management, there is a subtle, gradual shrinkage of the central soft callus bone with remodeling, consolidation of the fracture line, and maturation of hard bony callus.

Finally, Phase V structural remodeling is where there is gradual contraction and shrinkage of callus with resultant reorganization and configuration of normal bone anatomy and topography.

External Fixation and Fracture Repair

External fixators are used for a wide variety of clinical situations and allow for modification of stiffness and rigidity of fixation during fracture healing.[4,30]

The geometric composite construct of these elaborate frame configurations usually can be altered by several orders of magnitude. Several factors significantly contribute to the stability, rigidity, stiffness, and compression of the fracture site, as well as the mechanical properties of the frame.[30] The number of pins used; the length, diameter, and type of pin material; the number of side bars set in the spacing between pins; the spacing between side bars and bone surface; pin–bone contact; and proximal–distal pin spacing all contribute to the material characteristics: stability, stiffness, and compression of the fracture site.[8,30]

Fracture healing characteristics using external fixators depend on the rigidity obtained by the device. Overall, the more rigid the fixation, the earlier the radiographic confirmation of bone union. Less rigid fixators create greater periosteal callus formation, whereas rigid fixators characteristically stimulate direct primary cortical fracture healing.[8,30]

As stated, a unique advantage of external fixation is the ability to alter or modify rigidity during various stages of fracture healing. Several models demonstrate the effect of dynamization (mechanisms used to decrease stiffness of the fixation or mechanisms that allow for controlled micromotion between fracture fragments) on blood flow and bone callus formation.[8,20,25,30,35] A 25% increase in fracture site micromotion resulted in a 400% increase in regional blood flow and substantially more callus formation with animals receiving semirigid external fixators compared with rigid external fixation.[30]

Bone Fixation Devices

When caring for patients who have had fractures, the PTA must be aware of various methods used to immobilize or stabilize the fracture so a clear understanding of the extent of trauma can be appreciated. This also allows the PTA to understand the degree of tissue healing necessary before vigorous rehabilitation exercises can be undertaken.

The remarkable sensitivity of bone to normal biological stress is well-known.[1,22,27,33] After fractures, an attempt is made to stabilize the fracture, bring the fragments together by apposition (approximation) and alignment, and remove or minimize forces that may slow the normal healing process. Two general methods of immobilization are used in the treatment of fractures. In one method, the area is immobilized by external fixation devices. This method involves the use of casts, traction, splints, and braces and the external fixation devices employed with significant open (compound comminuted) fractures where the risk of infection is present (Fig. 9-10). These ominous-looking devices help fix the fracture site while allowing care of the open wounds with skin grafts, tissue flaps, or débridement. These are classified as external fixation devices because the pins used to immobilize the fracture do not contact the fragments directly, but are used to hold the bone segments in rigid alignment and anatomic apposition. With closed (simple) fractures, various rigid lightweight fiberglass casts, plaster casts, hinged-plaster casts, and adjustable-range hinged braces are used for immobilization.

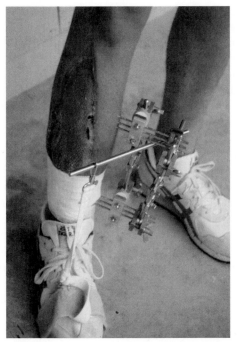

Fig. 9-10 External fixation device (external fixator).

The second method of immobilization uses internal fixation devices and is best for displaced fractures where external fixation does not provide the degree of immobilization necessary to effect healing. (See Box 9-1 for the background on the AO classification system, designed by the Association for the Study of Internal Fixation [ASIF or AO].) Internal fixation is called *open reduction with internal fixation (ORIF)* and involves surgically exposing the fracture site to reduce, approximate, and align the bone fragments. The materials used for ORIF procedures include metals (stainless steel and metal alloys of cobalt–chromium–molybdenum and titanium) and nonmetals (high-density polyethylene, polymethylmethacrylate, silicones, and ceramics). Metal internal fixation devices frequently are combinations of screws, staples, pins, nails, tension-band wires, and various plates. The placement of these materials can affect the delivery of certain therapeutic agents, such as ultrasound. Also, a hole or tunnel defect in a bone, with or without a screw in it, effectively reduces the overall strength of the bone up to 50%.[27] Even after screw removal, the bone will not regain normal strength for up to 1 year.[27]

Metal internal fixation devices occasionally loosen and can "back out," as is the case with screws. If the PTA notes signs of hardware loosening (pain, swelling, or crepitus), he or she must immediately consult with the supervising physical therapist (PT) and physician. Many metal fixation devices are designed to be left in place, as with most plates, but these devices should be removed if metal allergy reactions occur. Table 9-2 depicts the various internal fixation devices.

Table 9-2	*Internal Fixation Devices*
Type	**Use**
Compression plate	Diaphyseal fractures
Intramedullary rod	Lower extremity diaphyseal fractures (femur, tibia); removed at 1 or 2 years
Reconstruction plate	Used in pelvic and distal humerus fractures
Tension wires	Patella fractures and olecranon fractures
Sliding hip screws	Intertrochanteric hip fractures
Condylar screws	Distal femur fractures
Cannulated screws	Femoral neck fractures

From Miller M: *Review of orthopaedics*, Philadelphia, 1992, Saunders.

Factors Influencing Bone Healing

Several key factors are implicated in delayed biologic fracture repair. Tobacco smoke, malnutrition, inadequate reduction of the fragments, excessive motion from inadequate immobilization, poor vascular supply, soft-tissue interposition between fracture fragments, and infection significantly limit spontaneous fracture repair.[3,8]

Cigarette smoke is a vasoconstrictor that may reduce blood supply to the injury site. In addition, smoking directly interferes with osteoblast formation.[36] Protein, malnutrition, and calorie deprivation reduce skeletal muscle mass and may contribute to reduced periosteal and cortical bone formation.[8] Poor reduction of the fracture fragments and inadequate immobilization create excessive motion and reduced vascular supply to the bone (Box 9-2).[36] Occasionally a sleeve of soft tissue becomes interposed within the fracture site, significantly reducing both primary, cortical, and

BOX 9-2

Biological and Mechanical Factors Influencing Fracture Healing

BIOLOGICAL FACTORS	MECHANICAL FACTORS
Patient age	Soft-tissue attachments to bone
Comorbid medical conditions	Stability (extent of immobilization)
Functional level	Anatomic location
Nutritional status	Level of energy imparted
Nerve function	Extent of bone loss
Vascular injury	
Hormones	
Growth factors	
Health of the soft-tissue envelope	
Sterility (in open fractures)	
Cigarette smoke	
Local pathologic conditions	
Level of energy imparted	
Type of bone affected	
Extent of bone loss	

From Brinker MR, Miller MD: *Fundamentals of orthopaedics*, Philadelphia, 1999, Saunders.

secondary–periosteal bridging callus, and rendering the fragments devitalized.

Infectious organisms have many deleterious effects on both implants and the host bone environment. Orthopedic implant loosening, bone resorption, bone destruction, and reactive periosteal elevation can occur in the presence of infection.[8]

Stimulation of Fracture Repair

There are several methods available to augment, stimulate, or enhance fracture repair. Bone grafts are used to fill osseous defects and stabilize fractures. Bone autografts are taken from the same individual. Allograft bone tissue is used from the same species. An example of a fresh autograft is harvesting bone from the iliac crest to transpose (heterotopic transportation) to the lumbar spine for fusion.

Conversely, cadaveric bone allografts must be sterilized chemically. This process renders all cells nonviable. In both autografts and allografts, the implanted graft acts as a scaffold to support the growth of host bone tissue. This process is known as *passive osteoconduction*.[8] Gradually the implant bone tissue becomes revascularized with stimulation and transportation of osteoblasts into the new graft. This process is referred to as *osteoinduction*.[8] Although the sequence of events is similar (passive osteoconduction, gradual revascularization, and osteoinduction) with both graft materials, allogenic bone requires a longer time for creeping substitution to

take place. Additional materials used for osteoconduction that support vascular ingrowth, growth, attachment, division, and remodeling of bone include ceramics, bioactive glass, and synthetic polymers.[8]

Ceramic bone graft substitutes include hydroxyapatite and tricalcium phosphate. Some of these graft substitutes are formed from marine coral and crystalline hydroxyapatite. These bone substitutes generally have been shown to be as effective as autograft bone.[8]

Two clinically relevant methods of fracture healing augmentation are electromagnetic field application and low-intensity ultrasound. The use of exogenously applied pulsed electromagnetic fields over nonunion fractures is based on the piezoelectric effect in response to load deformation of crystalline–collagen component's of Wolff's law.[8] The use of specific electrical stimulation waveforms to induce bone formations is supported by scientific investigation and clinical observation that electric stimulation affects enchondral bone formation and connective tissue repair.

Basic science research suggests that the use of nonthermal, low-intensity ultrasound (30 mW/cm^2) has very strong biological value to bone healing due to signal transduction and gene expression; stimulation of chondroblasts and osteoblasts and increasing blood flow; and enhancement of greater mechanical and histologic influence on enchondral and periosteal bone healing.[16] Various studies have demonstrated that use of brief low-intensity ultrasound on the order of 20 minutes per day can reduce the time to fracture union.[8,14,19,24,29]

However, a recent systematic review[7] of the use of low-intensity pulsed ultrasound for fractures that assessed randomized controlled trials determined that many of the studies had only moderate to low quality evidence for its use. Studies rarely included functional endpoints, and two of the highest quality studies showed no difference in functional outcome with the use of ultrasound.

Clinical Application of Rehabilitation Techniques During Bone Healing

Immobilization after bone injury may not be total. Non-immobilized structures should be exercised throughout the period of immobilization. For example, a program of lower extremity strengthening and endurance activities (stationary cycle, treadmill, and leg extension) should be instituted for patients with upper extremity fractures. The same principle applies for patients with lower extremity fractures. Endurance activities can be either single-leg stationary cycling or upper body ergometer (UBE) exercises in these cases.

Specific exercises for the injured area frequently involve isometric muscle contractions. Therapeutic exercise programs during bone healing are designed to minimize muscle atrophy while maintaining or improving muscular strength. Muscle contractions provide forces acting to approximate fragments, improve circulation, promote motion to nonimmobilized body parts, and stimulate the piezoelectric effect.

The cast or brace serves as resistance in the initial phases of active range of motion (AROM) exercises involving the affected limb. Ankle weights can be applied to the cast or brace for added resistance in later stages. It is best to apply the external resistance superior to the injury site at first, such as in ligament injuries. A more distal application of external force may produce excessive, unwanted shearing, or torque through the fracture site.

Occasionally, electrical muscle stimulation (EMS) is used during cast immobilization to help retard atrophy and maintain strength. A small "window" is cut in the cast to allow the application of the electrodes. The patient is instructed to isometrically contract simultaneously with the electrically evoked muscle contraction. The benefits of electrical stimulation on muscle tissue during immobilization are controversial. The piezoelectric effect is enhanced by applying a negatively charged electrode to stimulate osteoblast activity, which is called *direct current* (any current in which electrons flow in one direction). An externally applied electrode with an external power source is called *inductive coupling*.[27]

Continuous passive motion (CPM) devices are used in some cases of intraarticular or extraarticular fractures of the tibia and femur.[13] Although this appears to conflict with the notion of secure immobilization leading to bone healing, Salter and colleagues[34] found positive effects of CPM on the development of chondrocytes and the reduction of intraarticular synovial adhesions when judiciously applied to healing intraarticular fractures.

The goals of rehabilitation programs during immobilization of healing fractures are as follows:
- Improve the overall fitness of the patient
- Promote motion of unaffected, nonimmobilized joints
- Minimize muscle atrophy (isometrics and muscle stimulators)
- Maintain or improve muscular strength
- Protect the healing structures; avoid unwanted, premature, or excessive motion
- Teach safe and effective transfers and gait activities (with cumbersome long-leg plaster casts or external fixators)

After immobilization, progressive exercise must be directed cautiously. Motion and circulation can be promoted by using various thermal agents. Strengthening exercises should systematically progress through isometrics, concentric and eccentric resistance, isokinetics, and CKC resistance exercises. Balance, coordination, and proprioceptive exercises are also included during the postimmobilization phases of rehabilitation. Stationary cycle ergometers, UBEs, stair climbers, and treadmills are tools that can enhance cardiorespiratory fitness both during and after immobilization.

❖ GLOSSARY

Bone matrix: Organic components—40% dry weight of bone, collagen, proteoglycans, glycoproteins, and phospholipids.

Bone types: Normal bone is lamellar. Immature or pathologic bone is woven, not stress oriented. Mature lamellar bone is cortical or cancellous.

Cancellous bone: Spongy or trabecular. Fractures generally progress at 6 weeks. Examples: calcaneus, vertebral body, radius, pelvis, and tibia.

Cortical bone: Eighty percent of adult skeleton.

Osteoblasts: Form bone. Increased endoplasmic reticulum, increased Golgi apparatus, and increased mitochondria.

Osteoclasts: Resorb bone. Bone resorption generally is more rapid than bone formation.

Osteocytes: Ninety percent of mature skeleton. Former osteoblasts that serve to maintain bone.

Piezoelectric effect: Compression side of bone is electronegative and stimulates osteoblasts. The tension side of bone is electropositive and stimulates osteoclasts.

Remodeling: Occurs long after the fracture has healed clinically. Woven bone formed during the repair phase is replaced with lamellar bone. Bone remodeling is affected by mechanical function according to Wolff's law. Removal of external stress can lead to significant bone loss. Bone remodels in response to stress and responds to piezoelectric charges.

Repair: Primary callus forms in about 2 weeks. Soft callus involving enchondral ossification occurs if fracture is not in continuity. Amount of callus is indirectly proportional to the degree of immobilization. Primary cortical healing occurs with immobilization and near anatomic reduction.

REFERENCES

1. Bassett C: Effect of force on skeletal tissue. In Downey JA, Darling RC, editors: *Physiological basis of rehabilitation medicine*, Philadelphia, 1971, Saunders.
2. Bennell K, Dannus P: Bone. In Kolt GS, Snyder-Mackler L, editors: *Physical therapies in sports and exercise*, London, 2003, Churchill Livingstone.
3. Bostrom MPG, Boskey A, Kaufman JK, et al: Form and function of bone. In Buckwalter JA, Einhorn TA, Simon SR, editors: *Orthopaedic basic science: biology and biomechanics of the musculoskeletal system*, Rosemont, Ill, 2000, American Academy of Orthopaedic Surgeons.
4. Brashear HR, Raney RB: *Fracture principles, fracture healing, Handbook of orthopaedic surgery*, St Louis, 1986, Mosby.
5. Buckwalter JA, Glimcher MJ, Cooper RR, et al: Bone biology, *J Bone Joint Surg Am* 77:1256–1277, 1995.
6. Busse JW, Bhandari M, Kulkarni AV, et al: The effect of low-intensity pulsed ultrasound therapy on time to fracture healing: a meta-analysis, *CMAJ* 166:437–441, 2002.
7. Busse JW, Kaur J, Mollon B, et al: Low intensity pulsed ultrasonography for fractures: systematic review of randomised controlled trials, *BMJ* 338:b351, 2009.

8. Day SM, Ostrum RE, Chao EYS, et al: Bone injury regeneration and repair. In Buckwalter JA, Einhorn TA, Simon SR, editors: *Orthopaedic basic science: biology and biomechanics of the musculoskeletal system*, Rosemont, Ill., 2000, American Academy of Orthopaedic Surgeons.

9. Einhorn TA: Enhancement of fracture-healing, *J Bone Joint Surg Am* 77:940–956, 1995.

10. Engles M: Tissue response. In Donatelli R, Wooden MJ, editors: *Orthopedic physical therapy*, New York, 1989, Churchill Livingstone.

11. Frankel VH, Nordin M: Biomechanics of bone. In Nordin M, Frankel VH, editors: *Basic biomechanics of the musculoskeletal system*, ed 3, Philadelphia, 2001, Lippincott Williams & Wilkins.

12. Frost HM: Mechanical determinants of skeletal architecture. In Albright JA, Brand RA, editors: *The scientific basis of orthopaedics*, ed 2, Norwalk, Conn, 1987, Appleton-Lange.

13. Hamilton HW: Five year's experience with continuous passive motion, *J Bone Joint Surg* 64B:259, 1982.

14. Heckman JD, Ryaby JP, McCabe J, et al: Acceleration of tibial fracture healing by non-invasive, low-intensity pulsed ultrasound, *J Bone Joint Surg* 76A:26–34, 1994.

15. Holtrop ME: In Hall BK, editor: *Bone, light and electron microscopic structure of bone-forming cells*, vol 1,Boca Raton, 1992, CRC Press.

16. Khan Y, Laurencin CT: Fracture repair with ultrasound: clinical and cell-based evaluation, *J Bone Joint Surg Am* 90:138–144, 2008.

17. Khan K, McKay H, Kannus P, et al: *Physical activity and bone health*, Champaign Ill, 2001, Human Kinetics.

18. Kisner C, Colby LA: *Therapeutic exercise: foundations and techniques*, Philadelphia, 1990, FA Davis.

19. Kristiansen TK, Ryaby JP, McCabe J, et al: Accelerated healing of distal radius fractures with the use of specific, low-intensity ultrasound. A multi-center, prospective, randomized, double-blind, placebo-controlled study, *J Bone Joint Surg* 79A:961–973, 1997.

20. Latta LL, Sarmiento A, Zych GA: Principles of nonoperative fractures. In Brown BD, Jupiter JB, Trafton PG, editors: *Skeletal trauma: fractures, dislocations, ligamentous injuries*, ed 2, Philadelphia, 1998, Saunders.

21. Lewis CB, Bottomley JM: *Geriatric physical therapy: a clinical approach*, New York, 1994, Appleton & Lange.

22. Li GP, Zhang SD, Chen G, et al: Radiographic and histologic analyses of stress fracture in rabbit tibias, *Am J Sports Med* 13:285–294, 1985.

23. Martin RB, Burr DB: *Structure, function, and adaptation of compact bone*, New York, 1989, Raven Press.

24. Mayr E, Rudzki MM, Rudzki M, et al: Acceleration by pulsed, low-intensity ultrasound of scaphoid fracture healing, *Handchir Mikrochir Plast Chir* 32:115–122, 2000.

25. Mazzocca AD, Caputo AE, Brown BD, et al: Principles of internal fixation. In Brown BD, Jupiter JB, Levine AM, et al, editors: *Skeletal trauma: fractures, dislocations, and ligamentous injuries*, Philadelphia, 1998, Saunders.

26. McRae R: *Practical fracture treatment*, New York, 1994, Churchill Livingstone.

27. Miller MD: *Review of orthopaedics*, Philadelphia, 1992, Saunders.

28. Morris JM: Fatigue fractures, *Calif Med* 108:268–274, 1968.

29. Nolte PA, van der Krans A, Patka P, et al: Low-intensity pulsed ultrasound in the treatment of nonunions, *J Trauma* 51:693–703, 2001.

30. Pollak AN, Ziran BH: Principles of external fixation. In Brown BD, Jupiter JB, Levine AM, et al, editors: *Skeletal trauma: fractures, dislocations, ligamentous bone injuries*, ed 2, Philadelphia, 1998, Saunders.

31. Rang M: *Children's fractures*, Philadelphia, 1974, JB Lippincott.

32. Rothstein JM, Roy SH, Wolf SL: *The rehabilitation specialists' handbook*, Philadelphia, 1991, FA Davis.

33. Salter RB: *Textbook of disorders and injuries of the musculoskeletal system*, ed 2, Baltimore, 1983, Williams & Wilkins.

34. Salter RB, Hamilton HW, Wedge JH, et al: Clinical applications of basic research on continuous passive motion for disorders and injuries of synovial joints. A preliminary report of a feasibility study, *J Orthop Res* 1:325–342, 1983.

35. Shenk RK: Biology of fracture repair. In Brown BD, Jupiter JB, Levine AM, et al, editors: *Skeletal trauma: fractures, dislocations, ligamentous bone injuries*, ed 2, Philadelphia, 1998, Saunders.

36. Steinburg FU: *The immobilized patient: functional pathology and management*, New York, 1980, Plenum.

37. Vernon-Roberts B: Morphological and functional interrelationships of bone cells and matrix, *Aust N Z J Med* 9:1–8, 1979.

REVIEW QUESTIONS

Short Answer

1. Name the two general methods used to immobilize fractures.
2. When treating a patient with an ORIF procedure in which a screw was used to stabilize a fracture, the PTA must be cautious of hardware loosening and "backing out." List three clinical signs of hardware loosening.

True/False

3. Compact bone heals faster than cancellous bone.
4. A reduced rate of bone healing (delayed union) can happen when physical therapy interventions are applied too soon or too vigorously.
5. When treating patients recovering from fractures, it is necessary to actively exercise all nonimmobilized joints.

10 Cartilage Healing

Erik P. Meira

LEARNING OBJECTIVES

1. Discuss the composition and function of articular cartilage.
2. Identify common causes of injury to articular cartilage.
3. Describe the sequence of healing and the extent of intrinsic repair of articular cartilage.
4. Define invasive and noninvasive techniques of stimulating articular cartilage repair.
5. Define and describe the composition and function of fibrocartilage.
6. Identify and discuss common mechanisms of injury to fibrocartilage.
7. Describe the mechanisms of intrinsic healing of the meniscus.

KEY TERMS

Angiogenesis

Articular cartilage

Chondrogenesis

Chondromalacia

Deep zone

Hyaline cartilage

Hydrophilic

Menisci (singular, meniscus)

CHAPTER OUTLINE

Learning Objectives

Key Terms

Chapter Outline

Articular Cartilage

  Composition

    Articular Cartilage Zones

    Collagen in Articular Cartilage

    Vascular Supply of Articular Cartilage

  Function

  Immobilization and Response to Healing

  Injury

  Healing and Repair

    Nonoperative Management for Articular Cartilage Pathology

    Operative Management for Articular Cartilage Pathology

Fibrocartilage

  Composition

  Function

  Injury

  Healing

Glossary

References

Review Questions

  Short Answer

  True/False

Understanding the mechanisms involved in the healing of articular (hyaline) cartilage and fibrocartilage guides the appropriate application of rehabilitation techniques. Proper rehabilitation techniques are based on the foundation of intrinsic cartilage repair (**chondrogenesis**), time necessary for healing, and extrinsic reparative interventions. Osteoarthritis, **chondromalacia** (softening of **hyaline cartilage**), meniscal lesions, labral tears, and many other cartilage pathologies are common problems the physical therapist assistant (PTA) sees clinically. Understanding the function, injury, and repair of articular cartilage and fibrocartilage helps the PTA execute appropriate rehabilitation techniques.

ARTICULAR CARTILAGE

Composition

Articular cartilage covers the ends of bones of synovial joints. It is composed primarily of water (approximately 65% to 80%),[11,13] which provides for load deformation of the cartilage surface.[16] The tensile strength of articular cartilage depends on type II collagen, which is approximately 20% of the total composition of articular cartilage.[19] Proteoglycans contribute 10% to 15% of the structure of articular cartilage. These proteoglycans are made up of glycosaminoglycans, which are in part responsible for bearing the compressive strength of articular cartilage. Finally, chondrocytes (mature cartilage cells) make up 5% of the articular cartilage.[16,19]

Articular Cartilage Zones

Articular cartilage is not homogeneous. The composition of articular cartilage varies considerably among four distinct zones. The superficial zone of articular cartilage is composed of water and parallel, highly organized collagen fibrils with very limited concentration of proteoglycans.[14] The middle or transitional zone of articular cartilage demonstrates randomly arranged, large diameter collagen and rounded chondrocytes.[14] The **deep zone** is rich in proteoglycans and lowest in water concentration. In this zone, collagen is large with a more organized structure that is arranged vertically.[14] The zone of calcified cartilage is the deepest zone that separates cartilage tissue from subchondral bone. This small distinct layer is composed mainly of cells, cartilage, matrix, and inorganic salts (Fig. 10-1 and Table 10-1).

Collagen in Articular Cartilage

Articular cartilage is an extremely unique biological tissue with both durable and permeable characteristics. Collagen represents more than 50% of the entire dry weight of articular cartilage.[14] The vast majority of collagen in articular cartilage is type II; however, the extracellular matrix also contains types IV, V, VI, X, and XL.

Clinicians must recognize the composition of various collagen types to fully appreciate the remarkable resilience of articular cartilage tissue. Collagen in general contains various amounts of proline, hydroxyproline, and hydroxylysine. The proline content of collagen provides a structure that is highly resistant to tensile forces. Conversely, hydroxyproline composition of collagen

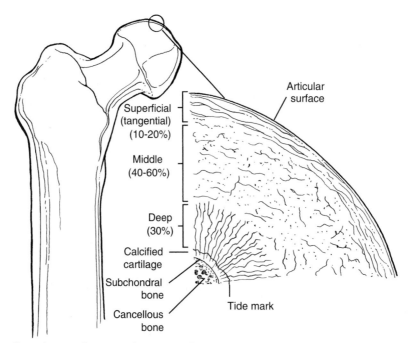

Fig. 10-1 Articular cartilage layers. (From Brinker MR, Miller MD, editors: *Fundamentals of orthopaedics*, Philadelphia, 1999, Saunders.)

Table 10-1	*Articular Cartilage Layers*			
Layer	Width (μm)	Characteristic	Orientation	Function
Gliding zone (superficial)	40	↓ Metabolic activity	Tangential	vs. Shear
Transitional zone (middle)	500	↑ Metabolic activity	Oblique	vs. Compression
Radial zone (deep)	1000	↑ Collagen size	Vertical	vs. Compression
Tidemark	5	Undulation barrier	Tangential	vs. Shear
Calcified zone	300	Hydroxyapatite crystals		Anchor

↑, Increased; ↓, decreased.
From Brinker MR, Miller MD: *Fundamentals of orthopaedics*, Philadelphia, 1999, Saunders.

Table 10-2	*Overview of Collagen Types*
Type	Location
I	Bone
	Tendon
	Meniscus
	Annulus of intervertebral disk
	Skin
II	Articular cartilage
	Nucleus pulposus of intervertebral disk
III	Skin
	Blood vessels
IV	Basement membrane
V	Articular cartilage (in small amounts)
VI	Articular cartilage (in small amounts)
VII	Basement membrane
VIII	Basement membrane
IX	Articular cartilage (in small amounts)
X	Hypertrophic cartilage
	Associated with calcification of cartilage (matrix mineralization)
XI	Articular cartilage (in small amounts)
XII	Tendon
XIII	Endothelial cells

From Brinker MR, Miller MD: *Fundamentals of orthopaedics*, Philadelphia, 1999, Saunders.

provides for the compressive stability of articular cartilage. Articular cartilage is composed of collagen types that are distinct in organization, structure, and fiber arrangement that are consistent with the zones of cartilage and their unique physiologic requirements of compression, tension, stiffness, strength, and durability (Table 10-2).[14]

Vascular Supply of Articular Cartilage

Vascularized tissues heal in an organized, predictable fashion. Trauma to vascular tissue incites an intense cascade of events characterized by hemorrhage, inflammation, and fibrin clot formation. **Angiogenesis,** or neovascularization, is the hallmark of intrinsic repair through mobilization of repair molecules and undifferentiated cells capable of synthesizing matrix and new tissue.[14]

Conversely, articular cartilage is a nonhomogeneous and avascular structure that lacks the ability to stimulate, regulate, or organize intrinsic repair.[1] Without an intense vascular response to injury, articular cartilage cannot form a fibrin scaffold or mobilize cells to repair the defect. Chondrocytes are essentially trapped within the dense extracellular matrix and are therefore incapable of traveling to the damaged site via a vascular access channel.[14]

This makes spontaneous healing of superficial wounds to articular cartilage limited. Since chondrocytes do not fill the defect, weak, fragile proteoglycans surround the injury. Deep injuries that communicate below the deep, calcified zone into subchondral bone produce a vascular inflammatory response to a limited extent. As expected, a fibrin clot forms a repairlike tissue but ultimately demonstrates a biochemically and mechanically weak scar.

Function

The viscoelastic structure of articular cartilage, by virtue of its component parts of collagen, water, and proteoglycans, makes articular cartilage incredibly durable.[16,19] Generally, articular cartilage is only 2 to 4 mm thick, yet it is capable of bearing compressive loads many times greater than body weight.[24] Articular cartilage is resistant to wear; has an extremely low coefficient of friction; and is responsible for influencing and dissipating compression, shear, and tension forces within synovial joints.[1,16,19,24]

Articular cartilage is also permeable. The chondrocytes within the cartilage must receive nutrition to remain viable. The synovial fluid surrounding the articular cartilage provides the necessary nutrients through diffusion, convection, or both.[19] Diffusion and convection are achieved through joint motion and normal physiologic weight bearing. Therefore normal joint motion is needed to maintain the cartilage integrity, fluid movement (lubrication between articulating surfaces), and nutrition of hyaline cartilage.[19]

Table 10-3	Biochemical Changes of Articular Cartilage	
Biochemical Structure	**Aging**	**Osteoarthritis (OA)**
Water content (hydration; permeability)	↓	↑
Collagen	Content remains relatively unchanged	Becomes disorderly (breakdown of matrix framework) Content ↓ in severe OA Relative concentration ↑ (because of loss of proteoglycans)
Proteoglycan content (concentration)	↓ (Also the length of the protein core and GAG chains decreases)	↓
Proteoglycan synthesis	↓	↑
Proteoglycan degradation	↓	↑
Chondroitin sulfate concentration (includes both chondroitin 4- and 6-sulfate)	↓	↑
Chondroitin 4-sulfate concentration	↓	↑
Keratin sulfate concentration	↑	↓
Chondrocyte size	↑	
Chondrocyte number	↓	
Modulus of elasticity	↑	↓

GAG, Glycosaminoglycan; ↑, increased; ↓, decreased.
From Brinker MR, Miller MD: *Fundamentals of orthopaedics*, Philadelphia, 1999, Saunders.

Immobilization and Response to Healing

Articular cartilage requires physiologic stress (e.g., cyclical compression) to maintain its unique environment as a strong, tough, fatigue-resistant, permeable, and low friction tissue.[14,15] The biochemical components of proteoglycans or glycosaminoglycans (GAGs), chondrocytes, matrix-molecules, and collagen significantly contribute to its structure, composition, and mechanical properties.[14,15]

Just as collagen is varied and distinct among the zones of articular cartilage, so are proteoglycans distributed in different concentrations between zones. Because these proteoglycan molecules—including chondroitin sulfate, keratan sulfate, and dermatan sulfate—bind and attract water (**hydrophilic**), their concentration and distribution among zones influence the various mechanical wear characteristics of articular cartilage.[14,15] The removal of normal physiologic loading, unloading, and joint motion have profoundly negative effects on the biochemical and mechanical characteristics of articular cartilage.[14,15]

The significance of articular cartilage atrophy and degeneration is related to the magnitude and duration of immobilization. Joint contact surfaces suffer greater degenerative changes than noncontact areas of articular cartilage (Table 10-3).[14,15]

Chondrocyte necrosis and subchondral bone degenerative lesions occur with prolonged rigid immobilization. Generally, immobilization and lack of physiologic stress cause a reduction in the synthesis and concentration of proteoglycans, which ultimately leads to surface fibrillation, fissures, and ulceration of the various zones of articular cartilage.[14,15]

Injury

Articular cartilage can be damaged in many ways.[1,19,24] Erosion and degeneration of the articular surface can be seen clinically in patients ranging from young athletes to the elderly. Causes of degenerative joint disease include related joint instability, blunt trauma, repetitive overloading, and immobilization.[24] Articular cartilage degeneration is generally characterized by three progressively overlapping degenerative events (Fig. 10-2).[24] Initially the hyaline cartilage begins to fray or fibrillate. Progressive destruction leads to blistering of the articular surface. Further joint deterioration leads to splitting or clefting (fissuring) of the surface. This affects the deeper layers of cartilage and eventually progresses to denuded bone.[24] Although blunt trauma, progressive friction abrasion, and a focal concentration of weight-bearing forces mechanically erode articular cartilage, joint immobilization does not cause these mechanical changes. However, joint immobilization may lead to loss of the load-bearing structural compression-resistant component GAGs.[19] Such loss is related to decreased normal joint loading and motion, which is needed for cartilage nutrition.

Articular cartilage erosion can occur after trauma, penetrating injury, infection, excessive shearing loads, joint immobilization, and/or reduction of normal joint mechanics. The therapeutic application of exercise and functional activities must be adjusted and modified to minimize the progressive destruction of tissue in patients who have a range of osteoarthritic changes to articular cartilage.

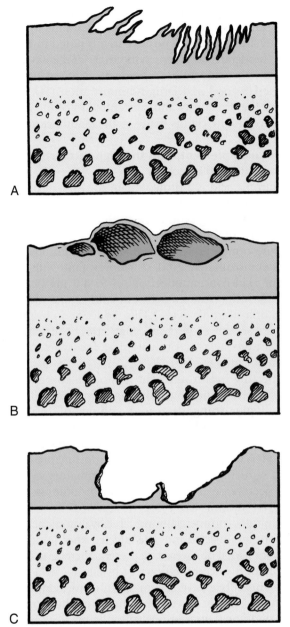

Fig. 10-2 Articular cartilage degeneration generally is characterized by three progressive overlapping stages: **A,** Fibrillation or fraying of articular cartilage. **B,** Blistering of articular surface. **C,** Splitting, clefting, or fissuring of articular surface.

Healing and Repair

Articular cartilage defects heal differently, depending on the extent or depth of the injury.[1,16,19,24] Less serious, more superficial lesions of articular cartilage do not spontaneously remodel or heal as well as deeper or full-thickness injuries due to the lack of vascularization. Healing of these superficial layers occurs through proteoglycans and limited chondrocyte proliferation, but the strength, composition, and durability of this healing tissue are inferior to those of normal articular cartilage.[19]

Superficial articular cartilage defects do not heal as well as deeper injuries because these injuries do not stimulate an inflammatory reaction.[19] The thickness of the articular cartilage (2 to 4 mm) forms a barrier between the superficial layers of the cartilage and subchondral blood vessels, effectively eliminating any contact among fibrin, fibroblasts, and inflammatory response cells (neutrophils, macrophages). In effect, the chondrocytes do not adhere to the defect and do not fill the injury site with new tissue.

Deeper wounds or full-thickness injuries expose subchondral bone blood vessels to the defect site, which stimulates the acute inflammatory response. Full-thickness cartilage injuries heal spontaneously with large amounts of Type I collagen. In fact, 1 year after injury, approximately 20% of the repaired defect remains type I collagen.[19] Although full-thickness injuries heal considerably better than superficial wounds, the quality of the scar formed within the defect remains inferior to normal articular cartilage because of the lack of type II collagen. The healed scar does not maintain its integrity over time.[19]

Nonoperative Management for Articular Cartilage Pathology

When treating patients recovering from injury, immobilization, or other damage to articular cartilage, appropriate physical therapy measures are those that stimulate cartilage repair.

Noninvasive therapeutic measures also are beneficial in the treatment of articular cartilage injury. Limited weight-bearing activities can arrest symptoms of pain and swelling in some cases of articular cartilage injury. Reducing vertical compressive loads (stair climbing, squats, and walking) is a critical first step in the care of tibiofemoral articular cartilage defects. Patients can maintain strength with isometric exercise or limited open kinetic chain (OKC) progressive–resistive exercise.

In cases of patellofemoral articular cartilage disease, vertical compressive loads generally do not negatively affect function. However, full range of motion (ROM) knee extension exercises may produce symptoms of pain, swelling, and crepitus (noise, grinding, and cracking). Limited ROM exercises that do not produce pain and crepitus, along with isometric exercises, are most appropriate with patellofemoral disease.

Continuous passive motion (CPM) is sometimes used in the care of articular cartilage injury. The benefits from the use of CPM appear to be limited to full-thickness hyaline cartilage defects.[21,22] Salter and colleagues[21,22] demonstrated that CPM used on full-thickness cartilage injury in rabbits showed healing of the defect with tissue resembling hyaline cartilage. Salter and associates,[20-22] who believe that CPM can help stimulate chondrocyte formation, also found that using CPM with full-thickness hyaline cartilage injuries improves articular cartilage nutrition by enhancing fluid mechanics, inhibiting adhesions, and clearing the joint of noxious material.

Maintaining near-normal joint motion through modified exercise regimens and weight-bearing activities (depending on the location and severity of the articular defect) is necessary for both healing of cartilage injuries and maintenance of hyaline cartilage nutrition.

Oral administration of glucosamine and chondroitin sulfate

Articular cartilage is composed of various collagen types and an extensive extracellular matrix of GAGs and proteoglycans. Major GAGs in human connective tissue are keratan sulfate, dermatan sulfate, heparin sulfate, chondroitin sulfate, and hyaluronic sulfate. Degenerative articular cartilage disease processes generally demonstrate an imbalance between production synthesis of proteoglycans and degradation of GAGs.

It should be recognized that proteoglycans and GAGs are extremely hydrophilic because of large negatively charged macromolecules referred to as *aggregates*. The binding and attraction for water contributes significant and important biochemical properties to articular cartilage to resist and influence compression and shear forces.

Catabolic processes involved with osteoarthritis (matrix metalloproteinases [MMPs], cytokines, and growth factors) create an imbalance between GAGs and proteoglycan synthesis and degradation. With reduction in proteoglycan content of articular cartilage (keratin sulfate, dermatan sulfate, heparin sulfate, hyaluronic acid, and predominantly chondroitin sulfate), the fluid-binding capacity of the large aggregate GAGs is lost. The result is a biochemically weaker structure that is increasingly vulnerable to compression, shear, and tensile loads, further stimulating the degradative processes of osteoarthritis.

The oral administration of two key constituents of articular cartilage proteoglycans and GAGs (glucosamine and chondroitin sulfate) may contribute to the reestablishment of fluid attraction, thereby reducing degenerative effects or preventing further erosion.

Generally, glucosamine is an amino saccharide that participates in the synthesis of GAGs and proteoglycans by chondrocytes.[6] Glucosamine is also an active substrate for the production of chondroitin sulfate, hyaluronic acid, and other proteoglycans in the articular cartilage matrix.[6]

Chondroitin sulfate is a GAG and significant constituent of large molecular mass proteoglycans referred to as *aggrecan*. The oral administration of glucosamine or chondroitin sulfate proposes a gradual "chondroprotective" role by reestablishing the water-binding nature of the articular cartilage matrix.

Clinical trials and commercial products recommend 500 mg three times daily as an effective regimen.[6] Glucosamine sulfate generally appears to have a more

rapid onset of effects (4 to 8 weeks), as compared with chondroitin sulfate (3 to 6 months).[6] Results in the literature are mixed with positive trends noted in patients with moderate to severe symptoms.[7] Because glucosamine is considered a supplement, it is not regulated by the US Food and Drug Administration (FDA). This means that the purity and concentration of the product can vary despite claims made by the manufacturer.

Viscosupplementation through intraarticular hyaluronic acid injection

Hyaluronic acid is a proteoglycan constituent of articular cartilage matrix and synovial fluid. Both fibroblasts and synoviocytes synthesize hyaluronic acid into the joint space of the knee.[26]

The normal, nonpathologic human adult knee contains approximately 2 mL of synovial fluid with a hyaluronic acid concentration of 2.5 to 4.0 mg per mL.[26] Osteoarthritis creates a deficit in volume and molecular mass of hyaluronic acid.[26] This reduction in hyaluronic acid causes lower viscosity, high stress concentration, and lowered elastic properties of the synovium and articular cartilage matrix.[26]

Injecting hyaluronic acid is thought to benefit the osteoarthritic knee by reducing pain and inflammation, replenishing decreased volume of hyaluronic acid, and stimulating intrinsic synovial synthesis of hyaluronic acid.[26] Hyaluronic acid injections are shown to reduce inflammation by limiting prostaglandins, reducing circulating proinflammatory cytokine, and decreasing the release of arachidonic acid from synovial fibroblasts.[26]

Typically, commercially available hyaluronic acid preparations are injected into the affected knee joint once a week for a total of 3 weeks. At present, there is no consensus about the clinical efficacy of hyaluronic acid intraarticular injections. Several clinical trials have demonstrated no increased joint function or pain relief when compared with traditional nonsteroidal antiinflammatory agents or intraarticular steroidal preparations. However, clinical trials of hyaluronic acid injections versus placebo favor its use. The rate of side effects is approximately 1% per injection. Local site reaction of pain, warmth, and swelling are most common and last 1 to 2 days.[26]

Operative Management for Articular Cartilage Pathology

Various surgical interventions are at the disposal of the surgeon that are designed to stimulate an intense inflammatory response or to débride and irrigate (lavage) cartilage debris from within the joint (Fig. 10-3).

Débridement

Short-term temporary relief of symptomatic articular cartilage lesions can be achieved with arthroscopic lavage or débridement of cartilaginous debris. Essentially,

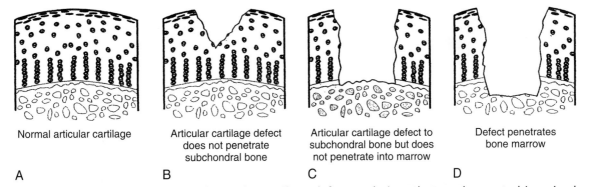

Normal articular cartilage	Articular cartilage defect does not penetrate subchondral bone	Articular cartilage defect to subchondral bone but does not penetrate into marrow	Defect penetrates bone marrow
A	**B**	**C**	**D**

Fig. 10-3 The various types and depths of articular cartilage defects or lesions that can be created in animal models to evaluate repair processes in articular cartilage. **A,** Normal articular cartilage is typically organized histologically into zones. **B,** A partial-thickness (superficial or shallow) defect penetrating to the middle zone is isolated from the blood supply and marrow space. Such a defect typically does not elicit or demonstrate a repair response. **C,** A lesion that penetrates to the subchondral bone but does not penetrate into the marrow space, if truly isolated from the marrow, will not repair. However, even a very small communication of the lesion with the marrow blood supply will elicit a repair response. Full-thickness lesions usually are in this category. **D,** A defect that penetrates through all zones of the articular cartilage and penetrates into the marrow space typically demonstrates a repair response that results in fibrocartilaginous tissue. (From Jackson DW, Scheer MJ, Simon TM: Cartilage substitutes: overview of basic science and treatment options, *J Am Acad Orthop Surg* 9:42, 2001.)

arthroscopic débridement removes particles of cartilage, degradative enzymes such as MMPs, and proinflammatory cytokines, all of which contribute to the painful disability of articular cartilage osteoarthritic lesions. The benefit of arthroscopic débridement is often temporary because of the lack of a true inflammatory response or cellular proliferation. Joint lavage (irrigation) with saline inflow provides a substantial isolated benefit by removing tissue debris and inflammatory cells even without surgical intervention of articular shavers with suction.[10]

Microfracture

Articular cartilage repair is promoted when the injury site can go through the inflammatory process and when factors lead to chondrocyte proliferation. With some cartilage defects, surgically abrading or fracturing multiple small holes through the cartilage layers down to bone stimulates bleeding and initiates the healing process (Fig. 10-4).[2]

Initially, the bleeding response produces a "superclot" over the chondral defect. The desired outcome of this penetrating technique is the development of fibrocartilage consisting of type I collagen, which attempts to fill the defect. Being different from the type II collagen of normal articular cartilage, the repair tissue that forms from microfracture is histochemically and biochemically fragile and weak when compared with structurally intact articular cartilage. The repair also lacks the anatomically distinct layers of differing collagen types characteristic of normal articular cartilage, which provide additional protection from compression, shear, and tensile loads.[2]

Microfracture has been shown to provide short-term functional improvement, but long-term efficacy is still

unknown.[17] Outcomes are highest when performed on younger patients with cartilage defects that are surrounded by normal articular cartilage.[2]

Arthroscopic osteochondral autografts

Full-thickness articular lesions (osteochondral) can be surgically filled with transplanted plugs of intact bone and articular cartilage using the technique of mosaicplasty or osteochondral autograft transplantation system (OATS) (Fig. 10-5).

The surgeon prepares the lesion by removing all nonviable surrounding tissue from the crater, thereby creating precise borders of the lesion. Multiple full-thickness bone plugs are surgically harvested from a relatively non–load-bearing surface of the femur, usually the superior lateral femoral condyle or, less often, the inferior condylar notch. Harvest site morbidity is a concern because full-knee ROM provides significant contact pressure of the mentioned harvest sites.[10] These cylindrical osteochondral plugs become revascularized (incorporated) into the lesion. These "press-fit" plugs contain viable hyaline cartilage, which tends to survive over time and remains structurally stable.[2,10]

Several key factors may compromise the outcome of the OATS technique. The convex geometry of the femoral condyles contributes to a relative joint incongruence because the shape of the plugs may not match the surrounding surface with anatomic precision. In addition, the depth placement of the chondral plugs is critical because the donor plugs may collapse or settle over time or may be inserted with too much "pride" (the surface of the plugs may sit too high above the horizon of the chondral plate).[10]

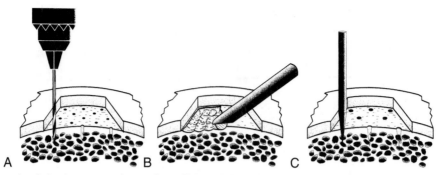

Fig. 10-4 Various methodologies currently used to elicit repair tissue in articular cartilage defects. **A,** Current methods involve penetrating the underlying bone endplate by drilling, as proposed in the Pridie procedure. Variations include abrasion **(B)** and microfracture **(C).** All these techniques penetrate the subchondral bond to open communication with a zone of vascularization to initiate fibrin clot formation and obtain the potential benefit of vascular ingrowth or migration of more primitive mesenchymal cells from the bone marrow. These communications open the defect to the migration of many types of cells, including fibroblasts and inflammatory cells. These cells may compete with a limited number of the primitive mesenchymal cells to occupy the fibrin matrix, contributing to a variety of repair scenarios. These methods penetrate the subchondral bone plate and tidemark, but the intent is not to disrupt the integrity of the subchondral bone. Large disruption or removal of the subchondral bone end plate may result in detrimental mechanical, structural, and biological changes. (From Jackson DW, Scheer MJ, Simon TM: Cartilage substitutes: overview of basic science and treatment options, *J Am Acad Orthop Surg* 9:45, 2001.)

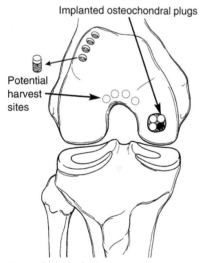

Fig. 10-5 Osteochondral plug transplantation technique. The lesion site is prepared by débriding any loose articular cartilage, and the number and size of the plugs to be used for repair are determined. The holes to receive the plugs are drilled in the floor of the lesion. With use of specialized harvesting instrumentation, the osteochondral plugs are procured from suitable sites so as to approximate the surface geometry of the lesion site. The plugs are then implanted to the appropriate depth into the holes placed in the lesion base. (From Jackson DW, Scheer MJ, Simon TM: Cartilage substitutes: overview of basic science and treatment options, *J Am Acad Orthop Surg* 9:48, 2001.)

Autologous chondrocyte implantation

Because of substantial variations in collagen types, orientation, proteoglycan content, extracellular matrix composition, and avascularity of the four anatomically distinct zones of articular cartilage, a tissue implantation procedure is available to generate a biologic substitute tissue.[2,10]

The autologous chondrocyte implantation (ACI) procedure calls for two separate surgical interventions. First the surgeon harvests articular cartilage from the superomedial edge of the trochlea or the lateral edge of the intercondylar notch. This harvested tissue is sent to a specific laboratory, where the chondrocytes are enzymatically separated from the extracellular matrix, cultured, and multiplied. The second procedure typically occurs 6 to 18 weeks after harvesting. At this time, a periosteal patch may be harvested from the proximal medial tibia.[2] However, concern regarding hypertrophy of the periosteum has lead to the development of second generation patches such as porcine derived collagen.[5,8] This patch is then secured with fibrin glue and sutures over the defect. The cultured chondrocytes are injected under the patch to fill the defect with biologically active viable chondrocytes (Fig. 10-6).

FIBROCARTILAGE

Understanding fibrocartilage injury and repair is a necessary foundation for the appropriate delivery of rehabilitation programs. The PTA also must be aware of the differences in healing between articular cartilage and fibrocartilage.

Composition

Fibrocartilage is found within the synovial joints of the shoulder, hip, and knee. A large percentage of fibrocartilage is water.[12] The collagen in fibrocartilage is

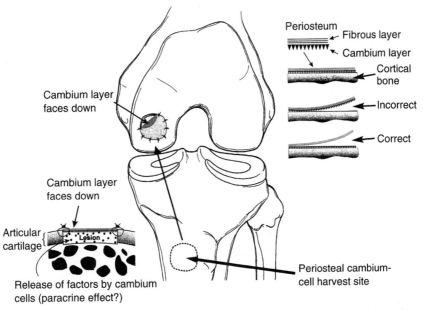

Fig. 10-6 Autologous chondrocyte implantation technique. Articular cartilage is procured, and its chondrocytes are enzymatically released and expanded in cell culture. When a sufficient number of cells are obtained, a second operation is performed for implantation of the cultured cells. A periosteal flap with matching geometry is harvested and sutured in place with the cambium cell layer facing the defect (down). Care must be taken to ensure that the cambium cells remain attached to the periosteal fibrous layer *(insets)*. (From Jackson DW, Scheer MJ, Simon TM: Cartilage substitutes: overview of basic science and treatment options, *J Am Acad Orthop Surg* 9:46, 2001.)

made up almost entirely of type I collagen. Proteoglycans and elastin (0.6%) complete the components of fibrocartilage.[3]

Function

The **menisci** of the knee are semilunar (C-shaped) fibrocartilage tissues that have several functions. Generally the meniscus dissipates extreme compressive (vertical) loads. By virtue of its anatomic position within the knee and its collagen makeup, the meniscus acts as a mechanical buffer between the load-bearing surfaces of the tibia and the femur. The meniscus of the knee also functions as a shock absorber.[3] Studies have shown that a knee without a meniscus has 20% less shock-absorbing capacity than normal knees.[25]

The meniscus may also function as a secondary restraint in joint stability. Several factors influence its effect, including ligament stability, joint surface congruency, and joint compression loads.[3] Significant joint instability does not occur with an isolated, total meniscectomy. However, a meniscectomy combined with anterior cruciate ligament injuries produces profound joint instability.[23]

The meniscus also limits knee hyperextension as a passive restraint and functions in joint lubrication and nutrition.[12] Normal physiologic joint motion promotes the lubricating effects of a thin layer of fluid between the joint surfaces. The meniscus may spread this lubrication medium during motion.[18]

The glenoid labrum of the shoulder and the acetabular labrum of the hip are also made up of fibrocartilage. It surrounds the glenoid and acetabulum respectively providing increased joint surface congruency. The role of the labrum is to provide stability to the joint through this increased congruency and as an anchor point for other structures.

Injury

Injuries to the meniscus can be traumatic or degenerative. Traumatic intraarticular fibrocartilage tears usually occur in a younger population (<40 years) and generally result from a combination of compression, torque, acceleration, or deceleration. These events usually occur during running, jumping, twisting, and dynamic change-of-direction activities.

Degenerative meniscal tears typically occur in an older population (>40 years). Patients with these injuries do not present with a history of sudden trauma, but rather with a minor event that precipitates complaints of pain and dysfunction.[3]

Injuries to the glenoid labrum often occur through direct trauma or repetitive stress. Detachment of the anterior-inferior labrum (Bankart lesion) is a common injury produced by anterior shoulder dislocation. The long head of the biceps tendon (LHBT) attaches to the superior labrum. Tears of the superior labrum, anterior to posterior (SLAP) lesions, are sometimes caused by trauma but are often caused by repetitive stress from the biceps tendon during throwing activities.

The most common injury to the acetabular labrum is through repeated bony contact seen in femoroacetabular impingement (FAI). The labrum can become torn or detached over time as the femur repeatedly makes contact during deep hip flexion or internal rotation. Traumatic tears also occur, typically in hip extension.

Healing

The vascular anatomy of fibrocartilage profoundly influences the type of healing that occurs and the degree of remodeling, such as with articular cartilage. The peripheral borders of the medial and lateral meniscus of the knee are vascularized between 10% and 30% of the width of the tissue.[3] If an injury occurs within a nonvascular region of the meniscus, spontaneous, intrinsic repair is not possible because no vascular supply communicates with the injury site. However, if the injury extends to the periphery where the cartilage is vascularized, healing is possible through the inflammatory–response mechanism.

Decisions regarding surgical repair or excision of meniscal tissue are based on the extent of the injury and location. If the tear is within the vascularized peripheral border (only 15% to 20% of all meniscal injuries occur within the vascularized bed of the meniscus), arthroscopic repair can be done by placing sutures in the meniscus to approximate the torn tissue.[3] Surgeons refer to the following zone system of evaluating meniscal injuries[9]:

■ Zone I: Both portions of the meniscus are torn within the vascularized periphery; "red-on-red"
■ Zone II: One portion of the meniscus is torn within the vascularized periphery, whereas the other portion is in the avascular region; "red-on-white"
■ Zone III: There is no blood supply on either side of the injury; "white-on-white"

Both red-on-red and red-on-white zones are considered reparable. When injuries occur in an avascular portion of the meniscus, the surgeon must perform either a partial or total meniscectomy. However, in animal studies,[4] when an injury was present within the white-on-white nonvascularized Zone III area of the meniscus, researchers surgically created a "vascular access channel" to connect the blood supply of the periphery to the area of injury without circulation.[3,4] These changes allowed blood vessels to migrate to the injury site and provided an avenue for repair.

In labral injuries of the hip and shoulder, torn or frayed fibrocartilage is similar to the white-on-white lesions in the meniscus. Because of a lack of blood supply, these are simply débrided. Labral detachments are more like the red-on-white lesions in the meniscus and usually respond well to surgical repair. Before reattachment, a bleeding bone bed is exposed in order to promote healing down of the labrum.

❖ GLOSSARY

Angiogenesis: The physiologic process during healing of bodily tissues in which new capillary blood vessels are formed from preexisting vasculature.

Articular cartilage: Concentration of collagen, proteoglycans, and water influences tensile forces, compression, shear, and permeability.

Chondrogenesis: Intrinsic cartilage repair.

Chondromalacia: Softening of hyaline cartilage.

Deep zone: Largest part of the articular cartilage. Contains the largest collagen fibrils and has the highest proteoglycan content and lowest water content.

Hyaline cartilage: A synonym for articular cartilage.

Hydrophilic: A quality of a molecule that causes it to bind to and attract water.

Menisci (singular, meniscus): Semilunar (C-shaped) fibrocartilage tissues in the knee that act as a mechanical buffer between the load-bearing surfaces of the tibia and the femur.

REFERENCES

1. Alford JW, Cole BJ: Cartilage restoration, part 1: basic science, historical perspective, patient evaluation, and treatment options, *Am J Sports Med* 33(2):295–306, 2005.
2. Alford JW, Cole BJ: Cartilage restoration, part 2: techniques, outcomes, and future directions, *Am J Sports Med* 33(2):443–460, 2005.
3. Arnoczky SP, Adams M, DeHaven K, et al: Meniscus. In Buschbacher JA, Woo SL-Y, editors: *Injury and repair of the musculoskeletal soft tissues*, Rosemont, Ill, 1988, American Academy of Orthopaedic Surgeons.
4. Arnoczky SP, Warren RF: The microvasculature of the meniscus and its response to injury. An experimental study in the dog, *Am J Sports Med* 11:131–141, 1983.
5. Bartlett W, Skinner JA, Gooding CR, et al: Autologous chondrocyte implantation versus matrix-induced autologous chondrocyte implantation for osteochondral defects of the knee, *J Bone Joint Surg Br* 87:640–645, 2005.
6. Brief AA, Maurer SG, Di Cesare PE: Use of glucosamine and chondroitin sulfate in the management of osteoarthritis, *J Am Acad Orthop Surg* 9:71–78, 2001.
7. Clegg DO, Reda DJ, Harris CL, et al: Glucosamine, chondroitin sulfate, and the two in combination for painful knee osteoarthritis, *N Engl J Med* 354:795–808, 2006.
8. Haddo O, Mahroof S, Higgs D, et al: The use of chondrogide membrane in autologous chondrocyte implantation, *Knee* 11:51–55, 2004.
9. Hammesfahr JR: Surgery of the knee. In Donatelli R, Wooden MJ, editors: *Orthopaedic physical therapy*, New York, 1989, Churchill Livingstone.
10. Jackson DW, Scheer MJ, Simon TM: Cartilage substitutes: overview of basic science and treatment options, *J Am Acad Orthop Surg* 9:37–52, 2001.
11. Jaffe FF, Mankin HJ, Weiss H, et al: Water binding in the articular cartilage of rabbits, *J Bone Joint Surg* 56A:1031–1039, 1974.
12. MacConaill MA: The function of intraarticular fibrocartilages, with special reference to the knee and inferior radio-ulnar joints, *J Anat* 66:210–227, 1932.
13. Mankin HJ: The water of articular cartilage. In Simon WH, editor: *The human joint in health and disease*, Philadelphia, 1978, University of Pennsylvania Press.
14. Mankin HJ, Mow VC, Buckwalter JA, et al: Articular cartilage structure, composition, and function. In Buckwalter JA, Einhorn TA, Simon SR, editors: *Orthopaedic basic science, biology, and biomechanics*, ed 2, Rosemont, Ill, 2000, American Academy of Orthopaedic Surgeons.

15. Mankin JH, Mow VC, Buckwalter JA, et al: Articular cartilage repair and osteoarthritis. In Buckwalter JA, Einhorn TA, Simon SR, editors: *Orthopaedic basic science, biology, and biomechanics*, ed 2, Rosemont, Ill, 2000, American Academy of Orthopaedic Surgeons.

16. Miller MD: *Review of orthopaedics*, Philadelphia, 1992, Saunders.

17. Mithoefer K, McAdams T, Williams RJ, et al: Clinical efficacy of the microfracture technique for articular cartilage repair in the knee: an evidence-based systematic analysis, *Am J Sports Med* 10(10):1–11, 2009.

18. Radin EL, Bryan RS: The effect of weight bearing on regrowth of the medial meniscus after meniscectomy, *J Trauma* 12:169, 1970.

19. Rosenberg L: Articular cartilage. In Woo SL-Y, Buckwalter JA, editors: *Injury and repair of the musculoskeletal soft tissues*, Rosemont, Ill, 1988, American Academy of Orthopaedic Surgeons.

20. Salter RB, Hamilton HW, Wedge JH, et al: Clinical application of basic research on continuous passive motion for disorders and injuries of synovial joints: a preliminary report of a feasibility study, *J Orthop Res* 1:325–342, 1984.

21. Salter RB, Mister RR, Bell RS, et al: Continuous passive motion and the repair of full-thickness articular cartilage defects: a one year follow-up, *Trans Orthop Res Soc* 7:167, 1982.

22. Salter RB, Simmonds DF, Malcolm BW, et al: The biological effect of continuous passive motion on healing of full-thickness defects in articular cartilage. An experimental investigation in the rabbit, *J Bone Joint Surg Am* 62:1232–1251, 1980.

23. Shoemaker SC, Markolf KL: The role of the meniscus in the anterior-posterior stability of the loaded anterior cruciate-deficient knee. Effects of partial versus total excision, *J Bone Joint Surg Am* 68:71–79, 1986.

24. Threlkeld JA: Electrical stimulation of articular cartilage. In Currier DP, Nelson RM, editors: *Dynamics of human biologic tissues*, Philadelphia, 1992, FA Davis.

25. Voloshin AS, Wosk J: Shock absorption of meniscectomized and painful knees: a comparative in vivo study, *J Biomed Eng* 5:157–161, 1983.

26. Watterson JR, Esdaile JM: Viscosupplementation: therapeutic mechanisms and clinical potential in osteoarthritis in the knee, *J Am Acad Orthop Surg* 8:277–284, 2000.

REVIEW QUESTIONS

Short Answer

1. Name the three classic surgical procedures used to correct tears of the meniscus.
2. The meniscus of the knee can be injured in two distinct ways. Name the two classifications of meniscal injuries.

True/False

3. If an injury were to occur to the central nonvascular portion of the meniscus, spontaneous intrinsic repair is not possible.
4. Normal joint motion and compressive loads are necessary for hyaline (articular) cartilage to remain viable.
5. The deeper and more extensive the damage to articular cartilage, the less "healing" occurs.
6. Superficial articular cartilage lesions heal much quicker and to a greater degree than significant wounds.
7. CPM is used to help stimulate cartilage nutrition in partial-thickness articular cartilage lesions.
8. The meniscus of the knee serves as a primary joint restraint.
9. The central portion of the medial and lateral meniscus is essentially avascular.

11 Muscle and Tendon Injuries

Jason Brumitt

LEARNING OBJECTIVES

1. Recognize the macrostructure and microstructure of muscle and tendon.
2. Describe the two main types of muscle fibers.
3. Describe the three mechanisms for a muscle injury.
4. Describe the injury mechanism's associated tendon pathology.
5. Name the functional unit of a tendon and its structural significance.
6. Describe the difference between a supraphysiologic and a subfailure load and how each type may contribute to an injury.
7. Define how a muscle strain differs from a ligament sprain.
8. Describe the differences between a tendonitis and a tendinopathy.
9. Describe the effects of aging on tendons.
10. Name and describe the three phases of connective tissue healing.
11. Describe the effects of immobilization on connective tissue.
12. Discuss clinical applications of therapeutic interventions based on the stages of connective tissue healing.

KEY TERMS

Endomysium

Epimysium

Perimysium

Muscle strain

CHAPTER OUTLINE

Skeletal muscles, and by extension their tendons, are responsible for human movement. Injury to a muscle or a tendon may significantly impact one's functional ability. One's experience after a muscle or tendon injury may range in severity from minor pain with minimal functional loss to severe pain with prolonged or permanent functional loss. A person who has sustained a muscle or tendon injury may benefit from a supervised clinical rehabilitation program.

For many patients who have sustained a muscle or tendon injury, or both, a conservative physical therapy treatment program may help reduce pain, increase range of motion (ROM) and strength, and restore functional abilities. To maximize a patient's recovery, communication between the physical therapist (PT) and the physical therapist assistant (PTA) is crucial. The PTA should be informed as to how and when the patient was injured and be able to integrate that knowledge to appreciate the patient's current stage of healing. Using this information is crucial to understanding why one patient is progressing and tolerating treatment, whereas a different patient's progress is plateauing or regressing.

The purpose of this chapter is to review the functional anatomy of the muscle and tendon, present the pathomechanics associated with common muscle and tendon injuries, identify the various types of muscle and tendon injuries, present an overview of the body's response to injury and the healing process, and present evidence-based and evidence-supported treatments to facilitate muscle and tendon healing.

MUSCLE AND TENDON FUNCTIONAL ANATOMY

Macrostructure of Muscle and Tendons

Functional movement of the human body is performed by the interaction of more than 600 skeletal muscles and their respective tendons. Skeletal muscles are complex tissues consisting of muscle fibers, connective tissue, blood supply, and innervating nerves. Tendons, fibrous connective tissue consisting of collagen fibers, extend from the skeletal muscle to provide an attachment to bone. The contraction of a muscle creates movement about a joint through the tension applied to the tendon.

The transition zone between the muscle and the tendon is known as the *musculotendinous junction*. The anatomic arrangement at the musculotendinous junction allows for the transmission of force from the muscle to the tendon. The attachment between a tendon and a bone is known as the *tendo-osseous junction*.

Microstructure of Muscle

The muscle consists of muscle fibers and connective tissue (Fig. 11-1). There are three layers of connective tissue: the **epimysium,** the **perimysium,** and the **endomysium.**

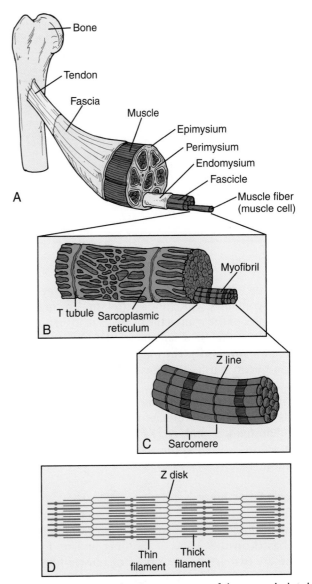

Fig. 11-1 Macro- and microstructure of human skeletal muscle. **A,** Skeletal muscle organ, composed of bundles of contractile muscle fibers held together by connective tissue. **B,** Greater magnification of single fiber showing small fibers, myofibrils, in the sarcoplasm. **C,** Myofibril magnified further to show sarcomere between successive Z lines. Cross striae are visible. **D,** Molecular structure of myofibril showing thick myofilaments and thin myofilaments. (From Cameron MH, Monroe LG: *Physical rehabilitation: evidence-based examination, evaluation, and intervention,* St Louis, 2006, Saunders.)

The epimysium surrounds the muscle and (along with the perimysium and the endomysium) is continuous with the muscle's tendons. Within the muscle, groups of muscle fibers (known as a *fasciculus*) are surrounded by the perimysium. Within each fasciculus, each individual muscle fiber is surrounded by the endomysium.

A muscle fiber (muscle cell) is further divided into myofibrils and myofilaments (see Fig. 11-1). Each muscle fiber is surrounded by a sarcolemma, the muscle fiber's

Table 11-1	Summary of Physical and Physiologic Differences Among the Three Most Common Skeletal Muscle Fiber Types		
Parameter	**Type I**	**Type IIA**	**Type IIB**
Cell body size	Small	Medium	Large
Conduction velocity	Slow	Fast	Fast
Number of muscle fibers	Few	More	Most
Rate of force development	Slow	Moderate	Fast
Absolute force generation	Low	Moderate	High
Resistance to fatigue	High	Moderate	Low
Mitochondrial density	High	High	Low
Aerobic capacity	High	Moderate	Low
Myoglobin content	High	Low	Low

cellular membrane. Within the muscle fiber, the myofibrils are contained within the sarcoplasm. The myofibrils are bundles of the contractile proteins myosin and actin grouped together as a sarcomere (the basic functional unit of the myofibril). The interaction between the myosin and actin during the muscle's contraction contributes to functional movement. The structural relationship between the contractile and noncontractile components allows skeletal muscles to perform both concentric (shortening) and eccentric (lengthening) muscle contractions as well as the ability to return to a resting position.[18]

Muscle Fiber Types

Several types of muscle fibers have been identified in skeletal muscle. The differences between muscle fibers are based on the shape of the fiber and its function. There are two general categories of muscle fiber types: fast twitch (FT) and slow twitch (ST). The "twitch" term relates to the time it takes muscle fibers (and its associated nerve) to contract and relax.

ST muscle fibers are also known as *type I muscle fibers*. The type I fibers appear red because of the presence of myoglobin, an oxygen-binding protein. This is an important feature of the type I muscle fiber because it is specifically adapted for continuous aerobic activity; therefore the type I muscle fibers are generally fatigue resistant. Examples of muscle groups consisting of a high number of type I fibers are the soleus and the erector spinae, postural muscles that must contract either repetitively or require being held for long durations.

Whereas the type I (ST) muscle fibers possess a high endurance capacity, the type II (FT) muscle fibers differ in that they are specialized for more anaerobic activities. There are several types of FT fibers that are differentiated by their resistance to fatigue, their functional use, and the type of myosin heavy chain (MHC) protein complex present (Table 11-1).[27]

Within the literature, there are at least eight types of named muscle fibers: I, IC, IIA, IIB, IIC, IID, IIX (IIB), and IIAX.[7,9,12,15,27,30,31,35] However, this does not mean that there are eight distinct fiber types. Rather, there appears to be an inconsistency in the literature as to how the fibers are named.[7,9,12,15,27,30,31,35] While the PTA can appreciate that there is variability among sources about the actual number of different fiber types, it is more important to appreciate the two broad categories of muscle fibers: type I and type II. Type I are the slow, oxidative fibers and type II are the fast, glycolytic fibers. There are significant differences between the two main types that have functional implications. The exercise prescription strategy used during different phases of the healing process should take into account the primary fiber composition of the injured skeletal muscle. The characteristics of the three most common fiber types in human skeletal muscle characteristics—types I, IIA, and IIB—will be compared in this chapter (see Table 11-1).[7,31,35]

Microstructure of Tendon

Tendons serve two functions: to facilitate movement or joint stability by transmitting forces between muscle and bone, and to store energy for later movement. An example of this is the energy created during plyometric exercises. The series elastic component stores elastic energy created during plyometric exercises in response to an eccentric stretch of the muscle. Tendons have the ability to withstand significant physiologic loads; however, they may be at risk of injury by either trauma, degeneration, or overuse. A tendon's structure is divided into three locations: the muscle–tendon junction, the midsubstance, and the bone–tendon junction.

Tendons are dense connective tissue consisting of fibroblasts (cells) and an extracellular matrix composed of collagen fibers, elastin, and ground substance (Fig. 11-2). The fibroblasts are responsible for synthesizing

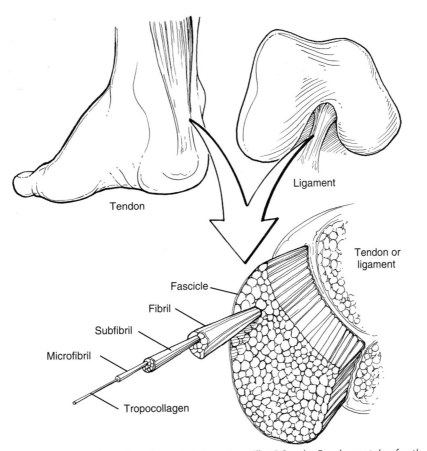

Fig. 11-2 Macro- and microstructure of tendon. (From Brinker MR, Miller DS, eds: *Fundamentals of orthopaedics*, Philadelphia, 1999, Saunders.)

components of the extracellular matrix.[28] The ground substance provides support to collagen fibers.[28] The collagen fibers, which are oriented in a parallel arrangement, provide strength to resist tensile forces.

The structural hierarchy of tendons is similar to skeletal muscle. Collagen fibrils are grouped together into the tendon's basic functional unit, the collagen fiber. Groups of collagen fibers (primary fiber bundle) form a subfascicle.[16] Several subfascicles grouped together form a fascicle (secondary fiber bundle).[16] Several fascicles grouped together form a tertiary bundle.[16] These three groups (bundles) are surrounded by a connective tissue called the *endotenon*.[16] The epitenon surrounds the entire tendon as a fine, loose connective tissue sheath.[16,28] Blood vessels and nerves are also contained within the epitenon.[28] The paratenon is a loose areolar connective tissue attaching to the outer portion of the epitenon.[16,28] The function of the paratenon is to allow gliding over adjacent structures.[16]

The transition from tendon into its osseous attachment site includes several connective tissue changes.[16] The first change is from the primary tendon structure into fibrocartilage. Next, the fibrocartilage converts into a mineralized fibrocartilage. The mineralized fibrocarti-

lage secures the attachment of the tendon to the bone. In addition to this arrangement, there are collagen fibers from the tendon that pass through these transition zones and attach to the bone. These fibers are known as *Sharpey's fibers*.

MUSCLE AND TENDON INJURIES

The human body experiences a range of physical loads and stresses during activities, work, and sports. These forces on the body, whether they are a onetime supraphysiologic load that is greater than a tissue's tolerance or a subfailure load that is experienced for a prolonged period of time, may contribute to a musculoskeletal injury.

Examples from the world of sports will help illustrate the significant loads and stresses that may be experienced by some athletes. During the deceleration phase of pitching a baseball, the pitcher's shoulder rotates up to 7000° per second with 400 newtons (N) of posterior shear forces, 300 N of inferior shear forces, and 1000 N of compressive forces experienced at the glenohumeral joint (Fig. 11-3, *A*).[20] Over time, these shear and compressive forces may increase the baseball pitcher's risk of sustaining a shoulder injury.[20,21,34] During the golf

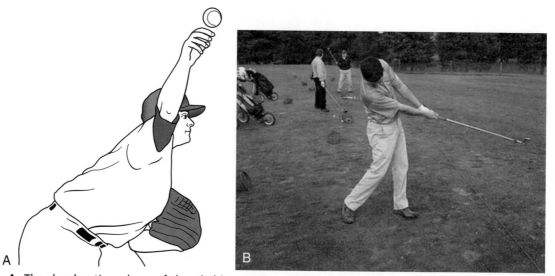

Fig. 11-3 A, The deceleration phase of the pitching motion. **B,** The follow-through phase of the golf swing. (**A,** From Ellenbecker T: *Clinical examination of the shoulder,* St Louis, 2005, Saunders.)

swing, a golfer may experience compressive loads in the lumbar spine that are eight times his or her body weight (Fig. 11-3, *B*).[11] To provide some perspective, a distance runner will experience compressive loads that are equal to three times his or her body weight during the run. To reduce the risk of injury, muscles and tendons must possess the ability to stretch or deform in response to the applied load. When an applied load supersedes the muscle or tendon's ability to resist tensile forces, the muscle or tendon is at a higher risk of injury.

Muscle and Tendon Injury Mechanisms

A patient's rehabilitation program will be developed by the PT based on the patient's medical history, the patient's subjective report, and the PT's physical evaluation of the patient. When guiding a patient through his or her treatment program, the PTA should be familiar with the patient's diagnosis and mechanism of the injury. Possessing this knowledge will help the PTA advance the rehabilitation program per the PT's plan and will alert the PTA to cease treatment and consult with the PT when the patient demonstrates a negative response to treatment.

A muscle injury may be caused by disease, a direct (external) mechanism, or an indirect (internal) mechanism. Some diseases may have profound effects on the muscular system and contribute to significant disability. Examples of diseases that weaken muscles include muscular dystrophy, multiple sclerosis (MS), Parkinson disease, and Huntington disease. Patients who have been diagnosed with a neuromuscular disease may benefit from treatment by the physical therapy team. However, for purposes of this chapter, the pathomechanics and only the rehabilitation strategies for direct and indirect muscle injuries will be addressed.

BOX 11-1

Sprain versus Strain

The terms *strain* and *sprain* are not the same thing. A strain refers to a muscle and/or tendon injury. A strain to the muscle, tendon, or musculotendinous unit may be caused by one of several mechanisms; direct impact, violent stretch or eccentric overload, or overuse. A sprain refers to an injury to a ligament. Ligament sprains occur in response to violent stretching mechanism above its physiologic capacity. A muscle and a ligament may be injured during the same mechanism; however they are two distinct entities.

A direct muscle injury will occur when an external force applied to the body results in a trauma. Examples of direct muscle injuries include a contusion caused by a blunt trauma or a deep laceration caused by a sharp implement. In each of these examples, the applied supraphysiologic load was greater than the muscle's maximum tissue tolerance. An indirect muscle injury occurs independent of an applied external force. Indirect muscle injuries are the result of either a supraphysiologic load (e.g., a violent or excessive muscular stretch or excessive muscular stretch combined with an eccentric muscular contraction) or repeated insults (e.g., overuse injury) to the tissue without proper time for recovery.[8,18] Indirect muscle injuries primarily occur at the musculotendinous junction; however, they may also occur in the belly itself.[18]

A **muscle strain,** frequently referred to as a muscle tear, is an indirect injury (Box 11-1). A pulled hamstring (or sometimes referred to as a *hammy*) is an example

Table 11-2	Characteristics of First Degree, Second Degree, and Third Degree Muscle Strains		
Parameter	**First Degree**	**Second Degree**	**Third Degree**
Extent of damage to the muscle	Tear of a few muscle fibers	Tear of approximately half of the muscle fibers	Tear (rupture) of the entire muscle
Muscle weakness	Minor	Moderate (significant)	Major
Loss of function	None to minor	Moderate	Major
Pain	Minor	Moderate to major	None (a lack of pain is associated with third degree strain because the nerve is often significantly damaged during the injury)
Swelling	Minimal to none	Noticeable degree of swelling	Significant degree of swelling

of a common muscle strain experienced in sports.[5,6,26] Muscle strains can cause significant pain and greatly reduce function.[5,6,26] Hamstring injuries can plague an athlete with a lengthy rehabilitation period and a slow return to sport.[25] Muscles that cross two joints, like the hamstrings, are frequently strained.[8,25] Sports medicine specialists believe that these muscles may become injured in response to an intense eccentric load.[8] Many of the most frequently strained muscles are composed of type II muscle fibers, the fibers that are least resistant to fatigue.[8]

Muscle strains are frequently described by the degree of damage to the muscle. Table 11-2 presents the characteristics associated with a first degree, second degree, or third degree muscle strain.

Because muscle attaches to bone via tendon, the two structures are interrelated and are frequently injured together (e.g., musculotendinous junction muscle strains). However, there are a number of injuries seen clinically that are specific to the tendon itself (e.g., tendinitis or Achilles tendon ruptures).

Tendon injuries range from acute tendinitis to chronic tendinopathy (Table 11-3). Tendinitis is an acute injury of the tendon associated with an inflammatory response. A patient with a "true" tendonitis may present to physical therapy with pain, functional loss, and signs associated with inflammation (pain, warmth, swelling, redness). A patient with tendinitis often describes performing an unfamiliar, repetitive activity from 1 day to a week before seeking medical attention. If a patient presents with a tendon injury that lacks inflammatory signs, it is likely that the patient has a tendinopathy. It is not uncommon to have a patient describe that he or she has experienced pain for many months to years before seeking medical attention. The Achilles tendon, the quadriceps tendon, and the supraspinatus tendon are common locations that one might develop a tendinopathy. The manner in which each condition is treated differs greatly. A tendon may also rupture, requiring surgical repair.

Table 11-3	Tendon Injury Classifications
Injury	**Classification**
Tendinitis	Acute injury to the tendon with associated inflammatory response
Tendinosis	Degeneration to the tendon, not associated with inflammatory process, due to one or more factors (e.g., microtrauma, age-related changes)
Peritenonitis	Inflammation of the peritenon only
Tenosynovitis	Inflammation of the tendon's synovial membrane
Tenovaginitis	An inflamed, thickened tendon sheath

When a tendon experiences strain levels that overload the tissue's tensile capabilities, microtrauma will result. A frequent, repeated strain to the tendon will continue the microtrauma (damage) to the microstructure of the tendon. An injury occurs when the rate of damage surpasses the tendon's ability to repair itself. Over time, if the tendon fails to heal, a tendinosis region will develop.

Some tendons may also be at risk for significant tearing or rupturing. In the event of a tendon rupture, surgical intervention is necessary to restore function. Orthopedic surgeons frequently perform tendon repairs to the tendons of the supraspinatus (in addition to the other rotator cuff muscles), extensor carpi radialis brevis, quadriceps tendon, and Achilles tendon.

Age Effects on Tendons

Over time, the aging tendon has an increased risk of sustaining an injury.[33] PTAs will frequently provide treatment for patients who are 40 years and older who have experienced a tendon injury. In some cases, patients will

Table 11-4	Timeline of Cellular Events Occurring During the Healing Process
Time Frame (Postinjury)	**Events**
Immediate to 48 hours	Rupture of blood and lymphatic vessels with initial vasoconstriction—coagulation
	Clot formation
	Vasodilation occurs shortly after the initial injury
	Immediate swelling—cellular (exudate) components from vessels fill wound site
	Patient experiences hallmark signs and symptoms of inflammation (redness, warmth, pain, swelling)
	Phagocytosis (process of removing injured/dead cellular material)
	Chemical mediators attracted to the area to control the inflammatory process
Day 2 to 4	Decrease in inflammation
	Decrease in clot size (reabsorption)
	Increase in granulation tissue (fibroblasts, myofibroblasts, and capillaries)
	Repair process initiated
	Angiogenesis: the process of developing a new blood supply to the injured region.
Day 4 to 21	Initiation of fibroplasia (scar formation)
	Fibroblastic activity (produces collagen, elastin, and ground substance)
	Growth of scar ceases at the end of the phase
Day 21 to 60	Remodeling of scar
	Collagen thickens and strengthens

receive conservative physical therapy treatment, whereas in other cases patients may require invasive procedures such as injections or surgical repair.

Pathomechanics Associated with the Aging Tendon

As one ages, the stresses that would have been tolerated in youth now can contribute to an overuse injury or a tendon rupture. The aging tendon is usually smaller in size (compared with its size during youth or when a young adult) with a decrease in total number of collagen fibers. In addition, the ability of the aging tendon to turn over collagen fibers decreases.[28,33] The inability to add new collagen fibers at the same rate, or at all, limits the body's effectiveness in repairing microtrauma. Over time, repeated subfailure loads to a tendon will result in a tendon rupture. In addition, because of the smaller overall size, the tendon will have a lower capacity to resist certain tensile loads.

INJURY AND HEALING

As an immediate response to a muscle or tendon injury, the human body will initiate the healing process. For a patient to optimally recover from a muscle and or tendon injury, his or her body must successfully complete the three stages of healing: acute, subacute, and chronic.[1,23,28] The events that occur during each of these three stages are fairly consistent among connective tissues. Table 11-4 provides a timeline overview of events that occur during the healing process. A chronic pain syndrome may develop if the body fails to appropriately progress through these three stages.

The Acute Stage (Inflammatory Phase)

The onset of the acute stage begins immediately in response to injury. Trauma incites a complex series of chemical events that mobilize cells and chemotactic agents to the injury site to stimulate coagulation (clot formation), control hemorrhage (bleeding), and to synthesize new collagen.

The inflammatory response, a hallmark sign associated with the acute stage, is the immediate physiologic response designed to protect the injured area, stop the progression of cellular damage, and stimulate the body's repair process. The signs and symptoms associated with an inflammatory response are redness (rubor), swelling (tumor), heat or warmth (calor), and pain (dolor). The redness and warmth of the injured site is due to the damage to blood and lymphatic vessels, dilation of the blood vessels, and increased permeability allowing exudate to fill the area. Swelling in the injured area is due to exudate. Exudate consists of plasma and serum proteins that have leaked out of the vessels and into the surrounding tissue. Their function is to repair the injured site, but excessive exudate can cause significant swelling. Swelling increases the pressure within the injured area and applies a mechanical stress to free nerve endings, causing pain.

It may take up to 6 days for the body to complete the cellular and vascular activity associated with the acute stage. However, the acute phase may continue for an additional period of time if the injured area is continually stressed (e.g., the football athlete who keeps playing despite pain).

The Subacute Phase (Repair and Healing)

Repair of the injured tissue (starting as early as the third day after the injury) is initiated and proceeds for up to 3 weeks. Growth of capillaries into the injured region and fibroblastic activity are initiated early in this phase. Fibroblasts are cells that synthesize new collagen. This new collagen, which replaces the clot material, is formed and oriented in haphazard fashion as it is first laid down. It is important to appreciate that this collagen, although new, is structurally immature (thin and weak). If this area is overstressed with activity or aggressive therapy it may be injured.

Angiogenesis begins during the subacute phase. Angiogenesis is the process of new growth of blood vessels supply to the injured area. This neovascularization is necessary for continued soft tissue injury healing. The new blood supply will carry oxygen and nutrients to the region.

The Chronic Stage (Maturation and Remodeling)

The scar tissue that was initially formed after the injury has stopped growing by the end of the third week. The body is now ready to enter the chronic phase of healing that is highlighted by tissue remodeling and strengthening. During this phase the collagen is remodeled along the line of forces that it experiences. Applying the appropriate volume of stress to the healing tissue will help to facilitate the functional growth of the collagen and the improvement in its tensile strength capability. This process may occur for 12 to 18 months after the date of originally injury.

Effects of Immobilization

After an injury, patients who have been immobilized for any period of time will experience significant changes to the muscle and tendon. Perhaps the most profound change in human skeletal muscle during immobilization is atrophy. The degree of atrophy depends on both the duration of immobilization and the position or stretch imposed on the muscle. If a muscle in a given joint is immobilized in a shortened position, the muscle fiber will decrease in length and there is an associated decrease in the number of sarcomeres. This muscle may atrophy more than a muscle that has been casted in a lengthened position. Muscles that are immobilized in a shortened position are also less extensible after cast removal than muscles that have been immobilized in a lengthened position.

Muscle fiber types are also affected by position during immobilization. When muscles are immobilized in a shortened position, type I muscle fibers atrophy (decrease in both number of fibers and fiber diameter)

BOX 11-2

Effects of Immobilization on Skeletal Muscle Tissue (Shortened)

- Muscle atrophy (type I)
- Sarcomeres decreased
- Increased protein breakdown
- Decreased muscle extensibility after immobilization
- Decreased muscle weight
- Decreased force generating capacity
- Increase in connective tissue
- Decreased anaerobic glycolytic enzymes
- Decreased aerobic oxidative enzymes

---

far more than type II fibers. When a large percentage of type I muscle fibers atrophy during periods of immobilization, the relative number of type II fibers increases.

Muscle atrophy also results in a decrease in muscle weight. Muscle that has atrophied and lost weight also loses its ability to generate force and tension. The greatest amount of atrophy occurs within the first week of immobilization, and muscle fiber size decreases by approximately 17% within 3 days of immobilization. Box 11-2 depicts the various physiologic changes that occur in skeletal muscle when immobilized in a shortened position.

If a tendon has to be immobilized because of injury or surgery, the collagen that is formed by the fibroblasts is oriented in a haphazard fashion. During immobilization the tissue lacks the stimulus to orient the new collagen fibers in a functional parallel orientation. There is also an increased risk of adhesion development between the disorganized collagen fibers. After immobilization, the tendon is at risk for reinjury for a period of time because of the limited tensile capacity of the repaired tissue. Failure to continue with a home exercise program after formal discharge from physical therapy can limit a patient's full return to function. Inactivity after an injury (or in general) can result in a decrease in quantity and size of collagen fibers.

Muscle Repair and Heterotopic Bone Formation

Can muscle cells be repaired after an injury? There is some debate within the scientific community; however, the current state of thought is that a special cell known as a *satellite cell* can increase in number and convert into muscle cells. Further research is necessary at this time to explain or refute this notion.

Occasionally, injury to a muscle (e.g., severe blunt injury, deep contusion, surgical exposures, and certain fractures) may result in heterotopic bone formation (ectopic bone formation). Heterotopic bone formation after blunt trauma to muscle is known as *myositis ossificans*.[22] Generally, if the contusion is severe (deep versus superficial), there may be a periosteal reaction that stimulates undifferentiated mesenchymal cells to proliferate during the first 3 to 4 days after the trauma. During the next 5 to 8 days, cartilage develops with gradual calcification and neovascularization with subsequent bone deposition.

EVIDENCE-BASED THERAPEUTIC INTERVENTIONS FOR INJURED MUSCLES AND TENDONS

No two muscle or tendon injuries should be rehabilitated the same. There is no "cookbook" or "one size fits all" approach to physical therapy. Instead, the PT must develop the patient's rehabilitation program based on several factors: the tissue (or tissues) injured, the severity of the injury, the current stage of healing, the findings from the patient's musculoskeletal exam, and the patient's short-term and long-term goals.

The function of this next section is to present evidence-based therapeutic interventions for both muscle and tendon injuries based on the stages of tissue repair. Evidence-based and evidence-supported rationales will be used when available.

Acute Stage: Immediate Response for a Muscle or Tendon Injury

A sports medicine team consisting of the PT, the PTA, or the PTA with a dual credential as a certified athletic trainer (ATC), will provide the first line of treatment once an athlete is injured. Many sports certified PTs who are dual-credentialed as an ATC or who are sports certified specialists (SCS, board certified sports physical therapist by the American Physical Therapy Association) provide game coverage within their community. The immediate treatment provided by the sports medicine team for the athlete who has been sidelined because of a sport-related injury will include protection, rest, ice, compression, and elevation (PRICE).

If an athlete sustains an injury that impairs function or if continued sports participation might worsen the injury, then the athlete should be removed from competition and allowed to rest the injured area. If possible, the injured region should be elevated. Elevation of the joint or extremity should be above the level of the heart (e.g., an athlete who has injured his leg should have the lower extremity elevated and supported while the athlete lies on his back). Elevating the extremity will reduce the swelling that occurs immediately post injury. Ice should be immediately applied to the injured area to reduce further inflammatory damage and control pain. Compression should be applied in conjunction with the ice for up to 20 minutes, every 30 minutes to 1 hour. Finally, the injured region should be protected

from further injury. For example, the athlete who has sprained an ankle might benefit from the use of bilateral crutches and decrease weight-bearing stress. Depending upon the severity of the injury, the athlete should be referred to the emergency room to rule out a fracture (if necessary) or to the appropriate sports medicine or orthopedic physician the following day.

Acute Stage: Treatment in the Physical Therapy Clinic

The clinical goals associated with this stage are to facilitate healing to the injured tissue, control or reduce the effects of the inflammation, decrease pain, initiate controlled movement to restore ROM, and reduce the loss of muscular strength

Physical agents are frequently used during the acute stage of healing to decrease pain, reduce inflammation, facilitate healing, and to restore muscular function. In addition, passive range of motion (PROM) and active assisted range of motion (AAROM) exercises are initiated to maintain or restore movement around the joint. Manual therapy techniques are performed to reduce pain and improve soft tissue and joint mobility. Isometric strengthening may also be performed during this phase to retard strength loss. Table 11-5 presents a list of evidence-supported treatments for patients in the acute stage of healing.

Patients should be provided with a home exercise program to perform between sessions. The effectiveness of each technique should be assessed during and between treatment sessions. Treatments that fail to impact the patient's recovery should be terminated. In addition, treatments that worsen the patient's state should be immediately stopped. A failure to remove stress to the injured tissue during the acute phase may increasing swelling, pain, and the length of this phase.

Subacute Stage: Treatment in the Physical Therapy Clinic

The clinical goals during the subacute phase are to restore full active and PROM, initiate muscular strengthening, continue to address residual swelling, reduce pain, and initiate functional movement tasks.

During the subacute phase of healing, the body deposits immature collagen fibers in the injured region. Prescribing therapeutic exercises that appropriately stress the injured region will help to promote the normal healing process and the development of a mobile scar. However, overstressing the area may injure the new collagen fibers. Pain during exercise should be avoided. Make it clear to patients that they should stop performing an exercise if it reproduces their pain.

A primary goal of this phase is to progress and restore range of motion. During the acute phase, PROM and AAROM exercises are prescribed. As tolerated, the patient should be progressed to active range of motion (AROM) techniques and static stretching exercises.

Table 11-5	*Evidence-Supported Treatments for Patients in the Acute Stage of Healing*

Goal	Treatment	Relevant Study
Facilitate healing of the injured tissue	Ultrasound	Noonan,[24] Reilly[29]
	Cryotherapy	Jarvinen,[13] Noonan,[24] Reilly,[29] Thompson[32]
Control or reduce the effects of inflammation	Ultrasound	Noonan,[24] Reilly[29]
	Cryotherapy	Jarvinen,[13] Noonan,[24] Reilly,[29] Thompson[32]
	Massage	Brumitt,[2] Reilly[29]
Decrease pain	Ultrasound	Noonan[24]
	Cryotherapy	Jarvinen,[13] Noonan,[24] Reilly,[29] Thompson[32]
	Massage	Brumitt,[2] Reilly[29]
	Joint mobilization	Brumitt[3,4]
Restore range of motion	PROM (manual or self techniques)	Brumitt,[4] Meier,[19] Noonan[24]
	AAROM (self techniques)	Brumitt,[4] Meier[19]
	Massage	Brumitt,[2] Reilly[29]
	Joint mobilization	Brumitt[3,4]
Restore muscular strength	Isometric exercises	Brumitt,[3,4] Frohm,[10] Jarvinen,[13] Meier,[19] Noonan[24]

Typically, multiple sets and repetitions of AROM exercises are prescribed. Manual therapy techniques (joint mobilization, massage) may continue to be necessary to restore joint and soft tissue mobility. Static stretching exercises should initially be performed gently, holding each stretch for 30 seconds.[13,24,37]

The prescription of resisted exercises will assist the collagen orientation and improve tensile capabilities. Initially, exercises should be performed with high repetitions and low weights. Performing a muscular endurance program will allow the patient to gradually gain strength while reducing the risk of damaging the new collagen fibers. Consider patients performing 15 to 25 reps of 1 to 2 sets per exercise. The initial number of exercises prescribed by the PT will be dependent upon the patient's presentation. The inclusion of neuromuscular electrical stimulation may further assist the restoration of muscular strength.[19]

Chronic Stage: Treatment in the Physical Therapy Clinic

During the chronic stage of healing, collagen aligns to the stresses applied and the tissue is maturing and remodeling. Physical therapy interventions should facilitate this through the continued prescription of therapeutic exercises.

Increasing the endurance capacity of the muscle may be continued as necessary, but now the therapy team should be able to progress strengthening as tolerated. Exercise prescription should be functional in nature and should account for muscle fiber structure within muscle groups. For example, muscles of the core (type I muscle fibers) should continue to be trained using endurance training strategies. Strength training variables may be applied to muscle groups containing higher percentages of type II muscle fibers. Once

the patient is pain free, plyometrics or power training may be initiated if functionally necessary (e.g., athletes, industrial workers).[4]

Special Considerations: Tendon Repairs and Tendinopathy

The patient who has been referred to physical therapy with a postoperative tendon repair requires special consideration. Failing to follow the physician's postoperative protocol may put the repaired tendon at risk for injury or rerupturing.

Patients who have been referred with a tendinopathy diagnosis will benefit from performance of eccentric exercises. There is a growing body of evidence that suggests the inclusion of eccentric exercises will help to reduce pain and restore function in individuals with either a tendinosis at the Achilles tendon or patella tendon.[10,14,17,36]

Summary

Successful rehabilitation after a muscle or tendon injury, or both, occurs when the rehabilitation team effectively communicates with one another regarding the patient's diagnosis and progression. When possible, the therapy team should use evidence-based rehabilitation interventions. If evidence-based rehab programs are not available in the literature, the rehabilitation professional should select interventions that are appropriate for the patient's current stage of healing.

❖ GLOSSARY

Endomysium: An internal connective sheathe that covers the muscle fibers. One of three layers of connective tissue that surrounds the muscle and is continuous with the muscle's tendons.

Epimysium: The outermost layer of tissue covering that becomes continuous with tendons. One of three layers of connective tissue that surrounds the muscle and is continuous with the muscle's tendons.

Perimysium: Covers groups of individual muscle fibers into bundles. One of three layers of connective tissue that surrounds the muscle and is continuous with the muscle's tendons.

Muscle sprain: An injury to a ligament.

Muscle strain: An injury to a muscle and/or tendon.

REFERENCES

1. Alaseirlis DA, Li Y, Cilli F, et al: Decreasing inflammatory response of injured patellar tendons results in increased collagen fibril diameters, *Connect Tissue Res* 46:3–8, 2005.
2. Brumitt J: The role of massage in sports performance and rehabilitation: current evidence and future direction, *N Am J Sports Phys Ther* 3(1):7–21, 2008.
3. Brumitt J, McIntosh L, Rutt R: Comprehensive sports medicine treatment of an athlete who runs cross-country and is iron deficient, *N Am J Sports Phys Ther* 4(1):13–20, 2009.
4. Brumitt J, Sproul A, Lentz P, et al: In-season rehabilitation of a division III female wrestler after a glenohumeral dislocation, *Phys Ther Sport* 10(3):112–117, 2009.
5. Cohen S, Bradley J: Acute proximal hamstring rupture, *J Am Acad Orthop Surg* 15(6):350–355, 2007.
6. Croisier JL: Factors associated with recurrent hamstring injuries, *Sports Med* 34(10):681–695, 2004.
7. den Hoed MD, Hesselink MKC, Westerterp KR: Skeletal muscle fiber-type and habitual physical activity in daily life, *Scand J Med Sci Sports* 19:373–380, 2009.
8. Dugan SA, Frontera WR: Muscle fatigue and muscle injury, *Phys Med Rehabil Clin N Am* 11(2):385–403, 2000.
9. Eriksson A, Kadi F, Malm C, et al: Skeletal muscle morphology in power-lifters with and without anabolic steroids, *Histochem Cell Biol* 124:167–175, 2005.
10. Frohm A, Saartok T, Halvorsen K, et al: Eccentric treatment for patellar tendinopathy: a prospective short-term pilot study of two rehabilitation protocols, *Br J Sports Med* 41(7):7, 2007.
11. Hosea TM, Gatt CJ Jr: Back pain in golf, *Clin Sports Med* 15(1):37–53, 1996.
12. Hostler D, Schwirian CI, Campos G, et al: Skeletal muscle adaptations in elastic resistance-trained young men and women, *Eur J Appl Physiol* 86:112–118, 2001.
13. Jarvinen TA, Kaariainen M, Jarvinen M, et al: Muscle strain injuries, *Curr Opin Rheumatol* 12(2):155–161, 2000.
14. Jonsson P, Alfredson H: Superior results with eccentric compared to concentric quadriceps training in patients with jumper's knee: a prospective randomized study, *Br J Sports Med* 39(11):847–850, 2005.
15. Kadi F: Adaptation of human skeletal muscle to training and anabolic steroids, *Acta Physiol Scan Suppl* 646:1–52, 2000.
16. Kannus P: Structure of the tendon connective tissue, *Scand J Med Sci Sports* 10:312–320, 2000.
17. Magnussen RA, Dunn WR, Thomson AB: Nonoperative treatment of midportion Achilles tendinopathy: a systematic review, *Clin J Sports Med* 19(1):54–64, 2009.
18. Matzkin E, Zachazewski JE, Garrett WE, et al: Skeletal muscle: deformation, injury, repair, and treatment considerations. In Magee DJ, Zachazewski JE, Quillen WS, editors: *Scientific foundations and principles of practice in musculoskeletal rehabilitation*, St Louis, 2007, Saunders.
19. Meier W, Mizner RL, Marcus RL, et al: Total knee arthroplasty: muscle impairments, functional limitations, and recommended rehabilitation approaches, *J Orthop Sports Phys Ther* 38(5):246–256, 2008.
20. Meister K: Injuries to the shoulder in the throwing athlete. Part one: biomechanics/pathophysiology/classification of injury, *Am J Sports Med* 28(2):265–275, 2000.
21. Meister K: Injuries to the shoulder in the throwing athlete. Part two: evaluation/treatment, *Am J Sports Med* 28(4):587–601, 2000.
22. Miller AE, Davis BA, Beckley OA: Bilateral and recurrent myositis ossificans in an athlete: a case report and review of treatment options, *Arch Phys Med Rehabil* 87(2):286–290, 2006.
23. Molloy T, Wang Y, Murrell G: The roles of growth factors in tendon and ligament healing, *Sports Med* 33(5):381–394, 2003.
24. Noonan TJ, Garrett WE Jr: Muscle strain injury: diagnosis and treatment, *J Am Acad Orthop Surg* 7(4):262–269, 1999.
25. Orchard J, Best TM, Verrall GM: Return to play following muscle strains, *Clin J Sport Med* 15(6):436–441, 2005.
26. Petersen J, Holmich P: Evidence based prevention of hamstring injuries in sport, *Br J Sports Med* 39(6):319–323, 2005.
27. Pette D, Staron RS: Transitions of muscle fiber phenotypic profiles, *Histochem Cell Biol* 115:359–372, 2001.
28. Platt MA: Tendon repair and healing, *Clin Podiatr Med Surg* 22:553–560, 2005.
29. Reilly T, Ekblom B: The use of recovery methods post-exercise, *J Sports Sci* 23(6):619–627, 2005.
30. Rodriguez LP, Lopez-Rego J, Calbet JAL, et al: Effects of training status on fibers of the musculus vastus lateralis in professional road cyclists, *Am J Phys Med Rehabil* 81:651–660, 2002.
31. Sciote JJ, Horton MJ, Rowlerson AM, et al: Specialized cranial muscles: how different are they from limb and abdominal muscles? *Cells Tissues Organs* 174:73–86, 2003.
32. Thompson C, Kelsberg G, St Anna L, et al: Clinical inquiries. Heat or ice for acute ankle sprain? *J Fam Pract* 52(8):642–643, 2003.
33. Thompson LV: Effects of age and training on skeletal muscle physiology and performance, *Phys Ther* 74:71–81, 1994.
34. Wang Q: Baseball and softball injuries, *Curr Sports Med Rep* 5(3):115–119, 2006.
35. Wang YX, Zhang CL, Yu RT, et al: Regulation of muscle fiber type and running endurance by PPARdelta, *PLoS Biol* 2(10):e294, 2004.
36. Woodley BL, Newsham-West RJ, Baxter GD: Chronic tendinopathy: effectiveness of eccentric exercise, *Br J Sports Med* 41(4):188–198, 2007.
37. Woods K, Bishop P, Jones E: Warm-up and stretching in the prevention of muscular injury, *Sports Med* 37(12):1089–1099, 2007.

REVIEW QUESTIONS

Short Answer

1. The process of new growth of blood vessels to an injured area is called: _____.
2. Name the three stages of healing: _____, _____, and _____.
3. The "R" in PRICE stands for: _____.
4. Name the three degrees of a muscle strain and provide characteristics for each type.
5. Describe the changes that occur in the aging tendon. How do these factors affect the ability of the body to repair itself?
6. Name the four cardinal signs of inflammation.

True/False

7. A tendon injury will result in a permanent functional loss.
8. The subfascicle is the basic functional unit of a tendon.

12 Neurovascular Healing and Thromboembolic Disease

Barbara Smith

LEARNING OBJECTIVES

1. Identify neural anatomy.
2. Discuss the vascular supply to nerve tissue.
3. Understand the mechanical behavior of nerve tissue.
4. Identify the causes and classification of nerve injury.
5. Discuss intrinsic nerve healing.
6. Describe methods of surgical repair of nerve injury.
7. Identify structure and composition of vascular tissue.
8. Discuss the vascular response to injury.
9. Explain the various signs and symptoms of vascular injury.
10. Discuss the pathophysiology of thromboembolic disease.
11. Recognize risk factors of deep vein thrombosis and pulmonary emboli.

KEY TERMS

Axonotmesis

Creep

Denervation

Neurapraxia

Neurotmesis

CHAPTER OUTLINE

PERIPHERAL NERVE INJURY

In general, peripheral nerves are traumatized by mechanical, thermal, chemical and ischemic injury. As an organ system, the peripheral nervous system (PNS) is highly vascularized. As such, a mechanical insult to nerve (e.g., compression, stretch, or severance) stimulates an intense inflammatory reaction.

Vascular Supply

Peripheral nerve has a complex and extensive blood supply. The PNS requires an ongoing nutritive energy supply for maintenance of nerve conduction. Longitudinal extrinsic vessels connect with regional feeding vessels that form a vascular plexus within the epineurium, perineurium, and endoneurium connective tissue network within the nerve fiber (Fig. 12-1).[2,9]

The initial response to nerve trauma is a predictable response like that seen after vascular tissue trauma. After a brief period of vasoconstriction, vascular permeability increases because of the release of potent chemical mediators such as serotonin and histamine.[11] The result is edema within the nerve fiber's connective tissue barriers (epineurium, perineurium, endoneurium). The dramatic change in fluid pressure and tissue edema adversely affects oxygen transport, nutrition, ion content of nerve cells, and conductivity of the traumatized nerve fiber.[9]

Mechanical Behavior of Nerve Tissue

Nerve tissue is highly deformable, expressing relatively similar viscoelastic mechanical behavior as other soft tissue. Essentially, two load deformation terms are used to quantify a tissue's ability to adapt structurally and mechanically to time-dependent forces. **Creep** is a term used to describe the tissue's ability to change or "creep" to a new length in response to a constant, applied load. The greater the load (stress), the faster the tissue will deform or creep. Stress relaxation is similar to creep, in that it is a time-dependent phenomenon. It occurs when a material is elongated (strained) to a given dimension and then maintained at that length. In this situation, there is a reduction in the amount of stress required to maintain the fixed length. Peripheral nerve tissue responds with this viscoelastic behavior by showing ultimate load-to-failure values of 20% to 60%. Although peripheral nerve tissue may tear when the nerve is elongated to approximately 20% more than its resting length, ischemic changes, which profoundly affect nerve function, may occur when a nerve is stretched less than or equal to 15% of its resting length.[1,12]

Causes and Classification of Nerve Injuries

Trauma to peripheral nerve comes from mechanical, thermal, chemical, and vascular injury. Mechanical sources cause contusion, concussion, stretch, compression, laceration, and transection.[8,9] Classification of nerve injury provides concise and anatomic descriptions. However, the clinical reliability of this system is debatable.[1,6,9] Many injuries cannot be classified into a single grade. The three most common categories of nerve injury are **neurapraxia, axonotmesis,** and **neurotmesis.**[6,8,9]

Neurapraxia is the reduction in nerve conduction at the site of injury, usually due to compression. The lesion is local, the axon's continuity is maintained, and all pathologic changes associated with neurapraxia generally are reversible if the cause is removed.[6,8,9] Functional recovery occurs within weeks or months.[9]

In axonotmesis, the epineurium remains intact, while damage to the perineurium and endoneurium occurs to varying degrees. Because the epineurium is undamaged, functional recovery without surgery may occur. However, as greater amounts of perineurium and endoneurium become involved, surgery is required to achieve the most functional recovery.[9]

Neurotmesis is diagnosed when the entire nerve trunk is transected or ruptured. The total loss of nerve continuity requires surgical adaptation and coaptation. Prognosis depends on the nature of the injury, as well as local and general factors, such as patient age and timing of the repair.[1,6]

In a very broad sense, a pure motor nerve is a greater risk for injury than a pure sensory nerve. A gross prediction is that peripheral nerves usually fail to conduct impulses related to motion (first), proprioception, touch, temperature and pain (last). Recovery of these abilities occurs in the reverse order.[1,8]

Compression and Traction Neuropathy

Nerve compression injuries are acute or chronic in origin. In both cases, the physiologic consequence of compression or traction on peripheral nerve tissue is mechanical disruption of the nerve fiber and ischemia (Fig. 12-2).[9] Anatomically, certain peripheral nerves are at risk for compression neuropathy because of the surrounding arrangement of soft tissue and bone, which limits the nerve's three-dimensional motion. Specifically at risk in the lower extremity are the common peroneal nerve behind the fibular head and the lateral femoral cutaneous nerve within the inguinal ligament (meralgia paresthetica).[1] In the upper extremity, nerves most susceptible to mechanical disruption are the radial nerve within the spiral groove of the humerus, and the median nerve within the soft tissue confines of the carpal tunnel arch. Spinal nerve roots are more susceptible to compression injury than peripheral nerves because spinal nerve roots have no epineurium.[9]

The biological responses of the PNS to acute and chronic compression include obstruction of intraneural blood vessels, tissue anoxia, local ischemia, nerve fiber deformation, increased vascular permeability, intraneural edema, and fibroblastic proliferation with resultant decreased nerve gliding.[9]

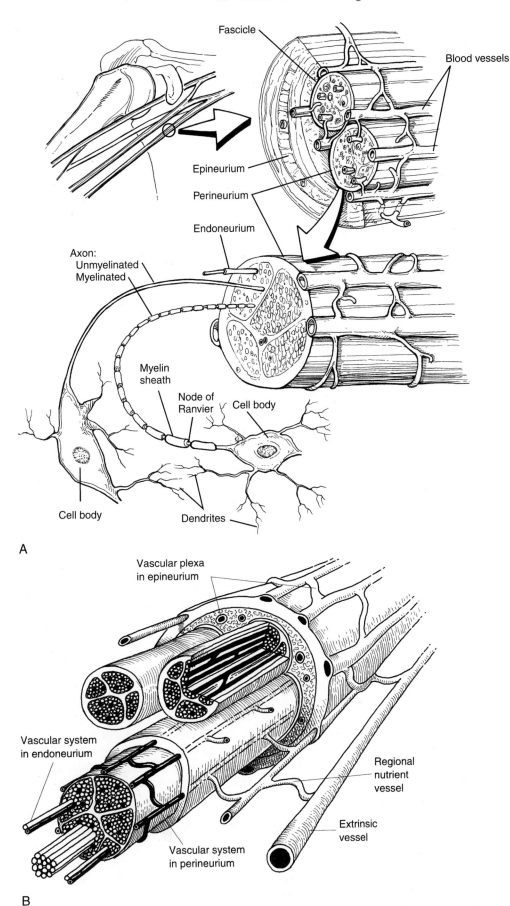

Fig. 12-1 **A,** Nerve architecture. **B,** Blood supply of a peripheral nerve. (**A,** From Brinker MR, Miller MD: *Fundamentals of orthopaedics*, ed 2, Philadelphia, 1999, Saunders; **B,** Adapted from Lundborg G: *Nerve injury and repair*, New York, 1988, Churchill Livingstone.)

Acute effects   **Chronic effects**

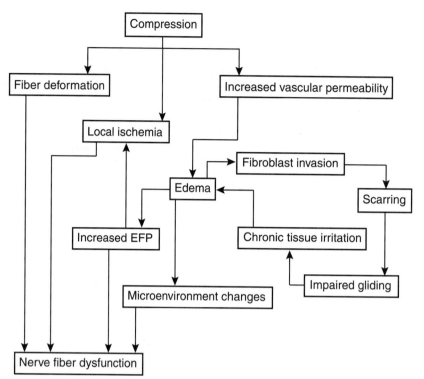

Fig. 12-2 Effects of compression on intraneural tissues. *EFP,* Effective filtration pressure. (From Lundborg G: *Nerve injury and repair,* ed 2, New York, 2004, Churchill Livingstone.)

Traction or stretch neuropathy is classified as acute or chronic with the magnitude of injury classified as neurapraxia, axonotmesis, and neurotmesis as described. A practical and common description of acute traction neurapraxia is the "burner" or "stinger" experienced by athletes, in which the shoulder is depressed with concomitant contralateral head and neck flexion that creates a brachial plexus stretch.[2]

Occasionally with lengthy surgical procedures, prolonged wide surgical field exposure leads to inadvertent stretch of surrounding peripheral nerve tissue. Surgical procedures may also require prolonged tourniquet application, with cuff pressures occluding neural blood supply.[8,9]

Physical therapy (e.g., range of motion [ROM] exercise) after prolonged joint immobilization may cause traction neurapraxia due to premature and intensive stretch. During the protection phase of postoperative care or during prolonged immobilization, slow, controlled stretch, devoid of high velocity or force protects nerve from unwanted injury.[8,12]

Some patients may experiences signs and symptoms of peripheral nerve compression or entrapment at more than one level of the same nerve. The term *double crush syndrome* is used to describe these signs and symptoms. The most common example is carpal tunnel median nerve compression neuropathy and cervical nerve root injury. Another example is nerve entrapment neuropathy at the elbow along with cervicothoracic root lesion. To explain this syndrome, it is hypothesized that a compression lesion at one level of the nerve makes the same nerve more susceptible to injury at another site.[1,9] It is suggested that compression reduces nerve conduction, blood supply, and the amount of plasma membrane proteins. These reductions adversely influence other segments, making them more sensitive to mechanical or compressive forces.[9]

Methods of Peripheral Nerve Repair

The term *neurorrhaphy* is synonymous with direct coaptation or surgical apposition of corresponding nerve stumps or fascicles.[8,9] This specific intervention is reserved for neurotmesis with complete disruption of nerve continuity. The basic objectives for surgical repair (neurorrhaphy) are to maximize the number of axons that regenerate across the lesion and to reinnervate distal sites accurately, for example, that proximal motor axons reach distal motor axons (Fig. 12-3).[1,8,9]

Skeletal stability and a well-vascularized tissue bed are essential for effective, direct coaptation. The procedure requires that appropriate tension be applied at the injury site.[8,9] Animal studies show that repairs subject to minimal tension produce better results than tension-free repairs.[8,9] Overall, four steps are identified

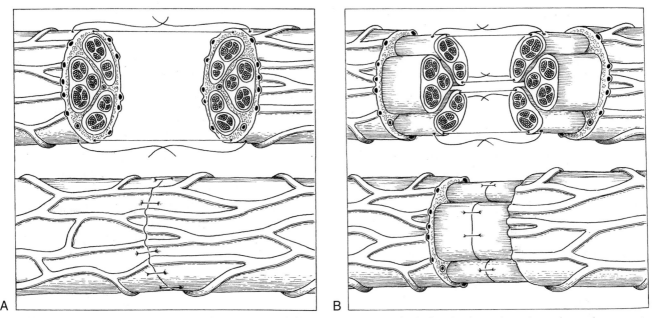

Fig. 12-3 **A,** Epineural suture. Coaptation is achieved by single epineural stitches in the epineurium along the nerve's circumference. A perfect superficial alignment can be achieved, but the internal orientation of fascicular abundance and individual fascicles may not be correct. **B,** Group fascicular suture. Epineural tissue has been resected, and fascicular groups are coapted with single sutures in the connective tissue between separate fascicles or in the outer layer of the perineurium. (From Lundborg G: *Nerve injury and repair*, ed 2, New York, 2004, Churchill Livingstone.)

as prerequisites for direct coaptation: clean preparation of traumatized nerve stumps, manual approximation of tissue stumps with correct tension, direct connection between nerve fascicles at both nerve endings or interposing nerve graft, and maintenance of coaptation with sutures, fibrin glue, or interstitial clot.[8,9]

When primary repair cannot be achieved without undue tension on nerve endings, autografts may be used for indirect coaptation. The most common autograft source for peripheral nerve repair is the sural nerve.[6,8,9] Other sources are the anterior branch of the medial antebrachial cutaneous nerve, the lateral femoral cutaneous nerve, and the superficial radial nerve. The use of autografts must be carefully weighed because their use sacrifices healthy nerves and puts the donor site at risk for morbidity and local disturbances of sensory function.[9]

Without repair, denervated tissues undergo many changes. Denervated bone becomes osteoporotic, joint capsule and periarticular soft tissues become fibrotic, and muscle atrophies leading to decreased muscle volume. During the first month after unrepaired nerve injury, muscle loses up to 30% of its weight, and approximately 60% is lost by the end of the second month of **denervation.**[8]

Currently, good to excellent results can be expected in approximately 50% of surgically repaired peripheral nerves. A few generalizations can be made concerning reconstruction. Better results occur in younger patients, patients with prompt repairs, more distal repairs, and those with shorter grafts.[8,9]

Recovery after Peripheral Nerve Injury and Repair

Repair site protection is the most important factor after peripheral nerve coaptation or autograft. Overzealous ROM exercise during early recovery can easily disrupt fragile healing of fascicle sutures and axonal regeneration. Typically, postoperative splinting is used to maintain appropriate tension and mechanical properties of the repaired nerve.[8,12] Compressive dressings help to decrease venous congestion and edema. ROM exercises, used cautiously, encourage venous return, muscle activation, and lymphatic flow, and reduce the potential for muscle and connective tissue adhesions.[8,12] Vascular supply to the healing and repaired nerve tissue must be continuously enhanced to influence axonal regeneration. Superficial heat application may encourage peripheral vascular blood flow to the healing tissues. Electrical stimulation may be of some benefit to initiate muscle contraction, increase blood flow, and stimulate removal of cellular debris.[9] Neuromuscular and sensory reeducation exercise are initiated early and progressed continuously during all phases of peripheral nerve recovery after injury, with or without surgical repair. Continuous stimulation of distal target sites of reinnervation is essential to redirect axonal regeneration and to facilitate reeducation. Various sensory stimulation tactics are used to decrease hypersensitivity. Reintroduction of light touch, pressure, vibration, thermal stimuli, texture, and stimulation of the mechanoreceptor system (proprioception and kinesthesia) are critical components of functional recovery of nerve injury or repair.[8]

Not only do changes occur at the site of injury and distal to it, but central changes also occur. The somatosensory cortex, even in adults, is rapidly altered after injury. Therefore the correct amount of sensory input from the affected area is necessary to reexpand cortical representation from the injured extremity. Animal studies show that the injured part needs repeated and substantial practice of functional movements to, perhaps, induce expansion of the contralateral cortical area that controls movement of the affected extremity.[9]

Assessment of Functional Recovery

To document the quality and quantity of motor and sensory nerve recovery after injury or surgical repair, an objective grading system is used to determine the level of functional recovery. The Mechanical Research Council Grading System is used for continued assessment of both motor and sensory recovery.[8,9] Motor recovery is graded M0 through M5, and sensory recovery S0 through S4. A parallel analogy is manual muscle strength testing:

- Trace, 1
- Poor, 2
- Fair, 3
- Good, 4
- Normal, 5

With an excellent result after nerve repair, a grade of M5, S4 describes full motor reinnervation and complete sensory recovery. A good result is described as M3, S3; a fair result is M2, S2; and a poor result is M0 to M1, S0 to S1.

By establishing objective documentation relating to functional motor and sensory nerve recovery after injury or surgical repair, appropriate physical therapy interventions can be explored to stimulate, regulate, or enhance specific motor or sensory functions. Patients should be encouraged to identify daily stresses that fall under a continuum of low to extreme stress on the injured or repaired extremity. Through activity modification, education, and physical therapy intervention, the patient may be able to achieve a better balance of stresses and improve functional recovery or prevent further injury or reinjury.[12]

VASCULAR INJURY

The peripheral vascular system frequently is damaged by trauma, surgery, or disease. The importance of bone and soft tissue vascularization after injury is well documented and firmly established. Bone and soft tissues become anoxic and necrotic, eventually ceasing to function, without a continuous supply of oxygen, red blood cells, and proliferative cells. The complex relationship between the causes of vascular tissue injury and the vascular response to injury is profoundly important for the patient's functional recovery.

Structure and Composition

Grossly, vessels consist of three basic components: endothelial cells, smooth muscles, and connective tissue. Arteries and veins consist of three identifiable concentric layers (lamina) that form the lumen or "walls." The innermost layer is the tunica intima (interna), consisting of connective tissue, endothelial cells, and a basement membrane. The middle layer is the tunica media, composed of smooth muscle cells and connective tissue. The outermost layer is the tunica adventitia (externa), made up of fibrous connective tissue that blends with loose surrounding connective tissue. Between the tunica media and externa is an external elastic membrane (elastic externa). The internal elastic lamina (elastica interna) lies between the internal and intermediate tunicae. The outermost walls of large vessels contain their own microvascular system. Nerves of the sympathetic nervous system innervate the arterial tunicae.[11]

Although veins contain the same three layers of tunicae, the relative percentage of smooth muscle and elastic components is less than that of arteries. In addition, the amount of connective tissue in veins is much greater than in arteries. These anatomic distinctions contribute to the vasomechanical differences between the highly elastic muscular arteries and the relatively less elastic veins. The biochemical composition within the vascular system varies greatly depending on regional requirements. Generally, the peripheral vascular system is composed of extracellular matrix, collagens, elastin, proteoglycans, squamous epithelial (endothelial), and smooth muscle cells.[11]

Vascular Response to Injury

As with other types of soft tissue, injuries to vessels incite an organized, predictable inflammatory response with distinct overlapping sequential events: coagulation, inflammation, fibroplasia, and remodeling and maturation. The most significant histochemical event in the vascular response is intimal hyperplasia, where smooth muscle cells proliferate after arterial injury. Depending on the nature and severity of injury, the cell proliferation of the damaged lumen may actual thicken vessel walls, reducing blood flow.[11]

Mechanisms of Injury

Vascular injury from traction, avulsion, compression or penetration can occur during orthopedic surgery (Table 12-1). Total knee arthroplasty (TKA) poses a risk to the popliteal artery as well. Total hip arthroplasty may put the common or external iliac artery at risk for injury. Identifiable arterial injury can occur because of shoulder dislocation and humeral neck fractures, resulting in axillary artery injury. Supracondylar humeral fractures

Table 12-1	*Arterial Injuries Associated with Orthopedic Operative Procedures*	
Body Area	**Orthopedic Procedure**	**Artery Injured**
Upper extremity	Clavicular compression plate/screw	Subclavian artery
	Anterior approach to the shoulder	Axillary artery
	Closed reduction humeral fracture	Brachial artery
Lower extremity	Total hip arthroplasty	Common or external iliac artery
	Nail or nail-plate fixation of intertrochanteric or subtrochanteric hip fracture	Profunda femoris artery
	Subtrochanteric osteotomy	Profunda femoris artery
	Total knee arthroplasty	Popliteal artery
	Anterior or posterior cruciate reconstruction	Popliteal artery
	External fixator pin	Superficial femoral, profunda femoris, popliteal, or tibial arteries
Spine	Anterior spinal fusion	Abdominal aorta
	Lumbar spine fixation device	Abdominal aorta
	Resection of nucleus pulposus	Right common iliac artery and vein, inferior vena cava

From Browner BD, Jupiter JB, Levine AM, et al: *Skeletal trauma*, ed 3, Philadelphia, 2003, Saunders.

Table 12-2	*Arterial Injuries Associated with Fractures and Dislocations*	
Body Area	**Fracture or Dislocation**	**Artery Injured**
Upper extremity	Fracture of clavicle or first rib	Subclavian artery
	Anterior dislocation of shoulder	Axillary artery
	Fracture of neck of humerus	Axillary artery
	Fracture of shaft or supracondylar area of humerus	Brachial artery
	Dislocation of elbow	Brachial artery
Lower extremity	Fracture of shaft of femur	Superficial femoral artery
	Fracture of supracondylar area of femur	Popliteal artery
	Posterior dislocation of the knee	Popliteal artery
	Fracture of proximal tibia or fibula	Popliteal artery, tibioperoneal trunk, tibial artery, or peroneal artery
	Fracture of distal tibia or fibula	Tibial or peroneal artery

From Browner BD, Jupiter JB, Levine AM, et al: *Skeletal trauma*, ed 3, Philadelphia, 2003, Saunders.

and elbow dislocation can lead to brachial artery injury. Posterior knee dislocation and supracondylar femoral fracture can result in popliteal artery injury (Table 12-2).[4]

Signs and Symptoms of Vascular Injury

General signs and symptoms of peripheral artery injury are classified either as "hard" or "soft." Hard signs and symptoms include the traditional indications of pulselessness, pallor, paresthesias, pain, and paralysis. Overt signs of bleeding and a rapidly spreading hematoma are additional signs that warrant immediate surgical repair.[4]

Soft signs include a possible history of arterial bleeding, hematoma over a peripheral artery, and a neurological deficit originating in a nerve adjacent to the injured artery. After specific fractures, dislocation, and selected surgical procedures (e.g., glenohumeral or posterior

knee dislocation, TKA), continuous reassessment of peripheral pulses (radial or dorsalis pedis) is essential to identify potential vascular injury. Also routinely assessed are skin color, temperature, presence of edema, and digital capillary refill.[4]

Diagnostic Studies

Noninvasive diagnosis of arterial occlusion uses Doppler flow detection or duplex ultrasonography. The latter is a combination of ultrasound imaging and pulsed Doppler flow detection. With Doppler flow, a comparison is made with the noninvolved extremity. In this way, an arterial pressure index (API) is calculated by dividing the Doppler systolic pressure of the involved extremity by that of the noninvolved extremity. Arterial injury can be predicted with 97% accuracy when the API is lower than 0.90.[3] Percutaneous arteriography is the gold standard and most commonly used invasive technique for diagnosis of suspected arterial injury. This technique requires injection of dye proximal (antegrade) or distal (retrograde) to the suspected injury, then multiple sequential plain film radiographs are taken of the area.[10]

Methods of Vascular Repair

An analogy of repair techniques can be drawn from peripheral nerve repair. Generally, direct vascular repair, including arteriorrhaphy or venorrhaphy or anastomosis, involves direct suturing of the traumatized vessel. Interpositional grafting uses an autograph or synthetic graft material (polytetrafluoroethylene [PTFE]) or Dacron).[10]

THROMBOEMBOLIC DISEASE

Thromboembolic disease, caused by a deep vein thrombosis (DVT) that may propagate to pulmonary embolism (PE), is one of the most common causes of mortality and morbidity in hospitalized patients. Hip and knee arthroplasties place patients at increased risk of developing thromboembolic disease. The probability of a TKA patient developing DVT, without additional risk factors or prophylactic anticoagulation, is between 40% and 70%.[7]

Risk Factors

Several intrinsic and extrinsic conditions are identified as additive risk factors in the potential development of thromboembolic disease. Surgery, trauma, obesity, pregnancy, age older than 40 years, use of oral contraceptives, and immobility are well-known causative factors. In addition, history of DVT and varicose veins, smoking, family history, and congestive heart failure contribute as risk factors for DVT development. The type of surgery has little effect on the incidence of DVT. Rather, it is other factors, such as heart disease and length of immobilization, that determine the incidence.[10]

Pathophysiology of Thromboembolism

Most thrombi start in the valve cusps of the deep lower leg veins. Critical components of the coagulation cascade are prothrombin, thrombin, fibronectin, and fibrin. The result of this cascade is stimulation of platelet adherence to vessel walls. Eventually, this buildup of blood cells creates a thrombus. A dislodged clot from the thrombus is referred to as an *embolus*. PE is a life-threatening consequence in which the lower lobes of the lungs are involved four times more often than the upper lobes.[11]

Virchow Triad

Three factors generally lead to DVT development. Categorically referred to as *Virchow triad*, the factors are hypercoagulability, venous stasis (caused by immobilization,

obesity, heart disease), and venous injury, especially with endothelial damage (caused by surgery, trauma, and previous DVTs). Damage exposes the vessel walls to collagen and basement membrane, and von Willebrand factor (vWF) increases platelet activity and number. The initial trauma shifts the balance more toward coagulation than fibrinolysis and ultimately DVT formation.[10,11]

Vessel wall injury and stasis are directly related to orthopedic surgical procedures, such as total joint arthroplasty (TJA), and repair of pelvic and femoral fractures. Once a DVT has formed, without treatment, one of three processes occurs. The thrombus undergoes partial or complete lysis with complete or near-complete recannulization of the thrombosed blood vessel. The thrombus becomes more organized, resulting in further proximal vessel occlusion. The thrombus dislodges, completely or partially escaping to a proximal site in the vascular system as an embolus.[10]

Signs and Symptoms of Deep Vein Thrombosis

Very high levels of suspicion must accompany all complaints of proximal thigh, inguinal and lower leg pain after TJA, pelvic or femoral fractures, spinal surgery, and general trauma. Some signs and symptoms are nonspecific, such as diffuse complaints of leg pain and tenderness. Others are more specific, including edema, palpable warmth, skin discoloration, prominent superficial veins, and presence of Homans sign (pain in the calf upon ankle dorsiflexion). Approximately 50% of DVT cases are asymptomatic. Both extremities require assessment because studies show that thrombosis is generally present bilaterally, even when injury is limited to only one lower extremity.[10]

Diagnostic Studies

Duplex ultrasonography is a common noninvasive diagnostic technique for suspected DVT. This test combines venous system Doppler flow detection and ultrasound imaging with manual compression of the suspected vein. Veins that do not easily compress with normal pressure on the transducer are considered positive for DVT. Clinical probability estimates of physical examination alone in the presence of Homans sign, edema, and palpable firmness are approximately 50% for incidence of DVT. Generally, thrombi in the inguinal area, deep proximal thigh, and popliteal area are considered more dangerous than deep calf vein thrombi, because distal clots are smaller and less frequently associated with major complications.[10]

Pulmonary Emboli

Pulmonary emboli are a result and complication of DVT. A dislocated deep vein thrombus may travel to the pulmonary artery or obstruct pulmonary blood supply. The result is hypoxia from constriction of the bronchioles, mediated by vasoactive substances such as serotonin, histamine, and prostaglandins. The effect is pulmonary infarction, shock, right heart failure, and occasionally, death.[5,10]

Signs and Symptoms

Generally, tachypnea (>18 breaths/minute) is the most common sign of PE. Dyspnea is the most frequent symptom. The patient may also complain of pleuritic pain, develop a cough or hemoptysis, or report feeling apprehensive. These signs and symptoms are usually related to the size of the embolus and the patient's cardiopulmonary status.[5,10]

Treatment of Thromboembolic Disease

Selective use of prophylactic anticoagulants decreases the incidence of DVT in elective surgery patients without altering the operative plan. Patients undergoing TJA are treated with heparin, or low-molecular-weight heparin (LMWH). The judicious use of LMWH has proven to be both safe and effective in DVT prevention and treatment. The patient's response to LMWH is more predictable than the response to heparin, and the rate of bleeding complications is less than with heparin.[10]

If prophylactic anticoagulants are not administered preoperatively, administration of anticoagulation medication begins 12 to 24 hours postoperatively. Warfarin (Coumadin), an oral anticoagulant, is used simultaneously with heparin or during the transition from intravenous or subcutaneous anticoagulation. Coumadin is indicated for prophylaxis and treatment of DVT or PE. The duration of therapy may be 3 to 6 months postoperatively, depending on patient's risk factors and possibility of recurrence.[5,10]

Nonpharmacologic treatment of DVT includes early mobilization and judicious exercise after surgery, use of antiembolism stockings, or intermittent pneumatic compression. Contraindications for use of antiembolism stockings are arterial compromise or peripheral neuropathy. Use of pneumatic compression devices is inadvisable in the presence of local ulceration, cellulitis, and arterial insufficiency. The bent knee and semisitting positions increase the incidence of postoperative thromboembolic complications. Patients should be as mobile as possible as early as possible after their surgery.[5]

✤ GLOSSARY

Axonotmesis: Loss of continuity of axons, with varying degrees of injury to the perineurium and endoneurium.

Creep: Tissue's ability to change or "creep" to a new length in response to a constant, applied load.

Denervation: Distal tissues undergo physiologic changes: bone becomes osteoporotic, joints become fibrotic, and muscles atrophy.

Neurapraxia: Axon maintains continuity, no distal degeneration, usually due to compression.

Neurotmesis: Complete physiologic disruption of nerve.

REFERENCES

1. Bodine SC, Lieber RL: Peripheral nerve physiology, anatomy, and pathology. In Buckwalter JA, Einhorn TA, Simon SR, editors: *Orthopaedic basic science, biology, and biomechanics of the musculoskeletal system*, ed 2, Rosemont, Ill, 2000, American Academy of Orthopaedic Surgeons.
2. Brinker MR, O'Connor DP: Basic sciences. In Miller MD, Hart JA, editors: *Review of orthopaedics*, ed 5, Philadelphia, 2008, Saunders.
3. Cole PA: Diagnosis and management of musculoskeletal trauma. In Swiontkowski MF, Stovitz SD, editors: *Manual of orthopaedics*, ed 6, Philadelphia, 2006, Lippincott Williams & Wilkins.
4. Feliciano DV: Evaluation and treatment of vascular injuries. In Browner BD, Jupiter JB, Levine AM, et al, editors: *Skeletal trauma: basic science, management, and reconstruction*, ed 3, Philadelphia, 2003, Saunders.
5. Goodman CG: The respiratory system. In Goodman CG, Fuller KS, Boissonnault WG, editors: *Pathology: implications for the physical therapist*, ed 2, Philadelphia, 2003, Saunders.
6. Gupta R, Mozaffar T: Neuromuscular diseases. In Einhorn TA, O'Keefe RJ, Buckwalter JA, editors: *Orthopaedic basic science: foundations of clinical practice*, ed 3, Rosemont, Ill, 2007, American Academy of Orthopaedic Surgeons.
7. Hyers TM, Hill RD, Weg JG: Antithrombotic therapy for venous thromboembolic disease, *Chest* 89(Suppl 2):26S–35S, 1986.
8. Lee SK, Wolfe SW: Peripheral nerve injury and repair, *J Am Acad Orthop Surg* 8(4):243–252, 2000.
9. Lundborg G: *Nerve injury and repair: regeneration, reconstruction, and cortical remodeling*, ed 2, Philadelphia, 2004, Churchill Livingstone.
10. Roberts CS, Gleis GE, Seligson D: Diagnosis and treatment of complications. In Browner BD, Jupiter JB, Levine AM, et al editors: *Skeletal trauma: basic science, management, and reconstruction*, ed 3, Philadelphia, 2003, Saunders.
11. Thibodeau GA, Patton KT: *Anatomy and physiology*, ed 6, St Louis, 2007, Mosby.
12. Topp KS, Boyd BS: Structure and biomechanics of peripheral nerves: nerve responses to physical stresses and implications for physical therapist practice, *Phys Ther* 86:92–109, 2006.

REVIEW QUESTIONS

Short Answer

1. Describe the gross anatomic connective tissue barriers of peripheral nerve tissue.
2. Outline and describe three classifications of peripheral nerve injury.
3. Certain peripheral nerves are at risk for compression because of surrounding soft tissue and bone that limit three-dimensional motion of nerves. Name four nerves.
4. Describe "hard" signs of vascular injury.
5. Name the components of Virchow triad.
6. List the risk factors for developing DVT.
7. Describe the signs of DVT.

True/False

8. Peripheral nerve tissue is avascular.
9. Peripheral nerve tissue is highly deformable, with viscoelastic properties similar to other soft tissue.

10. Peripheral nerve tissue healing is highly predictable.
11. Spinal nerve roots are more susceptible to compression injury than peripheral nerve tissue because spinal nerve roots have no epineurium or perineurium.
12. Anatomically, veins demonstrate more connective tissue than arteries, rendering veins less "elastic" than arteries.
13. Pulselessness, pallor, paresthesias, pain, and paralysis are examples of "soft" vascular signs of injury.
14. Approximately 10% of patients have asymptomatic DVT.
15. The presence of Homans sign, edema, and palpable soft tissue firmness is only 50% reliable for positive DVT.

PART III

COMMON MEDICATIONS IN ORTHOPEDICS

This section establishes an awareness of key elements, terms, and definitions involving antiinflammatory and antibiotic agents that provide the student physical therapist assistant (PTA) and practicing clinician with a cursory introduction to the basics of orthopedic pharmacology.

Orthopedic physical therapy interventions involving the PTA do not divest interest in or responsibility for the care of the whole patient. Knowledge concerning neurovascular anatomy and healing of various organ systems of the body play essential roles in the delivery of physical therapy procedures. Therefore an appreciation of antibacterial medications and antiinflammatory agents aids the PTA in understanding the complexity and interdependence of medications and orthopedic health care.

This section is presented as a means of broadening the focus of specific PTA education of exposing the student to concepts of prophylactic antibacterial medications used to treat orthopedic infections, classifications of antibiotic medications and related offending organisms, and introducing nonsteroidal antiinflammatory drugs (NSAIDs) and corticosteroids related to acute and chronic pain and inflammation.

In the day-to-day delivery of physical therapy, the PTA encounters many orthopedic afflictions requiring medications to target specific bacterial organisms, as well as antiinflammatory agents to control pain and swelling.

A basic understanding of drug administration routes and bioavailability, as well as the use of NSAIDs versus the use of corticosteroids, allows the student and clinician to more efficiently and effectively enhance patient care.

13 Orthopedic Pharmacology

LaDonna S. Hale

LEARNING OBJECTIVES

1. Discuss pharmacokinetic concepts, including absorption, distribution, metabolism, excretion half-life, and duration of action, and their relationship and significance to rehabilitation therapies.
2. Discuss pharmacodynamic concepts including the dose–response relationship, therapeutic window, adverse drug reactions, toxicity, tolerance, withdrawal, and addiction.
3. List the general principles of safe medication use and the physical therapist assistant's role in optimizing patient safety.
4. Discuss general principles of treatment and prevention of orthopedic infection including why such infections are difficult to treat and importance of antibiotic compliance.
5. Discuss the analgesics best suited for different types of pain.
6. Discuss how opioids work differently from antiinflammatory analgesics in the treatment of pain.
7. Discuss common side effects and precautions associated with opioids, acetaminophen, nonsteroidal antiinflammatory drugs, cyclooxygenase-2 inhibitors, and corticosteroids.
8. Discuss the risk of acetaminophen overdoses during pain management.

KEY TERMS

Absorption
Adverse drug reaction
Analgesic

Duration of action
Half-life
Neuropathic pain

Nociceptive pain
Pharmacodynamics
Pharmacokinetics

CHAPTER OUTLINE

BASIC PRINCIPLES OF PHARMACOLOGY AND SAFE MEDICATION USE

Knowledge concerning the interaction between medications and the treatment and maintenance of orthopedic health is essential for the safe and effective application of rehabilitation interventions. This chapter aids the student and practicing physical therapist assistant (PTA) in providing optimal patient care through an introduction to key concepts of orthopedic pharmacology. Infections, pain/inflammation, and osteoporosis can significantly affect recovery and optimal application of physical therapy.

Pharmacokinetics

Simply put, **pharmacokinetics** is a term used to describe what the body does to a medication. The four pharmacokinetic phases are (1) **absorption**, (2) distribution, (3) metabolism, and (4) excretion.[7]

Absorption describes how the medication moves from its site of administration into the systemic circulation (into the bloodstream). Some common routes of administration are shown in Table 13-1. Most medications must move from the site of administration into systemic circulation to be effective. Others, such as topical creams or inhalers, may provide therapeutic benefits through a localized effect. Although systemic absorption may not be necessary for effectiveness of topically applied medications, it can occur and result in side effects. For example, high dose, long-term use of inhaled corticosteroids to treat asthma has been shown to result in enough systemic absorption to increase the risk of developing osteoporosis.[12,15]

The rate and extent of drug absorption through the skin can be dramatically increased by application of heat; therefore heat generating modalities (e.g., heating pads, ultrasound, infrared lamps, and warm hydrotherapy) should not be applied near transdermal medication patches. Electromagnetic (e.g., ultraviolet radiation, lasers, and diathermy) and electrical current modalities (e.g., transcutaneous electrical nerve stimulation [TENS]) should also not be used near medication patches because many patches have metallic backings that conduct electric currents, leading to significant heat generation and burns.[3]

Distribution describes movement of the medication from the bloodstream into various areas of the body such as the central nervous system (CNS), breast milk, and adipose (fat) tissue. This concept can be helpful in understanding medication actions and side effects. For example, opioid pain relievers act on the CNS to relieve pain; therefore an opioid will be most effective if it can easily distribute into the CNS. Only antibiotics with good distribution into bone tissue will be effective in treating osteomyelitis.

Medications are cleared from the body through metabolism, excretion, or both. Metabolism is the biotransformation or chemical alteration of the medication. The byproduct of drug metabolism is called a *metabolite*. Through metabolism, some medications are inactivated, whereas others remain active (active metabolite) but are more water soluble for easier elimination by the kidneys. Generally, metabolism takes place in the liver but it can occur through enzymatic processes in the kidneys, lungs, and bloodstream. Differences in drug response, side effects, and safe dose can be greatly affected by genetic differences in drug metabolism.[21]

Excretion describes elimination of the medication without prior metabolism (excreted unchanged) or, more commonly, elimination of the metabolites. Generally, excretion takes place through the kidneys (renal excretion, urine) but also occurs through the gastrointestinal tract (feces), lungs (breath), and skin (sweat).

The rate at which a drug is cleared from the body is referred to as *half-life*. Technically speaking, half-life is the amount of time it takes to reduce the concentration of the drug in the body by half. Drug half-lives can range from seconds to days. Anything that slows a drug's clearance will lengthen its half-life. Liver metabolism and renal clearance are slower in older adults (>70 years) as compared with younger adults, and likewise for persons with acute or chronic liver or kidney disease.[7] The most common type of clinically significant drug-drug interaction occurs when the presence of one drug slows the metabolism of a second drug.[21] When drug clearance is decreased for whatever reason and the patient's daily dose is not also decreased, drug accumulation and toxicity can occur.

A medication's **duration of action** (the length of time it is active in the body) is related to its half-life. Drugs with a long half-life will have a long duration of action. Medications with a short duration of action usually require multiple daily administrations, three or four times daily, as compared to those with longer durations of action, which may only require dosing once or twice daily. One way medications can overcome a short duration of action is if they are formulated as a sustained release product. A sustained release product is usually in tablet or capsule form and is specially designed to dissolve very slowly in the intestines. By dissolving gradually over 12 or 24 hours, its effects will last longer. In general, sustained release products should not be chewed, crushed or broken open. Doing so can destroy the product's sustained release properties, causing the entire dosage to be released at once.

Pharmacodynamics

Simply put, **pharmacodynamics** is a term used to describe what the medication does to the body. It is a study of the relationship between the amount of drug in the body and the response observed.[7] Pharmacodynamics include a wide variety of principles, such as

Table 13-1	*List of Common Routes of Administration*	
Route	Description	Example Medication(s)
Oral (PO)	Swallowed; uses the gastrointestinal tract	Most commonly used route of administration in U.S.; tablets, capsules, oral liquids
Sublingual (SL)	Under the tongue; medication rapidly absorbs into systemic circulation	Nitroglycerin tablets for chest pain
Rectal	Administered through the rectum; some absorb into systemic circulation, others provide a local laxative effect	Glycerin suppositories (laxatives) Promethazine (Phenergan) for nausea
Inhalation	Into the lungs	Bronchodilators for asthma, such as albuterol inhalers Corticosteroids for asthma such as flunisolide (AeroBid) inhalers
Intranasal	Into the nose; some absorb into systemic circulation, others provide a local effect	Systemic absorption required for effectiveness: calcitonin (Miacalcin) nasal spray for osteoporosis Localized effect: intranasal decongestants (Afrin)
Intravenous (IV)	Directly into the veins; most rapid onset of action	Common route of administration in hospitals; morphine, antibiotics
Intramuscular (IM)	Into the muscle	Some vaccinations, penicillin G benzathine
Subcutaneous (SQ, SC, SubCut)	Into the subcutaneous layer of skin	Insulin Teriparatide (Forteo) for osteoporosis
Intraarticular	Into the joint space; causes a localized effect within the joint, some systemic absorption may occur	Triamcinolone, methylprednisolone, hyaluronic acid (Orthovisc, Hyalgan) for osteoarthritis
Epidural	Into the epidural space (within the spinal column but outside the dura mater)	Fentanyl, lidocaine, corticosteroids
Transdermal (TD)	Medication patches where the medication moves through the skin into systemic circulation	Patches including: nicotine, nitroglycerin, clonidine, contraceptives, fentanyl, and lidocaine
Topical	Creams and ointments applied to the skin with an expected localized effect; systemic absorption may or may not occur	Creams and ointments including BENGAY cream, capsaicin (Zostrix), hydrocortisone

the dose–response relationship, therapeutic window, adverse reactions, and toxicity.

The dose–response relationship describes the relationship between the amount of drug in the body and its expected effectiveness and likelihood and severity of side effects (e.g., the higher the dose, the more side effects seen). This is closely tied to the concept of therapeutic window. A drug's therapeutic window may be described as wide or narrow. The window is defined as the minimum drug concentration needed for the drug to show effectiveness, without causing toxicity in the patient. Penicillins and most cephalosporin antibiotics have wide therapeutic windows. Drugs with narrow therapeutic windows include the anticoagulant, warfarin (commonly used after orthopedic surgeries), and antiseizure medications (commonly used to treat

phantom pain after amputation or in diabetic **neuropathic pain**).

The term adverse drug reaction (ADR), also termed *side effect*, describes any unintended effect of the medication including an exaggerated medication response. An example of an exaggerated response is extreme hypotension after receiving a high blood pressure medication. Certain ADRs may be particularly problematic in the orthopedic population, including medications that may reduce safety or increase fall risk (e.g., orthostatic hypotension, dizziness, blurred vision, hypoglycemia, ataxia, gait abnormalities) or medications that affect cognitive function. There are also many medications that cause cardiovascular side effects that may complicate exertional activity by increasing heart rate (tachycardia) or blood pressure (hypertension), by

Table 13-2	*Helpful Drug Information Resources*
Name of Reference	**Description**
Epocrates Skyscape Medscape	Free online websites and free downloads for mobile devices. Source of general drug and disease information; some have information on drug costs.
Drugs.com	Free online website. Source of general drug information, a drug-drug interaction checker, and pill identifier.
Drug Information Handbook Publisher: Lexi-Comp, updated annually	For purchase in paperback and download for mobile devices. Source of comprehensive drug information.
Drug Facts and Comparisons Publisher: Facts and Comparisons	For purchase in hardbound and download for mobile devices. Source of comprehensive and very detailed drug information.

blunting the expected exercise-induced increase in heart rate, or by reducing heart rate (bradycardia). The term toxicity is often used interchangeably with ADR or side effect, but it is most accurate to reserve the term for situations where the serum concentrations have exceeded normal levels.

Tolerance occurs when the reaction to a drug diminishes over time. Tolerance can occur to both the benefits of a medication (making it less effective over time) and the ADRs (making it better tolerated over time).[4] Withdrawal symptoms indicate physical dependency and are expected to occur with certain medications when used over a prolonged period. Withdrawal symptoms are generally the opposite of the pharmacologic effects of the medication. For example, one withdrawal symptom of a medication used to lower blood pressure would be hypertension.

Psychological dependency, also called *addiction*, occurs with certain medications such as opioid **analgesics,** amphetamines, and benzodiazepine sleep aids, as well as other substances with abuse potential, including cocaine, heroin, alcohol, caffeine, and nicotine. Withdrawal symptoms do contribute to the development of addiction in that the patient continues to use the substance to avoid the unpleasantness of the withdrawal symptoms; but having withdrawal symptoms alone does not meet the definition of addiction. It is important to understand the difference between physical and psychological dependency.[4] Psychological dependency and addiction involve strong cravings and desires for the drug that overwhelm daily life. There is a loss of control over its usage and use continues despite its negative impact on quality of life.[4,6] Drug addiction is most strongly associated with medications that rapidly distribute into the CNS causing high levels of euphoria and dysregulation of the neurotransmitters involved in the body's natural reward and pleasure centers.

Principles of Safe Medication Use

Although PTAs are not involved in the decision-making process regarding prescription and over-the-counter (OTC) medication use, having a general understanding of commonly used medications and knowing where to look for more information can help the PTA identify medication-related problems that should be brought to the attention of the prescriber or other health care team members. PTAs often spend more time with patients during therapy sessions than a prescriber spends with the patient during a typical office visit. This may provide opportunities to identify problems with compliance, lack of medication knowledge, ADRs, and lack of drug effectiveness. A variety of drug information resources exist that can be helpful in providing information, such as mechanism of action, dosing, therapeutic uses, and ADRs. See Table 13-2 for a list of helpful drug information resources. Although such resources exist, the PTA must be cautious about providing specific information to the patient that would be considered outside the PTA's scope of practice.

The following general principles of safe medication use can be provided to any patient:

- Keep a current list of all medications including prescription, OTC, and herbal
- Keep medications in their original containers
- Never take some else's medication
- Take medications exactly as directed
- Do not start or stop medications without consulting the prescriber
- Report any new symptoms to the prescriber
- Don't chew, crush, or break any capsules or tablets unless instructed
- When measuring liquid medications, use only the measuring device provided
- Be knowledgeable about the medications
- Ask questions when things are unclear[10]

MEDICATIONS TO TREAT AND PREVENT ORTHOPEDIC INFECTIONS

Antibiotic use in the treatment and prevention of orthopedic related infections is common. Antibiotics are medications with the ability to kill or inhibit growth of bacteria. Common examples of antibiotics used in the

Table 13-3	Common Antibiotics Used to Treat and Prevent Various Types of Orthopedic Infections*
Drug Class	**Specific Antibiotics**
Penicillins	Amoxicillin (Amoxil) oral
	Dicloxacillin (Dynapen) oral
	Nafcillin (Nafcil, Unipen) injection
	Oxacillin (Prostaphlin) injection, oral
	Penicillin (various brands) injection, oral
Cephalosporins	Cefaclor (Ceclor) oral
	Cefadroxil (Duricef) oral
	Cefazolin (Ancef, Kefzol) injection
	Cefixime (Suprax) oral
	Cefpodoxime (Vantin) oral
	Cetazidime (Fortaz) injection
	Ceftriaxone (Rocephin) injection
	Cephalexin (Keflex) oral
Tetracyclines	Doxycycline (Vibramycin) oral
	Minocycline (Minocin) oral
	Tetracycline (Sumycin) oral
Antifolate (sulfonamides)	Sulfamethoxazole/trimethoprim (Bactrim, Septra) oral
Quinolones	Ciprofloxacin (Cipro) injection, oral
	Levofloxacin (Levaquin) injection, oral
	Ofloxacin (Floxin) injection, oral
Miscellaneous	Clindamycin (Cleocin) injection, oral
	Gentamicin (Garamycin) injection
	Vancomycin (Vancocin) injection

*This is not an all-inclusive list of antibiotics.

hospital and outpatient orthopedic settings are listed in Table 13-3. Orthopedic infections can result in slowed recovery, permanent joint damage, amputation, nonunion in cases of fracture, removal of implanted hardware, and death due to sepsis. Appropriate antibiotics are selected, taking into account the type of documented or suspected bacterial pathogens, the drug's ability to distribute adequately to the site of infection, patient allergy history, side effects, and cost. Because the risk of infection following orthopedic surgeries is high, antibiotics are routinely administered before the procedure to reduce the risk of infection-related complications. The use of antibiotics to prevent an infection is referred to as *prophylaxis*.

Compliance with the prescribed antibiotic regimen is essential to reduce the risk of bacterial resistance and to improve outcomes. Patients taking oral antibiotics should take the medication exactly as instructed for the full course of therapy. It is common for patients to stop taking their antibiotic when they start to feel better (e.g., fever resolves, pain at the site of infection is reduced). Stopping the antibiotic too early can allow the infection to return and/or increase the risk of developing bacterial resistance to that antibiotic. To assure optimal oral absorption, dosing instructions should be followed carefully. For example, some antibiotics should be taken on an empty stomach, defined as at least 1 hour before or 2 hours after a meal; others should be taken with meals to avoid stomach upset; others should not be taken within 2 hours of calcium-containing antacids or milk.

Another important concept regarding antibiotic compliance is around-the-clock dosing. To achieve steady blood levels of the antibiotic at the site of infection, antibiotics should be dosed at regularly spaced intervals throughout the day. For example, an antibiotic ordered to be taken three times daily should not be taken at breakfast, lunch, and supper but rather, divided evenly throughout the day every 8 hours. When the concentration of antibiotic falls below the minimum level needed to kill or inhibit bacterial growth, the weaker pathogen strains will be affected, leaving the strong pathogens to replicate and grow in numbers. This can quickly lead to bacterial resistance. Skipping doses creates a similar problem.

The PTA can improve outcomes by discussing the importance of following antibiotic instructions carefully, completing the full course of therapy as prescribed, and referring noncompliance issues to the appropriate health care provider. Antibiotic compliance is important for all orthopedic patients, but is especially important in those with reduced peripheral circulation, such as those with peripheral vascular disease (PVD) and diabetes. Delivery of antibiotics to the site of infection may be particularly reduced in these populations. The PTA can also help prevent the spread of infection through thorough hand washing and adequately cleaning rehabilitation equipment between patients.

MEDICATIONS TO TREAT PAIN AND INFLAMMATION

Effective treatment of pain and inflammation not only reduces suffering, but speeds healing following injury. Patients experiencing inadequately treated pain often have compromised mobility, restricted activities of daily living, disturbed sleep, and reduced quality of life. As a result, they may not be able to participate in beneficial physical therapy to the fullest potential.

Pain is often undertreated. Pain management is heavily associated with biases related to socioeconomic status, race, culture, age, and gender. Some prescribers do not understand treatment of different types of pain; pain is not always considered to be a treatment priority; and there are misperceptions regarding the risk of opioid addiction and side effects.

The Joint Commission has emphasized pain treatment as a responsibility of health care providers and a patient's right by requiring routine pain assessment as the "fifth vital sign." It is recommended that regular assessment and documentation of pain severity, functional ability, progress towards achieving therapeutic goals, and presence of ADRs occur in both children and adults.[1,6]

An analgesic is any medication that reduces pain. There are three broad categories of oral and IV analgesics: (1) opioids, (2) acetaminophen, and (3) antiinflammatory agents. Appropriate analgesics are chosen based upon the type of pain (acute/chronic, nociceptive/neuropathic, inflammatory/noninflammatory), level of pain, side effects, and cost.

Types of Pain

Nociceptive pain results from actual tissue damage. Nociceptive pain may be inflammatory or noninflammatory or both. Examples include osteoarthritis, bone pain, muscle sprains, and postsurgical pain. This type of pain responds well to opioid analgesics, acetaminophen, and antiinflammatory agents. Nociceptive pain specifically caused by inflammation is referred to as *inflammatory pain*. As expected, inflammatory pain responds best to the antiinflammatory agents, including corticosteroids, nonsteroidal antiinflammatory drugs (NSAIDs), and cyclooxygenase-2 (COX-2) inhibitors. Examples of inflammatory pain include rheumatoid arthritis, muscle aches and sprains, and bursitis.

Neuropathic pain results from damage to or dysfunction of nerves. Examples include nerve compression, fibromyalgias, diabetic neuropathy, postherpetic neuralgia, spinal cord injuries, and phantom pain following amputation. Neuropathic pain is relatively resistant to opioids, acetaminophen, and antiinflammatory agents, although they may be helpful in certain cases. The most effective medication to treat neuropathic pain will vary by patient. The medications that tend to be most effective in treating neuropathic pain are medications that slow or block nerve conduction. Antidepressants such as duloxetine (Cymbalta), amitriptyline (Elavil), desipramine (Norpramin), venlafaxine (Effexor), and others are commonly used, as are anticonvulsants such as pregabalin (Lyrica), gabapentin (Neurontin), carbamazepine (Tegretol), and others. Effective topical products include lidocaine (Lidoderm) patch and capsaicin (Zostrix) cream.[13,19,20] The opioid analgesic, tramadol (Ultram), is also often used to treat neuropathic pain because it is an opioid analgesic with additional antidepressant-like properties on nerve conduction.

Acute pain occurs following injury to the body and generally disappears when the injury heals. Chronic pain continues past the normal time of expected healing, which is assumed to be about 3 months.[6,11] Persistent pain, whether acute or chronic, generally responds better to around-the-clock dosing rather than on demand dosing (also called *prn dosing* or *as needed dosing*). Many types of inflammatory pain as well as neuropathic pain are chronic rather than acute. Opioids, acetaminophen, and NSAIDs have quick onsets of action, within minutes to hours, whereas drugs for neuropathic pain, such as antidepressants and anticonvulsants, generally are not effective for several weeks. Ideally, when treating persistent chronic pain, patients are prescribed medications with a long duration of action and/or sustained release products to prevent the need for frequent daily administration. Patients may then take a shorter-acting analgesic or immediate release product for breakthrough pain. *Breakthrough pain* is pain that occurs despite the use of regularly scheduled pain medications.[6]

Opioid Analgesics

Opioid analgesics are all chemically related to opium. Commonly used prescription opioid medications include morphine, oxycodone, hydrocodone, and codeine. See Appendix A for others. Opioid analgesics work within the CNS to block the transmission of pain and create a feeling of euphoria. It is important to note that although pain is relieved, the underlying disease process or cause of the pain is not altered. Opioids are the most powerful medications available for treatment of nociceptive pain; they are also effective for some patients with neuropathic pain. IV opioids are more commonly used for inpatient settings for moderate to severe acute pain. Oral agents can be used for mild, moderate, or severe acute or chronic pain in any setting. Opioids are sometimes administered epidurally to provide highly effective pain control directly upon the spinal cord. Fentanyl (Duragesic) is available as a transdermal patch that provides control of severe, chronic pain.

Side effects of the opioid analgesics include nausea and vomiting (take with food to minimize risk), allergic reactions, sedation, drowsiness, dizziness, constipation, hypotension and orthostatic hypotension, slowed heart rate, slowed respiration, impaired judgment, physical dependence, and addiction.[14] Several of these side effects reduce the patient's safety and may increase risk of falls and injury. Constipation caused by chronic opioid use is extremely common but can be treated and prevented with over-the-counter stool softeners and mild laxatives including senna, docusate (Colace), and bisacodyl (Dulcolax) tablets.

Health care providers and patients alike may overestimate the risk of developing addiction when managing pain with opioids. This misperception can lead to inadequate pain control through underprescribing or underdosing, and patients skipping doses or "taking as little as possible." The actual risk of developing opioid addiction following chronic use for medical management of pain is difficult to assess, but has been estimated at approximately 0.2% (2 in 1000) for persons with no prior history of substance abuse, and 3.3% (33 in 1000) for the general population.[8]

Tolerance and physical dependency are likely to occur with chronic use and are not equivalent to addiction. Although certain behaviors may seem like warning signs of addiction, the PTA should not make assumptions. Behaviors such as aggressively complaining about pain, occasionally taking more than prescribed, drug hoarding during periods of reduced pain, openly acquiring similar drugs from other medical resources, reporting unintended psychiatric effects, and resistance to changes in therapy are not necessarily signs of addiction. These behaviors are equally likely to occur in nonaddicted patients experiencing tolerance, an increase in pain level, poorly controlled pain, and anxiety related to a return of pain.[18] Prescribers must balance the legitimate medical need for opioids in patients with chronic pain with the possibility of addiction and abuse.[6]

Acetaminophen

Acetaminophen is the most commonly used OTC fever reducer and analgesic. It is effective for a variety of non-inflammatory, mild to moderate, acute, and chronic types of pain, including headaches, toothaches, sinus pain, back pain, osteoarthritis, and many others. Its mechanism of action is somewhat unclear but likely involves inhibition of prostaglandins and cyclooxygenase (COX) and some CNS activity.[2] Although it affects prostaglandins and COX, it does not have strong antiinflammatory properties and is not an NSAID.

Many oral opioids also contain acetaminophen. Acetaminophen tablets come in regular strength (325 mg per tablet) and extra strength (500 mg per tablet). Per OTC package instructions, the typical adult dose is two tablets every 6 hours.[14] For the regular strength tablets, this dose will equal 2600 mg/day; for the extra strength tablets, this dose will equal 4000 mg/day.

Acetaminophen has a strong record of safety when used at normal doses in healthy people. As compared to NSAIDs, acetaminophen is the safest OTC analgesic in patients with a history of gastrointestinal bleeding, congestive heart failure, hypertension, and patients taking the oral anticoagulant, warfarin (Coumadin). The major health concern with chronic acetaminophen use is hepatotoxicity (liver toxicity). Analysis of various national databases estimates that acetaminophen overdoses cause 56,000 emergency department visits, 26,000 hospitalizations, and 460 deaths annually in the United States, and the number of fatalities is growing rapidly.[16] In 2009, the US Food and Drug Administration (FDA) convened a special meeting to discuss how to address this growing public health problem.[17]

The cause of liver toxicity involves its metabolism. When used at normal dosages, the majority of acet-aminophen is metabolized into a nontoxic metabolite and only 5% is metabolized into a liver toxic metabolite. Under normal circumstances, the body is able to quickly detoxify this metabolite and no liver damage occurs. When used in excessive dosages or in the presence of preexisting liver impairment, the body cannot detoxify quickly enough.[7]

Patients taking acetaminophen chronically should be asked about alcohol use. Package instructions state: "If you consume three or more alcoholic drinks per day, ask your doctor whether you should take acetaminophen or other pain relievers/fever reducers."[14] The reason for this warning is that heavy, chronic alcohol use shifts the metabolism of acetaminophen, resulting in a higher percentage of toxic metabolite production. Again, the body cannot detoxify quickly enough and the risk of liver damage increases.

To minimize the risk of liver toxicity, dosages should not exceed 4 gm/day (4000 mg/day) for most healthy adult patients. This maximum "safe" dose may be too high for frail older adults, persons who chronically use alcohol, and those with impaired liver function.[17]

More than 100 prescription and OTC products contain acetaminophen, including cough and cold products and some sleep aids (e.g., Tylenol PM). Patients prescribed opioids containing acetaminophen must be cautioned to check the labels of all prescription analgesics and OTC products to avoid accidental overdose. Some prescription analgesics use the abbreviation APAP (N-acetyl-para-aminophenol) on the label rather than acetaminophen. Although this may save space on prescription labels, it can be confusing for patients. For example, a prescription bottle labeled as "hydrocodone/APAP" contains both hydrocodone and acetaminophen.

Nonsteroidal Antiinflammatory Drugs

Four NSAIDs are available OTC: aspirin, ibuprofen, naproxen, and ketoprofen. The others are available by prescription only. Two NSAIDs are available in injection form, ketorolac and ibuprofen. NSAIDs are very commonly used OTC as fever reducers and analgesics. NSAIDs are effective for a variety of noninflammatory, mild to moderate, acute and chronic pain, including headaches, back pain, and osteoarthritis, and are especially effective for inflammatory pain, including rheumatoid arthritis, carpal tunnel syndrome, acute gout, lateral and medial epicondylitis (tennis elbow and golf elbow), and bursitis.[5,7] NSAIDs can be found in a variety of OTC products, including cough and cold products and some sleep aids (e.g., Advil PM). A few prescription opioid analgesics contain ibuprofen or aspirin (see Appendix A).

Aspirin is an NSAID, although it is often described separately because its therapeutic uses and side effect profile are somewhat different from the other NSAIDs. Aspirin should not be used in children because it can cause a rare, but potentially fatal illness of childhood known as *Reye syndrome*. Aspirin has strong antiplatelet effects, and is therefore used in low dosages, 81 to 325 mg/day, to prevent ischemic strokes. Higher dosages (650 mg/dose) are required to achieve analgesic benefits.[14]

The mechanism of action of NSAIDs involves inhibition of prostaglandins and cyclooxygenase type 1 and COX-2. Because of side effects, NSAIDs are not appropriate for all patients. NSAIDs should be avoided in persons with difficult to control hypertension, congestive heart failure, kidney disease, stomach ulcers, bleeding disorders, alcoholism, and patients taking anticoagulants (e.g., warfarin).[7,14]

Cyclooxygenase-2 Inhibitors

Currently, celecoxib (Celebrex) is the only COX-2 inhibitor on the market. Available by prescription only, celecoxib is used to treat the same types of pain as NSAIDs but with a lower risk of certain side effects. Like the NSAIDs, celecoxib also inhibits the production of prostaglandins by inhibiting the COX enzyme; however, it inhibits COX-2 but not COX-1. Inhibition of COX-2 results in the same antiinflammatory benefits as the NSAIDs and side effects related to fluid accumulation (avoid in persons with hypertension, congestive heart failure, and kidney disease). Because celecoxib does not inhibit COX-1 to a large degree, it has fewer bleeding-related and stomach-related side effects, so it is safer than other NSAIDs in persons at risk for gastrointestinal bleeding, including persons over 65 years of age, with bleeding disorders, alcoholism, and taking anticoagulants.[5] Because of potential cross-sensitivity, persons allergic to sulfonamide antibiotics (e.g., sulfamethoxazole/trimethoprim [Bactrim and Septra]) should not be prescribed celecoxib.

Corticosteroids

Corticosteroids (also called *glucocorticoids*) are produced naturally by the adrenal cortex and are involved in regulating metabolism of carbohydrates, proteins, and fats; inflammation; immune function; wound healing; and a wide number of other body systems. When used medically, corticosteroids have powerful antiinflammatory and immunosuppressant effects, making them useful in treating conditions such as rheumatoid arthritis, osteoarthritis, carpal tunnel syndrome, acute gout, lateral and medial epicondylitis, bursitis, and systemic lupus erythematosus (SLE). Corticosteroids may be administered orally, intravenously, or intraarticularly (into the joint). Commonly used corticosteroids are listed in Appendix A.

Intraarticular injections of corticosteroids (mainly methylprednisolone and triamcinolone) can provide excellent pain relief for joints with the advantage of local drug delivery and possibly fewer systemic side effects. After injection, the patient should minimize activity and stress on the joint for several days. Pain generally begins to decrease within 24 to 72 hours after injection, with maximum benefits in about 1 week. The analgesic and antiinflammatory benefits from a single injection may last for up to 4 to 8 weeks.[7] The most commonly injected joint is the knee. Other joints may include the shoulder, wrist, temporomandibular joint, ankle, and elbow. Even localized drug delivery results in some systemic absorption.[9] Side effects from intraarticular administration are similar to those seen with oral and intravenous administration, but are less frequent and also include local side effects, such as osteonecrosis (loss of blood supply to the bone, resulting in tissue death), tendon rupture, and skin atrophy at the injection site.[7,9]

Because corticosteroids have such wide effects on body systems, the side effects are broad and often significant, somewhat limiting their use. Corticosteroids can increase the risk for developing osteoporosis (loss of bone density). Therefore calcium and vitamin supplementation are suggested for persons receiving long-term systemic corticosteroids, and depending upon the patient's bone mineral density and other risk factors, medications to treat or prevent osteoporosis may also be prescribed. Most commonly these would include the bisphosphonates once weekly or once monthly (e.g., alendronate [Fosamax], risedronate [Actonel], ibandronate [Boniva]).

Corticosteroids can increase blood glucose (sugar) levels, especially in persons with diabetes or at high risk of diabetes. Because of their effects on metabolism of carbohydrates, proteins, and fats, high-dose corticosteroids can cause muscle myopathy, manifested as muscle weakness as well as abnormal fat distribution to the abdomen (potbelly), face (moon face), and upper back (buffalo hump). Other corticosteroid side effects include edema, cataracts, glaucoma, stomach ulcers, insomnia, risk of infection, mood changes, and even serious psychiatric disturbance.[7,9,14]

Summary

Persons receiving rehabilitation therapy frequently take prescription and OTC medications to treat infection, pain, inflammation, and a variety of other medical conditions. The PTA is not expected to be intimately familiar with the hundreds of commonly used medications on the market; however, knowledge of the medications discussed in this chapter will be particularly applicable to the orthopedic setting. It is important to be aware of the potential impact that medications can have on rehabilitation and to understand the general principles of safe medication use. Because PTAs spend a significant amount of one-on-one time with patients, they can be important patient advocates in detecting medication-related problems, including noncompliance, lack of effectiveness, and side effects. There are a number of easily accessible drug information resources as well as other members of the health care team who can assist in clarifying potential medication issues.

❖ GLOSSARY

Absorption: Manner in which a medication moves from its site of administration into the systemic circulation (into the bloodstream).

Adverse drug reaction: Any unintended effect of the medication including an exaggerated response; also termed *side effect.*

Analgesic: Any medication that reduces pain.

Duration of action: Length of time a drug is active in the body.

Half-life: Rate at which a drug is cleared from the body. Technical definition is the amount of time it takes to reduce the drug's blood concentration by half.

Neuropathic pain: Pain resulting from damage to or dysfunction of nerves.

Nociceptive pain: Pain resulting from tissue damage.

Pharmacodynamics: What a medication does to the body.

Pharmacokinetics: What the body does to a medication.

REFERENCES

1. American Academy of Pediatrics Committee on Psychosocial Aspects of Child and Family Health and American Pain Society Task Force on Pain in Infants, Children, and Adolescents: *The assessment and management of acute pain in infants, children, and adolescents* (website) www.ampainsoc.org/advocacy/pediatric2. htm. Accessed March 23, 2010.
2. Anderson BJ: Paracetamol (acetaminophen): mechanisms of action, *Paediatr Anaesth* 18:915–921, 2008.
3. Ball AM, Smith KM: Optimizing transdermal drug therapy, *Am J Health Syst Pharm* 65:1337–1346, 2008.
4. Ballantyne JC, LaForge KS: Opioid dependence and addiction during opioid treatment of chronic pain, *Pain* 129:235–255, 2007.
5. Chen YF, Jobanputra P, Barton P, et al: Cyclooxygenase-2 selective non-steroidal anti-inflammatory drugs (etodolac, meloxicam, celecoxib, rofecoxib, etoricoxib, valdecoxib and lumiracoxib) for osteoarthritis and rheumatoid arthritis: a systematic review and economic evaluation, *Health Technol Assess* 12:1–278, iii, 2008.
6. Chou R, Fanciullo GJ, Fine PG, et al: Clinical guidelines for the use of chronic opioid therapy in chronic noncancer pain, *J Pain* 10:113–130, 2009.
7. DiPiro JT, Talbert RL, Yee GC, et al: *Pharmacotherapy: a pathophysiologic approach*, ed 7, New York, 2008, McGraw-Hill.
8. Fishbain DA, Cole B, Lewis J, et al: What percentage of chronic nonmalignant pain patients exposed to chronic opioid analgesic therapy develop abuse/addiction and/or aberrant drug-related behaviors? A structured evidence-based review, *Pain Med* 9: 444–459, 2008.
9. Habib GS: Systemic effects of intra-articular corticosteroids, *Clin Rheumatol* 28:749–756, 2009.
10. Institute for Safe Medication Practices (ISMP): *General advice on safe medication use* (website) www.ismp.org/consumers/brochure. asp. Accessed March 23, 2010.
11. International Association for the Study of Pain, Subcommittee on Taxonomy: Classification of chronic pain. Descriptions of chronic pain syndromes and definitions of pain terms, *Pain Suppl* 3: S1–S226, 1986.
12. Israel E, Banerjee TR, Fitzmaurice GM, et al: Effects of inhaled glucocorticoids on bone density in premenopausal women, *N Engl J Med* 345:941–947, 2001.
13. Kroenke K, Krebs EE, Bair MJ: Pharmacotherapy of chronic pain: a synthesis of recommendations from systematic reviews, *Gen Hosp Psychiatry* 31:206–219, 2009.
14. Lacy CF, Armstrong LL, Goldman MP, et al: *Drug information handbook 2008 – 2009*, ed 17, Hudson, Ohio, 2008, Lexi-Comp Inc.
15. Lipworth BJ: Systemic adverse effects of inhaled corticosteroid therapy: a systematic review and meta-analysis, *Arch Intern Med* 159:941–955, 1999.
16. Nourjah P, Ahmad SR, Karwoski C, et al: Estimates of acetaminophen (Paracetomal)-associated overdoses in the United States, *Pharmacoepidemiol Drug Saf* 15:298–405, 2006.
17. Organ-specific warnings; internal analgesic, antipyretic, and anti-rheumatic drug products for over-the counter human use; final monograph. Final rule, *Fed Regist* 74(81):19385–19409, 2009.
18. Portenoy RK: Opioid therapy for chronic nonmalignant pain: current status. In Fields HL, Liebeskind JC, editors: *Progress in pain research and management*, (vol 1) *Pharmacological approaches to the treatment of chronic pain: new concepts and critical issues*, Seattle, 1994, IASP Publications, pp 247–287.
19. Saarto T, Wiffen PJ: Antidepressants for neuropathic pain, *Cochrane Database Syst Rev* (4):CD005454, 2007.
20. Wiffen PJ, Collins S, McQuay HJ, et al: Anticonvulsant drugs for acute and chronic pain, *Cochrane Database Syst Rev* (3):CD001133, 2005.
21. Wilkinson GR: Drug metabolism and variability among patients in drug response, *N Engl J Med* 352:2211–2221, 2005.

REVIEW QUESTIONS

Short Answer

1. Describe the difference between absorption and distribution.
2. What are several ways in which medications are removed or cleared from the body?
3. List three common routes of drug administration.
4. Why would a patient be given a drug with a wide therapeutic window?
5. What types of problems occur as the result of orthopedic infections?

PART IV

MOBILIZATION AND BIOMECHANICS

In this section, the physical therapist assistant (PTA) is introduced to rudimentary concepts and compulsory scientific principles related to biomechanics, gait, and peripheral joint mobilization techniques.

The study of biomechanics supports the application of principles of kinesiology when providing therapeutic interventions. The utility of biomechanics in all clinical settings is demonstrated in the daily provision of gait analysis, manual muscle testing, goniometric assessments, therapeutic exercise modifications, facilitated balance and coordination activities, posture assessment, application and adjustment of prosthetic devices, recognition of abnormal movement patterns, and use of rehabilitation strategies to correct aberrant mechanics.

A basic, yet essential, component of orthopedic physical therapy management is the instruction and application of proper gait techniques after injury or disease of the musculoskeletal system. To safely and properly instruct patients in the use of assistive devices and effectively apply fundamental gait techniques, the PTA must understand the components of the gait cycle and be able to instruct patients in appropriate gait patterns and identify deviations in gait. This section clarifies and describes the gait cycle and introduces basic terms, definitions, and concepts. In addition, the PTA is introduced to proper gait-pattern instruction, weight-bearing status, and the identification of gait abnormalities.

It is clinically relevant to clearly state that the delegation of selected mobilization techniques is entirely at the discretion of the physical therapist, and the application of peripheral joint mobilization is not universally accepted as a routine domain of clinical practice for the PTA. Therefore the information concerning peripheral joint mobilization is provided as a means of stimulating the PTA's awareness of the rationale for improving motion and for the reduction of pain as identified and prescribed by the physical therapist.

This section's presentation of introductory mechanics precedes orthopedic pathologies and therapeutic interventions by pulling together essential basics of anatomy, physiology, tissue healing, kinesiology, and principles of therapeutic exercise, thereby providing the student PTA and practicing clinician a sound practical and scientifically based understanding of the essentials of human movement.

14 | Gait

Thomas W. Kernozek
John D. Willson

LEARNING OBJECTIVES

1. Define and describe basic components of the gait cycle.
2. Discuss the two phases of gait.
3. Identify and describe each component of the two phases of gait.
4. Define and describe common gait deviations.
5. Define and instruct appropriate gait patterns.
6. Outline and describe terms used to define weight-bearing status during gait.
7. Identify and discuss the appropriate use of assistive devices.

KEY TERMS

Antalgic gait
Stance phase
Step

Stride
Swing phase
Trendelenburg gait

Trendelenburg sign
Vaulting

CHAPTER OUTLINE

Rehabilitation professionals should understand the terminology and the requirements of what is described as normal locomotion or gait. Gait is often evaluated in a clinical setting as an important activity of daily living skill that links musculoskeletal or neurologic impairment with a functional movement performance. Gait is a repetitive and cyclical movement pattern. The joints that make up the lower extremities and pelvis work together as a series of linked segments or kinetic chain. As with any linked system, the motion at one segment can greatly influence the motion of another. For example, a lack of knee extensor strength may lead to performance change during gait such as an avoidance of knee flexion that could be perceptible to the observer.

Rehabilitation professionals who have an awareness of what constitutes a normal gait pattern will recognize this gait deviation and plan effective interventions.

GAIT CYCLE TERMINOLOGY AND PHASES OF GAIT

The definition of the gait cycle is based on a reference extremity (for example, the right foot) from a defined event such as heel contact until the next occurrence of that event (contact with the heel of that same foot). The gait cycle is often based on 100% and can be further broken down into the **stance phase** and the **swing phase** (Fig. 14-1). The stance phase is defined as the portion

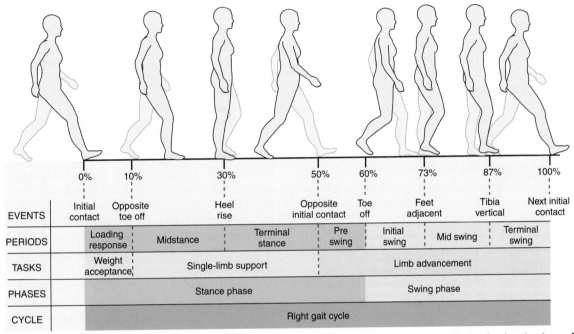

Fig. 14-1 Terminology to describe the events of the gait cycle. Initial contact corresponds to the beginning of stance when the foot first contacts the ground at 0% of gait cycle. Opposite toe off occurs when the contralateral foot leaves the ground at 10% of gait cycle. Heel rise corresponds to the heel lifting from the ground and occurs at approximately 30% of gait cycle. Opposite initial contact corresponds to the foot contact of the opposite limb, typically at 50% of gait cycle. Toe off occurs when the foot leaves the ground at 60% of gait cycle. Feet adjacent takes place when the foot of the swing leg is next to the foot of the stance leg at 73% of gait cycle. Tibia vertical corresponds to the tibia of the swing leg being oriented in the vertical direction at 87% of gait cycle. The final event is, again, initial contact, which in fact is the start of the next gait cycle. These eight events divide the gait cycle into seven periods. Loading response, between initial contact and opposite toe off, corresponds to the time when the weight is accepted by the lower extremity, initiating contact with the ground. Midstance is from opposite toe off to heel rise (10% to 30% of gait cycle). Terminal stance begins when the heel rises and ends when the contralateral lower extremity touches the ground, from 30% to 50% of gait cycle. Pre swing takes place from foot contact of the contralateral limb to toe off of the ipsilateral foot, which is the time corresponding to the second double-limb support period of the gait cycle (50% to 60% of gait cycle). Initial swing is from toe off to feet adjacent, when the foot of the swing leg is next to the foot of the stance leg (60% to 73% of gait cycle). Mid swing is from feet adjacent to when the tibia of the swing leg is vertical (73% to 87% of gait cycle). Terminal swing is from a vertical position of the tibia to immediately before heel contact (87% to 100% of the gait cycle). The first 10% of the gait cycle corresponds to a task of weight acceptance—when body mass is transferred from one lower extremity to the other. Single-limb support, from 10% to 50% of the gait cycle, serves to support the weight of the body as the opposite limb swings forward. The last 10% of stance phase and the entire swing phase serve to advance the limb forward to a new location. (From Neumann DA: *Kinesiology of the musculoskeletal system: foundations for physical rehabilitation*, ed 2, St Louis, 2010, Mosby.)

of the gait cycle where the foot is in contact with the ground whereas the swing phase is the portion where the foot is off the ground. A **step** is defined as contact on one foot until contact with the other (right to left or left to right). A **stride** is defined as contact with the one foot until contact with the same foot (right to right or left to left). The stance phase of the gait cycle is typically about 60% of the gait cycle, whereas the swing phase is about 40% (see Fig. 14-1). The reason why the stance and swing phases are not 50% is due to the relatively short period of double support (10%) within the gait cycle. This small portion of support phase is the period where the weight is transferred from one limb to the other.

The stance phase has been described as having two basic functions: weight acceptance and single limb support; whereas the swing phase has one primary function: limb advancement.[16] Figure 14-1 depicts the phases within the stance and swing phases of the gait cycle. Contact with the floor is often made with the heel (often called *heel contact* or *initial contact*). Perry[16] has described the first 15% of the gait cycle portion as when the foot functions as a heel rocker or first rocker. During this part of the gait cycle, impact forces tend to be large at 1 to 1.5 times body weight, depending on the speed of locomotion. Once the foot becomes flat on the ground the tibia advances forward over the stance foot. Perry[16] has described this as the ankle rocker or second rocker. This phase of the gait cycle is also called *midstance phase*. The terminal stance phase begins when the heel is raised off the ground (about 40% of the stance phase) until the opposite foot makes ground contact. The final phase of stance phase of the gait cycle is the pre-swing phase, which begins with heel strike of the contralateral limb and ends with toe off. When the heel is lifted from the floor (heel off), this can also be described as the toe rocker or third rocker.

The swing phase of the gait cycle has three portions: pre-swing, mid-swing and terminal swing phases. The pre-swing phase begins with double limb support and ends with toe off. This phase is primarily made up by the foot moving off the ground and is critical for limb advancement. This phase takes place as the gait cycle is 60% and 75% complete. Mid-swing phase is from 75% to 85% of the gait cycle, when the swing limb advances in front of the stance limb. The terminal swing phase completes the remainder of the swing phase until heel contact.

CHARACTERISTICS OF NORMAL GAIT

Many factors can influence gait, such as age, pain, strength, range of motion (ROM), walking speed, and fitness level. The extent of the influence of such factors can be quantified by taking simple measurements to characterize and assess a person's walking performance with a tape measure, goniometer, and stop watch. The measures are stride or step length, step width (walking base),

foot progression angle, walking speed, and cadence. Typical stride length reported from the literature has a range of 1.33 to 1.63 m in healthy individuals.[4,5,7,9-12,15,18] Males generally have a greater step length than females. Step width or the horizontal distance between feet while walking has a range of 0.61 to 9.0 cm.[11,12,17,20] Foot progression angle or angle of toe out has been reported to range between 5.1° and 6.8°. Various definitions for foot placement can be seen in Figure 14-2. The average typical walking speed is 1.49 m/sec for men and 1.40 m/sec for women, ranging between 3 to 4 miles per hour for both genders.[2-4,14,18,21] Average walking speed can be measured over a specific distance with a stop watch. Speed can be calculated by taking the distance over the elapsed time taken to walk the prescribed distance. Walking speed is based on cadence (number of steps per minute) and step length. Average cadence has a range of 107 to 125 steps per minute.[2-4,14,18,21] To increase walking speed, one can increase cadence or step length. Self selected walking speed is typically slower for women than in men. With the slower gait speed there appears to be a shorter step length and faster cadence for women than men. Keep in mind that all measurements of gait are largely dependent on walking speed.

As walking speed increases, stance time generally decreases in comparison to swing time. Most of the reduction in stance time comes from a reduction in double support time (due to the reduction in stance time on both limbs). Overall, these simple measures of gait can give the clinician an impression of the overall gait pattern. These measures are often called the *temporal spatial measures of gait*.

Normal gait is not entirely symmetrical.[18] Small asymmetries in gait are often considered typical. With slower walking speeds, greater amounts of asymmetry have been observed in healthy individuals with normal gait. Thus one must be able to identify if these subtleties in normal gait have clinical relevance.

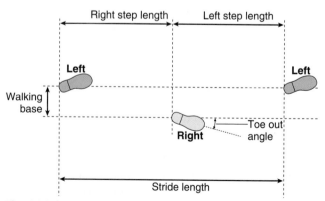

Fig. 14-2 Terms used to describe foot placement on the ground. (From Whittle MW: *Gait analysis: an introduction,* ed 4, St Louis, 2008, Butterworth-Heinemann.)

Movement patterns of the joints can provide additional insight to an individual's gait. Researchers in motion analysis laboratories have provided detailed three-dimensional data on the range of joint motion during walking. Sagittal plane motion patterns are the largest motions and represent the most studied parameters, whereas frontal plane and transverse plane motion patterns are smaller motions that have been less studied. Estimations of these motions can be visually observed by the health professional at a distance from the side for sagittal motions or from the front or behind for frontal plane motions as the patient is walking. Pure transverse plane rotation is difficult to observe in a clinical setting because an aerial perspective is required. One likely has to combine side and front views to estimate transverse plane motion.

Motions of the Foot, Ankle, Knee, Hip, and Pelvis

Foot

There are several joints within the foot, with some motion occurring at each of the joints during gait. However, most of the required motion at the foot is from the first metatarsophalangeal joint. At the instant of heel off during the terminal stance phase of gait, the first metatarsophalangeal joint typically hyperextends 45° to 55° as the ankle actively plantarflexes. The first metatarsophalangeal joint then returns to nearly 0° during the remainder of the gait cycle. A limitation in this passive hyperextension may cause compensations in other joints in the chain.[19]

Rearfoot motion is movement based on the motion of the posterior aspect of the heel relative to the posterior aspect of the lower leg in the frontal plane. This has been used as an estimation of the triplanar motion of pronation that occurs during the stance phase of gait when the foot everts, abducts, and dorsiflexes. When the posterior aspect of the heel is more everted relative to the lower leg the foot is considered to be in a more pronated position. With foot contact, the rearfoot is slightly inverted and immediately begins to evert or pronate until the midstance phase. At the instant of heel off during the beginning of terminal stance phase, the rearfoot is nearly neutral and then begins to invert until toe off. This inversion of the rearfoot is thought to describe the triplanar motion of supination during terminal stance when the foot inverts, adducts and plantarflexes.

Ankle

At ground contact, the ankle is primarily in a neutral position (0°, at a right angle to the tibia, neither plantarflexed nor dorsiflexed). After contact, the ankle plantarflexes about 5° so that the foot becomes flat on the ground.[16] This motion is controlled eccentrically by the ankle dorsiflexor muscles. Next, the tibia rotates over the stance foot resulting in maximum ankle dorsiflexion. This motion is generally controlled eccentrically by the ankle plantarflexor muscles. During the pre-swing phase of gait, the ankle plantarflexes to propel the person forward. An inadequate amount of plantarflexion may be due to a lack of ankle power, resulting in a reduction in step length during gait. During swing, the ankle must dorsiflex to allow for foot clearance as that leg steps forward for ground contact.

Knee

The knee is close to full extension at ground contact. The knee flexes 10° to 15° as the foot becomes flat on the ground during the initial 15% of the gait cycle. Knee flexion facilitates the absorption of forces during impact as the quadriceps muscles function eccentrically. After foot flat, the knee extends until about 40% of the gait cycle. As the ankle plantarflexes during terminal stance phase, the knee flexes to about 35° at toe off. Knee flexion during this phase reduces the overall length of the limb allowing for adequate foot ground clearance. The knee continues to flex to its maximum at about 60° during mid swing. Later in mid and terminal swing, the knee extends to nearly full extension in preparation for ground contact.[16] The knee motion reported during gait in the frontal plane is minimal (within 10° of abduction and adduction during the entire gait cycle) and appears to be quite variable.[1,3,8] A small amount of medial rotation of the knee that occurs during early stance and appears to be linked with foot pronation has been reported.[8] During midstance and throughout the swing phase the knee appears to laterally rotate back to neutral. Rearfoot pronation is accompanied by tibial medial rotation with knee flexion. This is thought to be important for shock absorption occurring with foot impact with the ground. Tibial lateral rotation occurs later in stance with foot supination and is accompanied by knee extension.

Hip

The hip is flexed to about 30° at ground contact. This is typically the maximum amount of hip flexion observed during normal gait. After this the hip extends to a hyperextension angle of about 10° at about 50% of the gait cycle. Hip flexion is started at pre-swing and continues until nearly ground contact.[16]

Pelvis

There is a small amount of pelvic motion apparent during the gait cycle. During the gait cycle, the pelvis goes through a symmetrical pattern of excursion twice. In general, the pelvis tilts anterior and the pelvis on the swing leg rotates forward whenever either hip extends. The pelvis also has a considerable amount of oscillating motion in the frontal and transverse planes (up to 10° of total motion). During the first 10% to 15% of the gait cycle the pelvis rotates and laterally tilts toward the swing leg contributing to hip adduction on the stance leg. From about 20% to 60% of the gait cycle, the pelvis rotates and tilts away from the swing leg contributing to hip abduction.[16]

Joint Motion and Energy Expenditure

Coordinated lower extremity movement patterns are thought to minimize the vertical oscillation of the body center of mass (COM). The body COM is nearly at the height of a person's navel and is in the center of the body anterior to the sacrum. Movement of the COM oscillates up and down and from side to side during normal gait (Fig. 14-3). Vertical oscillation of the COM has been related to energy expenditure. Greater energy expenditure is thought to be related to greater oscillation of the body COM. In general, the COM oscillates nearly 5 cm in the vertical direction and horizontally toward the stance limb.[6] The COM is typically highest during midstance and lowest during double support phases of gait. Lower extremity gait deviations may result in excessive COM motion, resulting in greater fatigue due to the higher metabolic cost.

Muscle Activation

Timing of muscle activation appears to be critical; generally occurring in short bursts during gait (Fig. 14-4). Much of the muscle action within the gait cycle is eccentric. Eccentric forces by the muscles are used control the rate of joint motion.

Foot and Ankle

The tibialis anterior is active eccentrically at heel contact to control the rate of ankle plantar flexion until the foot is flat on the ground. A second period of activity by the tibialis anterior is during early swing phase when it dorsiflexes the ankle to allow for foot clearance. The extensor digitorum and extensor hallucis longus have a similar role in helping control the rate of plantar flexion during the loading response. They may also be activated during the late mid-swing and terminal swing for propulsion in combination with the ankle plantar flexors. The ankle plantarflexors (gastrocnemius and soleus) are active most of the stance phase; eccentrically during the

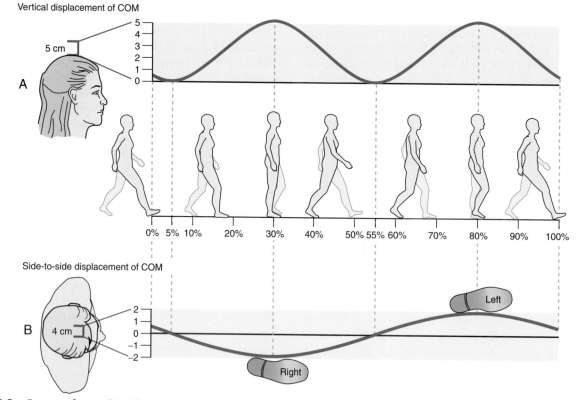

Fig. 14-3   Center of mass (COM) displacement during gait. The vertical and the medial-lateral displacements of the COM are illustrated in **A** and **B,** respectively. The COM is at its lowest and most central position, in the medial-lateral direction, in the middle of double-limb support (5% and 55% of the gait cycle)—a position of relative stability with both feet on the ground. Conversely, the COM is at its highest and most lateral position at midstance (30% and 80% of the gait cycle)—a position of relative instability. During single-limb support, the trajectory of the COM is never directly over the base of support. This factor is illustrated in **B,** with the vertical projection of the COM always medial to the footprints. (From Neumann DA: *Kinesiology of the musculoskeletal system: foundations for physical rehabilitation,* ed 2, St Louis, 2010, Mosby.)

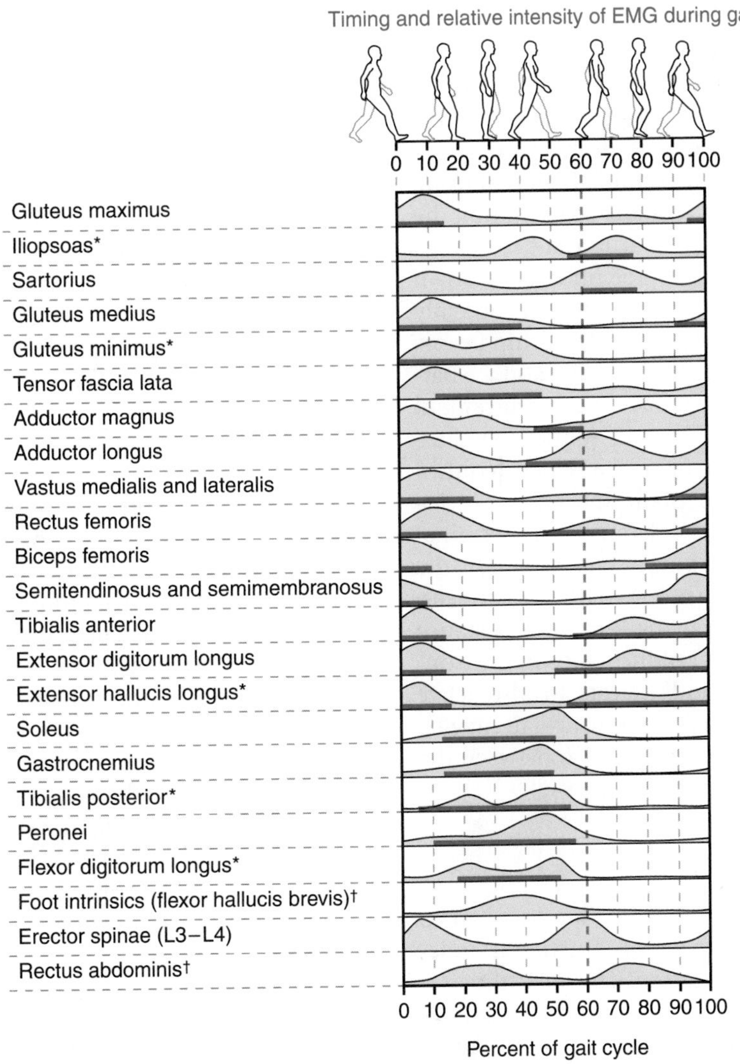

Timing and relative intensity of EMG during gait

Gluteus maximus
Iliopsoas*
Sartorius
Gluteus medius
Gluteus minimus*
Tensor fascia lata
Adductor magnus
Adductor longus
Vastus medialis and lateralis
Rectus femoris
Biceps femoris
Semitendinosus and semimembranosus
Tibialis anterior
Extensor digitorum longus
Extensor hallucis longus*
Soleus
Gastrocnemius
Tibialis posterior*
Peronei
Flexor digitorum longus*
Foot intrinsics (flexor hallucis brevis)†
Erector spinae (L3–L4)
Rectus abdominis†

Percent of gait cycle

Fig. 14-4 Timing *(dark red bars)* and relative intensity of muscle activation *(light red shading)* during gait. (Muscle timing data from Knutson LM, Soderberg GL: EMG: use and interpretation in gait. In Craik RL, Oatis CA [eds.]: *Gait analysis: theory and application,* St Louis, 1995, Mosby. Relative intensity of muscle activation data from Winter DA: *The biomechanics and motor control of human gait: normal, elderly and pathological,* ed 2, Waterloo, Canada, 1991, University of Waterloo Press; *Bechtol CO: Normal human gait. In Bowker JH, Hall CB [eds.]: *Atlas of orthotics: American academy of orthopaedic surgeons,* St Louis, 1975, Mosby; †Carlsoo S: *How man moves: kinesiological methods and studies,* New York, 1972, Crane, Russak & Company. Figure from Neumann DA: *Kinesiology of the musculoskeletal system: foundations for physical rehabilitation,* ed 2, St Louis, 2010, Mosby.)

first 10% to 40%, when they control the rate for tibial advancement over the foot, to a high burst of concentric activity at pre-swing (at heel off) until inactivity at toe off.[13] The tibialis posterior is primarily active between 5% and 35% of the gait cycle and is thought to limit excessive foot pronation. Later in stance, the tibialis anterior and posterior function concentrically to help supinate the foot to create a rigid lever for effective push off by the ankle plantarflexors.[19]

Knee

During terminal swing the quadriceps muscle group begins to become activated in preparation for weight acceptance during stance. At the instant of heel contact,

the quadriceps is highly active eccentrically to control the rate of knee flexion and absorb impact forces during the loading response phase. Later during midstance while in single limb support, the quadriceps act concentrically to extend the knee. During pre-swing, there may be some quadriceps activity to help flex the hip. The hamstrings are most active near the instant of heel contact and through approximately the first 10% of the stance phase. Before heel contact, the hamstrings slow the rate of knee extension, and early in stance, assist with hip extension and enhance knee stability with coactivation with the quadriceps. Minimal activation of the hamstrings is necessary during pre-swing and swing.[13,16,19]

Hip

The gluteus maximus is active during terminal swing to slow the rate of hip flexion and to prepare for weight acceptance during stance. This muscle becomes most active at the instant of heel contact for hip extension with assistance from the hamstrings and to prevent trunk flexion. The gluteus maximus remains active during the first 30% of the gait cycle.[16] The iliacus and psoas muscles are active eccentrically during toe off to slow down the rate of hip extension, and then are concentrically active to flex the hip during pre-swing. These hip flexors are active only during the first 50% of swing and are partially assisted by the quadriceps for limb advancement and foot clearance. The hip abductors (gluteus medius, gluteus minimis, and tensor fascia lata) help control pelvis motion in the frontal plane during single leg stance.[19] The gluteus medius is also active in terminal swing in preparation for heel contact. It is assisted by the gluteus minimus during the first 40% of the gait cycle to control pelvis tilt toward the swing limb during stance and may control the alignment of the femur in the frontal plane. The hip adductors and rotators are also active during stance. The hip rotators' role during gait may be important to enable control of the motion between the pelvis and femur during stance.[13]

GAIT ABNORMALITIES

The ability to move our bodies from one location to another is an important aspect of functional independence. The normal gait pattern described thus far is the method many of us choose to use to achieve this end. However, pain during gait or a variety of permanent or temporary neurological or musculoskeletal impairments will affect normal gait. The consequence of nearly every deviation from normal gait is increased energy consumption to move a given distance, decreased gait speed, abnormal joint loading, and in some cases, decreased safety. For some people, the additional energy required for ambulation may be so great that frequent rests are necessary even over relatively short distances. The health professional must be able to identify and describe gait abnormalities in order to make appropriate recommendations to the patient or other health care professionals to minimize the impact of the gait abnormality on functional independence.

Just as normal gait is a complex interaction of musculoskeletal and neuromuscular systems, adaptations or compensations in response to pain or limitations in either system are frequently equally complex. Indeed, there may be many ways for a person to compensate for or adapt to a given impairment. As a consequence, the same impairment may not result in the same gait abnormality among different people. Further, the way that a person compensates for a musculoskeletal or neuromuscular limitation may change, leading to different gait abnormalities over time for one person with the same limitation.

The clinical presentation and potential causes of several common gait abnormalities are briefly discussed in the remainder of this chapter. As previously noted, it is important to remember that the joints that make up the lower extremities work together as a series of linked segments or kinetic chain. As with any linked system, motion at one segment can greatly influence the motion of another. Therefore observed gait abnormalities may be due to pain or a limitation in any portion of the kinetic chain.

Antalgic Gait

Antalgic gait is a general term used to describe a gait pattern accompanied by pain. It can take on a number of forms, but generally there will be an observable reduction in motion at the painful joint as well as asymmetry in temporal–spatial gait parameters, with a reduction in stance time on the involved limb and a rapid swing phase of the uninvolved limb being most common. Patients who experience pain during walking as a consequence of weight bearing frequently find it more comfortable to walk if they reduce the magnitude of the loads delivered to the painful leg during the stance phase of gait. This is typically accomplished by leaning the trunk toward (hip pain) or away (knee or ankle pain) from the side of the painful lower extremity joint during the stance phase.

Lateral Trunk Bending

As described, lateral trunk bending may be observed among patients attempting to minimize joint compression loads and pain during ambulation. Lateral trunk bending may also be observed as a compensation for weakness of the hip abductors. During the stance phase of walking, patients with marked hip abductor weakness may lean toward the stance leg of the weak abductors in order to minimize the force required of these muscles to prevent downward movement of the pelvis on the side of the swing leg (contralateral pelvis drop). This lateral trunk bending is a compensation for ipsilateral hip abductor weakness and is most commonly referred to as *Trendelenburg gait*. Among people who have bilateral hip abductor weakness, the clinician may observe lateral trunk bending toward each side during the single leg stance phase of each leg, a presentation most commonly referred to as *waddling*. People who walk with a wide step width (walking base) or have unequal leg length may also demonstrate increased lateral trunk bending.

Contralateral Pelvis Drop

Excessive downward movement of the pelvis for the swing leg may also occur during walking. This is most frequently observed as a consequence of a musculoskeletal impairment, such as hip abductor weakness, or a neuromuscular disease affecting gluteus medius recruitment. Specifically, this occurs when the hip abductors do not produce enough force to resist the torque created by the weight of the trunk acting medially to the hip joint during the single leg stance phases of the gait cycle. This gait deviation is known as *increased contralateral pelvic drop* or as the **Trendelenburg sign**.

Posterior Trunk Lean

Patients who demonstrate a posterior trunk lean may do so during either the early stance or early swing phase of the gait cycle. During early stance, a patient may lean posteriorly in order to move the line of gravity of the trunk behind the hip joint. This tends to reduce the demands placed on the hip extensors to resist hip flexion during the loading phase and, as such, is a gait deviation frequently employed by individuals with weak hip extensors. Conversely, individuals may lean posteriorly during early swing in an effort to pull the femur anteriorly and advance the swing leg as a compensation for hip flexor insufficiency or hip extensor spasticity.

Anterior Trunk Lean

Anterior trunk lean is most commonly observed during the stance phase of gait. However, timing of the anterior trunk lean may vary according to the impairment causing this gait abnormality. Anterior trunk lean during early stance is often a compensation for quadriceps weakness. Shortly after heel strike, the magnitude and direction of the reaction force from the ground is posterior to the knee joint, which tends to produce knee flexion under the eccentric control of the knee extensors. If the knee extensors cannot generate enough force to resist knee flexion, a person may lean forward to move the ground reaction force anterior to the knee joint (Fig. 14-5). Moving the

ground reaction force anterior to the knee joint changes the effect of the ground reaction force to one that tends to cause knee extension rather than knee flexion, therefore diminishing the need for knee extension strength to resist knee flexion. Quadriceps weakness is a common consequence of poliomyelitis. Therefore this compensation is a common gait deviation among such individuals.

Anterior trunk lean during midstance or terminal stance is often a compensation for decreased ankle dorsiflexion range of motion. In order to continue to ambulate forward, the ankle typically dorsiflexes before initial contact of the contralateral leg to allow the person's COM to pass anterior to the stance leg base of support. Among individuals with ankle plantarflexor spasticity, a plantarflexor contracture, or pes equinus deformity, the ankle may not permit sufficient dorsiflexion at this stage of the gait cycle and the person may need to lean the trunk forward to move their COM anterior to the foot (Fig. 14-6).

Excessive Ankle Plantarflexion

Increased ankle plantarflexion is frequently observed in both the stance and swing phase of the gait cycle. Increased ankle plantarflexion during and after midstance of the stance leg is commonly referred to as *vaulting* (Fig. 14-7). This is frequently a compensatory mechanism intended to increase ground clearance for

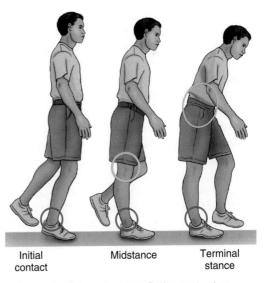

Initial contact   Midstance   Terminal stance

○ Impairment: ankle plantar flexion contracture
○ Compensations: knee hyperextension (midstance); forward trunk lean (terminal stance)

Fig. 14-6 Individuals with an ankle plantar flexion contracture will make initial contact with the ground with the forefoot region. At midstance, bringing the heel to the ground will result in knee hyperextension. Forward lean of the trunk occurs in terminal stance as a strategy to maintain forward progression of the center of mass. (From Neumann DA: *Kinesiology of the musculoskeletal system: foundations for physical rehabilitation*, ed 2, St Louis, 2010, Mosby.)

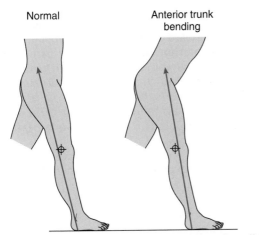

Normal   Anterior trunk bending

Fig. 14-5 Anterior trunk bending: in normal walking, the line of force early in the stance phase passes behind the knee; anterior trunk bending brings the line of force in front of the knee, to compensate for weak knee extensors. (From Whittle MW: *Gait analysis: an introduction*, ed 4, St Louis, 2008, Butterworth-Heinemann.)

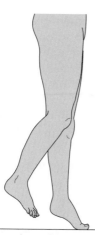

Fig. 14-7 Vaulting: the subject goes up on the toes of the stance phase leg to increase ground clearance for the swing phase leg. (From Whittle MW: *Gait analysis: an introduction*, ed 4, St Louis, 2008, Butterworth-Heinemann.)

the swing leg and is common among individuals with an impairment that prevents shortening of the swing leg during the swing phase, such as an ankle plantarflexion contracture, ankle dorsiflexor weakness, knee or hip extensor spasticity, or hip flexor weakness. Ankle plantarflexion of the stance leg may also be an indication of decreased ankle dorsiflexion ROM, particularly if the person demonstrates heel rise very shortly after contralateral toe off (early in midstance). In either case, the effect is a characteristic bouncing appearance, indicative of large vertical oscillations of the person's COM.

Increased ankle plantarflexion may also be observed in the swing phase of the gait cycle. This gait deviation is frequently the result of injury to the common fibular nerve, weakness of the ankle dorsiflexors, or spasticity or contracture of the ankle plantarflexors (Fig. 14-8, *A*). Compensations for increased swing phase ankle plantarflexion are typically necessary to avoid tripping due to toe drag during contralateral leg stance phase. These compensations often include vaulting on the stance leg, increased hip or knee flexion of the swing leg (steppage gait) (Fig. 14-8, *B*), or hip circumduction of the swing leg (described later). A combination of these compensations may also be used in order to increase ground clearance during the swing phase.

Hip Circumduction

Individuals who advance the swing leg in a lateral semicircular pattern rather than in a straight plane from posterior to anterior are said to be circumducting the hip. Hip circumduction is a common compensation used to advance the swing leg if a person lacks hip flexion, knee flexion, or ankle dorsiflexion ROM, because ground clearance is increased using this swing pattern. Individuals may also circumduct the hip if they lack hip flexion strength to swing the leg forward. In this case, the swing leg may be advanced by first externally rotating the hip

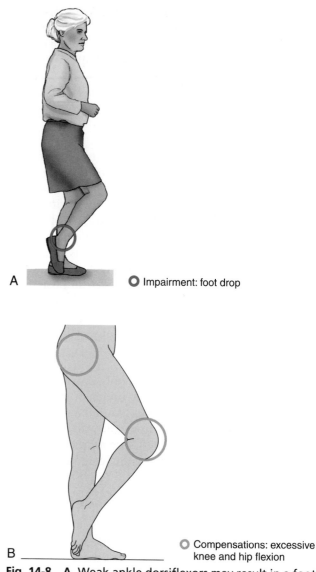

A ○ Impairment: foot drop

B ○ Compensations: excessive knee and hip flexion

Fig. 14-8 **A,** Weak ankle dorsiflexors may result in a foot drop during swing phase, requiring excessive hip and knee flexion for the toes to clear the ground as the limb is advanced forward during swing. **B,** Steppage: Increased hip and knee flexion improve ground clearance for the swing phase leg; in this case, necessitated by a foot drop. (**A,** From Neumann DA: *Kinesiology of the musculoskeletal system: foundations for physical rehabilitation*, ed 2, St Louis, 2010, Mosby. **B,** Modified from Whittle MW: *Gait analysis: an introduction*, ed 4, St Louis, 2008, Butterworth-Heinemann.)

and using the hip adductors rather than the hip flexors to pull the femur forward.

Increased Knee Flexion

Excessive knee flexion is most noticeable during either the loading response or terminal stance phase of the gait cycle, when the knee would normally be nearly fully extended. Increased knee flexion at initial contact will almost certainly be accompanied by initial contact with the midfoot or forefoot rather than the heel. As the

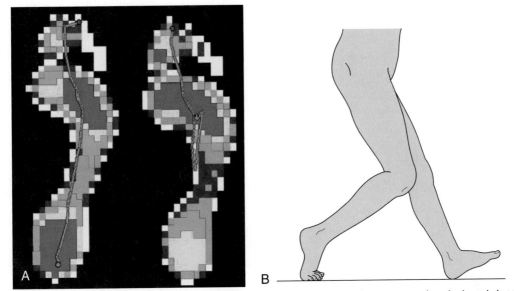

Fig. 14-9 **A,** The typical progression of the center of pressure is from the heel (starting at the *dark red dots*) to the fore-foot and toes (at the *light red dots*) as on the left figure. This was obtained with a pressure platform while walking bare-foot. Ground contact with the forefoot as on the left figure shifts the center of pressure largely anterior where it then travels posterior toward the heel before moving anterior again toward the forefoot and toes. **B,** Excessive knee flexion: in late stance phase there is increased knee flexion, caused by a flexion contracture of the hip. (**B,** From Whittle MW: *Gait analysis: an introduction*, ed 4. St Louis, 2008, Butterworth-Heinemann.)

remainder of the foot comes in contact with the ground, the center of pressure first moves posteriorly and finally anteriorly during stance rather than the typical posterior to anterior progression (Fig. 14-9, *A*). One consequence of this is that much of the forward momentum of the COM may be lost during early stance, minimizing the gait economy normally preserved by the foot and ankle rockers. Increased knee flexion during stance phase may be the consequence of a number of impairments including a knee flexion contracture, knee pain or knee joint effusion, or a hip flexion contracture (Fig. 14-9, *B*).

Increased knee flexion and hip flexion during gait is referred to as *crouch gait* and is commonly observed among individuals with spastic diplegia as a consequence of cerebral palsy (Fig. 14-10). Among such individuals, increased knee flexion may be due to spasticity of the hamstrings, hip flexors, or both. Careful gait and clinical analysis is required in order to develop the best course of surgical or conservative treatment for these patients.

GAIT PATTERN INSTRUCTION

Instructing patients in the proper use of assistive devices and identifying appropriate gait patterns are relevant clinical tasks for the physical therapist assistant (PTA). Several patterns are outlined here.

A four-point gait pattern is describe as advancing the crutch opposite the uninvolved limb first, followed by the involved limb, then advancing the crutch toward the

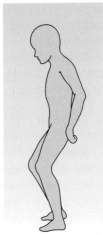

Fig. 14-10 Position of body at midstance in a 12-year-old child with crouch gait, following Achilles tendon lengthening for spastic diplegia. (Adapted from Sutherland DH, Cooper L: The pathomechanics of progressive crouch gait in spastic diplegia, *Orthop Clin North Am*, 9:143-154, 1978. In Whittle MW: *Gait analysis: an introduction*, ed 4, St Louis, 2008, Butterworth-Heinemann.)

uninvolved limb, then finally advancing the uninvolved limb (Fig. 14-11). If the injured limb is the left leg, the four-point gait pattern looks like this:

Right crutch × left foot × left crutch × right foot

The four-point gait pattern attempts to duplicate the normal reciprocal motion that occurs between the upper extremities and the lower limbs during normal gait.

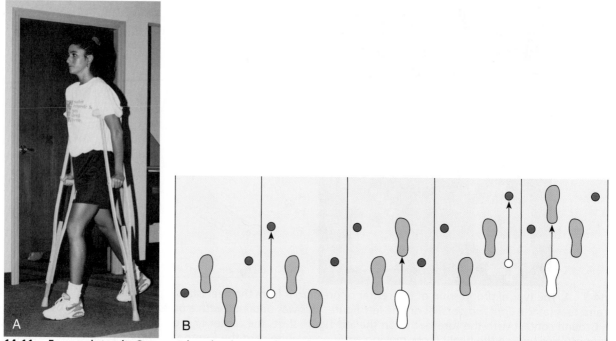

Fig. 14-11 Four-point gait. One crutch or leg is moved at a time in the pattern: left crutch—right leg—right crutch—left leg. (**B,** From Whittle MW: *Gait analysis: an introduction*, ed 4, St Louis, 2008, Butterworth-Heinemann.)

A three-point gait pattern is commonly taught using bilateral axillary crutches (Fig. 14-12). The sequence of events begins by advancing both crutches and the involved limb first followed by the uninvolved.

A two-point gait pattern is described as advancing the left crutch and right lower extremity at the same time, then advancing the right crutch and left lower extremity together. This gait pattern is similar to the four-point gait pattern in which normal reciprocal motion and walking rhythm is encouraged.

A tripod gait pattern is used for bilateral nonfunctioning limbs. Crutches are advanced, then the lower body is advanced. With a tripod gait, the body can be lifted and advanced to the crutch or swung through and beyond the crutches.

Weight-Bearing Status

Depending on the healing constraints of injured tissues (bone, ligament, tendon, cartilage, and muscle), certain weight-bearing restrictions are imposed to protect the injured tissues from excessive stresses and loads, as well as to promote normal physiologic healing. If an injured limb is unable to support any weight, non–weight bearing (NWB) status is assigned until sufficient healing has taken place to allow the limit to safely accept some degree of weight. Partial weight bearing (PWB) is frequently graded in a percentage of the patient's weight (20%, 40%, 50%, etc.) or in pounds of pressure applied to the floor from the involved limb. When teaching PWB with orders to apply a certain amount of weight (such as 20 pounds or 50 pounds), a bathroom scale can acquaint the patient with exactly how much weight is necessary to bear on the injured limb. The terms touch down weight bearing (TDWB) and toe touch weight bearing (TTWB) can be used synonymously to describe minimal contact of the involved limb with the ground. Generally, TDWB is used for balance purposes initially. As healing and pain allow, progressive weight bearing can be instituted. Weight bearing as tolerated (WBAT) is assigned to patients in whom pain tolerance is the predominant limiting factor. Then the patient is allowed to bear as much weight on the injured limb as is comfortable. When a patient no longer requires an assistive device to accommodate pain or healing of injured tissues, full weight bearing (FWB) status is generally allowed.

Weight-bearing status is a progressive process that involves constant assessment and reassessment of pain, joint stability, tissue healing constraints, and function. A patient with severe injuries progresses through each designation of weight bearing as follows:

$$\text{NWB} \times \text{TDWB} \times \text{PWB} \times \text{WBAT} \times \text{FWB}$$

Less severe injuries may begin anywhere along the continuum and progress from there.

Negotiating Stairs with Assistive Devices

Ascending and descending stairs, steps, or curbs requires prudent instruction and careful supervision with necessary tactile and verbal cueing. The safety of the patient is the principal concern. Perhaps no other gait training technique elicits as much anxiety as negotiating stairs.

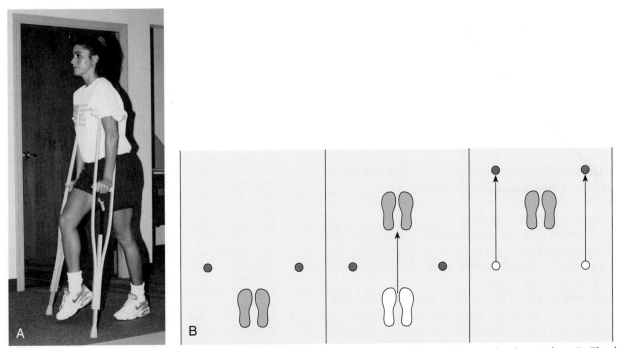

Fig. 14-12 Three-point gait. **A,** Three-point step-through gait in someone taking weight on both crutches. **B,** The legs are advanced together (weight bearing on uninvolved limb), in front of the line of the crutches, then the crutches are advanced together, in front of the line of the legs. (**B,** From Whittle MW: *Gait analysis: an introduction*, ed 4, St Louis, 2008, Butterworth-Heinemann.)

Therefore the PTA must accept the responsibility of clearly articulating the fundamentals of climbing and descending the stairs while both validating the patient's fears and providing confidence, encouragement, and a safe environment for instruction.

When instructing patients to ascend stairs using bilateral axillary crutches, the first step is to encourage the use of a handrail, if one is available. As the patient uses the handrail, both crutches are placed in the hand opposite the handrail. If at all possible the patient should be instructed to use the handrail on the side of the injured limb. This may provide an added sense of stability and support. Ascending a step requires the uninvolved leg to step up first. Then the involved limb and crutches are advanced up to the same step.

When descending steps, the same instructions about the use of the handrail next to the injured limb should be repeated. The first step when descending stairs is to advance the crutches or cane to the step. The injured limb is then advanced down to the step, followed by the uninjured limb. It may help patients to remember, "up with the good, down with the bad," when cueing them as to which limb to advance up or down the stairs. When providing support for the patient during stair climbing, the PTA should stand behind the patient while giving appropriate verbal cues and physical support at the waist. As a safety precaution, an interlocking gait belt should be applied and used during all phases of gait training. When instructing patients during stair descent, it is best to stand in front of the patient. However, enough space must be allowed between the therapist and patient to permit a technically correct and safe descent.

When no handrail is available the patient should follow the same steps, except that both crutches are used as with normal walking with crutches.

Selection of Assistive Devices

The initial selection of assistive gait devices depends largely on the age and activity level of the patient, the severity of the injury, and the weight-bearing status. Walkers can be prescribed for an elderly person because a walker is inherently more stable and easy to use. Children may find using a pediatric walker easier and safer than axillary crutches.

Axillary crutches provide less stability than a walker, but compensate with greater mobility. Canes provide the least support of all assistive devices. However, some types of canes provide more support than others. For example, a wide-based quad cane (four points) allows more stability than a narrow-based quad cane or a single-point cane. A hemi-walker provides a wider, more stable base of support than a wide-based quad cane. Hemi-walkers and quad canes are frequently used by patients who have had a cerebrovascular accident with resultant hemiparesis.

As with weight-bearing status, patients may progress from one form of assistive device to another. As pain, healing, and function allow, a patient may move from using an axillary crutch to a cane or from a walker to a set of axillary crutches. Constant reassessment of a patient's balance, coordination, strength, endurance, weight-bearing status and function will guide the PTA in consulting with the physical therapist concerning appropriate gait devices.

❖ GLOSSARY

Antalgic gait: A general term used to describe a gait pattern accompanied by pain.

Stance phase: The portion of the gait cycle during which the foot is in contact with the ground.

Step: Contact on one foot until contact with the other (right to left or left to right).

Stride: Contact with the one foot until contact with the same foot (right to right or left to left).

Swing phase: The portion of the gait cycle during which the foot is off the ground.

Trendelenburg gait: Lateral trunk bending as a compensation for ipsilateral hip abductor weakness.

Trendelenburg sign: A term used to refer to contralateral pelvic drop.

Vaulting: Increased ankle plantarflexion during and after midstance of the stance leg.

REFERENCES

1. Apkarian J, Naumann S, Cairns B: A three dimensional kinematic and dynamic model of the lower limb, *J Biomech* 22:143–155, 1989.
2. Auvinet B, Berrut G, Touzard C, et al: Reference data for normal subjects obtained with an accelometric device, *Gait Posture* 16:124–134, 2003.
3. Chao EY, Laughman RK, Schneider E, et al: Normative data of knee joint motion and ground reaction forces in adult level walking, *J Biomech* 16:219–233, 1983.
4. Cho SH, Park JM, Kwon OY: Gender differences in three dimensional gain analysis in 98 healthy Korean adults, *Clin Biomech (Bristol, Avon)* 19:145–152, 2004.
5. Hageman PA, Blanke DJ: Comparison of gait of young women and elderly women, *Phys Ther* 66:1382–1386, 1986.
6. Inman VT, Ralston HJ, Todd F: *Human walking*, Baltimore, 1989, Williams and Wilkins.
7. Kadaba MP, Ramakrishman HK, Wooten ME, et al: Repeatability of kinematic, kinetic and electromyographic data in normal adult gait, *J Orthop Res* 7:849–860, 1989.
8. Lafortune MR, Cavanaugh PR, Sommer HJ, et al: Three dimensional kinematics of the human knee during walking, *J Biomech* 25:347–357, 1992.
9. Larsson LE, Odenrick P, Sandlund B, et al: The phases of the stride and their interaction in human gait,, *Scand J Rehabil Med* 12:107–112, 1980.
10. Menz HB, Latt MD, Tiedemann A, et al: Reliability of the Gaitrite walkway system for the quantification of temporal-spatial parameters of gait in young and older people, *Gait Posture* 20(1):20–25, 2004.
11. Murray MP, Drought AB, Kory RC: Walking patterns of normal men, *J Bone J Surg Am* 46:335, 1964.
12. Murray MP, Kory RC, Sepic SB: Walking patterns of normal women, *Arch Phys Med* 51:637, 1979.
13. Oatis CA: *Kinesiology: the mechanics and pathomechanics of human movement*, ed 2, Baltimore, 2009, Lippincott Williams & Wilkins.
14. Oberg T, Karszina A, Oberg K: Basic gait parameters: reference data for normal subjects, 10-79 years of age, *J Rehabil Res Dev* 30:210–223, 1993.
15. Ostrosky KM, VanSwearingen JM, Burdett RG, et al: A comparison of gait characteristics in young and old subjects, *Phys Ther* 74:637–646, 1994.
16. Perry J: *Gait analysis: normal and pathological function*, Thorofare, NJ, 1992, Slack.
17. Sekiya N, Nagasaki H, Ito H, et al: Optimal walking in terms of variability of step length, *J Orthop Sports Phys Ther* 26:266–272, 1997.
18. Senden R, Grimm B, Heylingers IC, et al: Acceleration-based gait test for healthy subjects: reliability and reference data, *Gait Posture* 30:192–196, 2009.
19. Simoneau G: Kinesiology of walking. In Neumann DA, editor: *Kinesiology of the musculoskeletal system: foundations for physical rehabilitation*, St Louis, 2002, Mosby.
20. Stolze H, Kuhtz-Buschbeck JP, Mondwurf C, et al: Retest reliability of spatiotemporal gait parameters in children and young adults, *Gait Posture* 7:125–130, 1998.
21. Winter DA, Patla AE, Frank JS, et al: Biomechanical walking changes in the fit and healthy elderly, *Phys Ther* 70:340–347, 1990.

REVIEW QUESTIONS

Short Answer

1. What is the term used to describe linear distance between right and left feet during gait?
2. Name the two phases of gait.
3. Name the components of the stance phase of gait.
4. Name the components of the swing phase of gait.
5. Name a primary action of the foot-flat period of the stance phase of gait.
6. A single crutch or cane should be used on which side of the injured limb?

True/False

7. During gait, an individual's center of gravity displaces both vertically and horizontally.
8. Non–weight bearing status allows the patient to place minimal weight on the involved limb.
9. Partial weight bearing status allows the patient to place a prescribed amount of resistance on the involved limb. The amount of weight is determined by the physician and is carried out in physical therapy by grading the resistance by a percentage of the patient's weight (20%, 30%, 50%, etc.).

15 Concepts of Joint Mobilization

Robert C. Manske
Justin Rohrberg

LEARNING OBJECTIVES

1. Discuss the general and applied concepts of peripheral joint mobilization.
2. Define terms and principles of peripheral joint mobilization.
3. Define and describe the convex–concave rule.
4. Define the five grades of mobilization.
5. Identify and describe terms of joint end-feel.
6. Define and describe capsular and noncapsular patterns.
7. Identify common indications and contraindications for mobilization.
8. Discuss the clinical basics and applications of peripheral joint mobilization.
9. Identify and discuss the role of the physical therapist assistant in assisting the physical therapist with the delivery of peripheral joint mobilization.

KEY TERMS

CHAPTER OUTLINE

Providing comprehensive musculoskeletal rehabilitation requires that the physical therapist assistant (PTA) understand the basic concepts related to joint **mobilization.** He or she must be able to accurately and skillfully apply the mobilization techniques as delegated by the physical therapist (PT). This chapter focuses primarily on concepts, definitions, and general rationales for peripheral joint mobilization, including mobilization theory and compulsory scientific principles.

FUNDAMENTAL PRINCIPLES OF MOBILIZATION

A healthy joint is one that moves without limitation. In synovial joints, movement stimulates biological activity by moving synovial fluid to areas of avascular articular cartilage. Additionally, strength and resiliency of capsular tissue and periarticular tissue is maintained via joint movement. Immobilization causes a host of negative consequences such as fatty infiltration, articular adhesions, and physiologic changes to the strength and tolerance of ligaments, tendons, and capsular tissue. The term mobilization refers to an attempt to restore joint motion or mobility, or decrease pain associated with joint structures using manual, passive accessory-joint movement.[4,21]

Joint mobilizations are passive, skilled manual therapy techniques applied to joints and related soft tissues at varying speeds and amplitudes using physiologic or accessory motions for therapeutic purposes.[1] Range of motion (ROM) involves physiologic movements which are active/passive motions at a given joint through one of the traditional cardinal planes of flexion, extension, abduction, adduction, or internal and external rotation. Physiologic movements are sometimes called *osteokinematic*, classical, or traditional movements because they are movements of the actual bones of a given joint system. These motions can be visualized by the naked eye and are commonly measured by goniometric assessment. Osteokinematic motions occur in the cardinal planes of movement such as frontal, sagittal, and transverse. Hip, knee, and shoulder flexion movements are examples of osteokinematic movements. These are all movements that can occur under volitional control. Arthrokinematic movements are those that occur at the bone ends, without regard to the movement. These movements are not under volitional control. These types of movements are known as *accessory movements* involving motions specific to articulating joint surfaces.[4,21] These accessory joint motions are referred to as *glide or slide, spin, and roll*.[4,14] Because these are passive movements at the actual joint level, they are sometimes referred to as *arthrokinematic motions*. Accessory and physiologic joint motions occur together during active ROM. If full accessory motion does not occur, there will be a limitation in normal physiological cardinal plane movements. However, accessory joint motion cannot be selectively recruited, meaning that a patient cannot selectively perform joint roll, glide, or spin independently on their own.[4] The application of accessory joint motion is defined as "joint play" or "motion that occurs within the joint as a response to an outside force but not as a result of voluntary movement."[4]

An arthrokinematic glide and an arthrokinematic slide movement are essentially the same. Gliding and sliding occurs as a specific point on one portion of the articular surface comes into contact with a series of locations on the corresponding joint surface. An analogy of this would be a car wheel sliding on ice when brakes are pushed. One part of the tire glides or slides across a series of locations of the ice surface. When the elbow is flexed doing a biceps curl, the convex olecranon rolls anteriorly and glides or slides posteriorly on the relatively fixed concave trochlea of the distal humerus.

The arthrokinematic movement termed *spin* occurs when a portion of one joint spins or rotates, clockwise or counterclockwise, around a stationary longitudinal axis. An example of this is when a forearm goes through the motion of supination and pronation. At the radiohumeral joint, the radial head will spin on the capitellum of the distal humerus.

Rolling occurs when multiple points of contact on one joint surface come into contact with multiple points of contact on the corresponding joint surface. The analogy for this movement would be a car tire driving normally where the tire surface makes contact with a different portion of the road. In the human, this occurs as the convex distal femur rolls forward and glides on the concave tibia when the person moves from a seated to a standing position.

JOINT CONGRUENCY AND POSITION

The concept of joint congruency and the terms *close-packed* and *loose-packed*, referring to joint position, are pertinent to the discussion of various grades of mobilization. Congruence refers to articular position with regard to concave and convex joint surfaces. A joint is congruent when both articulating surfaces are in contact throughout the total surface area of the joint.[4,14] However, the study of **arthrokinematics** (joint movement) states that joints are rarely in total congruence. As joints move, the accessory motions of glide or slide, spin, and roll alter total joint congruence.

MacConaill and Basmajian[14] have described close-packed positions as the most congruent positions of a joint,[4,14] where the joint articular surfaces are aligned and the capsule and ligaments are taut and joint volume is minimal (Fig. 15-1). Generally, a close-packed position is used for testing the integrity and stability of ligaments and capsular structures. However, the close-packed position described by MacConaill and Basmajian[14] is not used for mobilization techniques.

The close-packed position is one of stability. When the elbow and knee are fully extended, the ligaments and joint capsule are taut, allowing no freedom of movement. Therefore the knee and elbow in extension serve as two excellent examples of joints in the close-packed position.

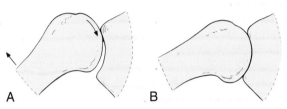

Fig. 15-1 The congruence of articular surfaces: **A,** Loose-packed position. **B,** Close-packed position. (From Gould JA: *Orthopaedic and sports physical therapy,* ed 2, St Louis, 1990, Mosby.)

Any joint position c   tion is a loose-packed p   the joint capsule and ligame   and allow the maximum amou   to as the joint's *resting position.*[4]   flexed to 30°, the intracapsular spa   supporting ligaments become more re   packed position is ideal for applying join   techniques, but painful, stiff, and dysfunc   are rarely in ideal resting positions for the ap   of joint mobilization. Table 15-1 lists resting and   packed positions of major joints in the human bod   If a joint has a limitation of arthrokinematic movemei   in which the close-packed position cannot be achieved, ground reaction forces and gravitational forces are not distributed through the joint in an optimal manner, thus additional stress and work has to be taken up by the periarticular muscles. If this dysfunctional

Table 15-1 Resting (Loose) and Closed-Packed Position of Joints

Joint	Resting Position	Closed-Packed Position
Facet (spine)	Midway between flexion and extension	Extension
Temporomandibular	Mouth slightly open (freeway space)	Clenched teeth
Glenohumeral	55° abduction, 30° horizontal adduction	Abduction and lateral rotation
Acromioclavicular	Arm resting by side in normal physiologic position	Arm abducted to 90°
Sternoclavicular	Arm resting by side in normal physiologic position	Maximum shoulder elevation
Ulnohumeral (elbow)	70° flexion, 10° supination	Extension
Radiohumeral	Full extension, full supination	Elbow flexed 90°, forearm supinated 5°
Proximal radioulnar	70° flexion, 35° supination	5° supination
Distal radioulnar	10° supination	5° supination
Radiocarpal (wrist)	Neutral with slight ulnar deviation	Extension with radial deviation
Carpometacarpal	Midway between abduction-adduction and flexion-extension	
Metacarpophalangeal (all)	Slight flexion	
Metacarpophalangeal (fingers)		Full flexion
Metacarpophalangeal (thumb)		Full opposition
Interphalangeal	Slight flexion	Full extension
Hip	30° flexion, 30° abduction, slight lateral rotation	Full extension, medial rotation
Knee	25° flexion	Full extension, lateral rotation of tibia
Talocrural (ankle)	10° plantarflexion, midway between maximum inversion and eversion	Maximum dorsiflexion
Subtalar	Midway between extremes of range of motion	Supination
Midtarsal	Midway between extremes of range of motion	Supination
Tarsometatarsal	Midway between extremes of range of motion	Supination
Metatarsophalangeal	Neutral	Full extension
Interphalangeal	Slight flexion	Full extension

From Magee DJ: *Orthopedic physical assessment,* ed 5, St Louis, 2008, Saunders.

NICS

describe the degree of force and rate of motion used during any of the grades of mobilization, as follows:

- Grade I mobilization: A small oscillation or small amplitude joint motion that occurs only at the beginning of the available ROM.
- Grade II mobilization: A larger amplitude motion occurring from the beginning of the ROM to near midrange.
- Grade III mobilization: A large amplitude motion that occurs from midrange of motion to the end of the available range.
- Grade IV mobilization: A small oscillation or amplitude of motion that occurs at the very end range of the available joint motion.
- Grade V mobilization: "A high velocity thrust of small amplitude at the end of the available ROM."[4] This grade is not applied to mobilization techniques used by PTAs and is not addressed in this text.

In general terms, a grade I or II small amplitude oscillation is used to treat pain or when joint motion produces pain.[4,21] Therefore mobilization in grades III and IV are used to treat joint restrictions.[4,21]

Translational movements during joint mobilization techniques can be performed in one of two planes. Joint mobilizations can be performed perpendicular or parallel to the treatment plane. The treatment plane is described as a line running perpendicular to, or at a right angle to, a line running from the axis of joint rotation in the convex surface to the center of the concave articular surface.[12] A translational joint mobilization technique (glide) is one in which the

mobile, the gliding motion occurs in the same direction as the bone movement.[4] This occurs because the convex bone surface always maintains an axis of rotation during joint motion (Fig. 15-2). The concept of accessory joint motions (glide or slide, spin, and roll), as they apply to joint congruency and the convex–concave rule, is clearly illustrated by MacConaill's classification of accessory movements (Fig. 15-3).

MOBILIZATION GRADES

Maitland[17] describes five grades of physiologic and accessory joint motions used in mobilization (Fig. 15-4). The terms velocity, oscillation, and amplitude of movement

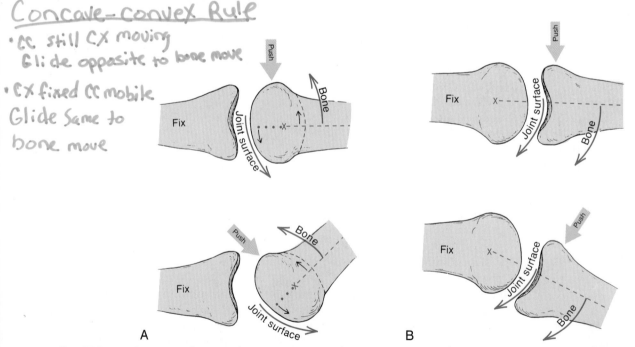

Fig. 15-2 **A,** Convex surface moving on concave surface. **B,** Concave surface moving on convex surface with a combination of roll, spin, and glide occurring in both simultaneously. (From Gould JA: *Orthopaedic and sports physical therapy*, ed 2, St Louis, 1990, Mosby.)

articulating surface glides along a line parallel to the treatment plane.

Traction also is used as a manual therapy technique either by itself or along with various mobilization techniques (Fig. 15-5). A traction technique is a joint mobilization technique that translates one articular surface in a perpendicular direction away from the treatment plane. Traction can be classified in grades or stages.[12,17] Generally, grade I or stage I traction is used for relief of pain and to minimize compressive joint forces during mobilization. The term *piccolo traction* describes a stage I traction technique. The force used to deliver grade I traction is not enough to actually separate the joint surfaces, but rather only neutralizes joint pressure.[4]

As a general rule, distraction techniques cannot stretch or increase length of any specific portion of a joint cavity; rather they are for general overall mobility. Translational glide techniques are used to specifically treat a single portion or restricted joint capsule or tight structure. The term *slack* refers to the amount of normal looseness found in nonpathologic joint capsules and describes various degrees of joint tightness with stage II and III traction. Stage II traction is defined as being able to "take up the slack" in the capsule of the joint being stretched; it is commonly used to treat pain. Stage III traction is more substantial and actually involves stretching of the soft tissues. These techniques are performed to stretch out joint tightness.

JOINT END-FEEL

There are various qualities of joint tightness or "play" during the application of passive joint movements. Three types of end-feel have been defined in normal, nonpathologic joints.[7,16] Bone to bone end-feel refers to a sudden, hard, nonyielding sensation felt at the end ROM. Generally, the end-feel is not painful. Terminal elbow extension in which the olecranon process contacts the olecranon fossa provides an example of a sudden bone-to-bone end-feel.

Another normal end-feel is soft-tissue approximation. This type of joint end-feel is characterized by a "yielding **compression**" typically encountered with knee or elbow flexion.[16] The end-feel that occurs with soft tissue approximation results from muscular tissue compression during joint flexion. The hamstring and calf muscles buttress and compress against each other during knee flexion, delivering a soft-tissue approximation end-feel.

The third normal joint end-feel is described as a hard or springy-tissue stretch. The characteristic feature of this end-feel is "elastic resistance" or "rising **tension**."[16] This type of end-feel is the most common normal feel at the end range of joints. Terminal knee extension and wrist flexion provide a springy stretch that defines tissue stretch.

The PTA must experience normal joint end-feel and be able to accurately identify distinguishing characteristics between bone-to-bone end-feel, soft-tissue approximation, and tissue stretch.[7] The PTA performing mobilization will undoubtedly encounter abnormal joint end-feel, and its precise identification requires considerable didactic and hands-on experience.[7]

The first type of abnormal end-feel is muscle spasm. The major component is pain accompanied by a sudden halt of movement that prevents full ROM.[4,7,16]

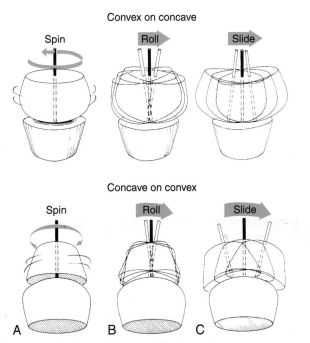

Fig. 15-3 MacConaill's classification of accessory movements: **A,** Spin. **B,** Roll. **C,** Glide. (From Gould JA: *Orthopaedic and sports physical therapy,* ed 2, St Louis, 1990, Mosby.)

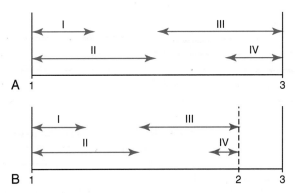

Fig. 15-4 **A,** Grades of oscillations used in manual therapy. **B,** Grades of oscillations used in manual therapy in relation to a joint with limited motion. *1,* Starting position of movement; *2,* point of limitation of movement; *3,* anatomical limit of movement. (From Gould JA: *Orthopaedic and sports physical therapy,* ed 2, St Louis, 1990, Mosby.)

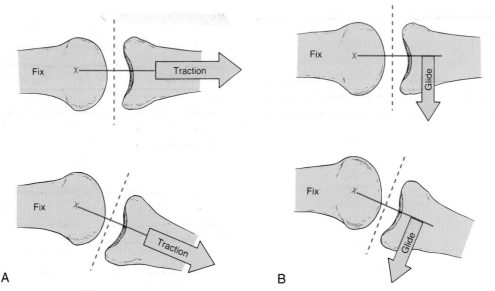

Fig. 15-5 **A,** Traction. **B,** Glide. (From Gould JA: *Orthopaedic and sports physical therapy*, ed 2, St Louis, 1990, Mosby.)

Table 15-2	*Normal and Pathologic End-Feels*	
	End-Feel	**Description and Example**
Normal	Capsular	Firm, forcing the shoulder into full external rotation
	Bony	Abrupt, moving the elbow into full extension
	Soft-tissue approximation	Soft; flexing the normal knee or elbow
	Muscular	Rubbery; tension of tight hamstrings
Pathologic	Adhesions and scarring	Sudden; sharp arrest in one direction
	Muscle spasm	Rebound; usually accompanies pain felt at the end of restriction
	Loose	Ligamentous laxity; a hypermobile joint
	Boggy	Soft, mushy; joint effusion
	Internal derangement	Springy; mechanical block such as a torn meniscus
	Empty	No resistance to motion

From Andrews J, Harrelson G, Wilk K: *Physical rehabilitation of the injured athlete*, ed 3, St Louis, 2004, Saunders; source material from Cyriax JH: *Textbook of orthopedic medicine*, vol 1, ed 6. Baltimore, 1975, Williams & Wilkins.

In springy block, or internal derangement, full motion is limited by a soft or springy sensation occasionally accompanied by pain. If a meniscus is torn in a knee, frequently the cartilage becomes caught in the joint, preventing terminal knee extension and its characteristic normal tissue stretch and feel.

In an empty end-feel, motion is very limited by significant pain without muscle spasm. Clinically, this end-feel is not characterized by any mechanical block or restriction.

Another abnormal end-feel is described as loose end-feel.[4] Its primary feature is joint hypermobility, with no resistance typically felt at the end ROM that signifies extraordinary joint looseness.

A capsular end-feel[16] is analogous to a normal tissue stretch, but the elastic resistance is encountered before the normal ROM. This end-feel is related to a capsular restriction.[16]

Table 15-2 lists various normal and pathologic end-feels and examples of each.[2]

CAPSULAR AND NONCAPSULAR PATTERNS

The PTA must be aware that certain limitations of motion can be caused by lesions specific to the capsule or synovial tissues of a joint. All joints controlled by muscle activity possess a characteristic "**capsular pattern** of proportional limitation."[16] Each joint has its own capsular pattern, which is generally universal among all. For example, in the shoulder joint, the capsular pattern "involves external rotation as the most limited movement,

Table 15-3	*Joint Restrictions from Noncapsular Pattern*
Type	**Description**
Ligament adhesions	These occur when adhesions form around a ligament after an injury and may cause pain or a restriction of mobility. Some movements will be painful, some are slightly limited, and some are pain free.
Internal derangement	Restriction in joint mobility is the result of a loose fragment within the joint. The onset is sudden, pain is localized, and movements that engage against the block are limited, whereas all others are free.
Extraarticular limitation	Loss in joint mobility results from adhesions in structures outside the joint. Movements that stress the adhesions will be limited and painful.

From Andrews J, Harrelson G, Wilk K: *Physical rehabilitation of the injured athlete*, ed 3, St Louis, 2004, Saunders.

abduction as less limited, internal rotation still less limited, and flexion as the least limited movement."[4,7] Any "characteristic pattern of limitation" is called a *capsular pattern*.

If a lesion causes a restriction of movement that does not correspond to a characteristic, predetermined capsular pattern, it is called a *noncapsular pattern*.[4,16] Cyriax[7] has identified three possible causes of noncapsular pattern restrictions:

1. Ligamentous adhesions: Frequently cause pain and limitation of motion. A noncapsular pattern exists when injury to the capsule or accessory ligaments causes a restriction in one direction, although other motions remain unaffected and pain free.
2. Internal derangements: A displaced or loose cartilaginous or bony fragment within the joint. The limitation of movement will depend on where the fragment is located and how large it is. If the medial meniscus becomes wedged in the joint, knee extension is affected although flexion remains normal.
3. Extraarticular lesions: Adhesions resulting from injury outside the joint. Muscular adhesions or acutely inflamed structures are examples. Causes of this can be bursitis, muscle strains, neural tissue irritation, and so on.

Table 15-3 lists joint restrictions from noncapsular patterns.[2]

INDICATIONS AND CONTRAINDICATIONS FOR MOBILIZATION

Patient safety should always be considered when applying joint mobilization or **manipulation** techniques. Cautions or contraindications for joint mobilization and manipulation are listed in Table 15-4 and Box 15-1.[15] Extreme caution must be employed before applying mobilization techniques in the early stages after trauma or surgery or during times of immobilization. Although pain is an indication for the use of mobilization, care must be taken to avoid retarding or impairing the sequence of tissue healing during the acute inflammatory phase.

Pain and joint restrictions are rarely separated completely. In many instances of severe joint limitations there may be only mild complaints of pain. Conversely, there may be little or no joint restriction but significant pain. Naturally there are varying degrees of pain and joint limitations occurring as either major or minor components. Therefore pain is a relative indication for joint mobilization, depending on which stage of tissue healing is present. If an injury is acute or a patient is recovering immediately after a surgical procedure, mobilization may not be indicated because it is best not to disturb the immature scar. Healing that proceeds in an organized fashion encourages mature collagen formation. When injured tissues have progressed from the acute, intense inflammatory phase to fibroplasia and scar maturation, mobilization is warranted to stress and remodel the scar.[21]

There are a few relative and absolute contraindications to the application of joint mobilization. Extreme caution is needed when considering mobilization in cases of osteoporosis, rheumatoid arthritis, joint hypermobility, and the presence of neurologic symptoms; all are therefore considered relative contraindications.[4,21] In cases of spinal mobilization, pregnancy and spondylolisthesis are relative contraindications. Some absolute contraindications include bone diseases of the area treated, malignancy of the area treated, acute inflammatory and infectious arthritis, central nervous system (CNS) disorders, and vascular disorders of the vertebral artery.[4,21]

CLINICAL APPLICATION OF JOINT MOBILIZATION

Safe and effective joint mobilization requires the patient to be placed in a very comfortable position and the specific joint to be mobilized to be placed in a maximal resting or loose-packed position.[14] Before mobilization is applied, patient compliance and relaxation can be facilitated by the judicious use of moist heat,

Table 15-4	Factors Involving the Patient's Anatomy or Physiology to Consider as a Caution or Contraindication for Mobilization or Manipulation
Type of Element	**Description**
Bony elements	Fractures (presently healing)
	Dislocations (presently healing)
	Past or present cancers that metastasize to bone (e.g., breast, bronchus, prostate, thyroid, kidney, bowel, lymphoma)
	Active bone infection (cautionary with past bone infections; e.g., osteomyelitis, tuberculosis, congenital anomalies)
	Gross foraminal or spinal canal encroachment on radiograph or other imaging examination
Vascular elements	Vertebral artery insufficiency
	Vascular disease (e.g., aneurysm, atherosclerosis)
	Signs of vascular insufficiency in that region
	Bleeding disorders
	Aortic graft
Neurological elements	Central nervous system disease or signs and symptoms of its injury
	Spinal cord disease or signs and symptoms of its injury
	Cauda equina disease or signs and symptoms of its injury
	Multiple/bilateral level nerve root involvement
Soft tissue elements	Collagen disease (e.g., Ehlers-Danlos syndrome)
	Connective tissue instability
	Acute posttraumatic stage of healing
Metabolic disease	Bone disease, such as osteoporosis
Systemic disease/condition	Asthma, hemophilia, pregnancy
Inflammatory diseases	Acute active inflammation such as rheumatoid arthritis or inactive inflammatory disease
Medications patient may be taking	Anticoagulants (e.g., heparin/caution with aspirin)
	Any medication that affects collagen (e.g., corticosteroids or tamoxifen or any medication that is linked to osteoporosis)
	Antidepressants

From Maffey LL: Arthrokinematics and mobilization of musculoskeletal tissue: the principles. In Magee DJ, Zachazewski JE, Quillen WS, editors: *Scientific foundations and principles of practice in musculoskeletal rehabilitation*, St Louis, 2007, Saunders.

ultrasound, transcutaneous electrical nerve stimulation (TENS), electrical muscle stimulation, ice, exercise, and the timely use of any physician-prescribed analgesics or muscle relaxant medications. If pain is the predominant feature of the joint to be mobilized, grade I and II mobilization can be employed safely.

Oscillations help modulate or minimize pain when using grade I and II mobilization. Manually applied joint oscillations occur at a rate of 1 to 3 per second, or 60 to 180 per minute.[4,17] Typically, a mobilization grade technique is applied for 20 to 60 seconds only four or five times. This is recommended for the treatment of painful conditions on a daily basis or until pain is reduced. These smaller amplitude mobilization techniques are used to stimulate mechanoreceptors within the joint that can limit pain perception transmission at the spinal cord or brainstem level through a hypoalgesic response mediated by the noradrenergic descending pain pathways from the periaqueductal gray area.[22]

It is not uncommon to perform grade I and II mobilizations to a joint for purposes of decreasing pain before more aggressive mobilization techniques to gain motion. Some irritable conditions require a short bout of smaller oscillation techniques before techniques designed to gain mobility.

A program of mobilization is carried out two to three times per week for the treatment of joint restrictions.[4] Piccolo or stage I traction can be used simultaneously with grade I or II mobilization or by itself to reduce pain and neutralize joint pressure. When the limitation of joint motion is greater than the complaints of pain, grade III and IV mobilization can be used to help stretch the capsule and soft tissues around the joint.

The pathologic condition of the joint to be mobilized must be thoroughly understood before applying

Factors Involving the Clinician and Patient Relationship to Consider as a Contraindication for Mobilization or Manipulation

- Insufficient subjective assessment of the patient; that is, inadequate information about coexisting conditions, disease, and/or medication, or in general the patient has an inability to communicate or is an unreliable historian
- Poor appraisal of the patient as a reliable historian
- Patient is intoxicated or heavily medicated
- Patient age: children (skeletal maturity, consent issues) or elderly (tissue health/integrity issues)
- Failure to discuss the assessment findings and treatment options with patient
- Failure to receive or to agree with patient consent
- Insufficient scanning examination or detailed biomechanical examination
- Inappropriate findings, end-feel, or patient response with the following:
  - Scanning examination
  - Biomechanical testing
  - Stress testing (positive for level desire to treat or cautionary if above or below joint/level treating)
  - Dizziness reproduction testing
- Clinician's insufficient awareness of contraindications and conditions requiring extra care and gentleness
- Clinician's physical limitations for the technique (e.g., their size, strength, speed, fatigue)
- Lack of clinician's confidence for the technique
- Lack of proper equipment for the technique (e.g., not using a high/low plinth)
- Pain in the position of the technique
- Patient's joint placed in a fully close-packed position

From Maffey LL: Arthrokinematics and mobilization of musculoskeletal tissue: the principles. In Magee DJ, Zachazewski JE, Quillen WS, editors: *Scientific foundations and principles of practice in musculoskeletal rehabilitation*, St Louis, 2007, Saunders.

any mobilization technique. For example, it is critical to avoid stressing the anterior capsule of the shoulder after an anterior dislocation, although mobilization to improve shoulder abduction may be warranted.[21]

In every case of joint mobilization, the PTA must constantly observe and document the patient's tolerance, pain response, and swelling to determine whether to halt the procedure, reduce the grade of motion, or consult with the PT about advancing the grade of mobilization.

As stated in the beginning of this discussion, the PT is responsible for delegating selected peripheral joint mobilization techniques to the PTA. Although peripheral joint mobilization beyond active and passive ROM is an area of treatment not usually delegated to the PTA,

understanding peripheral joint mobilization techniques and having an awareness of rudimentary concepts and principles of mobilization provide the PTA with a broad understanding of the rationale for the application of certain techniques.

MOBILIZATION EVIDENCE

When assessing the medical literature, there is very little in regard to high-level evidence via randomized controlled clinical trials (RCTs) assessing effectiveness of joint mobilization techniques. The studies that are described next are those that have a higher level of evidence via either number of participants, prospective, randomized designs, and described inclusion/exclusion criteria.

There are mixed reviews in the ankle. Lin and colleagues[13] recently reported that incorporation of large amplitude grade III anterior-posterior glides to the talus for 4 weeks did not enhance their outcomes at 24 weeks following ankle fractures. This is in direct contradiction to Green and coworkers[8] who used an experimental group given anteroposterior joint mobilizations to the talus following an acute ankle sprain and a control group that was treated with rest, ice, compression, and elevation (RICE). Following the intervention period the experimental group required fewer treatments, had greater improvements in ROM at the ankle, and greater increases in stride speed, indicating that the addition of joint mobilizations had a positive impact on outcomes.

In the hip, Hoeksma and associates[10] proved in a single-blind, RCT of 109 patients with osteoarthritic hips that manual therapy resulted in 81% success rates for the experimental group as compared with only 50% in the control group. The experimental group demonstrated better outcomes in regard to pain, stiffness, hip function, and ROM following 5 weeks (9 sessions) of manual therapy treatments of hip joint distraction followed by a hip traction manipulation. These beneficial changes remained even after 29 weeks.

In the shoulder, Senbursa and colleagues[19] used a RCT to compare effectiveness of two treatments for shoulder impingement—soft tissue and joint mobilization or independent exercise program. Thirty patients with impingement were randomized into one of the treatment approaches and followed for 3 months. The manual therapy group received a prescription of 12 sessions of joint mobilization. The experimental group demonstrated significant decreases in pain and increases in ROM. Conroy and Hayes[6] examined the usefulness of joint mobilizations on 14 patients with impingement syndrome. Random assignment was to an exercise program alone or an exercise program with joint mobilizations. The results were mixed, with the mobilization group demonstrating less 24-hour pain, and less pain with a subacromial compression test, but no differences in ROM and function.

Bang and Deyle[3] assessed the comparison of supervised exercise versus supervised exercise combined with manual therapy to the upper quarter in those with impingement syndrome. The manual therapy approach they used consisted mainly of grade I to V oscillatory caudal glides of the glenohumeral joint in varying degrees of flexion and abduction. Bang and Deyle[3] found significant improvement in pain reduction, function, and strength in those that received manual therapy in addition to supervised exercises. More recently, Manske and colleagues[18] used an RCT of stretching versus stretching plus posterior shoulder capsular mobilizations to assess for efficacy in treating a tight posterior shoulder. The main outcome measure was internal rotation motion loss. Using 39 randomly assigned subjects with at least a 10° loss of internal rotation, it was found that the addition of posterior shoulder joint mobilization to a stretching program resulted in trends towards increased motion.

A Cochrane review performed by Gross and colleagues[9] assessed mobilization and manipulation in patients with mechanical neck disorders. Outcomes were based on pain relief, functional improvement, or overall disability improvement. Studies including single session and multiple session manipulative therapy. Some in the presence of other treatment modalities showed little to no benefit for patients with acute, subacute, and chronic neck disorders. Mobilization alone was found to have similar results based on four randomized controlled trials in which mobilization was tested against cold pack, TENS, and ultrasound, among others. Mobilization and manipulation combined in a treatment approach also found little evidence to support their use for pain relief and improvement in function. Mobilization and manipulation with the addition of exercise was found to have positive results for the three outcome criteria. Though this is encouraging for those patients suffering with acute to chronic pain in the cervical spine, the authors also noted studies that compared manipulation plus exercise to exercise alone with little difference noted between these groups.

A review of literature done by Hurwitz and associates[11] looked at studies examining the use of mobilization and manipulation in the management of neck pain and headaches. Neck pain was broken down into acute, and subacute or chronic neck pain. In the studies reviewed, the authors found that mobilization provided some statistically significant decreases in pain when compared with other treatment options. Manipulation of the cervical spine in patients experiencing subacute and chronic neck pain as well as tension-induced headaches showed subjective improvements compared with other therapies, however; the authors

also noted the risks involved with cervical manipulation. These risks included paralysis and even death, with rates of injury occurring in 5 to 10 per 10 million manipulations.

In a study investigating the safety of mobilization to the thoracic spine, Sran and coworkers[20] used 12 cadavers to determine the in vitro effects of spinal mobilization to the sixth thoracic vertebra. Loading of the spinous process of T6 was performed using mechanical compression to the point of failure. The average amount of force to failure in the cadaver models was 479 ± 162 newtons (N). These results varied significantly when compared to the in vivo effects of mobilization, where two physiotherapists applied an average load of 145 ± 38 N. The amount of force then applied in this study showed that posterior to anterior mobilization when applied with care has a fairly significant margin of error before fracture occurs. The authors summarized the findings to be clinically relevant in cases where the patient needing mobilization, at least in the thoracic spine, may have bone density issues leading to use of decreased force of mobilization or mobilization being contraindicated.

Management of low back pain is difficult and a very common problem in the patient population of the PT or PTA. The use of manipulation or mobilization to address the dysfunction associated with the low back is becoming increasingly popular. A systematic review of literature provided by Bronfort and colleagues[5] showed that manipulation and mobilization of the spine did have some evidence to support its use in the management of acute and chronic low back pain. In acute episodes the authors were able to conclude manipulation was better suited to relieve pain than other treatment techniques, including mobilization and diathermy. For chronic low back pain the authors were able to conclude that manipulation with the addition of strengthening exercises had evidence to support its use in the reduction of pain and disability.

❖ GLOSSARY

Arthrokinematics: Study of motion within the joints. Description of joint typography.

Capsular pattern: Limitation of movement or a pattern of pain at a joint that occurs in a predictable pattern.

Compression: Occurs when two forces or loads are applied toward each other.

Manipulation: Passive intervention motion of high velocity at end ranges of available joint motion.

Mobilization: Passive intervention motion within and at end range of joint motion with varying degrees of speed and amplitude.

Tension: Occurs when two forces are applied in opposite directions.

REFERENCES

1. American Physical Therapy Association: Guide to physical thera-pist practice. Second edition. American Physical Therapy Associa-tion, *Phys Ther* 81:9–746, 2001.
2. Andrews J, Harrelson G, Wilk K: *Physical rehabilitation of the injured athlete*, ed 3, St Louis, 2004, Saunders.
3. Bang MD, Deyle GD: Comparison of supervised exercise with and without manual physical therapy for patients with shoulder impingement syndrome, *J Orthop Sports Phys Ther* 30:126–137, 2000.
4. Barak T, Rosen ER, Sofer R: Basic concepts of orthopaedic manual therapy. In Gould JA, editor: *Orthopaedic and sports physical therapy*, ed 2, St Louis, 1990, Mosby.
5. Bronfort G, Haas M, Evans RL, et al: Efficacy of spinal manipula-tion and mobilization for low back pain and neck pain: a system-atic review and best evidence synthesis, *Spine* 4:335–356, 2004.
6. Conroy DE, Hayes KW: The effect of joint mobilization as a com-ponent of compressive treatment for primary shoulder impinge-ment syndrome, *J Orthop Sports Phys Ther* 28:3–14, 1998.
7. Cyriax J: *Textbook of orthopaedic medicine*, vol 1, *Diagnosis of soft tissue lesions*, ed 8, London, 1982, Baillière Tindall.
8. Green T, Refshauge K, Crosbie J, et al: A randomized controlled trial of passive accessory joint mobilization on acute ankle inver-sion sprains, *Phys Ther* 81:984–994, 2001.
9. Gross AR, Hoving JL, Haines TA, et al: A Cochrane review of manipulation and mobilization for mechanical neck disorders, *Spine* 29:1541–1548, 2004.
10. Hoeksma HL, Dekker J, Ronday HK, et al: Comparison of manual therapy and exercise therapy in osteoarthritis of the hip: a ran-domized clinical trial, *Arthritis Care Res* 51:722–729, 2004.
11. Hurwitz EL, Aker PD, Adams AH, et al: Manipulation and mobi-lization of the cervical spine: a systematic review of the literature, *Spine* 21:1746–1759, 1996.
12. Kaltenborn F: *Mobilization of extremity joints: examination and basic treatment techniques*, Oslo, 1980, Olaf Norlis Bokhandel.
13. Lin CWC, Moseley AM, Haas M, et al: Manual therapy in addi-tion to physiotherapy does not improve clinical or economic out-comes after ankle fracture, *J Rehabil Med* 40:433–439, 2008.
14. MacConaill MA, Basmajian JV: *Muscles and movements: a basis for human kinesiology*, Baltimore, 1969, Williams & Wilkins.
15. Maffey LL: Arthrokinematics and mobilization of musculoskeletal tissue: the principles. In Magee DJ, Zachazewski JE, Quillen WS, editors: *Scientific foundations and principles of practice in musculosk-eletal rehabilitation*, St Louis, 2007, Saunders.
16. Magee DJ: *Orthopedic physical assessment*, ed 5, St Louis, 2008, Saunders.
17. Maitland G: *Peripheral manipulation*, ed 2, Newton, Mass, 1978, Butterworth-Heinemann.
18. Manske RC, Meschke M, Porter A, et al: A randomized, controlled, single-blinded, comparison of stretching versus stretching and joint mobilization for posterior shoulder tightness measured via internal rotation motion loss, *Sports Health* 2(2):94–100, 2010.
19. Senbursa G, Baltaci G, Atay A: Comparison of conservative treat-ment with and without manual physical therapy for patients with shoulder impingement syndrome: a prospective, random-ized clinical trial, *Knee Surg Sports Traumatol Arthrosc* 15:915–921, 2007.
20. Sran MM, Khan KM, Zhu Q, et al: Failure characteristics of the thoracic spine with a posteroanterior load: investigating the safety of spinal mobilization, *Spine* 29:2382–2388, 2004.
21. Wooden MJ: Mobilization of the upper extremity. In Donatelli R, Wooden MJ, editors: *Orthopaedic physical therapy*, New York, 1989, Churchill Livingstone.
22. Wright A: Hypoalgesia post-manipulative therapy: a review of a potential neurophysiological mechanism, *Man Ther* 1:11–16, 1995.

REVIEW QUESTIONS

Short Answer

1. When the concave surface is stationary and the convex surface is moving, the gliding movement in the joint occurs in a direction _____ to the bone movement.
2. When the convex surface is fixed, whereas the concave surface is mobile, the gliding motion occurs in the _____ direction as the bone movement.

True/False

3. When performing joint ROM, the physical therapist assistant should encourage the patient to perform all accessory joint motions.
4. The "close-packed" joint position is best used for determining joint stability.
5. The "loose-packed" position is best used for joint mobilization techniques.
6. A patient is being seen immediately after surgery when pain may be significant. If joint mobilization is an appropriate treatment method it is always appropriate to use grades I and II mobilization to help decrease pain.

16 Biomechanical Basis for Movement

Mitchell A. Collins
Michael Hales

LEARNING OBJECTIVES

1. Define and apply biomechanical concepts in the description of rudimentary movement patterns.
2. Discuss the difference between the kinematics and kinetics of movement.
3. Identify and discuss the kinematic principles as related to movement in a rehabilitation setting.
4. Discuss both the linear and angular kinematics and kinetics of movement, and explain how angular motion translates to linear movements.
5. Describe the differences among the different levers, and explain the concept of mechanical advantage as related to levers.
6. Describe Newton's laws of motion.
7. Identify and discuss the different forces that act on objects and how the forces affect movement.
8. Discuss the concepts of mechanical loading, and describe how loading is associated with different types of injuries.
9. Discuss the principles of mechanical energy.
10. Describe the concept of equilibrium and identify the factors that contribute to stability.

KEY TERMS

Force	Friction	Stress
Force couple	Inertia	Velocity

CHAPTER OUTLINE

Biomechanics is the study of the internal and external forces acting on the body and the effects these forces produce. The data obtained from biomechanical research provide a great deal of insight into human movement interactions in fields such as physical and occupational therapy, sports medicine, human factors, prosthetics, orthotics, and ergonomics.[12,31] Clinical biomechanics, a subdiscipline, provides direct measures of human motion which influence our knowledge of injury mechanics, rehabilitation, treatment, and prevention. This information can directly affect how a physical therapist assistant (PTA) rehabilitates a patient, an orthopedist repairs a broken limb or ruptured ligament, an athletic trainer implements modalities for treatment, or a clinician evaluates an individual's gait.[19,21,24]

The field of biomechanics combines the study of applied human anatomy with that of mechanical physics. These combined sciences allow for detailed descriptions of how and why the human body moves the way it does and why a person may or may not have sustained an injury. Understanding the neuromuscular and mechanical factors associated with human movement provides the PTA with the knowledge and skills necessary for administering rehabilitative techniques correctly and performing patient assistive lifting tasks safely. These biomechanical descriptions influence health professionals to refine their knowledge and, therefore, their approach to injury rehabilitation as well as to consider new and innovative techniques that may lead to improved rehabilitation processes. This information also provides insight into the mechanical causes of injuries, potentially leading to safer participation as individuals interact with the environment.

Biomechanics can provide the health professional with a better understanding and a broadened knowledge of the causes and degrees of severity associated with an injury. In order to improve upon a current rehabilitative technique, repair procedure or treatment process, the mechanics associated with the causation of the injury must be fully understood. To help the health professional accomplish this task, several factors need consideration when determining the cause and severity of an injury[36]:

- How much force was applied? (magnitude)
- Where on the body was the force applied? (location)
- Where was the force directed? (direction)
- How long was the force applied? (duration)
- How often was the force applied? (frequency)
- Does the force application vary in magnitude? (variability)
- How quickly is the force applied? (rate)

The major role of a PTA revolves around both the causes and effects of human motion and therefore it is imperative to have a fundamental understanding of the mechanical basis for whole body or segmental movement. Since biomechanics is concerned with the effects of forces on the human body, biomechanical principles are involved when a force is present. The following chapter will offer an overview of the science of biomechanics with practical applications for the PTA.

REFERENCE TERMINOLOGY

To facilitate the process of describing human movement, standardized terminology has been adopted to identify body positions and directions of motion (Box 16-1). Movements are defined based on a reference or starting position often referred to as the *anatomic position* (Fig. 16-1, *A*), which is a standing position with arms at one's side and palms facing forward. From the anatomic position, three imaginary cardinal planes bisect the body along three dimensions (Fig. 16-1, *B*). The transverse or horizontal plane segments the body into upper and lower parts; the frontal or coronal plane separates the body into front and back parts; and the sagittal or anteroposterior plane divides the body into right and left parts. It is important to note that the planes do not necessarily divide the body into equal parts. However, when the segments are equal, the mid-intersection point of the transverse, frontal, and sagittal planes is referred to as the *center of mass* (COM) or *center of gravity* (COG). Although human movement is not restricted to a single plane, most named movements (e.g., flexion and abduction) are described based on the three cardinal planes.

Movements in the transverse plane occur around the longitudinal axis, which runs superiorly–inferiorly while perpendicularly intersecting the transverse plane. These movements include medial and lateral rotation of the leg, thigh, and shoulder; supination and pronation of the forearm; and horizontal abduction and adduction of the shoulder. Movements in the frontal plane occur around the sagittal axis, which runs

---

BOX 16-1

Basic Directional Terms Used to Describe Body Parts or Other Objects in Relation to the Body

- Anterior: Toward the front of the body
- Posterior: Toward the back of the body
- Deep: Toward the inside (core) of the body
- Superficial: Toward the surface (skin) of the body
- Distal: Away from the body or torso
- Proximal: Closer to the body or torso
- Inferior: Toward the feet
- Superior: Toward the head
- Lateral: Away from the midline of the body
- Medial: Toward the midline of the body

anteriorly–posteriorly while perpendicularly intersecting the frontal plane. These movements include abduction and adduction of the shoulder and hip, lateral flexion of the neck and trunk, elevation and depression of the shoulder girdle, and inversion and eversion of the foot. Movements in the sagittal plane occur around the frontal axis, which runs from left to right while perpendicularly intersecting the sagittal plane. These movements include flexion and extension of the knee, hip, trunk, elbow, shoulder, and neck; and dorsiflexion and plantar flexion of the foot as well as hyperextension movements. A key role of the PTA is to facilitate patient rehabilitation through the incorporation of various exercises using basic movement patterns. Therefore it is important to be familiar with the appropriate terminology for these movements (Fig. 16-2).

BASIC CONCEPTS

To facilitate the discussion of biomechanical principles, a working understanding of various rudimentary concepts is essential. The following are definitions of some common terms along with their appropriate unit of measure. Most of these terms will be discussed in more detail as various biomechanical concepts are introduced.

Mass (m) is the amount of matter an object possesses within its physical boundaries; generally, the denser the material that comprises the object, the greater the mass. For example, muscle tissue is denser than fat tissue; therefore, two persons of equal size or volume may differ in mass if one is more muscular than the other.

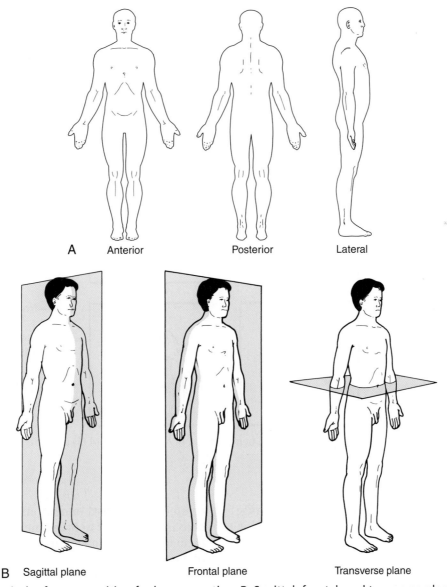

A   Anterior   Posterior   Lateral

B   Sagittal plane   Frontal plane   Transverse plane

Fig. 16-1 **A,** Anatomical reference position for human motion. **B,** Sagittal, frontal, and transverse planes. (From Cameron MH, Monroe LG: *Physical rehabilitation: evidence-based examination, evaluation, and intervention,* St Louis, 2006, Saunders.)

Wrist—sagittal

Flexion
Exercise: wrist curl
Sport: tennis serve

Extension
Exercise: reverse wrist curl
Sport: racquet backhand

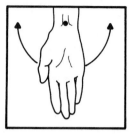

Wrist—frontal

Ulnar deviation
Exercise: specific wrist curl
Sport: baseball batting

Radial deviation
Exercise: specific wrist curl
Sport: golf backswing

Elbow—sagittal

Flexion
Exercise: arm curl
Sport: rowing

Extension
Exercise: triceps pushdown
Sport: boxing jab

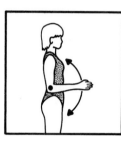

Shoulder—sagittal

Flexion
Exercise: medium-grip military press
Sport: softball pitch

Extension
Exercise: narrow-grip row
Sport: freestyle swimming

Shoulder—frontal

Adduction
Exercise: wide-grip pulldown
Sport: gymnastic rings

Abduction
Exercise: wide-grip military press
Sport: springboard diving

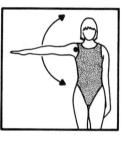

Shoulder—transverse

Internal rotation
Exercise: arm wrestle movement (with dumbbell or cable)
Sport: baseball pitch

External rotation
Exercise: reverse arm wrestle movement
Sport: karate block

Shoulder—transverse
(upper arm 90° to trunk)

Adduction
Exercise: wide-grip bench press
Sport: boxing hook

Abduction
Exercise: row (elbows high)
Sport: tennis backhand

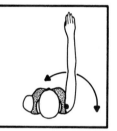

Neck—sagittal

Flexion
Exercise: neck machine
Sport: somersault

Extension
Exercise: neck machine
Sport: wrestling bridge

Neck—transverse

Left rotation
Exercise: neck machine
Sport: wrestling

Right rotation
Exercise: neck machine
Sport: wrestling

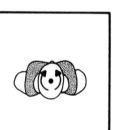

Neck—frontal

Left tilt
Exercise: neck machine
Sport: wrestling

Right tilt
Exercise: neck machine
Sport: wrestling

Fig. 16-2 Major movements of body segments. (With permission from *NSCA Journal* 14 (1) by Harman, Johnson, and Frykman, pp 47-54.)

Inertia is the resistance an object offers to a change in its state of motion (**velocity**) or direction of motion and is directly related to its mass. The greater the mass of the object, the more resistance it offers to any attempt at changing its velocity or direction of motion.

Force (F) is a push or pull acting on an object. A force will have both direction and magnitude, and it is commonly expressed in newtons (N). Forces applied to objects, if sufficient to overcome their inertia, will cause them to accelerate in direct proportion to the magnitude of the force.

Friction is created when two objects are in direct contact with one another and a force acts to impede motion of the objects. Frictional force can be increased

Lower back—sagittal
Flexion
Exercise: weighted sit-up
Sport: somersault

Extension
Exercise: reverse sit-up
Sport: rowing

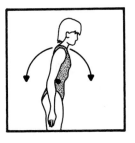

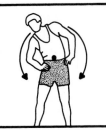

Lower back—frontal
Left tilt
Exercise: side bend
Sport: gymnastics side aerial

Right tilt
Exercise: side bend
Sport: gymnastics side aerial

Lower back—transverse
Left rotation
Exercise: torso machine
Sport: baseball batting

Right rotation
Exercise: torso machine
Sport: baseball batting

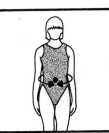

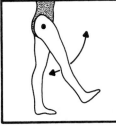

Hip—sagittal
Flexion
Exercise: leg raise
Sport: football punt

Extension
Exercise: squat
Sport: jumping

Hip—frontal
Adduction
Exercise: adduction machine
Sport: lateral movement

Abduction
Exercise: abduction machine
Sport: skating

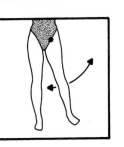

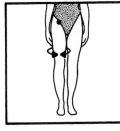

Hip—transverse
Internal rotation
Exercise: friction rotation
Sport: pivot movement

Extension
Exercise: friction rotation
Sport: pivot movement

Hip—transverse
(upper leg 90° to trunk)
Adduction
Exercise: adduction machine
Sport: karate in-sweep

Abduction
Exercise: abduction machine
Sport: karate out-sweep

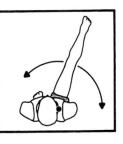

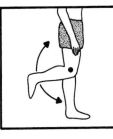

Knee—sagittal
Flexion
Exercise: leg curl
Sport: sprint running

Extension
Exercise: leg extension
Sport: bicycling

Ankle—sagittal
Dorsiflexion
Exercise: dorsiflexion
(weight-resisted)
Sport: running

Plantarflexion
Exercise: calf raise
Sport: jumping

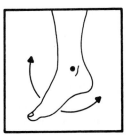

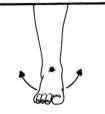

Ankle—frontal
Inversion
Exercise: inversion
Sport: ice skating

Eversion
Exercise: eversion (friction resisted)
Sport: ice skating

Fig. 16-2, cont'd

or decreased by adding substances between the two surfaces, such as the installation of tennis balls on the rear support for walkers. Joint damage (osteoarthritis) caused by chronic exposure to high frictional forces can lead to arthroplasty.

COM or COG is the point within which the weight and mass of an object is equally distributed or balanced in all directions. The COM is important because when a force is applied to an object, the movement pattern will vary based on the relation of the point of force application to the COM.

Kinetic energy (KE) is energy by virtue of an object's motion. The units for KE are typically expressed as a joule (J), however, one may also see units of newton-meters (N-m), which is an equivalent unit (i.e., 1 N-m = 1 J). An injury mechanism is predominantly due to the transfer of KE to the body arising from different sources under a variety of conditions: from blunt trauma (impact of object's colliding with the body), penetrating trauma, acceleration/deceleration motion (rapidly moving forward and backward), and crushing weight (high compression forces).

Potential energy is energy generated by virtue of the position or shape of an object. Potential energy may be affected by how much elastic energy is generated by either stretching or compressing the object (e.g., cartilage, tendon, connective tissue) such that, if the distorting force is removed, the object will recoil to its resting length. The units for potential energy are typically expressed as a J; however, one may also use units of N-m.

Torque (T) is the product of the force and the perpendicular distance from the line of action to the axis point, also called *lever arm length*. Torque is considered a rotary force, but more specifically a measure of the ability of a force to cause rotation. Consequently, torque can be increased or decreased easily by altering the length of the moment arm of the force. A **force couple** is formed in situations where there are two torques that are equal in magnitude but opposite in direction. The resultant action of a force couple is rotation without any translation. Torque is typically expressed in units of N-m.

Work (W) is the product of force and the distance the object moves. If no displacement of the object occurs, even though force may have been applied to the object, no work was done. The unit of measure is a N-m or a J.

Power (P) is the rate of performing work, and can be expressed algebraically as the product of force and displacement over time. If work is accomplished very quickly (i.e., in a very short amount of time) then a higher magnitude of power is generated as compared to the same amount of work being done over a longer interval of time. Given this explanation, power is work divided by time. Power is expressed in watts (w), and 1 w is equal to 1 J of work per second.

Pressure (p) is a measure of the distribution of a force over a given area (force/area), and it is expressed in newtons per meter^2 (N/m^2). An example of the concept of pressure in a rehabilitation setting is the development of decubitus ulcers that commonly occur among diabetics.[3,32,38] Innovations in shoe design help dissipate the forces applied to the foot over a larger area (e.g., reduced pressure) during locomotion, thus minimizing soft-tissue damage and the incidence of ulceration.[6,10,35]

Momentum is the product of mass and velocity used to determine the outcome of collisions between two objects of mass as well as to determine the ease with which one can stop or change the direction of travel when velocity is present. A motionless object has no momentum. The unit of measure is kilogram × meters/second (kg × m/sec).

Impulse is the product of the force magnitude and the force application time interval expressed in newton × seconds. The direct relationship between an applied force and the change in momentum it creates is known as the *impulse-momentum principle*. Consider a high force applied to the musculoskeletal system over a very short duration, as is often the case in force related injuries.

BIOMECHANICAL PRINCIPLES

Statics and Dynamics

Statics is the branch of mechanics concerned with the analysis of loads (force, torque/moment) on physical systems in static equilibrium. In biomechanics, statics is the study of the body under conditions where no accelerations or velocity changes are occurring. When acceleration of the body occurs, as is required if a person is to change positions, static conditions would no longer be present. Static conditions are common when considering the immobilization of a joint or when an individual is in traction to immobilize a body segment. Quite often, a PTA will incorporate proprioceptive neuromuscular facilitation (PNF) stretching exercises to help a patient regain normal range of motion (ROM) to a joint postinjury. During PNF stretching a static (isometric) contraction is performed by a patient and health practitioner.

Dynamics is the study of a body segment experiencing accelerations. As a result, body segments are increasing and decreasing in velocity as a particular skill is performed. This requires varying levels of force to produce these accelerations. Depending upon the intensity of the exercise, these forces and accelerations may range from very small to very large in magnitude. The legs in walking and running, and the arms in wheelchair propulsion are examples of dynamic segments used in performing human activities. A quantified movement analysis can clarify which muscles should be active during a posture or movement in the context of several external forces acting on the body.

Linear and Angular Motion

Linear motion is the point-to-point, straight-line movement of a body in space. The motion is generally measured in either a two-dimensional or three-dimensional system depending on the complexity of the activity being monitored. These measures are made in the geometric planes established by the Cartesian coordinate system, which are oriented to the human body (local) and/or Earth (global) such that anteroposterior, vertical, and mediolateral measures of motion are described linearly. Forces applied by or on the body in these respective directions lead to accelerations or velocity changes of these body points. Linear forces may be applied by muscles, gravity, the ground, or any number of other animate or inanimate objects.

Angular motion is the measurement of rotation about an axis of a rigid lever and is quantified through the use of a polar coordinate system. This is generally represented in the human body by body segments; an example is the upper arm rotating about a joint (axis of rotation) such as the shoulder. By tracking over time how the lever, as established by its endpoints (for the upper arm these would be represented by a line connecting the shoulder and elbow), rotates around its proximal joint (the shoulder), one can determine angular positional changes of the lever, rotational velocities of the lever about the joint, and increases/decreases in rotational velocity. These angular measures describe the quality of motion generated angularly by an individual performing an activity of daily living (ADL), occupational activity, or exercise. This is important because there is a direct link between the quality of angular motion of body segments or levers and the potential for overuse injuries to the subsequent joints. For example, the faster the forearm/racket combination is rotating or extending about the elbow at the instant before impact in a tennis serve, the faster the racket is moving linearly at the moment of impact with the ball. The faster the racket head is moving linearly at impact, the greater the momentum or force imparted to the tennis ball by the athlete. Conversely, because of the high action force and moment, the greater the reaction force and moment imposed on the joints, which could lead to inflammation of the lateral epicondyle (tennis elbow) if poor service mechanics are demonstrated.[22] The rotation of the forearm about the elbow is due in part to the contraction of the muscles (triceps group), which causes acceleration in the direction of elbow extension. The linear force of the triceps tendon pulling on the ulna generates a torque or rotational force. The greater the torque produced by the muscles, the greater the angular acceleration generated, leading to changes in angular velocity that lead to changes in angular position.

Kinematics and Kinetics

Kinematics is the description of human motion in terms of position, velocity, and acceleration. These three variables describe the quality of the motion resulting from forces produced by the muscular system or forces external to the body, such as gravity, other persons, and inanimate objects (ground, implements, and so on). However, the study of kinematics is not concerned with force measurements, therefore the magnitude or type of force responsible for generating these human motions is disregarded.

An understanding of kinematic principles is extremely important to PTAs. Analysis of motion can facilitate the determination of the etiology of injury, extent of damage, and assessment of the effectiveness of treatment. Historically, researchers have studied injuries in sport settings, but the same applications are pertinent to nonathletic settings, such as gait analysis of individuals with lower extremity joint injury or joint replacement.[7,9,11,16,27,28] Thus it is imperative for PTAs to be knowledgeable about normal movement patterns from a kinematic perspective to facilitate the recognition of abnormal movements of rehabilitating patients.

Kinetics is concerned with the forces responsible for maintaining equilibrium and the sources of motion generating the kinematic qualities described earlier. The various forces applied on or by a system can be quantified to determine why a body sustains an injury. This information can lead to very detailed analysis of movement mechanics and injury potential, because these forces lead directly to accelerations that cause increases and/or decreases in velocity, which in turn lead to changes in body position over time.

Newton's Laws of Motion

Much of the basis for kinetics originates from the laws of motion introduced by Sir Isaac Newton (1642-1727) in 1687. Although Newton's theories date back more than 300 years, the basic concepts introduced continue to be used today by biomechanists to provide the explanation for the factors that cause an object to move in a specific manner.

Newton's first law of motion is commonly referred to as the *law of inertia*, which states:

"A body remains in a state of rest, or of uniform motion in a straight line, unless it is compelled to change that state by forces impressed on it."[5]

Inertia of an object is used to describe the reluctance of an object to change its movement pattern; that is, to stay motionless or to move in a linear path unless a force is applied. The amount of inertia an object possesses is related to the mass of the object. As a result, the larger the mass or inertia of an object, the more difficult it is to alter its motion. We can observe the concept of inertia by examining events that occur during car accidents. If an automobile is struck in the rear by another vehicle, the head of the passenger tends to remain at rest momentarily as the body is thrust forward. Whiplash is the term used to describe the injury mechanism of the anterior longitudinal ligament.[37] Conversely, when a car strikes an object and is suddenly forced to stop, the passenger continues to move forward because of the person's inertia. This forward motion continues to occur until a force is applied (hopefully seat belts and air bags) to counteract the inertia. However, if the passenger is wearing a seat belt but an air bag is either not present or fails to deploy, the head tends to continue moving forward as the body stops. Basilar skull fractures are a common cause of death among race car drivers when their vehicle collides head-on with the race track concrete barrier at extremely high speeds.[24]

Newton's second law of motion is commonly referred to as the *law of acceleration,* which states that the change of motion is proportional to the force impressed and is made in the direction of the straight line in which that force is impressed.[5]

This law can be expressed algebraically with force (F), mass (m), and acceleration (a):

$$F = m \times a$$

When the equation is rearranged, it yields a useful expression:

$$a = \frac{F}{m}$$

which mathematically illustrates that the acceleration of an object is directly proportional to the force applied and inversely related to mass of the object. Newton's second law is relatively simple, but it has many applications to physical therapy. Because acceleration (motion) is inversely related to mass, it is clear that basic weight-bearing movements tend to be more challenging for larger patients. In addition, a greater force application is needed for these patients to accomplish said movement. The difficulty in locomotion is compounded if larger mass of a patient results from too much fat, because fat does not contribute to force production.

Newton's third law of motion is commonly referred to as the *law of reaction,* which states that to every action there is always opposed an equal reaction; or, the mutual action of two bodies upon each other are always equal and directed to contrary parts.[5]

The concept of reaction can be more difficult to visualize than inertia and acceleration, but when a force is applied to an object such as a wall, there is a force opposite in direction and equal in magnitude to the force applied. As the applied force increases, the reaction force likewise increases. From a clinical perspective, reaction forces are of interest during gait analysis. When a patient walks or runs, clinicians may analyze the differences in gait patterns among individuals with varying levels of disability and the subsequent ground reaction forces that occur when the foot strikes the floor. These forces can achieve three times one's body weight during running, and patterns vary based on running style. Physicians and therapists use devices such as orthotics to alter ground reaction force patterns to help minimize foot injuries.[33]

ADVANCED BIOMECHANICAL CONCEPTS

The following advanced concepts highlight several of the major areas that must be considered when evaluating movement skills. These biomechanical principles have direct implications on rehabilitation based on injury causation and level of severity: reaction forces, levers and resistive torque, kinetic link principle, and balance and stability.

Reaction Forces

Reaction forces are forces applied on a person by a surface with which the person's body is in contact. These forces are applied as an equal and opposite reaction force to the force applied to the surface by the person. The more force generated by the person onto the contact surface, as a result of their body weight and musculoskeletal activity, the more force the surface returns to the performer. When analyzing gait abnormalities, ground reaction forces (GRFs) should be measured in relation to a fixed three-dimensional coordinate system oriented at the surface of the platform.[30] The GRF planes of motion are termed anteroposterior, which describes forces imposed horizontally directed forward or backward; mediolateral, which describes forces generated horizontally side to side; and vertical, which describes forces directed upward or downward. In other words, if the person pushes downward on the surface the surface reacts by pushing upward with equal force. If the person pushes backward on the surface the surface pushes forward with an equal force. If the person pushes rightward on the surface the surface pushes leftward with equal force. Other sources for force application are wheelchair pushrims, which are referred to as *pushrim reaction forces.* These multidirectional forces are applied to the hand when in contact with the wheelchair pushrim in an equal and opposite manner. The forces specific to a pushrim are termed *tangential,* which describes forces applied tangent to the pushrim (causes motion); *radial,* which describes the forces directed toward the axis of rotation (frictional force); and *mediolateral,* which describes forces directed parallel to the axis of rotation. The forces imposed at the pushrim are transferred to the hand and used to determine subsequent upper extremity joint forces and moments during wheelchair ambulation. Chronic and acute shoulder pain of manual wheelchair users is one of the foremost issues facing PTAs.[2,4,8]

Levers and Resistive Torque

The human body consists of a very poor leverage system when one considers its need to generate large, forceful movements against heavy objects. Humans are designed, however, with leverage, which allows us to generate high speeds and produce large ROM. In more meaningful terms, because of the musculoskeletal system's structure with muscle tendon insertion attachment sites occurring very close to the proximal joint of the segment to which they apply force, the human body has very short force lever arms for the muscle to produce torque around the joint. The resistive forces that the muscle must compete against, the weight of a body segment and/or external object, often have much longer lever arm lengths with which to generate resistive torques. The muscles, therefore, must be very strong to overcome their poor mechanical leverage when dealing with objects which have great weight or momentum. This is the case when the external object contacts a body segment distal to the body's major torque producing joints (hip, knee, shoulder, and elbow).

With regard to the ability of the human body to generate speed and ROM, the close attachment of the inserting tendon to the proximal joint of a segment means that a small amount of muscle shortening through a concentric contraction will generate a relatively large rotation of the segment. Were the tendon to attach farther away from the joint, the same amount of muscle shortening would result in a lesser rotation around the joint. When the force production of the muscle is rapid, the large amount of angular displacement generated and the small time in which this displacement occurs means a fast angular velocity for the segment. Therefore the linear velocity generated at the end of the lever (i.e., the feet or hands) may be quite large in magnitude.

A lever system includes a fulcrum, which is the point or axis of rotation; an applied force; and a resistance (resistive force). The perpendicular distance from the line of action of the force to the fulcrum is termed the moment arm of the force (MF). Likewise, the perpendicular distance from the line of action of the resistance is termed the moment arm of the resistance (MR). This is important because a lever may be evaluated based on the computation of its mechanical advantage (MA).

$$MA = \frac{MF}{MR}$$

In a first-class lever, when the fulcrum is located halfway between the point of force and point of resistance on the lever, the MA is equal to 1 (e.g., MF = MR). If the fulcrum is closer to the point of the resistance than the point of force (e.g., MF > MR), the MA becomes greater than 1; thus a smaller force is necessary to overcome a constant resistance. In the opposite scenario where the MF is less than the MR, the MA is less than 1 and a larger force is necessary to move a given resistance. The head tilting backward, initiated by a concentric contraction of the extensor neck muscles (splenius capitis, semispinalis capitis, suboccipitals, trapezius) to overcome the resistive force imposed by the weight of the cranium where the fulcrum is the atlanto-occipital joint, is an example of a first-class lever system (Fig. 16-3, *A*).

In a second-class lever, the point of resistance is located between the fulcrum and the point of force. The MF is always greater than the MR, yielding a MA greater than 1. Hence this arrangement favors the effort of force, because less force is necessary to cause movement of a given resistance. Performing a toe raise exercise demonstrates a second-class lever. The plantar and dorsiflexion movement can be employed by the PTA to regain ankle ROM due to injury or surgery. Resistance

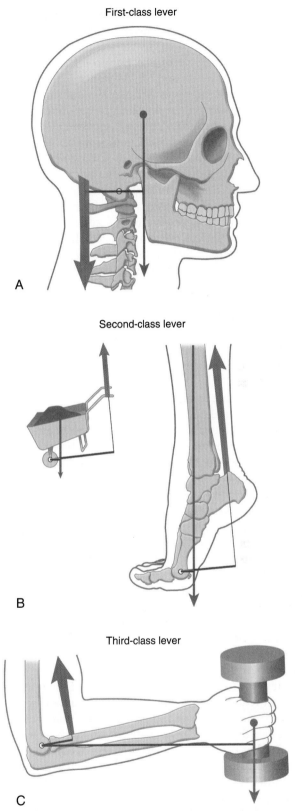

Fig. 16-3 Anatomic examples are shown of first-class **(A)**, second-class **(B)**, and third-class **(C)** levers. The muscle activation (depicted in red) is isometric in each case, with no movement occurring at the joint. (From Neumann DA: *Kinesiology of the musculoskeletal system: foundations for rehabilitation*, ed 2, St Louis, 2010, Mosby.)

can be added to create an exercise designed to strengthen the calf muscles (soleus and gastrocnemius), which represents a second-class lever system (Fig. 16-3, *B*).

In a third-class lever, the point of force is located between the fulcrum and the resistance. The MF always is less than the MR, yielding a MA less than 1. Therefore this arrangement favors the effort of resistance, because more force is necessary to cause movement of a given resistance. This is the more common type of lever found within the human body (Fig. 16-3, *C*). Therefore muscles within the body tend to work under a mechanical disadvantage, resulting in larger internal muscular forces than the mass of the external object (resistance) being moved. It is also important to realize that within some joints of the skeletal system, the actual fulcrum point changes through the ROM. Consequently, mechanical advantage and muscle force vary as the length of the moment arm changes. A person performing elbow flexion during a bicep curl exercise depicts a third-class lever system. The olecranon represents the axis of rotation where the biceps muscle group (biceps brachii, brachioradialis, brachialis) exerts a force to overcome the mass of the forearm or any additional resistance held in the hand.

The resistive force, or more specifically the resistive torque, encountered during movements varies based on the length of the resistance arm (moment arm of the resistance). During the performance of a bicep curl exercise, length of the resistance arm is maximized when the elbow is at a 90-degree angle (Fig. 16-4). As the angle increases or decreases, the length of the resistance arm shortens, thus reducing the magnitude of the resistive torque.[26] Therefore it is important to realize that less force is necessary to lift a given resistance when the resistance is closer to the fulcrum (e.g., the resistance arm is reduced). This basic biomechanical principle has numerous applications, including the mechanical function of exercise equipment. Various manufacturers use a pulley system consisting of cam-based pulleys. The unique advantage of a cam compared with a traditional round pulley is the variation in the length of the resistance and force arms during rotation of the pulley. By simply increasing the length of the resistance arm or reducing the length of the force arm, the resistive torque can be increased to provide a variable resistance through the ROM. This relatively simple alteration in design has enhanced the effectiveness of exercise equipment to provide proper loading on muscles throughout the full ROM.

Kinetic Link Principle

The coordination of body movements in sporting activities, occupational skills, or ADLs is critical for success. Many terms are used to refer to these coordinated movement patterns, such as perfect timing, fluid motion, natural, and graceful. Each of these terms means

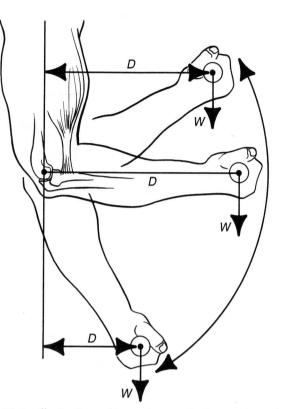

Fig. 16-4 Illustration of how changes in the angle at the elbow alter the length of the resistance arm, thus modifying the resistive torque. *D*, Distance; *W*, weight. (Redrawn from Baechle TR: *Essentials of strength training and conditioning*, ed 3, Champaign, Ill., 2008, Human Kinetics.)

simply that the body's nervous system is finely tuned for stimulating the body's musculature to contract with appropriate intensity or to relax at just the right time to produce the necessary joint rotations required for a successful performance. Without this timing between the nervous and muscular systems, the skeletal system motions that result would be less than effective or efficient.

Body segments are connected in more ways than most individuals realize. When there is a perpetual orthopedic problem in one area of the body, chances are the problem is related to another area of the body in some form or fashion. For example, if patients complain their ankles or knees hurt when they walk, it could be linked to an orthopedic issue with their feet. The foot pain could be directly associated with a problem in the calf region. A taut gastrocnemius–soleus muscle group can often lead to problems in the knees, hips, and lower back area. If this is ignored, the problem can migrate to the upper back, shoulders, and neck. In a sense, everything in the body is connected, in other words, it is a kinetic chain. When a part of this chain is weak or damaged, it will affect other parts of the kinetic chain (Box 16-2).

BOX 16-2

Sequential Kinetic Chain

Common reasons for these issues are:

■ Compensation due to another injury. An example would be putting more weight on one leg to take pressure off of the injured leg.

■ Muscular imbalances around a joint. This occurs frequently in the shoulder. In many people the internal rotators are overdeveloped or overactivated, whereas the external rotators are left weak or under-activated. Many people have muscular imbalances all over the body that can cause many issues.

■ Scar tissue build up or adhesions from previous injury. Most active people have some scar tissue somewhere in the body due to a previous injury. The scar tissue can cause an obvious limit in ROM, thus causing improper joint mechanics.

■ Improper movement patterns. If a person swings a tennis racket incorrectly for long enough, not only will his or her tennis game suffer, but bad motor patterns or mechanics will quickly develop. This in time will lead to imbalances of strength and flexibility, pain, injury, and overcompensation patterns. Bad movement patterns can occur in anything a person does, whether it is as simple as walking or as complex as throwing a baseball.

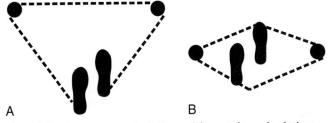

Fig. 16-5 A person ambulating with crutches, depicting stable **(A)** and unstable **(B)** positions.

The kinetic link principle is typically subdivided into two categories. First, the sequential kinetic link principle basically means segmental motions or joint rotations occur in a specific sequence such that time elapses occur between the peak rotational velocities of each involved segment. This coordinated effort typically leads to high velocity or momentum of the last segment involved in the performance. This principle is often observed in sports skills where the sequential kinetic link is employed for success, the energy or momentum flows from the core of the body (typically the trunk) distally to the appendages of the body (the leg segments to the foot or the arm segments to the hand). This flow is from the body's more massive segments to its least massive segments. The building of momentum in the bigger, slower segments (trunk and upper legs) of the body leads to effective transference of momentum to the smaller, faster moving segments. In other words, failure to use the trunk appropriately adversely affects the velocity with which a ball is thrown; a club, bat, or racket is swung; or a ball is kicked. Running and wheelchair propulsion demonstrate sequential movement patterns. It is extremely important for individuals with spinal cord injuries to develop core muscle strength because they do not have lower body muscle force contributing to the kinetic chain. For example, wheelchair racing athletes rely on a strong core region in which to transfer momentum generated by the abdominals to the upper extremities.

Second, the simultaneous kinetic link principle states that primary segmental and/or joint movements occur within the same time period where no visible difference in time exists between the contributions of the involved segments and/or joints during the activity. This type of movement is generally employed when an individual is required to move objects, or even their own body, which offer great resistance, such as wheelchair propulsion.

Squat lifting is an example of movement requiring force generation by several muscle groups simultaneously. These types of movements generally need high force magnitudes to overcome relatively high inertial conditions.[25]

Balance and Stability

Realize that biomechanically, stability and mobility are inversely related. A health professional can apply the principle of balance to provide a patient with an appropriate mix of stability and mobility for a particular activity or skill. Three biomechanical factors directly affect an individual's balance for improving stability: body mass, COG reference height, and base of support area.[1,17] The stability of the human body with respect to the base of support depends on the overall size of the base of support and the height of the body's COG above the base of support. For example, a person recovering from a lower extremity injury may use crutches or a walking cane in order to relieve the load on the injured limb. The use of crutches also increases the area of the base of support and makes it easier for the user to maintain stability (Fig. 16-5).[29,34] Postural sway is normally under the control of automatic neuromuscular mechanisms that dictate the adequate base of support area. However, those mechanisms are diminished in patients with a muscle atrophy disease or neurological disorder. The use of crutches would greatly increase the stability of these individuals.[29,34]

BASIC BIOMECHANICAL ANALYSES OF INJURY MECHANISMS

Mechanical Loading

Load is defined as an outside force or group of forces that act on an object. For example, when a patient performs an exercise with sandbags on the foot, a load is being applied to the muscles that cause knee extension. Although loads apply to the point of contact (e.g., use of compression bandage), other loads are applied away from the point of contact, as described. Depending on the magnitude of the load **(stress)**, there is a deformation in the object, termed a mechanical strain.

There are three types of stresses: compression, tension, and shear (Fig. 16-6). Compression occurs when two forces or loads are applied toward each other. A common example is the compression stress on the vertebral column during standing while supporting an object (e.g., dumbbell). Excessive compression stress can lead to contusions, fractures, or herniations.[23,25] Tension occurs when two forces or loads are applied in opposite directions. This type of loading is commonly applied to muscles and tendons during stretching activities to improve flexibility.

When the loading exceeds the ability of the object to resist the stress, injuries such as strains, sprains, and avulsion fractures commonly occur.[20] Figure 16-7 illustrates the tension stresses acting on the Achilles tendon during movements of the foot. Injuries associated with tension are more common during activities that utilize the stretch-shortening cycle most often observed during actions that require fast, quick, change in direction movements. Shear occurs when there are two parallel forces or loads in opposite directions, causing adjacent points on the surface to slide past each other. Injuries such as vertebral disk problems, femoral condyle fractures, and epiphyseal fractures of the distal femur in children occur as a result of shear stress acting on the body.

The resulting action of compression, tension, and shear forces is dependent on how these forces are distributed, a concept called *mechanical stress*. Force applied over a smaller surface area results in a greater mechanical stress than force applied over a larger surface area. Given that the lumbar vertebrae typically are more load bearing than the vertebrae in the upper back, one notices that the load-bearing surface area in the lumbar vertebrae is greater than that found in the upper vertebrae.[18] Accordingly, the greater surface area for the thoracic vertebrae translates into a lower mechanical stress for a given load.

Another type of loading on an object, called *bending*, occurs when nonaxial forces are applied, resulting in compressive stress on one side and a tension stress on the other. When an object is forced to twist along the longitudinal axis, a load called *torsion* is produced. Injuries commonly occur because of torsion in activities such as skiing, when a foot is planted and the body begins to twist.[11,16] Another example is an anterior cruciate ligament (ACL) injury, which commonly occurs during a running activity when one suddenly stops and then turns, thereby causing a deceleration of the lower limb, a forced hyperextension of the knee, or a forced tibial rotation (Fig. 16-8). Other injury mechanisms include an internal rotary force applied to a femur on a fixed weight-bearing tibia, an external rotation force

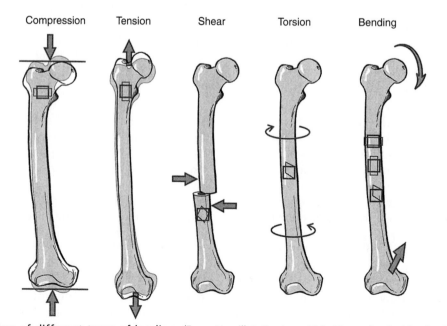

Fig. 16-6 Illustration of different types of loading. (From Hamill J, Knutzen KM: *Biomechanical basis of human movement*, Baltimore, 1995, Williams & Wilkins.)

with a valgus (outward) force, or a straight anterior force applied to the back of the leg, forcing the tibia forward relative to the femur.

Deformation or a change in shape can occur when an object is loaded. The load–deformation curve describes the relationship between the loading and corresponding degree of deformation (Fig. 16-9). Within the elastic region, the object deforms in direct relation to the force, and returns to the beginning shape once the force is removed. However, at the elastic limit point, the response becomes plastic, resulting in some degree of permanent deformation, even when the force is removed. Also within the plastic region, excessive loading can result in a point of failure. For a bone, this is the point where a fracture occurs. Although excessive acute loading as described can result in damage to the object, the effect of chronic or repetitive loading that commonly occurs in occupational settings is equally problematic.[31] Repetitive loading can result in microtrauma to the point of stress. If this persists long enough, a chronic wound, termed a stress-related injury, may occur.[26]

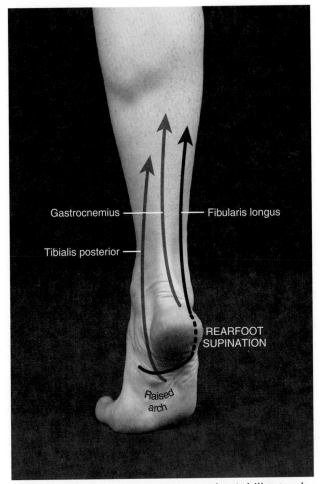

Fig. 16-7 Tension stresses acting on the Achilles tendon during foot movements. (From Neumann DA: *Kinesiology of the musculoskeletal system: foundations for rehabilitation*, ed 2, St Louis, 2010, Mosby.)

Another important consideration in predicting injury potential is the rate of loading. This variable reflects how rapidly an external force's load is transmitted to an internal musculoskeletal tissue. There is a period of time during which muscles are incapable of producing tension to resist forces applied to the body. This period of time, referred to as passive loading, is approximately 50 ms (0.05 second). If a large force is applied to the body such that it reaches a very high magnitude within this 50 ms or passive period, the muscles are not able to resist the force and other musculoskeletal tissues must assume this role. These other tissues, such as bone, ligaments, cartilage, and tendons, are less capable of enduring these forces. Should the forces be very high in magnitude and occur very rapidly an acute injury may occur. On the other hand, if the force peaks quickly, though not necessarily extremely high in magnitude, overuse injuries to the bone or connective tissues may occur if these forces are applied repetitively, such as in wheelchair propulsion activities. Therefore a goal in reducing injury would be to reduce either or both the magnitude of the forces applied to the body and the rate at which they are applied.

Common Musculoskeletal Injuries

Soft Tissue Strains and Sprains

Strain and sprain injuries are usually caused by trauma (slip, fall, collision). Strain refers to an injury to a muscle, occurring when a muscle–tendon unit is stretched or overloaded. Sports that incorporate a running component have a relatively high incidence of soft tissue strains, which are quite common injuries treated by PTAs. The injury mechanism begins just before ground impact of the foot; the hamstring muscles contract forcefully to halt the knee extension, which occurs at the end of the recovery phase.[20] The action of the hamstrings causes knee flexion to occur and this continues through the early portions of the ground phase. In combination with the hip extension, this knee flexion serves to reduce the braking force (decelerating force), which occurs when the foot strikes the ground. The braking force is a result of a forward moving foot at initial ground impact, analogous to kicking the ground. Hamstring (semitendinosus, semimembranosus, biceps femoris) muscle group injuries are quite common in running activities.[20] Hamstring injuries, such as strains or ruptures to soft tissues, result when the muscle concentrically contracts while the muscle continues to undergo stretching during heel contact. A non-sport related soft tissue strain often occurs during slips on surfaces with low coefficient fiction.

Sprain is an injury to a ligament when it is overstretched. The most commonly injured ligaments are located at the ankle, knee, wrist, and low back region. The purpose of ligaments is to hold the adjacent bones together in a normal alignment and prevent abnormal

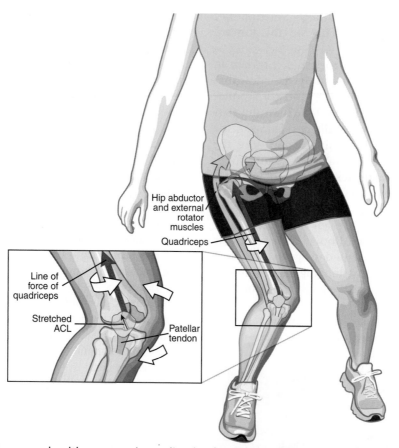

Fig. 16-8 An image of a young healthy woman immediately after landing from a jump. The inset on the left shows the increased tension in the anterior cruciate ligament (ACL) and the line of force of the quadriceps muscle. Note the relative lateral displacement of the patella relative to the intercondylar groove of the femur. (From Neumann DA: *Kinesiology of the musculoskeletal system: foundations for rehabilitation*, ed 2, St Louis, 2010, Mosby.)

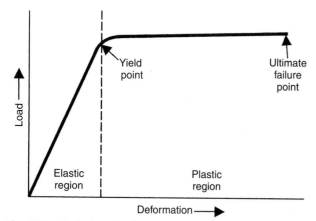

Fig. 16-9 Relationship between load and deformation of an object. (From Hall SJ: *Basic biomechanics*, ed 3, New York, 1999, McGraw-Hill.)

movements by the bones. However, when too much force is applied to a ligament, such as in a fall, the ligaments can be stretched or torn, leading to an injury. Back pain or injury is a leading cause of disability among warehouse and construction workers. The diagnosis of back sprain (whether lumbar or cervical) implies that the ligamentous and capsular structures connecting the facet joints and vertebrae have been damaged.[18,31]

Rotator Cuff Injury/Shoulder Separation

The primary biomechanical goal of the baseball overhand fastball pitch is to throw a ball at near maximum horizontal velocity with accuracy. Though there are numerous styles of pitching windups, the delivery phase of the overhand pitch (when the ball is accelerated to the release point) tends to have great similarity.[14] This complex series of body movements is characterized by the sequential nature in which the body segments contribute to the velocity of the ball. Basically, the lower body begins its contribution with the ground contact of the lead foot at the completion of the stride toward home plate. The forces created by the ground contact, when combined with the forward moving body, cause a rapid rotation of the lower trunk and pelvic area. This rotation is closely followed by the sequential movements of the upper trunk, the upper arm, forearm, and hand. When the hand reaches its maximum velocity the ball is released. The velocity of each successive segment exceeds that of its preceding segment. In other words, these successive segment rotations accept the momentum passed on by the preceding segments and add their momentum before passing it on to the next segment. As momentum builds with each successive segmental contribution, the kinetic energy of the ball increases and reaches a peak at the release point.[13]

One must consider the biomechanical issues associated with shoulder injuries in overhand baseball pitching. As a result of the very high shoulder rotational velocities attained during the acceleration of the ball toward the catcher, the pitcher must create tremendously large deceleration forces to stop this fast shoulder internal rotation. Relatively speaking, the pitcher spends much time building up shoulder internal rotation to throw the ball with high velocity to the batter, but must stop this motion in a very short time period in order to be ready to field his position. This very short time period for deceleration means the torques around the shoulder joint will be quite high.[13,14]

The rotator cuff muscles (supraspinatus, infraspinatus, teres major, and subscapularis) are a group of relatively small muscles that are challenged to maintain shoulder integrity and, particularly, to stop shoulder internal rotation and anterolateral distraction. Because the momentum for the shoulder with regard to both the internal rotation and the anterolateral distraction are high, this muscle group is challenged to the extreme with every ball thrown. With the onset of fatigue and the wear and tear of the forces associated with throwing a large number of pitches, injury to this muscle group occurs fairly frequently.[14] If the injury is severe, it may very well end a pitcher's career prematurely, much like an athlete suffering an ACL injury of the knee. Another common shoulder injury involves a disruption of the acromioclavicular (AC) joint. This joint is composed of the collar bone, or clavicle, and the highest portion of the shoulder blade, the acromion of the scapula. These two bones meet on top of the shoulder and form the AC joint, as mentioned earlier.[13,17] The most common cause of shoulder separation, or AC joint disruption, is a direct fall onto the shoulder. This fall injures the ligaments that provide stability to the joint. The laxity that results allows a degree of separation between the acromion and the clavicle. The degree of separation can range from mild to severe with a noticeable deformity depending on the momentum–impulse relationship. Treatment of this condition can vary from conservative management with a period of immobility followed by gentle shoulder strengthening, to surgery.

Low Back Injury

The two most serious leg or squat lifting errors are descending too rapidly and allowing the trunk to flex too far forward during the descent phase. Rapid descent should be avoided because it allows an excessive amount of momentum or kinetic energy to be generated, which

the muscles may not be able to overcome when challenged to halt and then reverse this motion. The faster an individual descends, the more muscle force required to reverse this direction. If the person is lifting at a resistance close to his or her maximum or is fatigued, it is likely at best that the ascent phase will not be successfully completed, or at worst an injury will occur.[15]

When the individual allows the trunk to flex too far forward, the forces occurring in the low back are greatly increased over those associated with a more upright posture. The reason for this is rather simple. The trunk can be considered a lever with a fulcrum or rotational axis formed in the lumbar area of the vertebral column. When this lever is rotated forward into flexion from a more vertical trunk posture, the line of action of the resistive force of the patient, not to mention the trunk weight itself, is moved from an orientation directly through the vertebral bodies to one very far forward of them.[15]

The shifting of the line of action of the resistive forces to this extreme position causes the torque (force of the weight of the barbell and trunk and head segment multiplied times the distance from this line to the lumbar vertebrae) to increase to very high levels. With the increased torque, the type and magnitudes of forces applied to the cartilaginous vertebral discs, which separate the bony vertebral bodies, are radically different from those applied while standing erect. Generally, the anterior portion of two adjacent vertebral bodies (i.e., L4-L5) are forced together, a compressive force, while the posterior aspect of these same bones are forced apart by a tensile force (Fig. 16-10).

The cartilaginous or intervertebral disc, which acts as a buffer between these bones, is greatly affected by this condition. The compressive force applied anteriorly forces its fluid core posteriorly toward the aspect of the disc that is allowed to bulge by virtue of the gap formed by the tensile force applied to the posterior aspect of the lower vertebral column. If the walls of this disc have been weakened as a result of cumulative trauma from poor biomechanics in lifting and other lumbar intensive activities, a bulge or rupture of the disc may occur. This may lead to moderate to severe low back pain and leg pain, because nerves are often impinged upon by the bulging disc. Often surgery is required to relieve the pain associated with a bulging disc.

ADVANCES IN BIOMECHANICS

Tremendous advances have been made in the area of rehabilitation and clinical biomechanics over the past 30 years. The surgical procedures for knee, hip, and ankle arthroplasty have improved with advancements in surgical instrumentation. The rehabilitation process has transformed as well, which has led to a shorter recovery period following joint replacement. The materials used

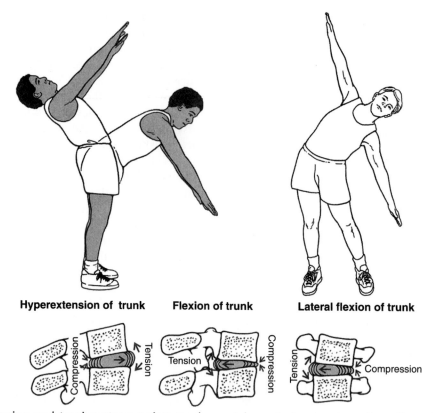

Hyperextension of trunk   **Flexion of trunk**   **Lateral flexion of trunk**

Fig. 16-10 Compression and tension stress acting on the vertebrae during trunk motion. (From Hamill J, Knutzen KM: *Biomechanical basis of human movement*, Baltimore, 1995, Williams & Wilkins.)

to construct the artificial joint have changed; titanium, the preferred metal, is more durable and lighter than stainless steel. Artificial joints can last for 25 to 30 years now, as opposed to 10 years when the procedure was first introduced.

Prosthesis design has made incredible advances in functionality. Today, an amputee who is physically active and participates in recreational sports may possess a variety of prostheses designed for a specific activity or sport. Today, prostheses are being fitted with microprocessors that produce a limb classified as artificial intelligence. The prosthesis has the ability to alter position based on feedback from the terrain. Springs and cables are being replaced with pneumatics and hydraulics. The combination of microprocessors and hydraulics produces a more efficient gait and improved balance characteristics compared with traditional prosthetic joints (Fig. 16-11).

Another area that has changed considerably is wheelchair design and wheelchair propulsion mechanics. Patented measuring devices are beginning to emerge in the field as a tool for physical therapy clinics to use for measuring upper extremity joint forces and muscle moments—tools that have been elusive in the past. With today's biomechanical instrumentation, a manual wheelchair user can visit a rehabilitation professional who has the ability to analyze the individual's propulsion technique

and make adjustments to the user's mechanics to reduce the force that contributes to acute and chronic shoulder pain or injury. Minor changes to wheelchair setup can impact the ease with which the user can propel the chair, ultimately resulting in improvements to well-being and possibly injury avoidance. During the wheelchair setup process, new instrumentation technology enables the clinician to measure and detect impact. Finally, the force sensor is used to teach a patient how to propel a wheelchair in the most efficient manner. Propulsion training is used to optimize pushing style by reducing the force and frequency of pushes.[8,22]

Summary

In this chapter, the internal and external forces affecting human movement characteristics were considered along with terminology used to describe injury causation and rehabilitation to the musculoskeletal system. The relationship between mechanical physics and injury was made clear. An understanding was provided of various injury mechanisms that occur to the musculoskeletal system and how these depend on the load characteristics. The chapter concluded with an explanation of specific injuries commonly associated with both chronic and acute loading rates.

Biomechanics is a science that considers the interaction of the body's anatomical structures and neuromuscular

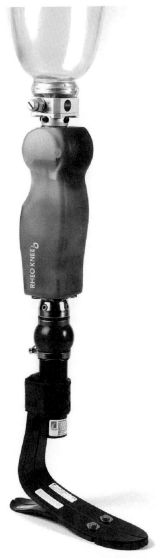

Fig. 16-11 Microprocessor-controlled knee unit. (Photo of RHEO KNEE courtesy Össur, Aliso Viejo, Calif.)

systems with the mechanics of motion as established by the principles of physics. By considering these two important areas, one can effectively evaluate human motion and establish principles upon which injuries can be repaired and rehabilitated. A knowledge base in biomechanics will definitely help the PTA student to understand the complexities involved in basic and advanced physical activities associated with sports, exercise, occupations, physical rehabilitation, and ADLs.

❖ GLOSSARY

Force: A push or pull acting on an object.

Force couple: A moment created by equal, noncollinear, parallel but opposite directed forces. The moment created is called a *couple*.

Friction: The result when two objects are in direct contact with one another and a force acts to impede motion of the objects.

Inertia: The resistance an object offers to a change in its velocity or direction of motion and is directly related to its mass.

Stress: A force required to maintain the deformation of viscoelastic material. Diminishes with time until equilibrium is reached.

Velocity: A change of position with respect to time. Velocity is also a vector, possessing both speed and direction.

REFERENCES

1. Bloem BR, Steijns JA, Smits-Engelsman BC: An update on falls, *Curr Opin Neurol* 16:15–26, 2003.
2. Boninger ML, Impink BG, Cooper RA, et al: Relation between median and ulnar nerve function and wrist kinematics during wheelchair propulsion, *Arch Phys Med Rehab* 85:1141–1145, 2004.
3. Boulton AJ, Kirsner RS, Vileikyte L: Neuropathic diabetic foot ulcers, *N Engl J Med* 351:48–55, 2004.
4. Burnham RS, May L, Nelson E, et al: Shoulder pain in wheelchair athletes: the role of muscle imbalance, *Am J Sport Med* 21:238–242, 1993.
5. Cajori F: *Sir Isaac Newton's mathematical principles* (translated by Andrew Motte, 1729), Berkeley, Calif., 1934, University of California Press.
6. Cavanagh PR, Ulbrecht JS, Caputo GM: New developments in the biomechanics of the diabetic foot, *Diabetes Metab Res Rev* 16(Suppl 1):S6–S10, 2000.
7. Chen CP, Chen MJ, Pei YC, et al: Sagittal plane loading response during gait in different age groups and in people with knee osteoarthritis, *Am J Phys Med Rehabil* 82:307–312, 2003.
8. Collinger JL, Boninger ML, Koontz AM, et al: Shoulder biomechanics during the push phase of wheelchair propulsion: a multisite study of persons with paraplegia, *Arch Phys Med Rehabil* 89:667–676, 2008.
9. Cooper RA, Quatrano LA, Stanhope SJ, et al: Gait analysis in rehabilitation medicine: a brief report, *Am J Phys Med Rehabil* 78:278–280, 1999.
10. Ctercteko GC, Dhanendran M, Hutton WC: Vertical forces acting on the feet of diabetic patients with neuropathic ulceration, *Br J Surg* 68:608–614, 1981.
11. DeVita P, Hortobagyi T, Barrier J: Gait biomechanics are not normal after anterior cruciate ligament reconstruction and accelerated rehabilitation, *Med Sci Sports Exerc* 30:1481–1488, 1998.
12. di Prampero PE, Narici MV: Muscles in microgravity: from fibres to human motion, *J Biomech* 36:403–412, 2003.
13. Dillman CJ, Fleisig GS, Andrews JR: Biomechanics of pitching with emphasis upon shoulder kinematics, *J Orthop Sports Phys Ther* 18:402–408, 1993.
14. Fleisig GS, Barrentine SW, Escamilla RF, et al: Biomechanics of overhand throwing with implications for injuries, *Sport Med* 21:421–437, 1996.
15. Garg A: Occupational biomechanics and low-back pain, *Occup Med* 7:609–628, 1992.
16. Georgoulis AD, Papadonikolakis A, Papageorgiou CD, et al: Three-dimensional tibiofemoral kinematics of the anterior cruciate ligament-deficient and reconstructed knee during walking, *Am J Sports Med* 31:75–79, 2003.
17. Hart-Hughes S, Quigley P, Bulat T, et al: An interdisciplinary approach to reducing fall risks and falls, *J Rehab* 70:46–51, 2004.
18. Hidalgo JA, Genaidy AM, Huston R, et al: Occupational biomechanics of the neck: a review and recommendations, *J Hum Ergol (Tokyo)* 21:165–181, 1992.
19. Kejonen P, Kauranen K, Ahsan R, et al: Motion analysis measurements of body movements during standing: association with age and sex, *Int J Rehabil Res* 25:297–304, 2002.

20. Kirkendall DT, Garrett WE Jr: Clinical perspectives regarding eccentric muscle injury, *Clin Orthop* 403(Suppl):S81–S89, 2002.

21. Koontz AM, Cooper RA, Boninger ML, et al: Shoulder kinematics and kinetics during two speeds of wheelchair propulsion, *J Rehabil Res Dev* 39:635–650, 2002.

22. Kraushaar BS, Nirschl RP: Tendinosis of the elbow (tennis elbow), *J Bone Joint Surg* 81:259–278, 1999.

23. Landers JE, Bates BT, DeVita P: Biomechanics of the squat exercise using a modified center of mass bar, *Med Sci Sports Exerc* 18:469–478, 1986.

24. McElhaney JH, Hopper RH, Nightingale RW, et al: Mechanisms of basilar skull fracture, *J Neurotrauma* 12:669–678, 1995.

25. McLaughlin T, Lardner T, Dillman C: Kinetics of the parallel squat, *Res Q* 49:175–189, 1978.

26. Nigg BM: *Biomechanics IX-B*, Champaign, Ill., 1985, Human Kinetics.

27. Nolan L, Kerrigan DC: Keep on your toes: gait initiation from toe-standing, *J Biomech* 36:393–401, 2003.

28. Perry J: The use of gait analysis for surgical recommendations in traumatic brain injury, *J Head Trauma Rehabil* 14:116–135, 1999.

29. Piirtola M, Era P: Force platform measurements as predictors of falls among older people – a review, *Gerontology* 52:1–16, 2006.

30. Riley PO, Kerrigan DC: Torque action of two-joint muscles in the swing period of stiff-legged gait: a forward dynamic model analysis, *J Biomech* 31:835–840, 1998.

31. Stock SR: Workplace ergonomic factors and the development of musculoskeletal disorders of the neck and upper limbs: a meta-analysis, *Am J Ind Med* 19:87–107, 1991.

32. Stokes IA, Faris IB, Hutton WC: The neuropathic ulcer and loads on the foot in diabetic patients, *Acta Orthop Scand* 46:839–847, 1975.

33. Tang SF, Chen CP, Hong WH, et al: Improvement of gait by using orthotic insoles in patients with heel injury who received reconstructive flap operations, *Am J Phys Med Rehabil* 82:350–356, 2003.

34. Thapa PB, Gideon P, Brockman KG, et al: Clinical and biomechanical measures of balance fall predictors in ambulatory nursing home residents, *J Gerontol* 51:239–246, 1996.

35. Veves A, Murray HJ, Young MJ, et al: Do high foot pressures lead to ulceration: a prospective study, *Diabetologia* 35:660–663, 1992.

36. Whiting WC, Zernicke RF: *Biomechanics of musculoskeletal injury*, ed 2, Champaign, Ill., 2008, Human Kinetics.

37. Yoganandan N, Pintar FA, Klienberger M: Cervical spine vertebral and facet joint kinematics under whiplash, *J Biomech Eng* 120:305–308, 1998.

38. Young MJ, Cavanagh PR, Thomas B, et al: The effect of callus removal on dynamic plantar foot pressures in diabetic patients, *Diabet Med* 9:55–57, 1991.

REVIEW QUESTIONS

Short Answer

1. What is the point called where the midtransverse, midfrontal, and midsagittal planes intersect?
2. What is the product of the force magnitude and the force application time interval called?
3. Which lever generally has the greatest mechanical advantage?
4. Which of Newton's laws of motion describes the relationship among force, mass, and acceleration?
5. What types of injuries commonly occur when tension loading exceeds the ability of the object to resist the stress?

True/False

6. Kinematics deals with the description of movements based on alterations in space and time.
7. The majority of human movements are restricted to a single plane of motion (e.g., abduction occurs only in the frontal plane).
8. There is a mechanical relationship between linear and angular motion.
9. A force couple is formed when there are two torques that are equal in magnitude and opposite in direction.
10. When the fulcrum is located somewhere between the point of force and point of resistance, the lever is termed *third class*.
11. Newton's third law is the law of inertia.
12. Pressure is a measure of the distribution of a force over a given area.
13. The speed of mechanical loading can influence the nature of different types of injuries (e.g., bone versus ligament).
14. Increased mass can contribute to the stability of an object.
15. As kinetic energy increases, there will be a proportional increase in potential energy.

PART V

MANAGEMENT OF ORTHOPEDIC CONDITIONS BY REGION

This section introduces the physical therapist assistant (PTA) to a variety of musculo-skeletal injuries. Each region's area of the body is discussed with specific soft-tissue injuries, fractures, and diseases defined. A problem-solving approach is described, and when available an evidence-based rehabilitation program is provided.

A more progressive way to manage rehabilitation is the criterion-based program, or critical mapping. This method, which is also known as critical treatment pathways, is "a description of the elements of care to be rendered… for a particular diagnosis. The pathway often takes the form of a chart or care path/care map that can be followed" by the clinician and patient.* Instead of using a timetable for progression, a set of criteria is developed that the patient must meet before progressing to the next phase of rehabilitation. These are based on tissue healing constraints and the patient's individual tolerance to the program. Therefore a criterion-based progression fosters close scrutiny of all objective and subjective data concerning the individual's performance.

The components necessary for effective management of orthopedic injuries by the PTA are knowledge of musculoskeletal tissue healing principles, familiarity with various rehabilitation programs, skillful application of rehabilitation techniques, and a fundamental understanding of common and uncommon soft-tissue injuries, fractures, and diseases of muscles, bones, and joints. Knowledge of specific indications and contraindications for certain therapeutic interventions also is helpful.

Orthopedic anatomy is not reviewed substantially in this section. Instead, chapters focus on mechanisms of injury, fracture classifications, clinical features of the injury, specific surgical procedures, and rehabilitation programs. Therefore the student clinician is strongly encouraged to review comprehensive musculoskeletal anatomy texts along with the study of each body part and disorder.

---

*American Physical Therapy Association guidelines for physical therapists facing changing organizational structures, American Physical Therapy Association Board of Directors, APP 3, 1995.

17 Orthopedic Management of the Ankle, Foot, and Toes

Walter L. Jenkins
D.S. Blaise Williams

LEARNING OBJECTIVES

1. Identify common foot and ankle ligament injuries.
2. Describe intervention methods for common foot and ankle ligament injuries.
3. Identify and describe common lower leg, ankle, and foot tendon injuries.
4. Outline and describe common methods of intervention for lower leg, ankle, and foot injuries.
5. Identify common foot and ankle fractures.
6. Discuss common methods of intervention for foot and ankle fractures.
7. Identify and describe common methods of intervention for toe injuries.
8. Describe common mobilization techniques for the ankle, foot, and toe.

KEY TERMS

Calcaneus fracture	Syndesmosis	Talus
Posterior tibialis tendon	Talar tilt test	Tibial nerve

CHAPTER OUTLINE

This chapter introduces the physical therapist assistant (PTA) to injuries affecting the lower leg, ankle, foot, and toes. Included in this chapter are repetitive motion injuries (overuse injuries) and traumatic injuries for the lower leg, ankle, and foot. Specific therapeutic interventions are described and detailed for each pathology. When possible, supporting evidence for specific interventions is outlined.

LIGAMENT INJURIES OF THE ANKLE

Injuries to the lateral ligament complex (the anterior talofibular ligament, fibulocalcaneal ligament, and posterior talofibular ligament) account for approximately 14% to 25% of all sports-related injuries.[34,62] Therefore inversion ankle sprains are among the most common sports and orthopedic injuries.[31,32,91] Studies report that approximately 95% of all ankle sprains occur to the lateral ligament complex.[92] Additionally, injuries to associated structures including articular cartilage and the synovial membrane have been identified on arthroscopy in individuals who had recurrent or recalcitrant lateral ankle sprains.[59] Untreated ankle sprains may lead to chronic pain, muscular weakness, and instability.[32] Ankle joint osteoarthritis has been observed in patients with chronic ankle instability.[108]

Lateral Ligament Injuries (Inversion Ankle Sprains)

Mechanisms of Injury

Ligament sprains of the lateral aspect of the ankle usually are caused by plantar flexion, inversion, and adduction of the foot and ankle (Fig. 17-1).[97] Large forces are not needed to produce an ankle sprain. Stepping off a curb, stepping into a small hole, or stepping on a rock can produce sudden plantar flexion and inversion motions. During athletic competition, stepping on an opponent's foot is a common occurrence that leads to lateral ligament sprains of the ankle. Most commonly ankle sprains occur with the foot is in an unloaded or non–weight-bearing (NWB) position before the injury.[104]

Classification of Sprains

Classifying inversion ankle sprains can be difficult and confusing.[97] The standard classification of ligament injuries (e.g., first-, second-, and third-degree sprains) requires elaboration when applied to inversion ankle sprains, specifically addressing grades, degrees, and descriptive severity of the injury (mild, moderate, or severe). A classification model described by Leach[64] is contrasted with the common standard classification of ankle sprains as a means of comparison and to illustrate the potential for confusion about classification of inversion ankle sprains.

■ First-degree sprain: Single ligament rupture.[64] The anterior talofibular ligament is completely torn. In the standard classification of ligament sprains a complete tear or rupture of a ligament is called a *grade III*, or *third-degree sprain* (Fig. 17-2, *A*).

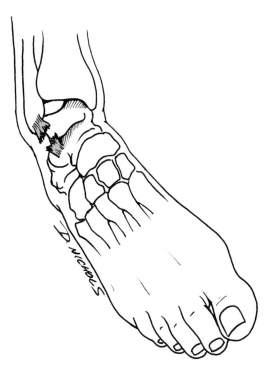

Fig. 17-1 Mechanism of injury to the lateral ligament complex of the ankle. Note the motion of plantar flexion, inversion, and adduction of the foot and ankle.

■ Second-degree sprain: Double ligament rupture.[64] Both the anterior talofibular ligaments and fibulocalcaneal ligaments are completely torn. The standard classification describes a partially torn single ligament as a grade II sprain (Fig. 17-2, *B*).

■ Third-degree sprain: All three lateral ankle ligaments (anterior talofibular, posterior talofibular, and fibulocalcaneal) are completely torn.[64] In the standard classification, a single ligament that is completely torn is defined as a grade III ligament sprain (Fig. 17-2, *C*).

Consequently, it is essential that the system of classification used to describe the severity or complexity of injury be accepted and understood and not confused with another system or model of classification.

Clinical Examination

The PTA must be aware of the organization and administration of examination procedures used to inspect inversion ankle sprains. Throughout rehabilitation, the assistant must communicate changes in the patient's status relative to initial evaluation data and make safe and appropriate modifications to the existing program based on consultation with the supervising therapist.

Testing

Ankle stability tests are used by the physician and the physical therapist (PT) to identify and quantify the integrity of the lateral ligament complex. Injury to the anterior

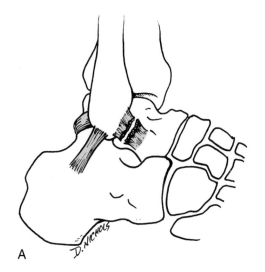

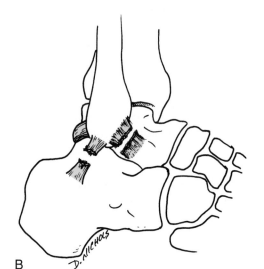

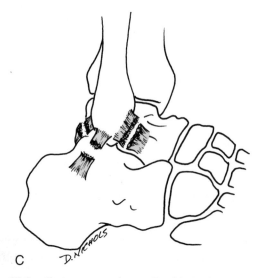

Fig. 17-2 First-, second-, and third-degree sprains. **A,** Tear of the anterior talofibular ligament. **B,** Tears of the anterior talofibular ligament and fibulocalcaneal ligament. **C,** Tears of the anterior talofibular ligament, fibulocalcaneal ligament, and posterior talofibular ligament.

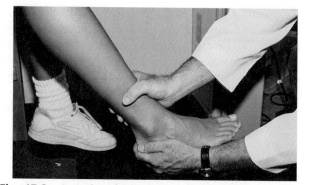

Fig. 17-3 Anterior drawer test of the ankle. With the affected foot slightly plantar flexed, the distal tibia is stabilized with one hand while the other hand grasps the calcaneus and directs an anterior force to manually displace the calcaneus to test the integrity of the anterior talofibular ligament.

talofibular ligament can be assessed clinically by performing the anterior drawer test (Fig. 17-3).[97] The patient must be in a relaxed seated or semirecumbent position with the involved leg flexed 90° at the knee and the involved ankle slightly plantar flexed. Stabilize the distal tibia and support it with one hand, while using the other hand to gently but firmly grasp the calcaneus and attempt to translate or pull the ankle forward. No excessive motion is seen or felt if the ligament is intact. However, the ankle demonstrates excessive forward or anterior motion if the anterior talofibular ligament is torn.

The **talar tilt test** or inversion stress test examines the ankle ligament's resistance to maximal inversion stress (Fig. 17-4).[97] The patient is in the same position used for the anterior drawer test, and the ankle is gradually stressed by exertion of constant pressure over the lateral aspect of the foot and ankle while counter pressure is applied over the inner aspect of the lower leg until maximal inversion is reached.[10] The severity of ligament injury should be graded according to the classification system used by the physician or the supervising PT.

Order of procedures
Table 17-1 outlines the procedure for evaluation of inversion ankle sprains. The mechanism of injury that produces an inversion ankle sprain also may cause other conditions that must be differentiated by the physician[91,97] and PT, such as fracture of the base of the fifth metatarsal, malleolar fractures, osteochondral fractures, osteochondritis dissecans, midfoot ligament sprains, and subluxing peroneal tendons.

Intervention
The specific rehabilitation program used to treat inversion sprains depends on the severity of sprain (first-, second-, or third-degree). Generally first- and second-degree sprains can be effectively managed non-operatively with a supervised rehabilitation program.[98]

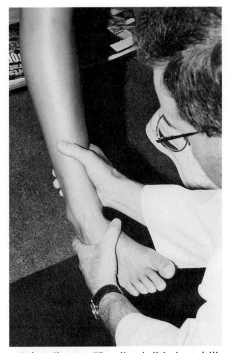

Fig. 17-4 Talar tilt test. The distal tibia is stabilized while the other hand tilts the talus to test the integrity of the lateral ligament complex.

Table 17-1	*Physical Therapist Initial Evaluation Outline for the Clinical Assessment of Inversion Ankle Sprains*
Order of Assessment	**Procedures**
History	1. How did the injury happen?
	2. Where is the pain located?
	3. Did you hear or feel a pop or snap?
	4. Have you had a similar injury previously? If yes, explain.
Observation	1. Note any obvious deformity suggesting a fracture or dislocation.
	2. Note the area and degree of swelling.
	3. Evaluate complaints of pain.
	4. Note any discoloration.
	5. Perform a bilateral visual comparison of symmetry.
Palpation	Always begin palpation by explaining the procedure, then initially performing the procedure on the uninvolved side.
	1. Distal tibia-fibula
	2. Lateral ligament complex
	3. Medial ligaments–deltoid ligament
	4. Base of the fifth metatarsal
	5. Peroneal tendons
	6. Achilles tendon
Range of motion	1. Active and passive
	2. Dorsiflexion
	3. Plantar flexion
	4. Inversion
	5. Eversion
Strength	1. Manual muscle testing
	a. Dorsiflexion
	b. Plantar flexion
	c. Inversion
	d. Eversion
Clinical stability tests	1. Anterior drawer test
	2. Talar tilt test

Initial management of acute inversion ankle sprains calls for rest, ice, compression, and elevation (RICE). Rest is a relative term used to define avoidance of unwanted stress; it does not necessarily require complete avoidance of all stress. The application of ice, compression, and elevation is directed at minimizing and reducing intense inflammatory response, hemorrhage, swelling, pain, and cellular metabolism to provide the most conducive environment for tissue healing.[91]

Clinically, the most effective means to reduce swelling are elevation and compression. Elastic compression bandages (Ace wraps) are applied while elevating the injured limb above the heart. A three-phase (phase I, maximum protection; phase II, moderate protection; phase III, minimum protection), criteria-based rehabilitation program is effective for the management of inversion ankle sprains. The maximum-protection phase calls for the RICE program to be used three to five times daily. Application of ice should be encouraged for 15 to 20 minutes, with a 1- to 2-hour rest period between applications. Protecting the torn ligaments from unwanted stress is the cornerstone of this phase. Joint protection and immobilization can be achieved through an array of commercial appliances, tape, casting, and braces; selection is left to the physician or PT. Some physicians choose to use a short-leg walking cast or posterior plaster splint. More commonly, a plastic shell brace with an inflatable air bladder or a leather semirigid ankle support is used. Tape can be used for both compression and ligament support, but it must be applied skillfully and reapplied daily to be effective. The ankle must be positioned correctly during the application and use of all support devices. It should be in a neutral position or slightly dorsiflexed and somewhat everted to closely approximate the torn ligaments. Weight-bearing status and ambulation with assistive devices are individualized to the patient's pain tolerance. Secondary to improved stability of the ankle during weight bearing, patients are commonly instructed to "weight bear as tolerated" during this phase.

An active range of motion (AROM) program must be used cautiously during the maximum-protection phase.

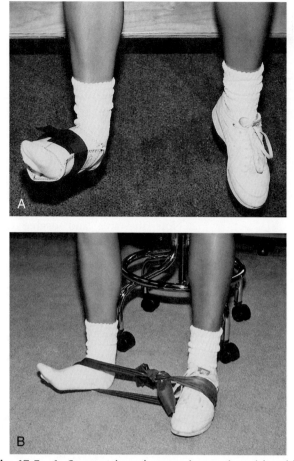

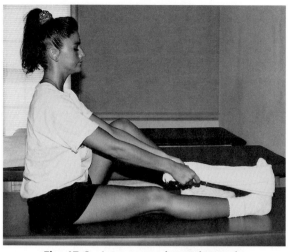

Fig. 17-6 Long-seated towel stretch.

Fig. 17-5 **A,** Concentric and eccentric exercise with ankle weights. As the weight is slowly elevated to a position of dorsiflexion and eversion, the patient is encouraged to emphasize the eccentric or lowering phase of the exercise. **B,** Thera-Band elastic band resistance for eversion and dorsiflexion.

It is imperative to avoid plantar flexion and inversion when instructing patients to perform range of motion (ROM) exercises. Excessive plantar flexion and inversion increase the load on the anterior talofibular and calcaneofibular ligaments leading to a disruption of the healing process in these ligaments.

Motion exercises are important to help reduce pain and swelling, as well as help increase function of the joint. However, if certain motions (e.g., plantar flexion or inversion) are employed too early in the rehabilitation period, these unwanted stresses can disrupt the normal healing process. Electrical galvanic stimulation also can help reduce pain and swelling.

Isometric strengthening exercises are initiated as soon as the patient's pain tolerance allows. Isometric dorsiflexion and eversion exercises are performed for two or three sets of 10 repetitions, holding each contraction for 10 seconds. Proximal leg-strengthening exercises (leg extension, hamstring curls, hip abduction and adduction, and hip extension exercises) and general full-body conditioning should be encouraged throughout the course of rehabilitation. Clinically it is vital to view inversion ankle sprains as injuries that affect the whole person, rather than just the injured extremity. Maintaining aerobic fitness and strength during recovery is particularly important in a population involved in sports.

The moderate-protection phase can begin once the patient can bear weight on the injured limb without crutches, perform all ROM and isometric exercises without undue complaints of pain, and control the swelling. This phase encourages the use of the RICE principle, full weight bearing (FWB), and continued ligament support with the use of braces or tape. More progressive exercises are initiated, including concentric and eccentric contractions (Fig. 17-5) (with ankle weights or latex bands), heel cord stretching (Fig. 17-6) (towel stretch, wall stretch, or prostretch), and standing toe and heel raises.

Gradually and cautiously, inversion and plantar flexion motions are added as pain allows. Stationary bicycling can be initiated with the seat height lowered slightly to encourage a more neutral ankle position instead of a plantar flexion position.

Proprioception exercises are commonly initiated during the moderate-protection phase. Protection of the ligament must be encouraged during these challenging exercises. Balancing on the injured limb on a flat surface is slowly progressed to a balance board, and then to a minitrampoline—all excellent exercises that stimulate balance, coordination, and muscular endurance (Fig. 17-7).

The minimum-protection phase can begin once the patient can perform all resistive exercises, (ankle weight, Thera-Band, and manual resistance) ambulate without pain or limping, and swelling is reduced. Although proprioception training is commonly used in practice there are few articles outlining its effectiveness in rehabilitation.[115]

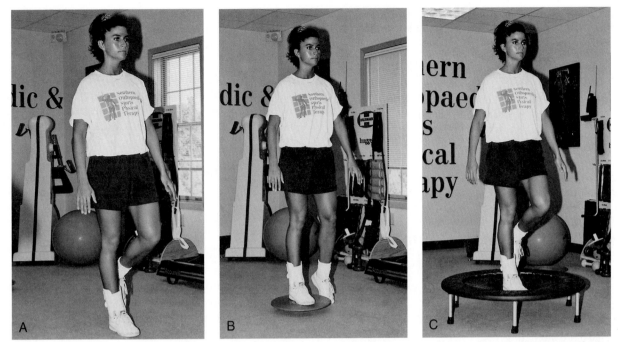

Fig. 17-7 A, Single-leg standing proprioception and balancing. Note the continued use of external support during the late stage of recovery. **B,** Single-leg standing proprioception and balancing with use of a wobble board or biomechanical ankle platform system (BAPS) board. **C,** Single-leg standing proprioception and balancing on a minitrampoline. The highly unstable surface provides a challenging balance activity.

From 4 to 8 weeks after injury, new collagen formation allows almost-normal stresses to be applied.[91] At this point, more functional activities are allowed, including straight-line jogging, large figure-of-eight running, jumping drills, and cutting activities.

The minimum-protection phase does not imply removal of all supportive devices. Maturation of the injured ligaments can take as long as 6 to 12 months.[91] Therefore it is critical to encourage patient compliance with the use of either tape or a semirigid brace during all running activities.

Box 17-1 outlines a general three-phase rehabilitation program for an inversion ankle sprain. In all instances, if pain, swelling, or irritation persists, the patient is not taken to the next phase until he or she is pain free in the present phase. The ankle must be securely taped or braced when running, jumping, or otherwise performing aggressive, ballistic motions.

The treatment of grade III ankle sprains (using the standard classification) is somewhat controversial.[91,98] At this time there are few, if any outcome studies that outline differences in conservative and surgical treatment for acute grade III injuries. Kerkhoffs and associates[56] concluded that "there is insufficient evidence available from randomized controlled trials to determine the relative effectiveness of surgical and conservative treatment for acute injuries of the lateral ligament complex of the ankle." Some authors[10,12,103] report that surgery is needed because "surgical exploration often reveals that the torn ends of the fibulocalcaneal

ligament are so widely separated that simple immobilization alone is not sufficient to allow the ligament to heal in a stable position."[10] However, other authors have found that "early controlled mobilization (functional treatment) was the method of choice and provided the quickest recovery in ankle mobility and the earliest return to work and physical activity without compromising the late mechanical stability of the ankle."[91] Therefore depending on the physician's choice of treatment, a grade III sprain can be treated either surgically or with early controlled motion and supervised physical therapy. A good to excellent long-term prognosis can be expected in 80% to 90% of patients with grade III ankle sprains regardless of the intervention.[54] However, if inadequate treatment is performed, chronic instability may occur leading to injuries to associated structures.[31] Secondary to the possibility of chronic instability Ferran and Maffulli[31] have proposed that athletes with acute grade III injuries be surgically treated.

Generally joint protection lasts longer with grade III ankle sprains than with grade I and II sprains. When these injuries are treated surgically, and postoperative immobilization is used, deleterious effects on muscle, bone, cartilage, tendons, and ligaments can be expected.[1]

Deltoid Ligament Sprains (Medial Ligament)

Acute isolated sprains of the deep and superficial layers of the deltoid ligament are rare, occurring in only 3% to 5% of all ankle sprains.[91,92] It is clinically important

---

BOX 17-1

General Three-Phase Intervention Program for Inversion Ankle Sprains

PHASE I: MAXIMUM-PROTECTION PHASE

1. Rest, ice, compression, and elevation (RICE)
2. Electrical galvanic stimulation (EGS)
3. Weight bearing as tolerated (WBAT)
4. Joint protection (plastic, hinged orthosis, tape, air cast, semirigid braces)
5. Active range of motion (dorsiflexion and eversion)
6. Isometric exercises
7. General fitness exercises

PHASE II: MODERATE-PROTECTION PHASE

1. RICE
2. FWB
3. Concentric and eccentric contractors (latex rubber band, ankle weights)
4. Continued joint protection
5. Heel cord stretching
6. Stationary cycling
7. Proprioception exercises
8. General fitness exercises
9. Avoidance of unwanted stresses (inversion and plantar flexion)

PHASE III: MINIMUM-PROTECTION PHASE

1. Joint protection during activities
2. Running
3. Jumping
4. Plyometrics
5. Proprioception exercises
6. General fitness exercises
7. Isotonic exercises
8. Isokinetic exercises

---

to recognize that "complete deltoid ligament ruptures occur in combination with ankle fractures."[91]

However, according to Hintermann and associates,[43] sprains of the deltoid ligament appear to be more frequent than commonly recognized, leading to problems with **posterior tibialis tendon** dysfunction and chronic medial ankle instability. Fractures of the medial or lateral malleolus may cause disruption of the deltoid ligament.[43]

Intervention

Partial tears of the deltoid ligament are managed nonoperatively with physical therapy. Because complete ruptures occur with fractures, many authorities advocate surgical repair and fixation of the fracture fragments.[14,20] However, some authors recommend casting, NWB for 6 weeks, then progressive weight bearing

and physical therapy.[38] In either case, rehabilitation focuses primarily on joint protection and the use of a semirigid orthosis.

The use of ice, compression, and elevation assists with pain and swelling. Progressive strengthening follows a three-phase plan of maximum, moderate, and minimum protection. Isometric exercises, latex rubber band strengthening exercises, AROM (carefully avoiding unwanted stresses), and progressive weight bearing are added as tolerated. Generally, a total body fitness program can be initiated during cast immobilization and NWB.

High Ankle Sprain or Ankle Syndesmosis Injury

When the ankle is forced into dorsiflexion or rotation with the foot in a weight-bearing position, injury to the ankle **syndesmosis** commonly occurs. This mechanism of injury is prevalent in skiing, football, soccer, and other sport activities.[68] Injury to the structures supporting the ankle syndesmosis, the anterior and posterior tibiotalar ligaments, the interosseus membrane, interosseus ligament, and the deltoid ligament, can result in an unstable distal tibiofibular articulation.[68,86,89] Diagnostic testing for the high ankle sprain include the external rotation and squeeze tests, and various forms of diagnostic imaging.

Intervention

Treatment of these injuries may include immobilization, limitation of weight bearing, and surgery.[68,86,89] A conservative approach to treatment and rehabilitation is necessary secondary to weight bearing being disruptive to the healing process for these ligaments. Chronic instability and arthritis commonly occur when this injury is mismanaged.[89]

Chronic Ankle Ligament Instabilities

The PTA, as an integral part of the rehabilitation team, must be aware of certain short- and long-term complications that may arise from acute or chronic ligament injuries of the ankle. Complications after surgical repair or conservative treatment of ankle sprains are common. Renstrom and Kannus[91] report that 10% to 30% of patients have chronic symptoms of weakness, swelling, pain, and joint instability after inversion sprains. There are two types of instabilities associated with chronic ankle sprains: mechanical and functional.

Mechanical Instabilities

Mechanical instability is defined as laxity of the ankle ligaments. With mechanical instabilities, surgery may be necessary to stabilize the ankle joint.[6] The Watson-Jones,[117] Evans,[30] Chrisman–Snook,[17] and Elmslie[17] procedures are common reconstructive surgical procedures used to help stabilize the lateral ligament complex

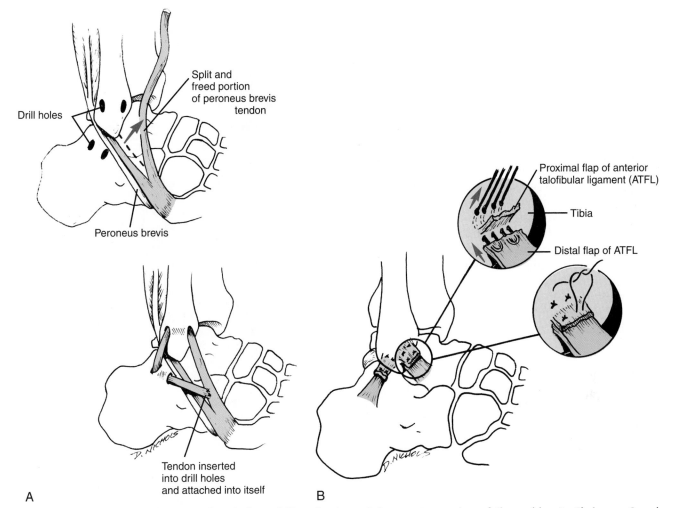

Drill holes

Split and
freed portion
of peroneus brevis
tendon

Peroneus brevis

Proximal flap of anterior
talofibular ligament (ATFL)

Tibia

Distal flap of ATFL

Tendon inserted
into drill holes
and attached into itself

A

B

Fig. 17-8 Surgical procedures used to help stabilize the lateral ligament complex of the ankle. **A,** Chrisman–Snook procedure. **B,** Direct delayed primary anatomic repair of torn ligaments.

of the ankle. In general, the peroneus brevis muscle is rerouted through a surgically constructed tunnel in the distal fibula (Fig. 17-8, *A*). The rerouting of the peroneus brevis dynamically stabilizes the lateral aspect of the ankle. Another method used to help stabilize chronic ligament laxity is a delayed anatomic repair of the ligaments. The ligaments are surgically cut, shortened, and reattached to the bone with this method (Fig. 17-8, *B*). Surgical repair has been gaining popularity among foot and ankle surgeons because of the failure of most reconstruction procedures to correct preinjury ankle biomechanics.[44,70]

Ankle arthroscopy has also been gaining popularity among foot and ankle surgeons secondary to the need to identify and treat intraarticular lesions at the time of surgery.[21,59,70] In particular, articular cartilage lesions can be identified and treated with arthroscopy.

Intervention

Perhaps secondary to the large number of surgical procedures the postoperative course of treatment after surgical correction of chronic ankle instability is variable.

Commonly rehabilitation involves some form of ankle immobilization for approximately 2 to 6 weeks depending on the surgeon. Passive dorsiflexion and plantar flexion exercises are begun after immobilization has ended. When reconstructive procedures involving the rerouting of the peroneus brevis tendon are utilized active motion is not permitted initially. Restriction of AROM allows for the reconstruction to stabilize. When tolerated, AROM exercises begin with careful avoidance of excessive plantar flexion and inversion motions. A general body fitness program is encouraged throughout the period of immobilization. The use of aerobic exercises (stationary bicycle), leg strengthening exercises (leg extensions and hamstring curls), and proprioception exercises is vital throughout rehabilitation.

In primary delayed repair or anatomic reconstruction, the ligament is surgically shortened and reinserted (imbricated). The healing time for ligaments is slightly longer and more tenuous than that for muscle and tendon reconstructions (tenodesis); therefore the period of immobilization may be prolonged. The progression of rehabilitation is the same as with a tenodesis. Active and passive ROM, control of swelling and pain, isometric and manual resistive exercises (being careful to avoid unwanted excessive plantar flexion and inversion motions), Thera-Band and isotonic exercises, and isokinetics are used.

Dynamic muscular support is the foundation of various surgical procedures to correct chronic ankle instabilities. Therefore careful and thorough consideration is given to isometric stabilization exercises, Thera-Band resistive exercises in all directions, manual resistance, isotonic resistance (with ankle weights), and isokinetic strengthening during the minimal-protective phase. In all cases, full ROM exercises with an emphasis on the eccentric contraction phase of each repetition should be encouraged.

Generally, proprioceptive exercises are used extensively. Single-leg standing exercises, balance board activities, minitrampoline exercises, and heel walking exercises are part of the moderate- and minimum-protection phases of rehabilitation. In all cases, joint protection with tape, braces, or a hinged orthosis is a rudimentary but critical principle throughout rehabilitation.

Functional Instabilities

Functional instability refers to a subjective feeling of giving way without affecting ligament laxity. Unlike mechanical instability, functional instability involves a host of factors, including strength, proprioception, and ligament stability. McVey and colleagues[77] report that up to 40% of patients with lateral ankle instability have functional instability.

Intervention

The primary components of rehabilitation for chronic functional instabilities are closed-chain resistance exercises, proprioception maneuvers, dynamic muscular exercises (concentric and eccentric loads), and bracing for support. Single-leg support proprioception exercises with external resistance (Fig. 17-9) provide dynamic support and balance training. Balance board activities, heel-toe walking, and minitrampoline activities are the cornerstones of proprioception exercises for the ankle throughout all phases of rehabilitation for functional ankle instabilities.

SUBLUXING PERONEAL TENDONS

The PTA must recognize that certain anatomic variations and acute injuries can result in instability of the peroneal tendons and ultimate disability. This injury is classified as acute or chronic. The mechanism of injury involves passive dorsiflexion with the foot slightly everted.[27,73] Acute subluxation of the peroneal tendons can be misdiagnosed as a lateral ankle sprain because of the close anatomic proximity of the tendons to the lateral ligament complex (Fig. 17-10). Patients suffering with peroneal tendon subluxation commonly describe

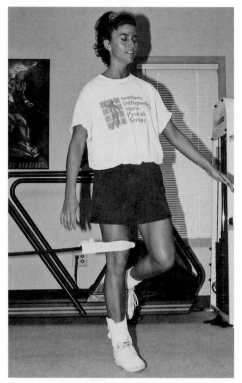

Fig. 17-9 Single-leg standing balance and proprioception exercise with the use of elastic cord to stimulate and encourage strength in a weight-bearing closed-chain functional position.

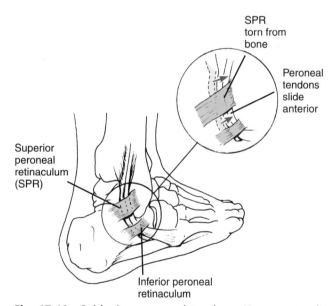

Fig. 17-10 Subluxing peroneal tendons. Note anatomic position of the peroneal tendons in relation to the lateral ligament complex of the ankle.

posterior ankle pain and may complain of a popping sensation in the lateral ankle. Active dorsiflexion with eversion of the ankle may reproduce the symptoms.[41]

Some patients who suffer dislocation of the peroneal tendons have a loose retinaculum (which supports the tendon within the peroneal groove) and also may have a very shallow peroneal groove.[33] Acute injuries to the ankle ligaments (grades I, II, and III, using the traditional classification of sprains) may also result in injury to the peroneal retinaculum. Misdiagnosis of an ankle sprain is quite common.[33] When subluxation occurs the peroneal tendons normally dislocate anteriorly over the lateral malleolus with ankle dorsiflexion.[27,33,73]

Intervention

Acute injuries usually are treated initially with conservative measures, including rigid-cast immobilization and NWB gait for approximately 6 weeks.[33,105] Ferran and associates[33] report that conservative management is successful in approximately 50% of cases. However, in some cases, patients ultimately require a surgical repair to correct the disability.[55,105] Many authorities still recommend cast immobilization and NWB for 6 weeks for acute injuries, but operative care is the treatment of choice for cases involving recurrent or chronic subluxing peroneal tendons.[55] Keene[55] reports the five basic types of surgical repair procedures for correction of chronic subluxing peroneal tendons:

■ Bone block procedures
■ Rerouting procedures
■ Periosteal flaps
■ Groove deepening procedures
■ Tendon slings

Postoperative Interventions

The postoperative care of subluxing peroneal tendons requires excellent communication among the PTA, PT, and surgeon. The exact procedure performed should be explained to the PT, who should articulate the key points of the surgery to the PTA and outline the indications and contraindications for rehabilitation. Usually postoperative care involves the use of immobilization for a few weeks and instruction in weight bearing as tolerated (WBAT). Keene[55] recommends plantar flexion and dorsiflexion exercises 3 weeks after surgery. Heckman and colleagues[41] suggest that patients remain non–weight bearing for 2 weeks followed by 2 to 4 weeks of immobilization in a cast or walking boot. ROM exercises are commonly initiated at 4 to 6 weeks postoperatively.

While immobilized, the patient progresses through a general body conditioning program of aerobic exercise and strengthening. After immobilization, AROM and isometric strengthening exercises are begun. As pain allows, manual resistive and Thera-Band strengthening exercises can be added. Care must be taken with extreme dorsiflexion and eversion maneuvers after surgery. Depending on which procedure was used, soft-tissue and bone healing constraints must be observed carefully to avoid placing excessive stress on the surgically repaired tissues.

Initially, limited ROM dorsiflexion strengthening exercises should be used. As pain, swelling, and strength improve, greater degrees of dorsiflexion motion can be added. Proprioception exercises on a flat surface can be initiated soon after immobilization ends. Progression to balance board activities and minitrampoline exercises depends on the patient's tolerance. Keene[55] recommends that a running program can begin when ROM has been achieved and the involved limb reaches 80% of the strength of the noninvolved limb.

At first, slow straight-line jogging is attempted. Longer distances are tried if there is no pain, swelling, or complaint of instability. As symptoms allow, sprints can be attempted with careful observation of symptoms.

Plyometric exercises and rapid cutting maneuvers can be included for the athletic patient. For example, jumping in place, side-to-side hops, and quick figure-of-eight sprints are progressive functional activities that involve rapid change of direction and ballistic concentric and eccentric open- and closed-chain loading. In most cases, full return to activity can be achieved about 16 weeks after surgery.

ACHILLES TENDINOPATHY

Achilles tendinopathy is an overuse injury resulting from repetitive microtrauma and accumulative overloading of the tendon (Fig. 17-11).[55] The primary feature of Achilles tendinopathy is localized pain at the midportion, distal third, and insertion on the calcaneus. It should be distinguished from other similar posterior foot and ankle disorders such as retrocalcaneal bursitis and Haglund disease.[101]

Many intrinsic and extrinsic factors can lead to Achilles tendinopathy. Decreased vascularity, malalignment of the hindfoot or forefoot, and issues with gastrocnemius–soleus flexibility are common intrinsic factors.[55,101] Extrinsic factors include variations in training, running surface changes, and poor or inappropriate footwear. The general features of Achilles tendinopathy include soft-tissue swelling, pain, and crepitus.

Intervention

Most cases of Achilles tendinopathy are managed conservatively with various physical agents, oral medications, relative rest, and progressive exercises. Initial management includes the use of ice massage or ice packs for 15 to 20 minutes, three to five times daily. The treating physician may prescribe a nonsteroidal antiinflammatory drug (NSAID) to help reduce swelling and pain. All aggravating motions must be stopped. For example, an athletic patient who runs must stop running temporarily until symptoms subside. A program of aerobic exercise using a stationary bicycle or a swimming program can take the place of the running program. Sometimes a small felt heel-lift can be placed in everyday shoes to

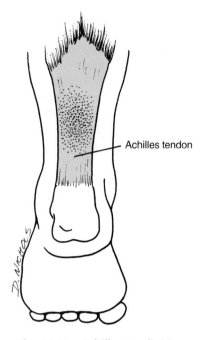

Fig. 17-11 Achilles tendinitis.

Achilles tendon

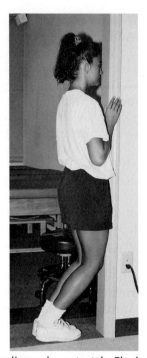

Fig. 17-12 Standing soleus stretch. Flexing the knees enhances the stretch to the gastrocnemius–soleus complex.

help reduce the stress on the tendon. Use of the heel-lift is gradually diminished as symptoms are reduced. It is not advisable to suddenly remove the heel-lift support when symptoms improve because pain and swelling return occasionally.

Ultrasound also can be used to help reduce pain and assist with collagen synthesis.[50] Generally, ultrasound can be used immediately before an exercise program to improve circulation, enhance relaxation of the soft tissues, and reduce pain. Occasionally phonophoresis (ultrasound used with a topical hydrocortisone cream) is used in cases of severe pain.

Flexibility exercises are used to increase dorsiflexion motion and reduce the effects of scarring in prolonged cases of Achilles tendinopathy. Researchers have pointed out that a lack of dorsiflexion is a common denominator for patients suffering from Achilles tendinopathy.[63]

Initially, active dorsiflexion exercises are used. Towel stretches are gradually added as pain allows. In many cases it may be helpful to apply ice packs or ice massage to the tendon before stretching and strengthening exercises. Standing heel cord stretches can be added to the flexibility program as soon as towel stretches do not cause pain or swelling. In all cases of stretching, it is advisable to avoid any ballistic motions, stretch gently and firmly, and hold each stretch for 10 to 30 seconds.

Standing heel cord stretches can be performed on a small block or with a commercial appliance to produce greater dorsiflexion motion. A soleus stretch is also used for Achilles tendinopathy. The patient faces a wall with his or her knees touching the wall while keeping the heels on the floor (Fig. 17-12).

Strengthening exercises often prove very beneficial for patients with Achilles tendinopathy. However, most full ROM strengthening and stretching exercises also cause complaints of pain. A safe and effective exercise program focuses initially on limited ROM and submaximal exercises. When the patient can perform all exercises without pain, the next phase of more vigorous exercise can begin.

Curwin and Stanish[23] advocate eccentric strength training exercises for treatment of many types of tendinopathy. When strengthening the gastrocnemius–soleus muscle group, standing heel raises are a preferred form of exercise. The patient is instructed to rise up on the balls of the feet using the uninvolved limb, then before the descent phase, body weight is transferred to the involved limb and slowly lowered using the ipsilateral gastrocnemius–soleus muscle. Several authors have strongly advocated the use of an eccentric only strength training program for Achilles tendinopathy.[3,58] Alfredson and associates[3] describes excellent clinical outcomes following a 12-week eccentric strength training program for Achilles tendinopathy. In their study subjects who performed the eccentric program were able to resume running in 12 weeks, whereas those who performed a more standard concentric rehabilitation program were not able to return to running during this same time frame.[3] Knobloch[58] reports that "daily eccentric training for Achilles tendinopathy is a safe activity without any evidence of adverse effects in either mid-portion and insertional Achilles tendinopathy."

In some severe cases of Achilles tendinopathy, physicians may prescribe rigid cast immobilization of the ankle for 10 days.[63] The entire program of rehabilitation after cast immobilization progresses at a slightly slower rate because of the ROM and strength loss associated with immobilization. In all cases of Achilles tendinopathy, the patient is instructed in a general body fitness program. Aerobic exercise can be achieved with an upper body ergometer (UBE), seated bicycle ergometer with the seat height corrected to prevent plantar flexion, or a swimming program. Upper- and lower-body stretching and strengthening exercises are encouraged as long as the tendon suffers no undue stress or pain.

RUPTURES OF THE ACHILLES TENDON

Complete ruptures of the Achilles tendon can occur with sudden eccentric-concentric contraction of the gastrocnemius–soleus (Fig. 17-13).[101] These ruptures usually involve the area "3 to 4 cm proximal to its insertion on the calcaneus, within the area of decreased vascularity" and occur mostly in men 20 to 50 years old.[55,101] Racquet sports and other activities requiring a deceleration to acceleration mechanism are often the mechanism of injury. Approximately 50% of Achilles tendon ruptures are secondary to degenerative changes in the tendon.[101] Corticosteroid injections or fluoroquinolone antibiotics are also responsible to weakening the tendon and predisposing an individual to rupture.[101]

In acute Achilles tendon rupture, palpation reveals a defect or gap in the continuity of the distal third of the tendon. The Thompson test clinically assesses the integrity of the Achilles tendon. To perform this simple test, the patient lies prone on an examining table with the feet extending off the end. The entire lower leg is exposed, from knee to toes. The belly of the calf of the uninvolved limb is grasped and squeezed so that the foot plantar flexes. If the tendon is ruptured on the involved limb when the calf is squeezed, no plantar flexion motion results (Fig. 17-14).

Intervention

A ruptured Achilles tendon can be treated surgically or with cast immobilization.[57,101] Nonoperative treatment of Achilles tendon ruptures requires the patient to be immobilized for as long as 8 weeks.[55,57,101] However, with nonoperative treatment, researchers have documented rerupture rates of 8% to 39%.[9,30,52,57] In addition, there is a greater loss of strength, power, and endurance compared with surgically repaired tendons.[9,49,52,55] Surgically repaired Achilles tendons have a much lower rate of rerupture (0% to 5%), and there is a significant increase in the ultimate recovery of muscular strength, power, and endurance.[57] However, Nistor[85] reports only minor differences between surgical and nonsurgical management. Some surgeons[85] prefer

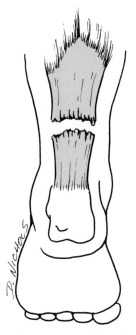

Fig. 17-13   Complete rupture of the Achilles tendon.

nonoperative management because there are fewer complications related to surgery, reduced complaints, no hospitalization, and no significant differences in function compared with surgically treated patients. There are numerous surgical techniques used to repair acute Achilles tendon ruptures, including end-to-end primary repair and direct repair and augmentation with tendon or synthetic grafts.*

The rehabilitation program used after nonoperative immobilization of an Achilles tendon rupture requires the PTA to appreciate the time-dependent nature of tendon healing and plastic and elastic deformation principles. Throughout the course of immobilization, the patient should be instructed in a general body conditioning program that does not stress the involved tissues. The muscles of the noninvolved limb (i.e., quadriceps, hamstrings, gastrocnemius–soleus) should be vigorously strengthened along with the thigh and hamstring muscles of the involved limb. Aerobic exercise is also encouraged. Stationary bike ergometers using only the uninvolved limb (a toe clip is necessary for single-limb cycling) and UBEs are appropriate and safe cardiovascular fitness tools. When the cast is removed and after the initial evaluation by the PT, the PTA proceeds with thermal agents as indicated. Moist heat can be used before ROM and flexibility exercises. If pain and swelling are present, a cold whirlpool or ice packs with compression can be applied.

---

*For more information on these techniques, please refer to the articles found in references 2, 15, 29, 36, 42, 45, 47, 48, 53, 55, 57, 60, 61, 69, 88, 99, 100, 106, 107, 111, and 113.

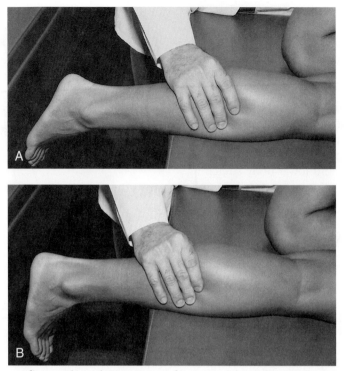

Fig. 17-14 Thompson test to confirm or deny the presence of a ruptured Achilles tendon. **A,** A negative Thompson test is demonstrated by observation of plantar flexion of the foot when squeezing the calf. **B,** A positive Thompson test reveals no plantar flexion of the foot when the calf is squeezed.

Regaining full dorsiflexion and plantar flexion motion is an exceedingly slow process after cast removal. Gentle active dorsiflexion and plantar flexion exercises are initiated immediately. Typically, a small heel-lift is used in everyday shoes to minimize stress on the healing tendon. Because the tendon was not surgically repaired, the process of regaining tensile strength and collagen alignment must be approached cautiously. Progressive active motion is an essential component for full return to function. However, if the tendon is stressed too soon or vigorously, it may rerupture. The heel-lift is commonly worn for 3 to 4 weeks and gradually reduced in size to prevent sudden excessive stress on the tendon.[55]

Progressive plantar flexion and dorsiflexion exercises using a latex band are encouraged as pain and motion allow. Proprioception exercises can be employed early, depending on the patient's tolerance. Generally, proprioception exercises begin with the patient in a seated position (Fig. 17-15) and progress as tolerated. If rerupture occurs, it is usually within 4 weeks after immobilization.[55] During this maximum-protection phase, the patient is encouraged to avoid sudden forceful plantar flexion or dorsiflexion motions.

As motion increases gradually, closed-chain resistive exercises can be initiated, based on the patient's ROM, pain tolerance, swelling, and the length of time after cast removal. Seated stationary cycling can be used for aerobic fitness, ROM, and local muscular endurance. The

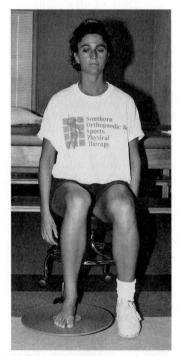

Fig. 17-15 Initial proprioception activities can begin in a seated position using a wobble board.

seat must be adjusted to avoid excessive plantar flexion or dorsiflexion, however. Step-ups can be used (with heel-lift) to encourage weight bearing eccentric loading.

Weight-bearing plantar flexion can begin gradually once the patient has successfully completed the prescribed program of ROM and strengthening exercises without complications. Standing plantar flexion is initiated without a block to stand on. The patient is instructed to gradually rise up on the toes using primarily the uninvolved limb, then lowers himself or herself using both feet. As strength improves, the patient gradually uses more of the involved limb to rise up on the balls of the feet. Adding a small block of wood on which to rise adds greater dorsiflexion stress and motion. Seated calf raises can be performed by modifying a leg extension machine (Fig. 17-16). The seated position may be more comfortable initially.

The PTA reassesses the patient's ROM, strength, pain, and swelling on a daily basis. Modifications are necessary if the patient is having undue pain with any phase of the program. Daily communication with the PT allows continuous restructuring of the rehabilitation plan based on the patient's needs as assessed by the PTA. Isokinetic testing for plantar flexion, dorsiflexion, ROM, strength, power, and local muscular endurance generally is reserved for the minimal-protection phase. However, isokinetic strengthening exercises can be employed early if done at higher speeds and performed submaximally under limited ROM conditions.

Rehabilitation following surgical repair or reconstruction of the Achilles tendon is quite variable. Secondary to the large number of procedures available, the timing of the surgery (acute vs. chronic), stability of the repair/reconstruction, and intrinsic patient variables the rehabilitation progression may be different from

surgeon to surgeon, and patient to patient. In particular the surgical variations are numerous with each having differing needs for immobilization and restriction of weight bearing during the immediate postoperative period. Variables such as ROM, weight bearing, and initiation of strength training are determined by the surgeon. Therefore each individual should be rehabilitated independently.*

Generally, rehabilitation following Achilles tendon repair or reconstruction follows a criteria-based rehabilitation program as described previously. Following a period of immobilization a gradual progression of weight bearing and ROM is pursued. Normally plantar flexion is less restricted than dorsiflexion during the early postoperative period. Strength training can begin as early as 2 to 4 weeks postimmobilization.[55]

Secondary to the large differences in Achilles tendon surgery and rehabilitation programs the return to full activity is also variable. At least one author believes that successful outcomes are dependent on tendon elongation. Kannas and Renstrom[54] report that improved outcomes occur when less elongation of the Achilles tendon occurs. Therefore symmetric ankle dorsiflexion ROM is a goal of treatment, and increased dorsiflexion beyond the contralateral side is discouraged. Generally most patients are able to return to full activity within 6 to 9 months. Surgical complications following Achilles tendon repair or reconstruction include sural nerve dysfunction, infection, skin sensitivity, adhesions, rerupture, and tendon necrosis.[57,61] The vast majority of patients appear to be satisfied with their results.[2,29,48,57,88]

COMPARTMENT SYNDROMES

Compartment syndromes of the lower leg are defined as either acute or chronic elevated tissue pressure within a closed fascial space, resulting in occlusion of vessels and compromised neuromuscular function.[4,35,93]

Acute compartment syndromes of the leg are most commonly associated with tibial fractures, direct trauma to the area, muscle rupture, muscle hypertrophy, and circumferential burns.[62,91] Acute elevated intracompartmental pressure within the lower leg is considered a medical emergency.[35]

Chronic compartment syndromes also are referred to as *exertional compartment syndrome* or *exercise-induced compartment syndrome*. Muscular contractions and exertion have been shown to cause increases in muscle size, leading to increased intracompartmental pressure.[62,91] This results in ischemia and reduced neuromuscular function. To understand this series of events, it is necessary to review pertinent anatomy of the lower leg.

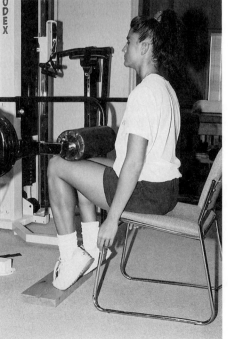

Fig. 17-16 Seated heel or calf raises are performed by modifying and adjusting a knee-extension machine with a range-limiting device.

*For more information on these techniques, please refer to the articles found in references 2, 15, 29, 36, 42, 45, 47, 48, 53, 55, 57, 60, 61, 69, 88, 99, 100, 106, 107, 111, and 113.

There are four well-defined compartments of the leg, divided by nonyielding fascia.[4,93] The anterior compartment of the lower leg contains the tibialis anterior muscle, anterior tibial artery and vein, and foot and toe extensor muscles. The lateral compartment contains the superficial peroneal nerve and short and long peroneal muscles. The superficial posterior compartment contains the soleus muscle and plantaris and gastrocnemius tendons. The deep posterior compartment contains the posterior tibialis muscle, the peroneal artery and vein, **tibial nerve,** and posterior tibial artery and vein. If swelling occurs in one or more of these compartments, reduced capillary blood perfusion results in neurovascular and muscular dysfunction.

Clinical symptoms of acute compartment syndrome include pain, palpable swelling or tenseness, and paresthesias.[4,93] The skin may be warm, shiny, and tense. Passive stretching of the muscles of the lower leg may produce severe pain.

Symptoms of chronic or exertional compartment syndromes include a dull aching pain within the muscle during and after long-term exercise. Paresthesias also may develop as the syndrome progresses. The sections most commonly affected with chronic exercise-induced compartment syndromes are the anterior and deep posterior compartments of the lower leg.

Intervention

Acute compartment syndrome is treated with a surgical procedure called a *fasciotomy.*[4,93] When nerve and muscle ischemia last longer than 12 hours, severe and irreversible damage occurs.[4] If, however, the ischemia can be reduced in less than 4 hours, usually no permanent damage occurs.[4]

A surgical fasciotomy is designed to relieve intracompartmental pressure by opening or releasing the fascial compartment, thus allowing the pressure to be reduced. It is interesting to note that the surgical incision is sometimes left open and is managed with sterile dressings.[4] Recently, less invasive techniques such as endoscopy have been utilized.[120] Immediately after surgery, ice packs and leg elevation are necessary to reduce swelling. Walking as tolerated and active and passive gentle ROM of the ankle and knee are begun 2 days after surgery. Early ROM is crucial in order to prevent contractures. Treatment with ice and leg elevation is continued after exercise. A general conditioning program can begin with strengthening exercises and aerobic exercises using a single-leg ergometer or UBE. Once the patient shows improved motion and reduced pain and swelling, light resistance exercises can begin for the involved leg. Close attention should be paid to foot structure because contractures may develop postsurgery, resulting in varying levels of equinus deformity in the foot.[109] However, very light resistance should be encouraged because heavy and intense exercise, which leads to muscular hypertrophy, is contraindicated after fasciotomy for acute compartment syndromes.

The management of chronic exercise-induced compartment syndromes is similar to that of acute compartment syndromes. However, chronic compartment syndromes do not always represent a surgical emergency. Conservative management should include relative rest, antiinflammatory drugs, stretching and strengthening of the involved muscles, and foot orthotic devices (if appropriate).[118] Subcutaneous fasciotomy should be used only when pain and symptoms affect function. The postoperative management of fasciotomy after chronic compartment syndromes parallels the rehabilitation program outlined for acute compartment syndromes.

ANKLE FRACTURES

The most widely accepted classification of ankle fractures is called the *Lauge–Hansen classification.*[76] Another type of classification, called *AO*, is based on principles, which are similar to, though slightly different from, the Lauge-Hansen (Fig. 17-7). The organization and classification of ankle fractures frequently involve the direction of force, which results in specific patterns of injury. For example, a Lauge–Hansen pronation-abduction or pronation–lateral rotation injury may result in a malleolar or bimalleolar fracture of the ankle (Fig. 17-18).

Ankle fractures include lateral malleolar fractures, medial malleolar fractures, bimalleolar fractures (combined medial and lateral malleolar fractures), and trimalleolar fractures (bimalleolar fractures plus the posterior margin of the tibia). Though simple malleolar fractures are managed initially with immobilization, many fractures are managed with an open reduction with internal fixation (ORIF) procedures. Typically, these fractures are fixed with various screws and plates to hold the fragments in place (Fig. 17-19).

In many cases of ankle fractures repaired with an ORIF procedure, the patient is in a semirigid postoperative removable splint for 2 weeks. This splint can be removed to allow for active dorsiflexion and plantar flexion ROM exercises. However, this is patient-specific and should be confirmed with the surgeon. Because of the mechanism of injury that caused the malleolar fracture and the position of the internal fixation devices, no inversion or eversion exercises are performed.

A walking cast is applied once the patient achieves full plantar flexion and dorsiflexion ROM. Before casting, the surgical wound must be fully closed, sutures removed, infection absent, and no drainage present. A general full-body conditioning program is prescribed throughout immobilization. Both aerobic fitness and strengthening exercises are advocated also. Further, strengthening of the uninjured limb has shown beneficial crossover results in strength of the injured limb.[114]

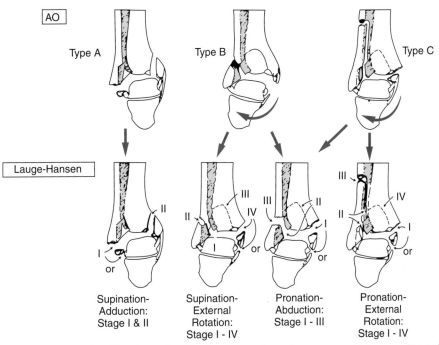

Fig. 17-17 AO and Lauge–Hansen classification of ankle fractures. (From Sangeorzan BJ, Hansen ST: Ankle and foot: trauma. In Poss R, ed: *Orthopaedic knowledge update III*, Park Ridge, Ill, 1990, American Academy of Orthopaedic Surgeons.)

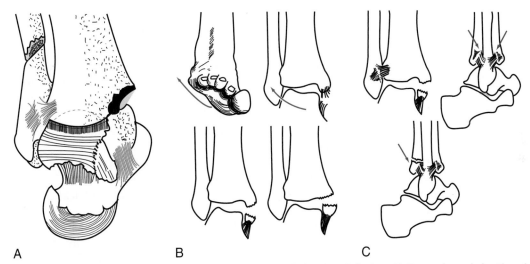

Fig. 17-18 **A,** Pronation–lateral rotation injury. **B,** Pronation-abduction injuries. **C,** Pronation-abduction injury. (From McRae R: *Practical fracture treatment*, ed 3, New York, 1994, Churchill Livingstone.)

ROM exercises, isometric strengthening, stationary cycling, and weight-bearing exercises are begun once the cast is removed. Progressive exercises employ latex rubber tubing or bands, manual resistive exercises, isoinertial/isotonic strengthening, and proprioception exercises. Return to function exercises should be incorporated as soon as the patient is able. Single limb activities, landing activities, and out of plane activities are important examples used for proprioceptive training and return to activity.

The PTA must be acutely aware of the signs and symptoms of possible hardware loosening (increased pain, swelling, crepitus, and motion) so as to swiftly inform the PT and make all necessary modifications in the present program. If, for example, after cast removal following an ORIF procedure for a medial malleolar fracture the PTA recognized increased swelling and complaints of crepitus when strengthening exercises were increased, stressing inversion of the ankle, the PTA should halt those particular exercises and inform the PT. Weight-bearing status; active, passive, and resisted ROM; and functional progression should be determined by the physician throughout rehabilitation.

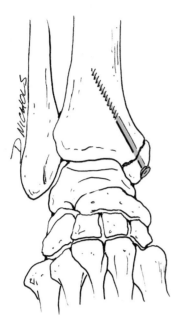

Fig. 17-19 Open reduction with internal fixation screw fixation for medial malleolar fracture.

Distal Tibia Compression Fractures (Pilon Fractures)

Distal tibia compression fractures (pilon fractures) occur as a result of vertical or axial loads that drive, or compress, the tibia into the **talus.** The initial management of these injuries usually involves an ORIF procedure, external fixation, or skeletal traction with a calcaneal pin.[76] If the fracture was managed with external fixation, special attention should be given to these individuals because malunion is more common with this type of fixation.[90] Because of the nature of these fractures, weight-bearing activities usually are deferred for as long as 12 or more weeks. Weight bearing creates vertical compression and compromises the natural course of healing needed for a stable outcome. Secondary osteoarthritis is a common complication with severe multifragmented compression fractures.[76] Typically throughout immobilization, a general conditioning program is allowed as long as no weight bearing occurs.

After immobilization, active motion and general ankle strengthening exercises are performed to the patient's tolerance. Care is taken to protect the articular surface of the distal tibia and talus. It is also important to recognize that hardware placed at or near the joint may provide rigid resistance to ROM activities. Initially, NWB strengthening exercises and ROM maneuvers are allowed. Progressive loading (compression) can proceed cautiously using latex surgical tubing or bands for long-sitting plantar flexion strengthening. Partial weight-bearing (PWB) repetitive motion activities, such as a stationary bicycle ergometer, can be used to enhance ankle motion and endurance. Weight-bearing

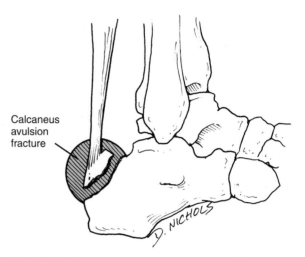

Calcaneus avulsion fracture

Fig. 17-20 Fractured calcaneus type II with avulsion.

activities generally are painful until satisfactory healing has occurred. However, toe-touch weight bearing progressing to PWB is well tolerated, helps restore proprioception, and assists with healing. Weight-bearing status; active, passive, and resisted ROM; and functional progression should be determined by the physician throughout rehabilitation.

Calcaneal Fractures

Calcaneal fractures are intraarticular depression fractures usually caused by falls from a height and resulting in compression of the calcaneus from the talus (Fig. 17-20). McRae[76] describes seven common patterns of calcaneal fractures:

1. Vertical fractures of the calcaneal tuberosity
2. Horizontal fractures
3. Fractures of the sustentaculum tali
4. Anterior calcaneal fractures
5. Fracture of the body of the calcaneus without involvement of the subtalar joint
6. Calcaneal fractures with lateral displacement and involvement of the subtalar joint
7. Central calcaneus crushing fractures

Each calcaneal fracture type has individual characteristics that allow the physician to determine the treatment options and the rehabilitation progression. Both conservative (casting) and surgical (ORIF) procedures are used with **calcaneus fractures.**[76] As with all fractures, specific rehabilitation procedures should be cleared by the physician before initiation. When possible early ROM activity is used in rehabilitation to reduce stiffness and prevent long-term ROM loss. Weight-bearing status; active, passive and resisted ROM; and functional progression should be determined by the physician throughout rehabilitation. Supportive measures to control pain and swelling are used as necessary.

In the long term, the cornerstone in recovering from a calcaneal fracture lies in regaining motion and

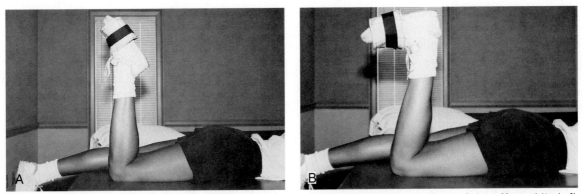

Fig. 17-21 Prone gastrocnemius–soleus strengthening. **A,** Starting position with the knee of the affected limb flexed to 90°. **B,** The patient actively plantar flexes the foot against gravity and the applied resistance.

strengthening the plantar flexors. Multiangle isometric plantar flexion can be initiated and progressed to full ROM manual resistance dorsiflexion and plantar flexion. The use of latex rubber tubing and bands for plantar flexion in a long-seated position is an appropriate and challenging calf-strengthening exercise during the moderate-protection phase of rehabilitation. Strengthening of the soleus can be achieved by having the patient lie prone with the affected leg flexed 90° at the knee and placing ankle weights around the foot of the affected leg (Fig. 17-21).

Gait examination and retraining will be necessary in this population, because initial contact during gait will be compromised. Patients are more likely to load on the midfoot or forefoot at initial contact. Training of a normal heel strike pattern on soft surfaces may be necessary to avoid long-term gait deviations.

Fractures of the Talus

The talus can be fractured by falling from a height and landing on the foot in a crouched position.[76] This produces an axial compression load between the talus and calcaneus. There are four classifications of talar fractures[76]:

■ Type I: Talar neck fracture without displacement
■ Type II: Talar fracture with subtalar subluxation (the incidence of avascular necrosis is as high as 50%)[76]
■ Type III: Talar fracture with further subtalar subluxation (the incidence of avascular necrosis is as high as 85%)[76]
■ Type IV: The talar head dislocates from the navicular in association with a type III injury

These fractures can be treated with closed reduction and cast immobilization or with an ORIF procedure. To allow for proper healing, these fractures require 3 months of NWB. The rehabilitation program can proceed during this immobilization period with single leg stationary cycling, aerobic training, UBE or contralateral limb strengthening. Strengthening exercises include knee extension and hamstring curl maneuvers and NWB hip abduction, adduction, flexion, and

extension. Usually the patient is immobilized in a posterior splint that can be removed for exercise periods. ROM exercises and supportive measures for pain and swelling control can be used during the maximum-protection phase of the rehabilitation program. Osteoarthritis is a common long-term complication with talar fractures because of the duration of immobilization and NWB status. As with all fractures weight-bearing status; active, passive and resisted ROM; and functional progression should be determined by the physician throughout rehabilitation.

STRESS FRACTURES OF THE FOOT AND ANKLE

A stress fracture is a partial or complete fracture of bone caused by unrelenting stress and force that do not allow for osteoblastic repair of bone and in turn cause accelerated bone resorption. Common sites for stress fractures in the foot and ankle are the metatarsals, lateral malleolus, os calcis, navicular, and sesamoid.

Clinically, pain is the predominant feature of a stress fracture. The pain usually increases with activity and subsides with rest. The incidence of stress fractures in the foot and ankle is related in part to participation in demanding physical activity. If stress and forces are applied to bone and are not removed to allow the bone to repair, osteoclast activity overtakes the rate of osteoblast activity and stress fractures occur.

The development of stress fractures can be viewed in part as resulting from a linear progression or continuum of excessive external forces that lead to intrinsic reactions of muscle, bone, and periosteum. For example, with increased muscular forces resulting from continued and excessive use (marathon running, recreational jogging, aerobic dance, or occupations that require standing or walking all day) there is an associated increased rate of bone remodeling around the area of increased stress.[102] If the stress is not removed, this increase in bone remodeling is followed by a greater rate of bone resorption. If the stress continues, the bone eventually responds by developing microfractures, periosteal inflammation, and resultant stress fractures.[102] If stressed further, and the bone and soft tissues are not allowed to recover fully and heal properly, the development of linear fractures and ultimately displaced fractures can occur.[102]

There are certain stress fractures that pose a greater risk of delayed union, nonunion, and displacement than others.[74] The base or proximal diaphysis of the fifth metatarsal is described as "no-man's-land" and is "at risk" for delayed union or nonunion after a stress fracture.[74,91] Usually, complete rigid-cast immobilization is indicated for 6 to 8 weeks when conservative, relative rest has failed to arrest symptoms of pain.[74,91,92] Other stress fractures termed at risk[22] are tarsal navicular fracture, sesamoid fractures, and all intraarticular fractures.

The management of not-at-risk[74] stress fractures of the foot and ankle can be effectively rehabilitated with activity modification; relative rest; therapeutic agents to relieve pain and swelling; and specific leg, ankle, and foot stretching and strengthening exercises. Low-impact aerobic exercise is useful in athletic patients who are extremely active. For example, instead of running, the patient can use a stationary cycle, recumbent cycle, elliptical trainer or run in a NWB manner under water.

For stress fractures of the foot and ankle that are at risk[74] (fifth metatarsal, navicular, sesamoids, and intraarticular fractures), more caution is necessary during the advancement of closed-chain activities to protect the healing bone from unwanted forces. With at-risk stress fractures, some form of external support can be used to brace the area. Usually some type of bracing, padding, casting, or orthosis is applied to control stress and forces to the healing bone.[74] The application of therapeutic exercises must be approached cautiously. Submaximal isometric exercises are encouraged initially. AROM and light concentric and eccentric loads are added as pain allows. Obviously, vertical compressive loads and shearing forces (i.e., jumping, running, cutting) are strictly prohibited to allow proper healing. Modifications in aerobic activity and general physical conditioning can allow the patient to continue to participate in strenuous physical conditioning, provided no stress is applied to the healing tissues. The initiation of closed-chain functional activities must be deferred until radiographic confirmation by the physician documents stable bone healing.

MEDIAL TIBIAL STRESS SYNDROME

Musculoskeletal overuse injuries of the lower leg involving the distal third of the posterior medial border of the tibia have historically been referred to as *shin splints*. This term has no place in orthopedic management and should be discarded as a nonspecific term used to describe any pain occurring in the lower leg.[4] A more precise and descriptive term is medial tibial stress syndrome (MTSS), which describes pain over the distal and middle thirds of the tibia along the posterior medial border.[10] Differential assessment by the physician and PT includes stress fractures of the tibia and fibula, ischemic disorders, and deep compartment syndromes of the lower leg.

The predominant feature of MTSS is tenderness over the distal, posteromedial tibia.[80] Traditionally a number of different structures are thought to cause these symptoms. Musculotendinous inflammation, periosteal inflammation of the muscle–tendon–bone interface at the posterior medial border of the tibia, injury to the tibia bone, the posterior tibialis muscle, and the medial origin of the soleus muscle have been identified as a primary source of pain in patients with MTSS.[4,7,25,78] More recent work has noted that a primary source of symptoms with MTSS is the tibial bone.[72,80]

Several studies have attempted to determine the etiology of MTSS.[8,28,46,80,112,121] Intrinsic factors for MTSS include overpronation of the foot, female sex, high body mass index, hip ROM (internal and external rotation), and ankle ROM loss (dorsiflexion). Hubbard and colleagues[46] report that a previous history of MTSS, previous history of stress fracture, and less than 5 years of experience in a sport predispose an athlete to MTSS. Runners, basketball and volleyball players, tennis players, and military recruits have a greater incidence of MTSS.[28,80] Diagnosis of MTSS is primarily made on physical exam, but diagnostic imaging including plain film radiographs, bone scans, dual energy x-ray absorptiometry (DEXA) scans, and magnetic resonance imaging (MRI) are also used.[72,80]

Because pain is the predominant feature of MTSS, it is helpful to classify and describe the severity of pain related to the patient's ability to perform activities.[51] Grade I describes pain that is experienced after activities. Grade II defines pain felt both during and after activities that does not affect the actual performance of activities. Grade III pain is felt before, during, and after activities and affects the patient's ability to perform activities. Grade IV pain is so significant that no activities can even be attempted.

In general, grade I pain refers to muscle soreness and minor soft-tissue inflammation. Grade II pain is viewed as a mild or moderate soft-tissue inflammation. Grade III pain involves significant soft-tissue inflammation and bone microfractures. Grade IV pain defines an actual stress fracture.

A patient experiencing minor pain (grade I) typically describes transient muscle soreness and general tenderness after activities.

Treatment generally consists of ice packs or ice massage, physician-prescribed NSAIDs, rest, and gradual stretching and strengthening exercises for the entire lower leg. However, treatment of MTSS is highly individualized and specifically related to the comprehensive evaluation performed by the PT. If the PT determines that the patient demonstrates excessive foot pronation, custom molded orthotics may be prescribed to relieve stress. Cryokinetics (ice packs or ice massage in conjunction with stretching and strengthening exercises) usually are advocated as a means to control pain and swelling and encourage motion and function. Relative rest is prescribed in most cases of MTSS. That is, instead of complete rest and immobilization, the patient's activity level is modified to accommodate the patient's complaints of pain and dysfunction. For example, a patient who is an avid jogger may be encouraged to jog in a pool instead. If a UBE is available, the patient can still actively perform aerobic conditioning activities without the associated stress on the lower leg.

Currently there is evidence to support the use of relative rest, foot orthotic devices, and stretching to improve symptoms in patients with MTSS.[80,112] However, a multimodal approach utilizing mechanical and therapeutic approaches appears to be most beneficial with this disorder.[28]

PLANTAR FASCIITIS (HEEL SPUR SYNDROME)

Chronic inflammation of the plantar aponeurosis, with or without an associated calcaneal heel spur, is called *plantar fasciitis* (Fig. 17-22). Leach and co-workers[65] describe plantar fasciitis as repetitive microtrauma leading to injury, attempted repair, and chronic inflammation. Brody[13] describes plantar fasciitis as an "inflammatory reaction due to chronic traction on the plantar aponeurosis (fascia) at its insertion into the calcaneus."

Although most authors and clinicians believe this pathology is an inflammation of the plantar fascia there are several authors who describe this disorder as a *plantar fasciopathy* or *plantar fasciosis*.[67,94] These authors believe that the pathology can be degenerative as well as inflammatory in nature, depending on the chronicity of the pathology. The same issue has been discussed with other overuse tendon injuries.

Patients with plantar fasciitis frequently complain of pain along the medial border of the calcaneus on the plantar surface. Many patients report that pain is worse in the morning when the foot contacts the floor in getting out of bed. Palpation of the plantar fascia usually reveals tenderness at the medial tuberosity of the os calcis or throughout the entire course of the fascia.[4] Palpation is performed with the toes flexed, which reduces tension on the fascia, or with the toes extended, which increases tension on the fascia.[11] Dorsiflexion of the ankle may also provoke symptoms.[16]

Intervention

Many patients respond well to conservative physical therapy procedures.[83,94] Relative rest, stretching, manual therapy, exercise, iontophoresis, arch taping, and foot

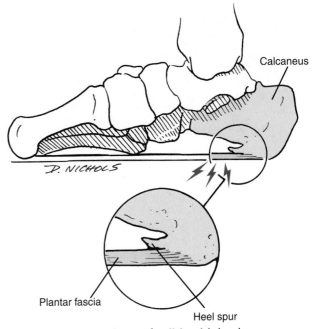

Fig. 17-22 Plantar fasciitis with heel spur.

orthotic devices have been shown to improve symptoms and function in patients with plantar fasciitis.* A specific physical therapy approach where the clinician treats impairments, functional limitations, and disabilities with interventions designed to improve each item observed in the examination appears to have the greatest impact on patients with plantar fasciitis.[75]

Specifically addressing ROM deficits at the ankle joint (dorsiflexion) with manual therapy and stretching exercises appears to be helpful in these patients. If indicated, both the gastrocnemius and soleus muscles should be stretched. However, if stretching of the gastrocnemius or soleus is painful in the area of the plantar fascia the clinician may want to decrease this activity.[16] In the author's experience if arch taping is helpful in reducing symptoms use of an over-the-counter foot orthotic device may be helpful. Custom-made foot orthotic devices may also be used in selected patients. In particular those patients who have a large arch deformity and did not respond favorably to an over the counter device may be good candidates for a custom-made foot orthoses.

Strength training for the musculature in the foot and lower leg may be indicated if specific weaknesses are observed during the examination. Inversion, eversion, dorsiflexion, and/or plantar flexion strength training is necessary when weakness occurs. Strength training for the intrinsic musculature in the foot may also be necessary. Activities such as toe curls, picking up marbles with the toes, or gripping a towel can be used to strengthen the foot intrinsic musculature (Fig. 17-23).

---

*For more information on these techniques, please refer to the articles found in references 5, 19, 26, 66, 75, 82, 87, 95, 116, and 122.

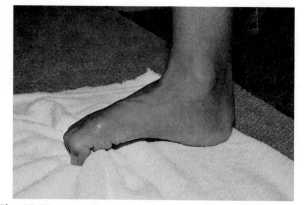

Fig. 17-23   Resistive toe curls are performed by gripping a towel.

The physician may inject a local steroid to help decrease pain and swelling in more severe cases. Because many patients complain that the most severe pain is in the morning, some physicians and PTs prescribe night splints to stretch the Achilles tendon and the plantar fascia. In an athletic population, plantar fasciitis occurs from running and competitive sports participation. During recovery from plantar fasciitis, it is imperative to maintain aerobic fitness and general body strength. Aerobic exercises can be performed without weight bearing in a pool or with a UBE to decrease repetitive loading on the plantar fascia. Stationary cycling is an excellent alternative.

Extracorporeal shockwave therapy has been used for several years to assist in the healing process in patient with plantar fasciitis. This modality attempts to break up adhesions and improve soft tissue extensibility of the plantar fascia. Several authors have shown good results with this form of treatment.[94,110,116]

With some patients who do not respond to conservative therapy, the physician may decide to correct the problem surgically. Surgical options include plantar fascia release (fasciotomy) and partial plantar fascia release. Rompe[94] states that conservative management is the first and best option, and should last approximately 6 months before other forms of treatment. If conservative management fails, then surgery is the next option.

ARCH DEFORMITIES (PES PLANUS AND PES CAVUS)

Pes planus (flatfoot) is a congenital or acquired deformity of the foot where the medial longitudinal arch of the foot is reduced, causing the medial border of the foot to contact the ground when a person is standing.[71] The usual cause of acquired pes planus is muscular weakness, laxity of ligaments that support the medial longitudinal arch, paralysis, or a pronated foot.[71] Pes planus deformity can be classified as mild, moderate, or severe.[81]

During the initial evaluation, the PT measures the degree of hindfoot and forefoot alignment in NWB. The hindfoot alignment is defined as the longitudinal bisection of the calcaneus relative to the long axis of the lower leg, and the forefoot alignment is defined as the metatarsal alignment relative to the perpendicular of the longitudinal bisection of the calcaneus. If the plantar surface of the distal segment is medial relative to the proximal segment, this is defined as a varus alignment. If the plantar surface of the distal segment is lateral relative to the proximal segment, this is defined as a valgus alignment. In addition, the PT assesses the deformity in a weight-bearing position.[92] With a rigid pes planus deformity, the foot appears to have an abnormally low arch in both weight-bearing and NWB positions.[92] With a flexible pes planus deformity, the foot appears to have a normal arch in a NWB position, but an abnormally low or flat arch in weight bearing.

No specific therapeutic interventions are necessary if there is no associated pain or dysfunction. However, because the area is a terminal component of the closed kinetic chain during weight bearing (the arch can affect the knee, hip, and spine in a closed kinetic chain), treatment that is specific to the arch may be indicated if associated pain and dysfunction are experienced in other joints along the kinetic chain. For example, pes planus can affect the normal neutral-to-pronation sequence of the foot during the gait cycle. Because the foot is already pronated (with pes planus), the reduced normalized motion from neutral to pronation is affected during gait. Therefore the knee and other joints along the kinetic chain must compensate for this reduced motion. If pain and resultant dysfunction occur in one or more of these associated joints, then corrective action is necessary to place the foot in a more neutral position to enhance the normal physiologic motion of the entire kinetic chain. Injuries common to those with pes planus occur more often to medial soft tissue structures of the knee.[119]

Usually the use of a custom-fabricated foot orthotic device is indicated to create a more normal mechanical arch. Materials used to fabricate foot orthotic devices include cork, leather, rubber, foam, felt, and plastic.[18] The rationale for the use of a custom-molded foot orthotic device to correct a symptomatic pes planus is supported in the literature.[24] Further, successful treatment of other lower extremity injuries commonly attributed to pes planus have been documented.[37] However, individual consideration should be given to each patient for prescription foot orthoses as lower extremity overuse injuries are always multifactorial.[84]

Pes cavus, on the other hand, describes an abnormally high arch.[71,91] Pes cavus usually is a result of neurogenic pathologic processes, muscle imbalances, and congenital abnormalities; both medial and lateral longitudinal arches can be affected. Clinically, patients may complain of painful calluses beneath the metatarsal heads because of the mechanical friction and pressure that occur with metatarsal heads. Osteoarthritic changes are not uncommon in the tarsal area because of the altered biomechanics of the foot. Mechanical compensation at proximal joints in the lower extremity is also common with injuries being more common to lateral bony structure of the foot and lower leg.[119]

Treatment for pes cavus is much more challenging than for pes planus and should be focused on pain and shock attenuation. Recent evidence supports the effectiveness of custom-made foot orthoses for treatment of pain related to pes cavus.[40] No treatment is indicated if no symptoms exist, although the PT may document this deformity during a lower-quarter evaluation.

MORTON NEUROMA (PLANTAR INTERDIGITAL NEUROMA)

Patients with a neuroma may complain of diffuse, occasionally radiating pain into the toes and proximally to the dorsal or plantar surface of the foot.[22] A neuroma usually occurs at the 3-4 interspace and less frequently at the 2-3 interspace (Fig. 17-24).[79] Morton neuroma occurs bilaterally only 15% of the time, with the patient complaining of a burning, cramping, or catching sensation.[22,79] A painful mass can be palpated in approximately one third of the cases.[79]

Intervention

Conservative care calls for the use of a metatarsal pad; change of footwear to a wider, softer shoe; and local corticosteroid injections. Surgical excision of the neuroma may be necessary when all attempts at conservative care fail to relieve pain. However, success of the surgical technique is around 83%.[39]

Postoperative physical therapy care involves early active motion of the involved metatarsal phalangeal joint to limit stiffness and fibrosis. Postoperative care dictates that the patient be WBAT and progressed to FWB as pain allows. Compression bandages are used with elastic tape to assist with swelling and pain management. Generally, physical therapy care begins 2 to 3 weeks after surgery, once the sutures are removed. Typically, however, patients are encouraged to perform active ankle, foot, and knee ROM exercises during the early healing phase before physical therapy is begun. Patients are likely to need a molded foot orthotic device after surgery. This device may be advanced to a custom molded device if the mechanics and morphology of the foot dictate.

Thermal agents used to reduce swelling and pain may include whirlpool baths and cryotherapy. In addition, ultrasound can be used under water in conjunction with active motion exercises to improve circulation, reduce tissue congestion, and improve motion. AROM exercises include ankle motion in all directions, knee flexion and

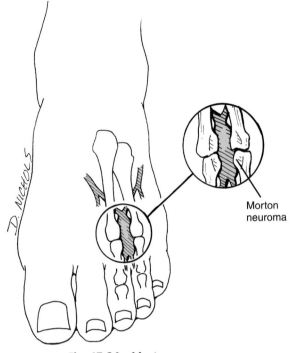

Fig. 17-24 Morton neuroma.

extension, and specific toe extension exercises with toe curls and splaying of the toes as tolerated. Occasionally, passive mobilization of the metatarsals may be needed to avoid the development of movement limitations. Strengthening exercises can be initiated as soon as the pain allows.

All strengthening exercises for the ankle and knee are included with specific intrinsic foot strengthening exercises. Resistive toe curls can begin as an open kinetic chain exercise and progress to a closed kinetic chain exercise as strength and patient tolerance allow.

HALLUX VALGUS

Hallux valgus is a lateral or valgus deviation of the great toe with both soft tissue and bony deformity (Fig. 17-25). This condition can be exacerbated by improper footwear (narrow toe box), and often the associated pain can be relieved by modifying or changing poor footwear. Examination should include assessment of the deformity in a standing position, which often accentuates the deformity,[22,79] and measurement of the hallux valgus angle (normal is <15 degrees) to determine the degree of deformity and angle of deviation. Hallux valgus is often associated with hallux rigidus. Therefore, first metatarsal phalangeal joint extension ROM should also be assessed. Further, it has been suggested that abnormal pronation is associated with the development of hallux valgus.[96]

Management options include both conservative care and operative procedures. Initial care is supportive, with a change in footwear to include a wider toe box (this alone can significantly reduce symptoms), over-the-counter or

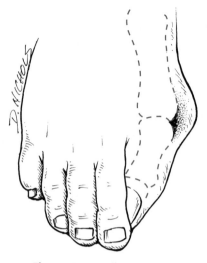

Fig. 17-25 Hallux valgus.

custom foot orthotic devices, or pads to dissipate stress and relieve pain. Modifications in activity may reduce symptoms profoundly. In an athletic population, changing from running activities to swimming or bicycling can reduce pain caused by the repetitive pounding of running. Ultimately, activity modification alone will not be enough to eliminate pain related to hallux valgus.

Many surgical options are available, depending on the severity of the deformity. General physical therapy management of postoperative bunionectomy is designed to reduce pain and swelling, improve first metatarsal phalangeal joint ROM, and increase strength to enable a return to normal daily activities. Initially after surgery, the patient wears a hard-soled shoe, progressing to walking boot, and then to shoes with a wide or open toe box. Gauze padding and toe spacers may be used to maintain proper alignment after the surgical procedure. Once the sutures are removed and the wounds closed, AROM exercises for both flexion and extension of the great toe can begin. Manual resistive toe extension and toe flexion exercises can begin as pain allows. Gait mechanics must be reviewed carefully and correct walking encouraged after bunionectomy. Usually weight-bearing patterns and restrictions of movement affect proper gait mechanics, especially the strength, power, and motion needed for toe-off. Restoration of joint motion and stability, and toe flexion and extension strength, form the foundation of the rehabilitation program.

LESSER TOE DEFORMITIES (HAMMER TOES, MALLET TOES, AND CLAW TOES)

Three distinct types of lesser toe deformities are hammer toes, mallet toes, and claw toes (Fig 17-26). All three deformities are worsened by wearing improper shoes (narrow toe box).

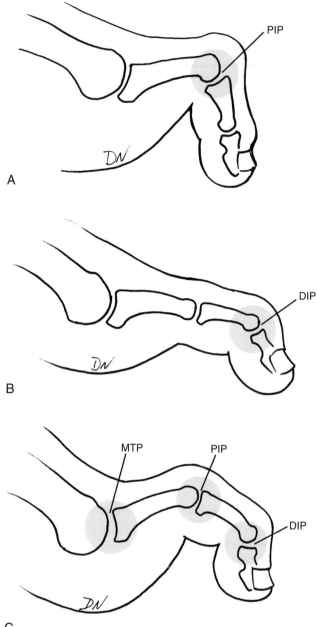

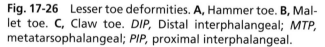

Fig. 17-26 Lesser toe deformities. **A,** Hammer toe. **B,** Mallet toe. **C,** Claw toe. *DIP,* Distal interphalangeal; *MTP,* metatarsophalangeal; *PIP,* proximal interphalangeal.

Hammer toe (see Fig. 17-26, *A*) is characterized by deformity of the metatarsophalangeal (MTP) joint, proximal interphalangeal (PIP) joint, and distal interphalangeal (DIP) joint. The MTP joint is either in neutral position or extension. The PIP joint is held in flexion with the DIP joint in either flexion or extension.

Mallet toe (see Fig. 17-26, *B*) is characterized by a neutral MTP joint, a neutral PIP joint, and a flexed DIP joint.

Claw toes (see Fig. 17-26, *C*) often are associated with neuromuscular disease and are similar in appearance to hammer toes. Claw toes are distinguished by MTP hyperextension, PIP flexion, and DIP flexion. This deformity usually results from "simultaneous contraction of the extensors and flexors."[79]

The physician or PT determines if the lesser toe deformity is either rigid (fixed) or flexible. Flexible deformities usually are correctable with conservative, passive measures, whereas fixed deformities may require surgery.

Intervention

Nonoperative conservative care of lesser toe deformities focuses on modifying activities that exacerbate pain, changing footwear to a wider, softer toe box (to avoid pressure and the occurrence of soft or hard callus formation over bony prominences), padding areas subjected to blistering and corn formation, and using supportive measures to reduce pain and swelling (such as over-the-counter or custom-molded foot orthotic devices). Ultrasound, stretching exercises for the toes, and foot and ankle strengthening exercises may help reduce pain and swelling.

Surgical repair is reserved for fixed or rigid deformities, although some flexible deformities also require operation. Typically, sutures and pins are removed about 3 weeks after surgery.[22] The patient is WBAT initially, with a progression to FWB as pain allows. The affected extremity is held in a rigid-solid open-toe postsurgical boot to protect the repair from unwanted excessive flexion and extension of the toes.

For approximately 6 weeks after surgery, taping, padding, and protecting the repair are emphasized before progressing to weight bearing toe-off proper gait mechanics. This time is necessary to protect the surgical repair and to allow for the healing of bone and tendons (tenotomies are done for flexible lesser toe deformities). Throughout the rehabilitation program, from the immediate postoperative period until discharge, maintain strength, flexibility, and aerobic fitness. The affected extremity may be strengthened with open-chain resistive exercises (knee extension and leg curls), and aerobic fitness can be achieved with a stationary bike ergometer with the seat height lowered to maintain a neutral ankle position at the bottom of the pedal stroke. If the patient cannot operate the bike in this fashion, the opposite, uninvolved extremity can be used alone (single-leg pedaling) using toe clips. A UBE also can be an effective aerobic conditioning tool during rehabilitation.

Once the pins and sutures are removed at 3 weeks, physical therapy management can begin. Ultrasound, AROM, and gentle stretching and strengthening exercises (open-chain progressing to closed-chain toe curls with a towel or marbles) can be employed. The toes must be protected from unwanted stress throughout the maximum-protection phase (6 to 8 weeks after surgery) of rehabilitation. Coughlin[22] recommends avoiding all running activities for 9 to 12 weeks after surgery to allow for proper healing.

COMMON MOBILIZATION TECHNIQUES FOR THE ANKLE, FOOT, AND TOES

Limitations of movement resulting from fibrosis after trauma, surgery, or disease of the foot, ankle, or toes frequently require specific mobilization procedures to regain normal joint function. Mobilization techniques typically are used in conjunction with thermal modalities to control pain and swelling and aid in relaxation; these modalities include hot packs, ultrasound, whirlpool baths, and ice packs. Active and passive exercises, specific stretching exercises, strengthening exercises (open progressing to closed chain), and proprioception tasks help the patient regain balance, coordination, and function. The choice of mobilization technique, direction of application, grades, amplitude of force, velocity, oscillations, and distractions is made by the PT based on the specific pathologic condition involved, tissue-healing constraints, and overall appropriateness with regard to the short- and long-term goals of the rehabilitation program.

The following techniques are general procedures used for a wide variety of specific joint limitations. These techniques can be modified by the PT depending on the specific nature of the limitations involved. This list is not intended to be a comprehensive review of all techniques for each joint of the ankle, foot, and toes. These methods are commonly used, easily practiced, effective procedures for treating a host of joint limitations. It is clinically relevant to restate that the delegation of selected mobilization techniques to be used by the PTA is entirely at the discretion of the PT, and peripheral joint mobilization is not universally accepted as a routine domain of practice of the PTA. Information concerning peripheral joint mobilization has been provided as a means to stimulate the PTA's awareness of the rationale for improving motion and for the reduction of pain as identified and prescribed by the PT.

Ankle Mobilization

Anterior and posterior glides are best performed with the patient in a supine or long-sitting position with the lower leg firmly and comfortably supported. For anterior glide of the calcaneus, the hand position, stabilization, and direction of force are similar to those for the anterior drawer test for ligament stability testing of the anterior talofibular ligament. One hand should be placed firmly on the distal anterior surface of the tibia and fibula. The application hand should be used to firmly cup the calcaneus and provide an anterior-directed force (Fig. 17-27).

The posterior glide technique is performed with the patient in the same position as the anterior glide. The distal tibia and fibula should be stabilized with the palm of one hand. The application hand should be placed on the dorsal surface of the talus to provide a posterior-directed force (Fig. 17-28).

Traction is achieved through long-axis distraction of the talus caudally from the tibia and fibula. The patient

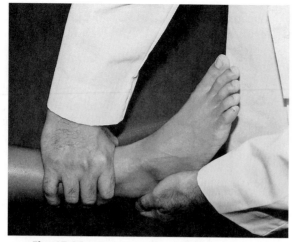

Fig. 17-27 Anterior glide of the calcaneus.

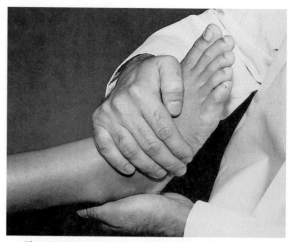

Fig. 17-29 Long-axis distraction of the talus.

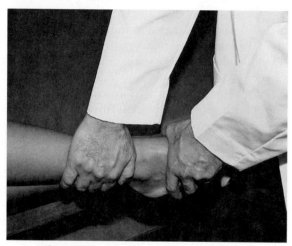

Fig. 17-28 Posterior glide of the talus.

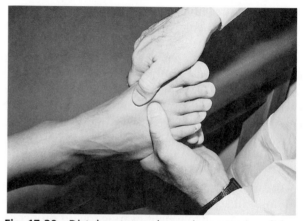

Fig. 17-30 Distal metatarsal anterior-posterior glides.

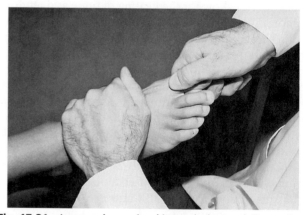

Fig. 17-31 Long-axis proximal interphalangeal distraction.

can be supine or prone with the lower leg firmly and comfortably supported. The dorsal surface of the talus should be firmly grasped with the open palm of one hand, while the other hand is used to firmly grasp and cup the calcaneus. The force should be applied simultaneously with both hands along the long axis of the tibia and fibula (Fig. 17-29), effectively distracting the talus from the mortise.

Metatarsal Mobilization

Distal metatarsal glides are performed while the patient is supine with the lower leg supported. The hand, thumb, and fingers of one hand should be used to stabilize the ray of the second metatarsal while the hand, thumb, and fingers of the application hand firmly grasp the first ray at the metatarsal head. Force should be applied in a plantar and dorsal direction (Fig. 17-30).

Proximal Interphalangeal Joint Mobilization

Long-axis distraction of the PIP joint is achieved by stabilizing the affected metatarsal ray with one hand while using the application hand to firmly grasp the affected

phalanx. The thumb and fingers apply long-axis traction (distraction) (Fig. 17-31).

Plantar and dorsal PIP glides are performed with the patient supine and the lower leg supported. One hand should be used to firmly grasp the first metatarsal ray at the metatarsal head. The thumb of the stabilizing hand must be placed on the dorsal surface of the metatarsal head. The application hand should be used to grasp the

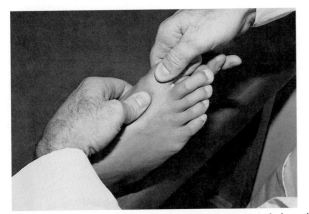

Fig. 17-32 Proximal interphalangeal plantar and dorsal glides.

proximal phalanx and apply a plantar and dorsal force while stabilizing the metatarsal head (Fig. 17-32).

❖ GLOSSARY

Calcaneus fracture: A calcaneus fracture that heals in a varus position locks the subtalar joint in inversion, creating a rigid transverse tarsal joint.

Posterior tibialis tendon: Rupture results in planovalgus, or flatfoot.

Syndesmosis: Ligaments responsible for maintaining stability of the distal tibiofibular articulation.

Talar tilt test: Tests integrity of both anterior talofibular ligament and calcaneofibular ligament. Both must be disrupted for a positive tilt.

Talus: No muscle attachment origin or insertion. Has a tenuous blood supply.

Tibial nerve: Passes behind the medial malleolus.

REFERENCES

1. Akeson WH, Amiel D, Abel MF, et al: Effects of immobilization on joints, *Clin Orthop Relat Res* 219:28–37, 1987.
2. Aktas S, Kocaoglu B: Open versus minimal invasive repair with Achillon device, *Foot Ankle Int* 30:391–397, 2009.
3. Alfredson H, Pietila T, Jonsson P, et al: Heavy-load eccentric calf muscle training for the treatment of chronic Achilles tendinosis, *Am J Sports Med* 26:360–366, 1998.
4. Andrish JT: In DeLee JD, Drez D, editors: *Orthopaedic sports medicine, principles and practice, The leg* vol 2, Philadelphia, 1994, Saunders.
5. Baldassin V, Gomes CR, Beraldo PS: Effectiveness of prefabricated and customized foot orthoses made from low-cost foam for noncomplicated plantar fasciitis: a randomized controlled trial, *Arch Phys Med Rehabil* 90:701–706, 2009.
6. Baumhauer JF, O'Brien T: Surgical consideration in the treatment of ankle instability, *J Athl Train* 37:458–462, 2002.
7. Beck BR, Osternig LR: Medial tibial stress syndrome. The location of muscles in the leg to symptoms, *J Bone Joint Surg Am* 76:1057–1061, 1994.
8. Bennett JE, Reinking MF, Pluemer B, et al: Factors contributing to the development of medial tibial stress syndrome, *J Orthop Sports Phys Ther* 31:504–510, 2001.
9. Beskin JL, Sanders RA, Hunter SC, et al: Surgical repair of Achilles tendon ruptures, *Am J Sports Med* 15:1–8, 1987.
10. Black HM, Brand RL: Injuries of the foot and ankle. In Scott NW, Nisonson B, Nicholas J, editors: *Principles of sports medicine*, Baltimore, 1984, Williams & Wilkins.
11. Bordelon RL: In DeLee JD, Drez D, editors: *Orthopaedic sports medicine: principles and practice, Heel pain* vol 2, Philadelphia, 1994, Saunders.
12. Brand RL, Collins MDF, Templeton T: Surgical repair of ruptured lateral ankle ligaments, *Am J Sports Med* 9:40–44, 1981.
13. Brody DM: Running injuries: prevention and management, *Clin Symp* 39(3):1–38, 1987.
14. Canale ST: Ankle injuries. In Crenshaw AH, editor: ed 7, *Campbell's operative orthopaedics* vol 3, St Louis, 1987, Mosby.
15. Ceccarelli F, Berti L, Giuriati L, et al: Percutaneous and minimally invasive techniques of Achilles tendon repair, *Clin Orthop Relat Res* 458:188–193, 2007.
16. Cheung JT, Zhang M, An KN: Effect of Achilles tendon loading on plantar fascia tension in the standing foot, *Clin Biomech (Bristol, Avon)* 21:194–203, 2006.
17. Chrisman OD, Snook G: Reconstruction of lateral ligament tears of the ankle: an experimental study and clinical evaluation of seven patients treated by a new modification of the Elmslie procedure, *J Bone Joint Surg Am* 51:904–912, 1969.
18. Clanton TO: In DeLee JD, Drez D, editors: *Orthopaedic sports medicine: principles and practice, sport shoes, insoles and orthoses* vol 2, Philadelphia, 1994, Saunders.
19. Cleland JA, Abbott JH, Kidd MO, et al: Manual physical therapy and exercise versus electrophysical agents and exercise in the management of plantar heel pain: a multicenter randomized clinical trial, *J Orthop Sports Phys Ther* 39:573–585, 2009.
20. Conrad JJ, Tannin AH: Trauma to the ankle. In Jahss MH, editor: *Disorders of the foot*, Philadelphia, 1982, Saunders.
21. Corte-Real NM, Moreira RM: Arthroscopic repair of chronic lateral ankle instability, *Foot Ankle Int* 30:213–217, 2009.
22. Coughlin MJ: In DeLee JD, Drez D, editors: *Orthopaedic sports medicine: principles and practice, Conditions of the forefoot* vol 2, Philadelphia, 1994, Saunders.
23. Curwin S, Stanish W: *Tendinitis: its etiology and treatment*, Lexington, Mass, 1984, Callamore Press.
24. D'Ambrosia RD: Orthotic devices in running injuries, *Clin Sports Med* 4:611–618, 1985.
25. Detmer DE: Chronic shin splints. Classification and management of medial tibial stress syndrome, *Sports Med* 3:436–446, 1986.
26. Digiovanni BF, Nawoczenski DA, Malay DP: Plantar fascia-specific stretching exercise improves outcomes in patients with chronic plantar fasciitis: a prospective clinical trial with two-year follow-up, *J Bone Joint Surg Am* 88:1775–1781, 2006.
27. Eckert WR, David EA: Acute rupture of the peroneal retinaculum, *J Bone Joint Surg Am* 58:670–673, 1976.
28. Edwards PH, Wright ML, Hartman JF: A practical approach for the differential diagnosis of chronic leg pain in the athlete, *Am J Sports Med* 33:1241–1249, 2005.
29. El Shewy MT, El Barbbary HM, Abdel-Ghani H: Repair of chronic rupture of the Achilles tendon using 2 intratendinous flaps from the proximal gastrocnemius-soleus complex, *Am J Sports Med* 37:1570–1577, 2009.
30. Evans DL: Recurrent instability of the ankle: a method of surgical treatment, *Proc R Soc Med* 46:343–344, 1953.
31. Ferran NA, Maffulli N: Epidemiology of sprains of the lateral ankle ligament complex, *Foot Ankle Clin* 11:659–662, 2006.
32. Ferran NA, Oliva F, Maffulli N: Ankle instability, *Sports Med Arthrosc* 17:139–145, 2009.
33. Ferran NA, Oliva F, Maffulli N: Recurrent subluxation of the peroneal tendons, *Sports Med* 36:839–846, 2006.

34. Fong DT, Chan YY, Mok KM, et al: Understanding acute ankle ligamentous sprain injury in sports, *Sports Med Arthrosc Rehabil Ther Technol* 30:1–14, 2009.

35. Frink M, Hildebrand F, Krettek C, et al: Compartment syndrome of the lower leg and foot, *Clin Orthop Relat Res* 468:940–950, 2010.

36. Gigante A, Moschini A, Verdenelli A, et al: Open versus percutaneous repair in the treatment of acute Achilles tendon rupture: a randomized prospective study, *Knee Surg Sports Traumatol Arthrosc* 16:204–209, 2008.

37. Gross ML, Napoli RC: Treatment of lower extremity injuries with orthotic shoe inserts. An overview, *Sports Med* 15:66–70, 1993.

38. Harper MC: The deltoid ligament: an evaluation of need for surgical repair, *Clin Orthop* 226:156–168, 1988.

39. Hassouna H, Singh D: Morton's metatarsalgia: pathogenesis, aetiology and current management, *Acta Orthop Belg* 71:646–655, 2005.

40. Hawke F, Burns J, Radford JA, et al: Custom-made foot orthoses for the treatment of foot pain, *Cochrane, Database Syst Rev* 16(3):CD006801, 2008.

41. Heckman DS, Gluck GS, Parekh SG: Tendon disorders of the foot and ankle, part 1: peroneal tendon disorders, *Am J Sports Med* 37:614–625, 2009.

42. Herbort M, Haber A, Zantop T, et al: *Arch Orthop Trauma Surg* 128:1273–1277, 2008.

43. Hintermann B, Knupp M, Pagenstert GI: Deltoid ligament injuries: diagnosis and management, *Foot Ankle Clin* 11:625–637, 2006.

44. Hintermann B, Renggli P: Anatomic reconstruction of the lateral ligaments of the ankle using a plantaris tendon graft in the treatment of chronic ankle joint instability, *Orthopade* 28:778–784, 1999.

45. Hohendorff B, Siepen W, Staub L: Treatment of acute Achilles tendon rupture: fibrin glue versus fibrin glue augmented with the plantaris longus tendon, *J Foot Ankle Surg* 48:439–446, 2009.

46. Hubbard TJ, Carpenter EM, Cordova ML: Contributing factors to medial tibial stress syndrome: a prospective investigation, *Med Sci Sports Exerc* 41:490–496, 2009.

47. Huffard B, O'Loughlin PF, Wright T, et al: Achilles tendon repair: Achillon system vs. Krackow suture: an anatomic in vitro biomechanical study, *Clin Biomech (Bristol, Avon)* 23:1158–1164, 2008.

48. Ibrahim SA: Surgical treatment of chronic Achilles tendon rupture, *J Foot Ankle Surg* 48:340–346, 2009.

49. Inglis AE, Sculco TP: Surgical repair of ruptures of the tendon Achilles, *Clin Orthop* 156:160–168, 1981.

50. Jackson BA, Schwane JA, Starcher BC: Effect of ultrasound therapy on the repair of Achilles tendon injuries in rats, *Med Sci Sports Exerc* 23, 271-176:1991.

51. Jackson DW: Shin-splints: an update, *Phys Sports Med* 6:101–161, 1978.

52. Jacobs D, Martens M, Van Audekercke R, et al: Comparison of conservative and operative treatment of Achilles tendon rupture, *Am J Sport Med* 6:107–111, 1978.

53. Kangas J, Pajala A, Ohtonen P, et al: Achilles tendon elongation after rupture repair: a randomized comparison of 2 postoperative regimens, *Am J Sports Med* 35:59–64, 2007.

54. Kannus P, Renstrom P: Current concepts review: treatment of acute tears of the lateral ligaments of the ankle, *J Bone Joint Surg Am* 73:305–312, 1991.

55. Keene JS: In DeLee JD, Drez D, editors: *Orthopaedic sports medicine: principles and practice, tendon injuries of the foot and ankle* vol 2, Philadelphia, 1994, Saunders.

56. Kerkhoffs GM, Handoll HH, deBie R, et al: Surgical versus conservative treatment for acute injuries of the lateral ligament complex of the ankle in adults, *Cochrane Database Syst Rev* 18(2):CD000380, 2007.

57. Khan RJ, Fick DP, Keogh A, et al: Interventions for treating acute Achilles tendon ruptures, *Cochrane Database Syst Rev* 21(1):CD003674, 2009.

58. Knobloch K: Eccentric training in Achilles tendinopathy: is it harmful to tendon microcirculation? *Br J Sports Med* 41:e2, 2007.

59. Komenda GA, Ferkel RD: Arthroscopic findings associated with the unstable ankle, *Foot Ankle Int* 20:708–713, 1999.

60. Labib SA, Rolf R, Dacus R, et al: The "Giftbox" repair of the Achilles tendon: a modification of the Karckow technique, *Foot Ankle Int* 30:410–414, 2009.

61. Lansdaal JR, Goslings JC, Reichart M, et al: The results of 163 Achilles tendon ruptures treated by a minimally invasive surgical technique and functional after treatment, *Injury* 38:839–844, 2007.

62. Lassiter TE, Malone TR, Garrett W: Injury to the lateral ligaments of the ankle, *Orthop Clin North Am* 20:629–640, 1989.

63. Leach RE, James S, Wasilewski S: Achilles tendinitis, *Am J Sports Med* 9:23–98, 1981.

64. Leach R: Acute ankle sprains: vigorous treatment for best results, *J Musculoskelet Res* 1:68–76, 1983.

65. Leach RE, Seavey MS, Salter DK: Results of surgery in athletes with plantar fasciitis, *Foot Ankle* 7:161–356, 1986.

66. Lee SY, McKeon P, Hertel J: Does the use of orthoses improve self-reported pain and function measures in patients with plantar fasciitis? A meta-analysis, *Phys Ther Sport* 10:12–18, 2009.

67. Lemont H, Ammirati KM, Usen N: Plantar fasciitis: a degenerative process (fasciosis) without inflammation, *J Am Podiatr Med Assoc* 93:234–237, 2003.

68. Lin CF, Gross ML, Weinhold P: Ankle syndesmosis injuries: anatomy, biomechanics, mechanism of injury, and clinical guidelines for diagnosis and intervention, *J Ortho Sports Phys Ther* 36:372–384, 2006.

69. Maffulli N, Ajis A: Management of chronic ruptures of the Achilles tendon, *J Bone Joint Surg Am* 90:348–1360, 2008.

70. Maffulli N, Ferran NA: Management of acute and chronic ankle instability, *J Am Acad Orthop Surg* 16:608–615, 2008.

71. Magee DJ: Lower leg, ankle and foot. *Orthopaedic physical assessment*, ed 2, Philadelphia, 1992, Saunders.

72. Magnusson HI, Ahlborg HG, Karlsson C, et al: Low regional tibial bone density in athletes with medial tibial stress syndrome normalizes after recovery from symptoms, *Am J Sports Med* 31:596–600, 2003.

73. Marti R: Dislocation of the peroneal tendons, *Am J Sports Med* 5:19–22, 1977.

74. McBryde A: In DeLee JD, Drez D, editors: *Orthopaedic sports medicine: principles and practice, Stress fractures of the foot and ankle* vol 2, Philadelphia, 1994, Saunders.

75. McPoil TG, Martin RL, Cornwall MW, et al: Heel pain-plantar fasciitis: clinical practice guidelines linked to the international classification of function, disability, and health from the orthopaedic section of the American Physical Therapy Association, *J Ortho Sports Phys Ther* 38:A1–A18, 2008.

76. McRae R: *Practical fracture treatment*, New York, 1994, Churchill Livingstone.

77. McVey ED, Palmieri RM, Docherty CL, et al: Arthrogenic muscle inhibition in the leg muscles of subjects exhibiting functional ankle instability, *Foot Ankle Int* 26:1055–1061, 2005.

78. Michael RH, Holder LE: The soleus syndrome: a cause of medial tibial stress (shin splints), *Am J Sports Med* 13:27–94, 1985.

79. Miller M: *Review of orthopaedics*, Philadelphia, 1992, Saunders.

80. Moen MH, Tol JL, Weir A, et al: Medial tibial stress syndrome: a critical review, *Sports Med* 39:523–546, 2009.

81. Myerson MS: In Jahss MH, editor: *Disorders of the foot and ankle: medical and surgical management*, ed 2, *Injuries to the forefoot and toes* vol 2, Philadelphia, 1991, Saunders.

82. Nawoczneski DA, Janisse DJ: Foot orthoses in rehabilitation—what's new, *Clin Sports Med* 23:157–167, 2004.

83. Neufeld SK, Cerrato R: Plantar fasciitis: evaluation and treatment, *J Am Acad Orthop Surg* 16:338–346, 2008.

84. Nigg BM, Nurse MA, Stefanyshyn DJ: Shoe inserts and orthotics for sport and physical activities, *Med Sci Sports Exerc* 31:S421–S428, 1999.

85. Nistor L: Surgical and nonsurgical treatment of Achilles tendon rupture, *J Bone Joint Surg Am* 63:394–399, 1981.

86. Norkus SA, Floyd RT: The anatomy and mechanisms of syndesmotic ankle sprains, *J Athl Train* 36:68–73, 2001.

87. Osborne HR, Allison GT: Treatment of plantar fasciitis by LowDye taping and iontophoresis: short term results of a double blinded, randomized, placebo controlled clinical trial of dexamethasone and acetic acid, *Brit J Sports Med* 40:545–549, 2006.

88. Pajala A, Kangas J, Siira P, et al: Augmented compared with nonaugmented surgical repair of a fresh total Achilles tendon rupture. A prospective randomized study, *J Bone Joint Surg Am* 91:1092–1100, 2009.

89. Porter DA: Evaluation and treatment of ankle syndesmosis injuries, *Instr Course Lect* 58:575–581, 2009.

90. Pugh KJ, Wolinsky PR, McAndrew MP, et al: Tibial pilon fractures: a comparison of treatment methods, *J Trauma* 47:937–941, 1999.

91. Renstrom PAFH, Kannus P: In DeLee JD, Drez D, editors: *Orthopaedic sports medicine: principles and practice, Injuries of the foot and ankle* vol 2, Philadelphia, 1994, Saunders.

92. Riddle DL: Foot and ankle. In Richardson JK, Iglarsh ZA, editors: *Clinical orthopaedic physical therapy*, Philadelphia, 1994, Saunders.

93. Riehl R: Rehabilitation of lower leg injuries. In Prentice WE, editor: *Rehabilitation techniques in sports medicine*, ed 2, St Louis, 1994, Mosby.

94. Rompe JD: Plantar fasciopathy, *Sports Med Arthrosc* 17:100–104, 2009.

95. Roos E, Engstrom M, Soderberg B: Foot orthoses for the treatment of plantar fasciitis, *Foot Ankle Int* 27:606–611, 2006.

96. Ross FD: The relationship of abnormal foot pronation to hallux abducto valgus–a pilot study, *Prosthet Orthot Int* 10:72–78, 1986.

97. Safran MR, Benedetti RS, Bartolozzi AR III, et al: Lateral ankle sprains: a comprehensive review: part 1: etiology, pathomechanics, histopathogenesis, and diagnosis, *Med Sci Sports Exerc* 31(7 Suppl):S429–437, 1999.

98. Safran MR, Zachazewski JE, Benedetti RS, et al: Lateral ankle sprains: a comprehensive review part 2: treatment and rehabilitation with an emphasis on the athlete, *Med Sci Sports Exerc* 31(7 Suppl):S438–47, 1999.

99. Sanchez M, Anitua E, Azofra J, et al: Comparison of surgically repaired Achilles tendon tears using platelet-rich fibrin matrices, *Am J Sports Med* 35:245–251, 2007.

100. Saxena A, Muffulli N, Nguyen A, et al: Wound complications from surgeries pertaining to the Achilles tendon: an analysis of 219 surgeries, *J Am Podiatr Med Assoc* 98:95–101, 2008.

101. Schepsis AA, Jones H, Haas AL: Achilles tendon disorders in athletes, *Am J Sports Med* 30:287–305, 2002.

102. Stanitski CL, McMaster JH, Scranton PE, et al: On the nature of stress fractures, *Am J Sports Med* 6:391–396, 1978.

103. Staples OS: Ruptures of the fibular collateral ligaments of the ankle. Result study of immediate surgical treatment, *J Bone Joint Surg Am* 57:101–107, 1975.

104. Stormont DM, Morrey BF, An KN, et al: Stability of the loaded ankle, *Am J Sports Med* 13:295–300, 1985.

105. Stover CN, Bryan D: Traumatic dislocation of peroneal tendons, *Am J Surg* 103:180–186, 1962.

106. Suchak AA, Bostick GP, Beaupre LA, et al: The influence of early weight-bearing compared with non-weight-bearing after surgical repair of the Achilles tendon, *J Bone Joint Surg Am* 90:1876–1883, 2008.

107. Suchak AA, Spooner C, Reid DC, et al: Postoperative rehabilitation protocols for Achilles tendon rupture: a meta-analysis, *Clin Orthop Relat Res* 445:216–221, 2006.

108. Suqimoto K, Takakura Y, Okahashi K, et al: Chondral injuries of the ankle with recurrent lateral instability: an arthroscopic study, *J Bone Joint Surg Am* 91:99–106, 2009.

109. Thati S, Carlson C, Maskill JD, et al: Tibial compartment syndrome and the cavovarus foot, *Foot Ankle Clin* 13:275–305, 2008.

110. Toomey EP: Plantar heel pain, *Foot Ankle Clin* 14:229–245, 2009.

111. Twaddke BC, Poon P: Early motion for Achilles tendon ruptures: is surgery important? A randomized, prospective study, *Am J Sports Med* 35:2033–2038, 2007.

112. Tweed JL, Campbell JA, Avil SJ: Biomechanical risk factors in the development of medial tibial stress syndrome in distance runners, *J Am Podiatr Med Assoc* 98:436–444, 2008.

113. Uchiyama E, Nomura A, Takeda Y, et al: A modified operation for Achilles tendon ruptures, *Am J Sports Med* 35:1739–1743, 2007.

114. Uh BS, Beynnon BD, Helie BV, et al: The benefit of a single-leg strength training program for the muscles around the untrained ankle, *Am J Sports Med* 28:568–573, 2000.

115 Valovich McLeod TC: The effectiveness of balance training programs on reducing the incidence of ankle sprains in adolescent athletes, *J Sport Rehabil* 17:316–323, 2008.

116. Wang CJ, Wang FS, Yang KD, et al: Long-term results of extracorporeal shockwave treatment for plantar fasciitis, *Am J Sports Med* 34:592–596, 2006.

117. Watson-Jones R: Recurrent forward dislocation of the ankle joint, *J Bone Joint Surg Br* 34:519, 1952.

118. Wilder RP, Sethi S: Overuse injuries: tendinopathies, stress fractures, compartment syndrome, and shin splints, *Clin Sports Med* 23:55–81, 2004.

119. Williams DS III, McClay IS, Hamill J: Arch structure and injury patterns in runners, *Clin Biomech (Bristol, Avon)* 16:341–347, 2001.

120. Wittstein J, Moorman CT III, Levin LS: Endoscopic compartment release for chronic exertional compartment syndrome, *J Surg Orthop Adv* 17:119–121, 2008.

121. Yates B, White S: The incidence and risk factors in the development of medial tibial stress syndrome among naval recruits, *Am J Sports Med* 32:772–780, 2004.

122. Young B, Walker Strunce J, Boyles R: A combined treatment approach emphasizing impairment-based manual physical therapy for plantar heel pain: a case series, *J Orthop Sports Phys Ther* 34:725–733, 2004.

REVIEW QUESTIONS

Short Answer

1. Chronic instability may follow an inversion ankle sprain. Name the two types of instabilities associated with chronic ankle sprains.

2. Name the three major ligaments that represent the lateral ligament complex of the ankle.

3. Name the pathology shown in the figure.

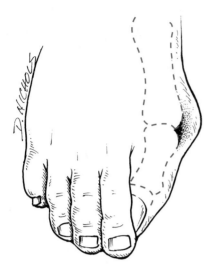

4. Match the following figures with the appropriate name of the deformity:
Claw toe _____ Hammer toe _____ Mallet toe _____

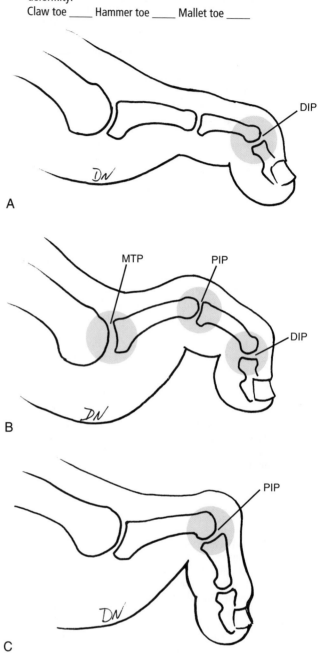

True/False

5. During the early recovery (acute phase) period of an inversion ankle sprain, it is imperative to instruct the patient to write the alphabet with the injured ankle.
6. Complete deltoid ligament sprains occur in combination with ankle fractures.
7. Mechanical instability may require surgery to stabilize the ankle.
8. Treatment for a ruptured Achilles tendon is always with surgery.
9. The loss of strength is less if the ruptured Achilles tendon is treated nonsurgically.

10. The initial management of pilon fractures usually involves an open reduction with internal fixation procedure, external fixator, or skeletal traction.
11. In severe cases of plantar fasciitis, the physician may inject a local corticosteroid to reduce pain and swelling.
12. In cases of plantar fasciitis where all conservative measures fail to bring significant results, the physician may elect to perform a fasciotomy or excision of a calcaneal exostosis.
13. Treatment of Morton neuroma is always with surgical excision.
14. The removal of tight shoes may significantly reduce painful symptoms associated with hallux valgus.
15. Lesser toe deformities are characterized as either rigid or flexible.

18

Orthopedic Management of the Knee

Kenneth Bush
Justin Rossetter
Matthew Smith
Michael Allen

LEARNING OBJECTIVES

1. Identify common ligament injuries of the knee.
2. Discuss general methods of management and rehabilitation of common ligament injuries of the knee.
3. Identify and describe common meniscal injuries of the knee.
4. Discuss common methods of management and rehabilitation of meniscal injuries of the knee.
5. Discuss surgical and postoperative management of articular cartilage injuries.
6. Describe common methods of management and rehabilitation of patellofemoral disease of the knee.
7. Identify and describe common patella, supracondylar femur, and proximal tibia fractures.
8. Describe common methods of management and rehabilitation of fractures around the knee.
9. Identify and describe methods of management and rehabilitation after knee arthroplasty and high tibial osteotomy.
10. Describe common mobilization techniques for the knee.

KEY TERMS

Anterior drawer test
Closed kinetic chain (CKC) exercises

Hughston jerk test
Lachman examination
Pivot shift test

Quadriceps angle (Q angle)

CHAPTER OUTLINE

The physical therapist assistant (PTA) is frequently challenged to safely and effectively manage acute, chronic, and postsurgical orthopedic conditions of the knee. This chapter presents common pathologic conditions of the ligaments, meniscus lesions, patellofemoral diseases, extensor mechanism disorders, and fractures of the knee, as well as rehabilitation procedures related to total knee joint replacement. This chapter gives the PTA an appreciation of various knee ailments, mechanisms of injury, and specific tissue healing constraints, and provides an introduction to the rationale behind criterion-based rehabilitation programs for the knee.

Although the knee at first glance appears to be a simple synovial joint, its position and ligamentous and soft tissue support actually reveal a very complex structure. Because of this complexity, the PTA is strongly encouraged to review pertinent knee joint anatomy and functional mechanics before and throughout this study.

LIGAMENT INJURIES

Ligament injuries of the knee refer to various degrees of sprains that may lead to ruptures of the ligament, manifested by loss of joint function. Knee ligament sprains and joint instability are complex problems involving various degrees of straight-plane or combined rotatory instability. Knee ligament sprains may be defined as follows:

■ Grade I: An incomplete stretching of collagen ligament fibers resulting in minimal pain, minimal or no swelling, no loss of joint function, and no clinical or functional instability.
■ Grade II (second degree): A partial loss of ligament fiber continuity. A few collagen ligament fibers may be completely torn; however, most of the ligament remains intact. This degree of sprain is characterized by moderate pain, moderate swelling, and some loss of joint function and stability.

■ Grade III (rupture): The entire collagen ligament fiber bundles are completely torn. There is no continuity within the body of the ligament. This is usually characterized by profound pain, intense swelling, loss of joint function, and instability.

Anterior Cruciate Ligament Injuries

The anterior cruciate ligament (ACL) primarily resists anterior tibial translation on the femur; it also prevents hyperextension and extreme varus, valgus, and rotational movements around the knee.[71] The cruciate ligaments are intracapsular structures, which can produce a joint effusion when injured. This anatomic relationship is contrasted with the medial and lateral collateral ligaments, which are extracapsular structures. When the medial collateral ligament (MCL) is sprained, there is generally less swelling and no intraarticular effusion because the resultant bleeding from the injured tissues can evacuate the area and the fluid is not restrained within the joint capsule.

Etiology

It is well published that female athletes tear their ACLs at a higher rate than their male counterparts.[1] The common mechanism for both contact and noncontact injuries results in a combined force of external rotation of the hip, valgus stress at the knee joint, and internal tibial rotation with or without knee hyperextension while the affected foot is planted (Fig. 18-1).[24,73,74,77,91,97]

Clinical Evaluation

The PTA must be aware of various clinical ligament stability tests to accurately and effectively communicate changes in a patient's stability to the supervising physical therapist (PT) and physician. Although ligament stability tests are part of the initial evaluation procedures used by the physician and PT, the PTA can better understand the static and dynamic restraints of the knee and develop a more comprehensive view of rehabilitation when exposed to the rudimentary concepts of ligament stability testing.

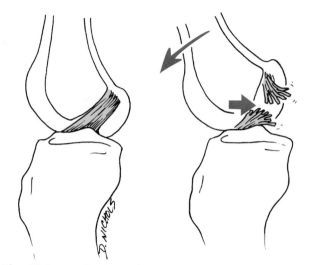

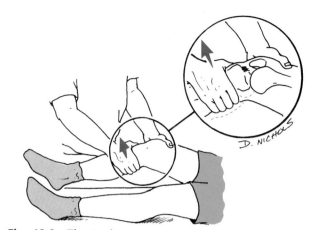

Fig. 18-1 Mechanism of injury to the anterior cruciate ligament (ACL). Typically, the ACL is injured in a noncontact deceleration mechanism of combined forces of external tibial rotation, valgus stress, internal tibial rotation, and knee hyperextension.

Fig. 18-2 The Lachman examination. This examination tests the stability of the anterior cruciate ligament (ACL) with the knee flexed 25° to 30°. If the tibia can be displaced anteriorly in reference to the stabilized distal femur, then an injured ACL should be considered.

Perhaps the most common, specific, and clinically useful ligament stability test for the ACL is the **Lachman examination** (Fig. 18-2).[47] The patient is supine on an examining table with the affected knee flexed to approximately 25° to 30°. One hand is used to stabilize the distal femur, and the other hand grasps the proximal tibia. An anterior and posterior force is gently directed to the proximal tibia. The integrity of the ACL should be observed, and the degree of anterior tibial translation should be noted.

The **anterior drawer test** (Fig. 18-3) is another clinical examination used to approximate the degree of anterior tibial translation relative to the fixed femur. This examination is a less sensitive test to challenge the integrity of the ACL, and is instead thought to assess the meniscotibial ligaments and the mobility of the menisci on the tibia.[47] The examination is performed with the patient supine and the affected knee flexed to approximately 90°. Stabilize the affected limb by sitting on the patient's foot. Both hands should be used to grasp the proximal posterior tibia, with the thumbs on the anterior joint line of the knee. An anterior and posterior force should be exerted to the proximal tibia, and the amount of joint separation of the tibia relative to the femur should be observed.

Other relevant tests for the stability of the ACL incorporate multidirectional rotation examinations to acknowledge the presence of anterolateral rotator instability (ALRI), anteromedial rotatory instability (AMRI), posteromedial rotatory instability (PMRI), and posterolateral rotatory instability (PLRI). ALRI is the more common multiplanar instability encountered.[47,91] The **Hughston jerk test** and **pivot shift test** are commonly used examinations to sublux and reduce the tibia relative to the femur.[47]

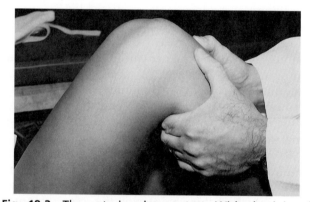

Fig. 18-3 The anterior drawer test. With the injured knee flexed to 90°, the clinician grasps the proximal tibia and provides an anteriorly directed force. If the tibia displaces anteriorly in reference to the stabilized distal femur, then the anterior cruciate ligament may be considered injured.

Throughout the performance of the examination, complete muscle relaxation of the hamstrings, quadriceps, and gastrocnemius–soleus muscle group must be maintained. Swelling, intraarticular effusion, and muscle spasm falsely stabilize the knee, rendering the examination meaningless.[51]

Operative Management

The PTA must recognize the various surgical procedures used to correct functional instabilities related to ACL injuries and be aware of the short- and long-term ramifications of ligament healing to more effectively deliver sound rehabilitation. Therefore this section provides a rudimentary description of the most common ACL surgical procedures as they relate to the scope and practice of the PTA.

An autograft reconstruction uses tissue from the body of the patient. Various tissues are used for grafts, including the gracilis tendon, fascia lata, semitendinosus tendon, and quadriceps muscle tendon. The bone–patellar tendon–bone (BPTB) autograft is a commonly used graft because of its boney anchor points. The BPTB and bundled gracilis and semitendinosus autografts have all been shown to have greater tensile strength to sheer forces than the original ACL.[20,72] An allograft refers to biologic tissue taken from a human cadaver. The major risks of using allograft involve disease transmission and problems with effective sterilization procedures that do not weaken the graft.[28]

The arthroscopic central one-third BPTB autograft procedure involves harvesting the graft from the involved knee (Fig. 18-4, A) and surgically routing this structure through tunnels placed in the femur and tibia in a way that duplicates normal ACL anatomy, then securing the graft to the bone to allow for stable healing (Fig. 18-4, B-C). A small incision is made in the knee, and a small diameter drainage tube is inserted to help evacuate the joint of residual bleeding, which may increase the risk of arthrofibrosis if allowed to accumulate. This small drain is usually removed after a few days when the bleeding is controlled. Even with the placement of the drain, postoperative arthrofibrosis is a clinically significant problem that can occur.[45] Sterile bandages are placed over the incisions, and the patient's leg is often placed in a hinged brace locked in 0° of flexion.

Healing of the graft after surgery

Ligament healing processes and revascularization of graft material are vital concerns in the prescribed rehabilitation program designed by the supervising PT. The appropriate progression of the rehabilitation program depends on the PTA's awareness of the various stages of healing after an autograft procedure. Once the graft is harvested and surgically routed within the knee, it begins a gradual process of avascular necrosis over the first 6 to 8 weeks.[28] The graft gradually loses strength and is quite fragile during the first 2 months after surgery, so excessive loads and forces that would compromise the healing of the graft must be avoided during this time period. The graft slowly revascularizes, and at approximately 3 months the tensile strength of the graft is less than 50% of its original strength.[28,75] Graft strength may take as long as a year to mature and may never reach preoperative tensile strength after the graft cell death and subsequent revascularization process.

Postoperative rehabilitation

The rehabilitation program after ACL reconstruction is designed to protect the graft; reduce pain and swelling; increase joint motion while improving strength, endurance (local muscular endurance, as well as aerobic fitness), flexibility, and proprioception; and ultimately return the

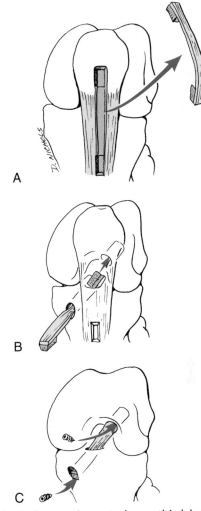

Fig. 18-4 Arthroscopic central one-third bone–patellar tendon–bone (BPTB) autograft procedure. **A,** BPTB harvest. A pedicle of bone from the tibial tubercle and patella is removed along with a full-thickness graft of the patellar tendon to be used to anatomically reconstruct the anterior cruciate ligament. **B,** The graft is placed within the knee joint, through tunnels drilled in the tibia and femur. **C,** The graft tissue and bone pedicles are secured with anchor screws.

knee to full function. This task is organized sequentially and is constantly modified, based on the patient's individual response to surgery and rehabilitation. The PT and PTA must work together to assess and adjust programs based on the individual's ability and goals.

In general terms, ACL reconstruction rehabilitation can be organized into three broad, interconnecting phases[91]:

1. Maximum-protection phase: From the first day postoperatively to approximately the sixth week after surgery.
2. Moderate-protection phase: From approximately the 7th to the 12th weeks after surgery.
3. Minimum-protection phase: From the 13th week after surgery until return to activity.

This section reviews each phase separately and introduces the PTA to the many variables and individual differences among patients. The importance of reassessment of initial evaluation data and the need for open communication and teamwork with the supervising PT cannot be emphasized too strongly.

Maximum-protection phase (0-8 weeks). As the graft slowly loses its strength (6 to 8 weeks after surgery), excessive loads and forces that stress the ACL must be avoided. These forces are controlled primarily by joint protection with range-limiting hinged braces and avoidance of anterior tibial translation, shearing forces, and rotational motions.

Control of swelling is important throughout each phase of rehabilitation. Postoperative swelling can have a profound negative effect on the progress of the patient, even with suction drains inserted at the time of surgery. Swelling inhibits muscle contractions, contributes significantly to pain, limits joint motion, and can stimulate arthrofibrosis.[85] Cryotherapy, elevation of the limb, and the use of a compression wrap help to minimize swelling.

The patient's ability to achieve early active range of motion (AROM) is an essential component of the maximum-protection phase. Patellar motion (caudal, cephalic, medial, and lateral glide) must be an immediate goal for the restoration of knee motion. Scarring from the graft harvest site and the suprapatellar pouch typically inhibits free patellar motion and full knee ROM.[85] Initially the PTA must provide gentle stretching of the patella (Fig. 18-5, A-C) and instruct the patient to perform these stretches two to three times daily. Generally, full knee extension is achieved soon after surgery; if not, passive prone or supine knee extension stretches can be used judiciously to gradually increase knee extension (Fig. 18-5, D). In addition to active and passive knee flexion and extension, some authors advocate the use of a continuous passive motion (CPM) device for a limited time very early in this phase.[28,76,91] The use of a CPM device has been suggested to help maintain a normal articular surface as well as to help evacuate synovial joint hemarthrosis and aid in the prevention of joint contracture.[28,76,91] The use of CPM generally is limited to the period immediately after hospitalization.[28]

Weight-bearing status remains a controversial subject in the literature. In general, weight bearing with crutches is allowed as tolerated immediately after surgery, and patients should be full weight bearing somewhere between 2 and 6 weeks from surgery.[21,28,91]

The primary focus of strengthening the postoperative ACL patient during the maximum-protection phase is to encourage quadriceps control and hamstring strength. Strengthening exercises during the maximum-protection phase focus on isometric co-contractions of the quadriceps and hamstrings. Hamstring strengthening is emphasized during this phase of maximum protection

because they act as dynamic stabilizers to limit anterior tibial shearing forces.[28,63,76,77,91] Both standing leg curls and supine leg curls can be initiated during this phase if a brace is used.

Exercises that do not strain the ACL include[10]:

■ Isometric hamstring muscle contraction exercises at 15°, 30°, 60°, and 90°
■ Isometric quadriceps contractions at 0° and 90°
■ Simultaneous contraction of the quadriceps and hamstring muscles at 60° and 90°
■ Active flexion-extension motion of the knee from 60° to full flexion[81]
■ Passive flexion-extension motion of the knee without muscle contraction

Open kinetic chain (OKC) active knee extension, with or without resistance, causes an anterior tibial translation force relative to the femur that stresses the new graft. The largest anterior tibial translational forces occur between the knee flexion angles of 30° to 50°.[81] This stated knee range of motion (ROM) should be completely avoided when performing OKC knee extension exercise in the early rehabilitation phases of ACL reconstruction.

Four-way hip (flexion, extension, abduction, and adduction) and calf-strengthening exercises as well as stationary bicycling are also encouraged during this phase. The criteria to be achieved by the patient before advancing to the moderate-protection phase include the following:

■ ROM from 0° extension to 120° of flexion
■ Full weight bearing (FWB) with normal gait mechanics
■ Quadriceps control
■ Hamstring control
■ Controlled pain and swelling
■ A minimum of 6 weeks from the day of surgery

Moderate-protection phase (6-12 weeks). To advance to this level the patient must be FWB and should be able to demonstrate proper gait mechanics. Immobilization is generally discontinued around the fifth or sixth week postoperatively.[21] Control of pain and swelling with the use of cryotherapy, compression, and elevation continues as indicated.

Closed kinetic chain (CKC) exercises are a system of interdependent articulated links in which motion at one joint produces motion at all other joints in the system in a predictable manner. CKC exercises and progressive proprioceptive tasks (to stimulate the afferent neural input system) are initiated and progressed throughout this phase. Gradual CKC progressive loads are essential to encourage functional muscle control, confidence in the use of the affected limb, and help stimulate neuromuscular coordination. Initial instruction in CKC exercises begins with the patient braced to protect the healing graft. Standing and shifting of body weight from the nonaffected limb to the affected limb is a safe and appropriate introduction to CKC exercises. Once the patient demonstrates confidence, muscle control, and stability, the brace is removed (with prior

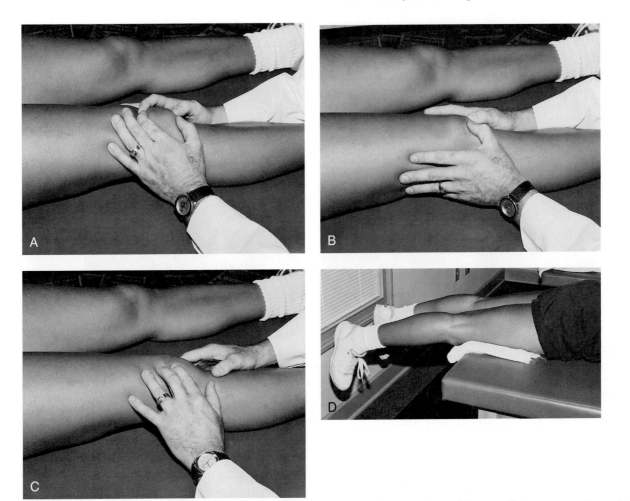

Fig. 18-5 Postoperative manual patellar stretching is used to enhance knee motion. If the patella becomes adhered to surrounding tissues, normal knee flexion and extension cannot occur. **A,** A caudal (inferior)-directed force applied to the patella. **B,** A cephalic (superior)-directed force. **C,** The patella being directed medially. **D,** Prone passive knee-extension stretch. Note the application of a folded towel under the thigh to elevate the leg and avoid compression of the patella and patellar tendon against the end of the table.

consultation and concurrence from the supervising PT) and the patient is allowed to shift weight without braced support. The leg press is used as a CKC exercise in a short-arc motion early in the moderate-protection phase while the patient is braced (Fig. 18-6). Progressive ROM exercises are allowed as tolerated. Standing wall slides also are introduced during the moderate-protection phase if the affected limb is braced and the tibia is kept vertical to avoid an anterior tibial translation force (Fig. 18-7). The short-arc step-up is an excellent exercise used to stimulate quadriceps control and strength. A biofeedback system can be used in conjunction with step-ups to encourage appropriate quadriceps firing patterns (Fig. 18-8).

Stationary cycling should be progressed with added time and resistance throughout this phase. The stationary bicycle is used initially to encourage ROM, but during the middle and later stages of this phase the bicycle can be used as an aerobic conditioning tool if the patient has achieved the required ROM, strength, and

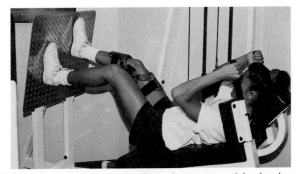

Fig. 18-6 Closed kinetic chain leg press with the knee braced. The uninvolved leg is used to support the weight and provide confidence during the application of the short-arc leg press.

stability to perform endurance activities. Stair-steppers and inclined walking can also be introduced during this phase if the ROM and intensity of the resistance on the apparatus are modified and controlled initially to allow for protected joint motion (Fig. 18-9). To stimulate

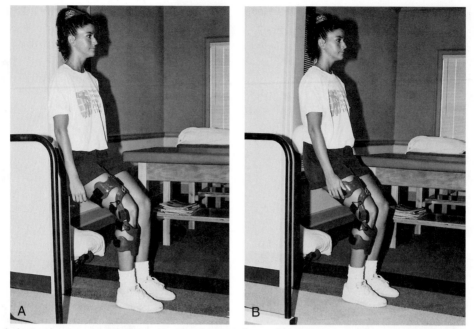

Fig. 18-7 Closed-chain short-arc wall slides. As the knee is braced to avoid unwanted anterior tibial translation, the patient is introduced to quadriceps strengthening (concentrically, eccentrically, and isometrically) in a vertical weight-bearing position. **A,** A partial wall slide with the patient holding an isometric position. **B,** Note the use of a small ball placed behind the patient to encourage greater balance and control.

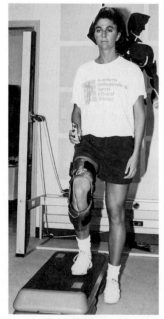

Fig. 18-8 The use of portable biofeedback or electrical muscle stimulation can be used to enhance greater quadriceps control during short-arc step-ups.

greater strength and local muscular endurance of the quadriceps, the patient can be instructed to perform the stair-stepper in a reverse manner.

Throughout this phase the patient is encouraged to maintain patellar, hamstring, and quadriceps-stretching exercises; normal gait mechanics; a general fitness

program of strength and endurance activities that do not stress the affected limb; ice application after exercises; and joint-protection principles.

Criteria that must be met by the patient before progressing to the next phase include the following:

■ Full ROM (flexion, extension, and patellar mobility)
■ Normalized FWB gait and removal of brace as indicated
■ Improved quadriceps strength
■ Improved hamstring strength
■ Continued control of pain and swelling
■ A minimum of 12 to 13 weeks from the day of surgery

Minimum-protection phase (12-24 weeks). The minimum-protection phase signals the return to more normalized activities and the introduction of more challenging functional activities. Isolated knee ligament stability tests (e.g., Lachman test, anterior drawer test, and pivot shift test) are performed at the discretion of the PT and physician, usually during the moderate-protection and minimum-protection phases of rehabilitation. Ongoing documentation of the stability of the affected limb is essential to justify progression to more challenging exercises and quantify the clinical results of the surgery. The use of isokinetic testing of the involved limb is also left to the judgment of the PT and physician. Generally, isokinetic examinations are reserved for the moderate-protection and minimum-protection phases. Certain precautions must be taken to minimize the tibial translation forces produced with isokinetic testing and training to protect the healing graft. Positioning the pad

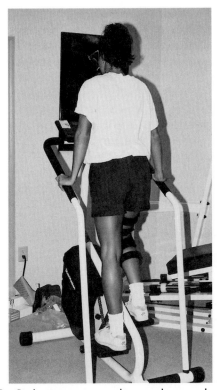

Fig. 18-9 Stair-steppers can be used as a closed-chain functional (stair climbing) exercise, provided the knee is braced and the intensity controlled to avoid excessive unwanted forces.

proximally on the tibia helps to protect the reconstructed ACL against excessive anterior tibial translation forces.[91]

More progressive proprioceptive exercises can be initiated when clinical testing demonstrates improved strength, neuromuscular control, and stability of the ligament. The use of a balance board and minitrampoline further challenges the mechanoreceptor system (Fig. 18-10). Standing knee extension with resistance provided by elastic tubing is an excellent CKC exercise that encourages quadriceps control in more functional positions (Fig. 18-11).

A pool running program progressing to a straight-line interval land running program can start later in this phase. Plyometric exercise is also suggested for individuals returning to athletic activities. The inclusion of bilateral ballistic movements, progressing to unilateral movement should be included in the rehabilitation of athletes in order to prepare these individuals for the demands of their sport. It is important to understand that strengthening and plyometric exercises in this phase should not only be progressed from bilateral to unilateral, but also progressed from sagittal, to frontal, to transverse planes of movement.

Progressive strengthening of the entire lower extremity includes isokinetic velocity spectrum training, and isotonic eccentric quadriceps strengthening. The PTA must be constantly aware that rehabilitation after ACL reconstruction involves the entire body and not just the affected limb. Care must be taken to involve all muscle

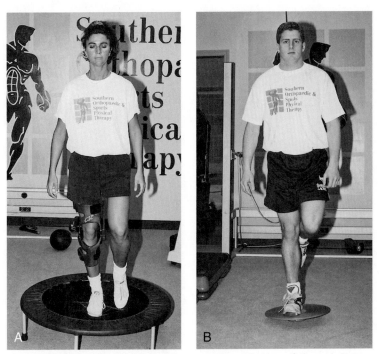

Fig. 18-10 Closed kinetic chain balance and proprioception exercises. **A,** Use of the minitrampoline is a challenging and effective balancing exercise. **B,** Single-leg standing on a wobble board.

groups, as well as the sensory input systems and aerobic system throughout each phase of rehabilitation. Returning the patient to functional activities is the primary focus of the rehabilitation team.

Frequently, other structures are injured along with the ACL. The rehabilitation plan outlined does not account for possible injury to the meniscus, posterior cruciate ligament (PCL), MCL, lateral collateral ligament (LCL), or joint capsule; associated fractures; or impaired neurovascular structures. The complex nature and vast array of combined injuries dictates modifications at each level of rehabilitation and prolongs the healing process. Common injuries associated with an ACL rupture include a concomitant MCL sprain with a lateral meniscus tear.[6,84] In regard to an injured MCL, or débrided meniscus, there will not be a large alteration to the rehabilitation process. In the case of a meniscus repair, it is common for the ACL reconstruction and the meniscal repair to be staged at different times ranging from 3 to 5 months apart. This is done to individually maximize the rehabilitation outcomes of the two surgeries. It has been found that surgical repair of both the ACL and meniscus at the same time yields poorer outcomes than staging the surgeries at separate healing intervals.[14]

Nonoperative Rehabilitation

The PTA also must be aware that isolated ACL injuries may dictate a nonsurgical course of treatment. The physician must decide if the patient is best suited for surgery or should be treated nonoperatively. If the patient is treated nonoperatively, the rehabilitation program progresses at a faster pace, although the injured knee must still be protected and allowed to heal from the trauma of the initial injury. The maximum-protection phase should range from 2 to 4 weeks, moderate-protection phase should range from 3 to 12 weeks, and minimum-protection phase ranging from 10 to 16 weeks from injury. The aforementioned time frames are approximate and should be based on each individual patient's prior level of function and current goals with rehabilitation. It is suggested that returning to running after an ACL injury treated nonoperatively should be approximately 12 weeks.[21]

Posterior Cruciate Ligament Injuries

The primary function of the PCL complex is to restrict posterior tibial translation. It acts as a secondary restraint to tibial varus, valgus, and external rotations.[100] Isolated PCL injuries occur less often than ACL injuries.[7,17,22] PCL injuries are most commonly the result of some sort of trauma to the knee. Although high-velocity knee injuries often result in PCL tears in combination with other ligamentous injuries, this chapter will deal only with isolated PCL injuries.[100]

Etiology

The most common mechanism of PCL injury is a fall on a hyperflexed knee that results in a posterior translation of the tibia on the femur (Fig. 18-12).[22,47,100] Other

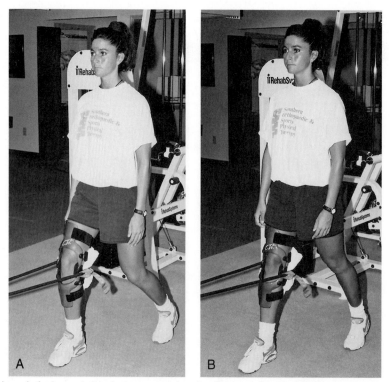

Fig. 18-11 Functional closed-chain resistive knee extension in the standing position. **A,** Starting position with affected knee flexed. **B,** End position with affected knee extended.

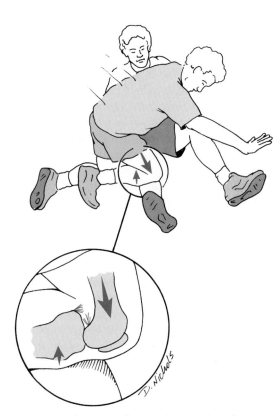

Fig. 18-12 Mechanism of posterior cruciate ligament injury. With the knee flexed, the proximal tibia is driven in a posterior direction.

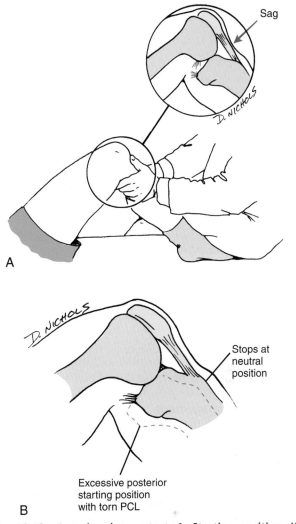

Fig. 18-13 Anterior drawer test. **A,** Starting position. If the posterior cruciate ligament injury is torn, the proximal tibia will be in a posterior tibial sag initial reference position. **B,** A false-positive anterior drawer test can be seen when the tibia translates forward during the drawer test because the torn posterior cruciate ligament (PCL) injury places the tibia posterior to the femur; therefore when the clinician directs an anterior force, the tibia appears to actually displace anterior to the femur.

mechanisms include a dashboard injury from a motor vehicle accident that also causes the tibia to translate posteriorly on the femur. Hyperextension injuries can also tear the PCL, however this commonly will result in a concomitant ACL injury.[100]

Clinical Evaluation

Clinical examination of the PCL may be very complex and begins with a careful history to determine the mechanism of injury. When eliciting a history from a patient with an acute, isolated PCL tear, unlike with an ACL tear, the patient will often not report feeling a pop or tear.[100] Patients with acute PCL tears will typically have mild to moderate knee effusion, a slight limp, pain in the back of the knee, and will often lack full flexion of the knee. More instability is experienced with combined injuries than with isolated tears. Patients with chronic PCL tears may complain more of disability, having difficulty doing things such as walking up or down inclines secondary to increased tibial movement on the femur.[100]

The most accurate test for the integrity of the PCL is the posterior drawer test.[100] This test is performed with the patient supine, the knee at 90° flexion, and the tibia in neutral, external, and internal rotations. As seen in Figure 18-13, *A,* a positive posterior drawer test is observed when the tibia sags, or subluxes, posteriorly

relative to the femur. In cases of isolated PCL tears, there is less posterior tibial translation with internal tibial rotation because the MCL and posterior oblique ligament contribute to this as a secondary restraint. Therefore there will be greater posterior tibial translation with the tibia in external rotation when the MCL and posterior oblique ligaments are not compromised. The examiner may produce a false-positive anterior drawer sign, where the posterior tibial sag actually is being reoriented to the neutral position rather than a true anterior translation occurring (Fig. 18-13, *B*).

Another PCL laxity test is the Godfrey posterior tibial sag test. The patient is supine with the hip and knee

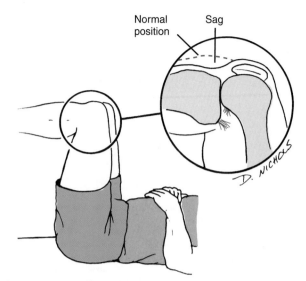

Normal position   Sag

D. NICHOLS

Fig. 18-14 Godfrey tibial sag test. This is a clinically sensitive test to view the reference of the proximal tibia in relation to the distal femur with the leg flexed to 90°.

of the affected limb held at 90°. Hold the heel of the affected limb and allow the tibia to translate, sublux, or sag posteriorly by gravity (Fig. 18-14).

Operative Management

Current surgical indications for PCL injuries include combined ligamentous injuries involving the PCL, symptomatic grade III laxity, and bony avulsion fractures.[100] There are a number of graft options for patients seeking a PCL reconstruction. Autologous tissues that are available include BPTB and hamstring and quadriceps tendons, of which the BPTB is the most frequently used. To decrease harvest site morbidity and surgical time, the Achilles allograft is an alternative to the autografts just listed.[22,29,100]

Postoperative rehabilitation

Postoperative treatment may begin as quickly as the day after surgery. Patients may present with use of a knee immobilizer or hinged knee brace most often locked in full extension and use of crutches to decrease stress placed through the surgically repaired knee. Weight-bearing restrictions after PCL reconstruction vary from immediate full weight bearing to partial weight bearing (PWB) for 4 to 6 weeks.[22,29]

Maximum protection phase. Early physical therapy will include quadriceps setting, multiplane straight leg raises, patella mobilization, and ROM exercises to gain full extension. Hamstring isometrics at angles greater than 30° have been shown to increase strain on the PCL, and therefore should be avoided in the maximum-protection phase.[63] Minimizing full knee flexion from 60° to 90° is necessary early in the rehabilitation to protect the healing PCL graft. Generally, full knee flexion ROM can be achieved by 2 months after surgery.[22]

Moderate and minimum protection phases. These phases of rehabilitation are similar to that of the postoperative ACL in terms of goals and time frames. Considered an agonist of the PCL, the quadriceps should be emphasized more than when rehabilitating a patient from an ACL reconstruction.[63] The goal of the moderate protection phase (6 to 12 weeks from surgery) of rehabilitation is to restore full ROM and progress strength of the affected leg. The minimum protection phase consists of progressing strengthening exercises from bilateral to unilateral. Running and plyometric exercises for the athletic patient should be progressed in a similar fashion to that of rehabilitating the postoperative ACL. Return to sport can range from 6 to 9 months from surgery.

Nonoperative Rehabilitation

Nonoperative treatment is indicated for patients with acute, isolated grade I or II PCL tears.[100] Patients may present with a knee immobilizer or hinged knee brace, along with crutches. Patients will begin physical therapy immediately to focus on decreasing inflammation, maintaining quadriceps tone, and restoring knee ROM. Rehabilitation exercises will include quadriceps isometrics, multiplane straight leg raises, and ROM. CKC strengthening may begin after 2 to 4 weeks as swelling, pain, and ROM improve. As mentioned previously, quadriceps strengthening should be emphasized because of the agonistic nature they have with the PCL to prevent posterior tibial translation.[26,63] Stationary bike, elliptical, or pool work may be implemented to increase cardiovascular fitness. Plyometric and sport specific training may be implemented once adequate strength is demonstrated and the patient shows no signs of pain or swelling. Typical return to sport is approximately 6 to 8 weeks with low grade PCL sprains.[100]

Medial Collateral Ligament Injuries
Etiology

Injuries to the MCL are the most common ligament injuries seen in the knee.[31,58,98] The MCL can be injured by direct contact to the lateral knee resulting in a valgus stress to the knee (Fig. 18-15, *A*). Uncommonly, a noncontact valgus or rotational stress to the knee can produce an isolated tear of the MCL when the lower leg is fixed and the tibia rotated externally (Fig. 18-15, *B*). Upon injury, patients may feel or hear a pop, but more commonly state they felt a tearing or pulling on the medial aspect of the knee. Patients will often present with swelling, and more severe sprains may present with ecchymosis. Patients will also walk with a limp; as they will be very hesitant to fully extend the knee because of increased stress and pain.

Literature shows the higher the grade of MCL lesion, the higher the incidence of an associated ligament injury; with grade III MCL injuries commonly associated with an ACL lesion.[30] Because of a high rate of associated injuries to an MCL sprain, one must also bear in mind the anatomical relationship between the MCL and medial meniscus of the knee. The MCL and medial meniscus are attached to one another (Fig. 18-16), which helps in understanding how a blow to the lateral aspect of the knee may also injure the medial meniscus. O'Donoghue[73] is credited with describing the unhappy triad as a combined injury to the MCL, ACL, and medial meniscus. However, as time has passed the more clinically common triad includes the MCL, ACL, and lateral meniscus.[6,25,67,84]

Clinical Evaluation

The most sensitive clinical test to describe the severity of an MCL sprain is the valgus stress test. This test is performed with the patient supine on an examining table while the examiner stands to the side of the affected limb at the level of the distal tibia and the affected knee flexed to 30°. The medial aspect of the distal tibia is firmly grasped with one hand, while the other hand is used to apply a valgus force to the lateral proximal joint line. The examiner's valgus force will cause the medial joint line to gap, or open, and place stress through the MCL. Gapping with the knee in full extension suggests there may be significant injury to multiple structures including the MCL, ACL, PCL, and posterior capsule.[47]

Rehabilitation

Consensus is that isolated grade I-III MCL injuries can be treated nonoperatively.[4,42,49,68] Patients will initially present with the use of crutches and a hinged knee brace to decrease valgus and rotational forces. In this early maximum-protection phase, the goal is to decrease inflammation, restore ROM, and increase quadriceps tone. Exercises will consist of knee ROM exercises, quadriceps setting, and multiplane straight leg raises without creating unnecessary valgus stress across the affected knee. Patients may progress to FWB within 1 to 2 weeks from injury as pain and quadriceps strength allows.

Unlike rehabilitating the cruciate ligaments, the moderate-protection phase of the MCL starts at 2 weeks. The goals of the moderate protection phase are the same:

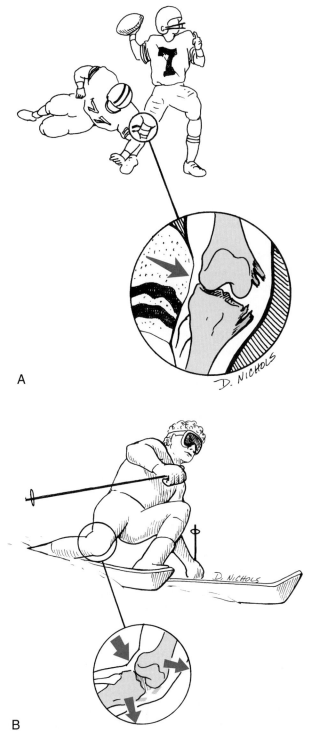

Fig. 18-15 Medial collateral ligament (MCL) sprains. **A,** MCL sprain caused by an external force contacting the lateral aspect of the knee, causing the medial knee structures to be torn. **B,** The MCL also can be sprained from noncontact forces.

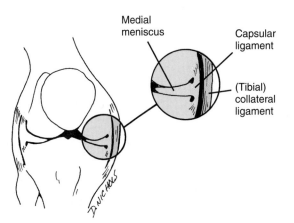

Fig. 18-16 The medial meniscus can also become injured in conjunction with the medial collateral ligament (MCL) because of its intimate anatomic relationship with the MCL.

(1) restore ROM; (2) progress strength of the affected limb; (3) continue protection of the involved tissues; and (4) continue use of antiinflammatory modalities as needed. CKC exercises should be progressed as mentioned earlier; from bilateral to unilateral, and from sagittal to frontal, to transverse plane in nature. If patients struggle to achieve full ROM without increased levels of pain, or struggle with full weight-bearing activities, reevaluation by the PT is advised.

If normal gait mechanics exist and strength and ROM allow, a running progression may start as early as 6 weeks from injury. Plyometric strengthening may start at the same time, progressing through different planes of movement as discussed previously. General return to sport will happen between 8 and 12 weeks from injury. A functional brace may be suggested to further protect the injured MCL when return to sport is permitted.[24]

MENISCUS INJURIES

The menisci are C-shaped or semicircular fibrocartilaginous structures with bony attachments at the anterior and posterior aspects of the tibial plateau, which contain primarily (90%) type I collagen.[3,37] The medial and lateral menisci of the knee serve as extensions of the tibia

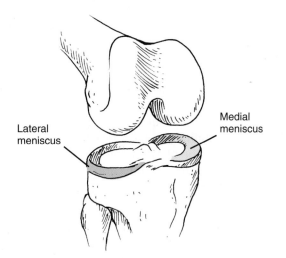

Fig. 18-17 Anatomic relationship of the medial and lateral meniscus to the tibia and femur.

and provide for reception of the femoral condyles onto the surface of the tibia (Fig. 18-17).[3] The menisci are important in many aspects of knee function, including stability, shock absorption, load transmission, nutrition, lubrication, joint stress reduction, increased congruity, and contact area.[15,37,40,44,48] Injury to the meniscus can result in many patterns of tears (Fig. 18-18). Five main types have been identified,[32] as follows:

■ Horizontal tears
■ Longitudinal (vertical longitudinal) tears
■ Degenerative (degenerative complex) tears
■ Flap (oblique) tears
■ Radial (radial) tears

The most common tears are flap (oblique) or vertical longitudinal, which occur in nearly 81% of meniscus tears. Vertical longitudinal tears can be complete (bucket handle tears) or incomplete and most often occur in younger individuals. Complex or degenerative tears are more common in individuals older than 40 years of age. Transverse or radial tears are often seen in isolated meniscus injuries or in conjunction with other meniscus tears. Lastly, horizontal tears are thought to be the result of shear forces generated by axial compression. They are very common in the lateral meniscus with runners.[37]

Etiology

The meniscus can be injured by sudden trauma or gradual degeneration.[3,15,32,44] As mentioned, traumatic meniscus injuries are most common in a younger population, whereas degenerative tears occur more frequently to individuals older than 40 years of age.[3,37] Noncontact, weight-bearing injuries to the meniscus usually involve combined forces of knee flexion, rotation, compression, and shear (Fig. 18-19).[3,15,32] Degenerative tears can be subtle and do not usually involve a history of sudden overt trauma. Generally with degenerative tears, some type of insignificant activity (squatting or getting out of a car) precedes the symptoms of pain, swelling, and locking of the knee.

Clinical Examination

A history of some type of twisting injury followed by symptoms of pain, swelling, locking, or catching may indicate meniscal injury. While assisting the PT during

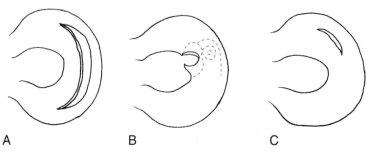

Fig. 18-18 Various patterns of tears can occur to the meniscus. **A,** Bucket-handle tear. **B,** Parrot-beak tear. **C,** Longitudinal tear.

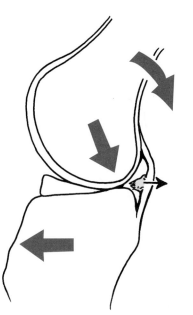

Fig. 18-19 Mechanism of injury to the meniscus. Combined forces of flexion, rotation, and compression can tear the meniscus.

the initial clinical examination, the PTA observes various manually applied stress tests to identify if a meniscal lesion is present.

Apley compression and distraction test is used to determine if the injury is ligamentous or meniscal.[83] To perform this test, the patient is prone with the affected knee flexed to 90°. The distal femur is stabilized with a strap or hand. The free hand is used to grasp the distal tibia and provide a distraction and internal-external rotation force to the tibia. Pain signifies the possibility of a ligament tear. The compression component of this examination is performed in the same manner, except that the free hand applies a compression and rotational force to the distal tibia. Pain with compression and combined internal and external rotation on the flexed knee suggests the presence of a meniscal lesion.

The McMurray test also is used to reproduce symptoms of a torn meniscus.[32,83] The patient is supine with the hip and knee of the affected limb fully flexed. To test for the presence of a medial meniscus lesion, a valgus force to the knee is applied with one hand while an external rotation force is applied and the knee is extended by holding the distal tibia with the other hand. To test for a lateral meniscus tear, a varus force with internal tibial rotation is provided. With either internal or external rotation of the knee, if a tear is present, the patient may experience pain and an audible or palpable snap or pop may occur.

The *bounce home* test is designed to determine if a torn meniscus is preventing knee extension.[83] The patient is supine with the affected knee flexed and supported by the examiner's hand. The knee is passively extended to full extension. If the meniscus is torn, the knee may not

fully extend because the torn tissue blocks extension and creates a rubbery, springy end-feel.[61]

The Thessaly test has been shown to be the most accurate clinical test to detect a meniscus tear.[52] The patient stands on the affected limb with the knee flexed 5° or 20°. The examiner supports the patient's outstretched arms while the patient rotates their knee internally and externally three times. Joint line discomfort or a sense of catching or locking of the knee is considered a positive test.[52]

Management

The rationale for treatment options is directly related to the location of the tear in the meniscus and the ability of the meniscus to repair itself. The vascular anatomy of the medial and lateral meniscus is reserved for the peripheral 10% to 30% of its width (Fig. 18-20, A).[3] The remaining portions are relatively avascular and aneural. Researchers and surgeons recognize a zone classification of injury related to the vascular supply of the meniscus.[3,40,44,83] The injured meniscus may or may not heal or repair itself, depending on the location of the tear. A zone I tear is recognized as *red-on-red* because the location of the tear is vascular on both sides (Fig. 18-20, B). Injuries in this area may heal better than those in other areas because of the blood supply. Because of this blood supply in the red-on-red area, some surgeons elect a nonsurgical course of treatment. A zone II tear is located in the *red-on-white* area of the meniscus (Fig. 18-20, C). A tear in this area has a vascular supply on only one side. These tears also may heal because of the communication with a blood supply. A zone III tear is located in the nonvascular central body of the meniscus called the *white-on-white area* (Fig. 18-20, D). An injury in this area does not heal because there is no blood supply to support the healing process.

Surgical indications for arthroscopic treatment of meniscal pathology include the following: (1) symptoms of meniscus injury that affect activities of daily living, work, or sports; (2) positive finding from clinical examination; (3) failure to respond to nonsurgical treatment; and (4) absence of other causes of knee pain identified in clinical examination or imaging studies.[66] The age of the patient, the stability of the knee, the location of the tear, and the integrity of the meniscus should all be considered when deciding on the course of treatment.[32]

Surgical options include total meniscectomy (removal of the entire meniscus), subtotal or partial meniscectomy (removal of only the torn portion of the cartilage), meniscal repair (suturing the torn meniscus together), or meniscal transplant.

Surgical Procedures

Although infrequent today, total meniscectomy was once a common procedure for meniscus injury. Joint space narrowing and osteophyte formation are

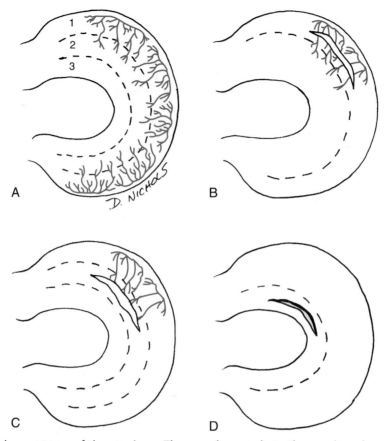

Fig. 18-20 **A,** The vascular anatomy of the meniscus. The vascular supply to the meniscus is reserved for the peripheral 10% to 30% of the meniscus. *1,* Red-on-red zone; *2,* red-on-white zone; *3,* white-on-white zone. **B,** Tear of the meniscus in the red-on-red zone of the meniscus. This zone I tear refers to the tear being vascular on both sides. This is a reparable tear. **C,** Tear of the meniscus in the red-on-white zone. This zone II tear refers to the tear being vascular on only one side. This is a reparable tear. **D,** Tear of the meniscus in the white-on-white zone. This zone III tear refers to the tear being avascular on both sides. This tear is considered not reparable.

common problems that have led to a decrease in total meniscectomy surgeries.[3,32,38,83] Current treatment of meniscal injuries is to maintain as much viable tissue as possible by avoiding total meniscectomy and investigating the possibility of surgical repair.

Subtotal or partial meniscectomy

To avoid the long term affects of total meniscectomy, partial meniscectomy is advised when a meniscus repair is not feasible. Preservation of the load-bearing functions of the meniscus is the foundation for a partial meniscectomy. The long-term consequences of subtotal meniscectomy must be clearly understood when addressing functional activities and return to athletics. Early degenerative changes are seen with both total and partial meniscectomy, and include narrowing of the tibiofemoral joint space, formation of bone spurs (osteophytes), and degeneration of the femoral articular surface on the side of the surgery.[3,32]

Counseling and education of the patient focus on modifying their activities of daily living (ADLs) related to stair climbing and repetitive vertical compressive loading.

Postoperative rehabilitation. The fact that many meniscal injuries occur in conjunction with injuries to other structures (ACL, MCL, or joint capsule) is significant and must be fully appreciated by the PTA. The rehabilitation program for combined subtotal meniscectomy and the presence of other joint pathologic conditions must be modified to account for the healing of other structures. The following is a general protocol for a partial or subtotal meniscectomy without concomitant injury.

Rehabilitation following subtotal meniscectomy should focus on reducing inflammation, normalizing patella mobility, and progressing to full ROM as soon as possible. Depending on the size of the meniscectomy and severity of degenerative changes in the knee, PWB should persist from 1 to 14 days. Progressive stretching and early strengthening exercises will begin about 2 weeks after surgery. At this time, the patient may progress to multiplane open- and closed-chain strengthening and stationary bicycling. Restoring the patient's joint and limb to normal functional status is the goal. If the patient is athletic, low-level plyometrics and running can start approximately 6 to 8 weeks after surgery. Return to competition may be seen between months 2 and 4. However, if a patient is diagnosed with a degenerative joint disorder during arthroscopic examination, a more conservative rehabilitation program will be more appropriate to decrease joint stress.

Meniscal repair

Multiple surgical options are available when considering meniscal repair, which include nonfixation healing enhancement (meniscal trephination or synovial abrasion), open repair, arthroscopic repair (inside-out, outside-in, all inside suture techniques), and nonsuture techniques (biomaterial). A review of the literature showed that meniscal repairs demonstrated greater potential for healing under the following conditions: (1) repairs involve the lateral meniscus; (2) meniscal injuries are acute; and (3) repairs are performed in conjunction with ACL reconstruction.[38,90]

Postoperative rehabilitation. Rehabilitation following meniscal repair remains controversial. Because many meniscal repairs are performed in conjunction with ACL reconstruction, postoperative protocols are quite varied. Thus it is important to communicate with the orthopedic surgeon and PT to fully understand the specific plan of care. The following will provide a general rehabilitation protocol of an isolated meniscal repair.

Physical therapy often begins in the maximum protection phase (weeks 0 to 6) with protective weight bearing, the use of a brace locked into extension, and restricted ROM to 90° flexion. Delaying FWB status until 4 to 6 weeks is recommended to avoid vertical compression forces into the repaired tissue.[48] Exercises include patella mobility, knee ROM limited to 90° of flexion, quadriceps setting, straight leg raises, and gait training. If the patient will be non–weight bearing, (NWB) it is important to include open-chain multiplane hip strengthening and ankle and foot strengthening. Progression of exercises into closed-chain strength training will be dependent upon the weight-bearing restrictions, which may remain until 4 to 6 weeks after surgery.

The moderate protection phase begins between 4 and 6 weeks when the patient is allowed FWB status. Exercises during this phase include bilateral CKC strengthening advancing to single leg as tolerated, and stationary cycling progressing to weight-bearing cardiovascular exercises such as the elliptical trainer and stair-climber. CKC exercises should be progressed with caution so that the repaired meniscus does not experience an overload

of compression forces. Progressing CKC exercises within the pool reduces compression through the knee secondary to the buoyancy of the patient.

The goals of the minimum-protection phase vary based on the patient's goals to achieve prior levels of function. At this point the patient should demonstrate full ROM, normal gait mechanics, and fairly good strength compared with the uninvolved limb. Light plyometric progressions may start at 4 months after surgery, beginning bilaterally and progressing to unilaterally. As mentioned with strengthening, progressing plyometrics in the pool first helps reduce the compression forces throughout the knee. Jumping rope is a simple way to introduce more impact throughout the knee before progressing into higher level plyometrics.

Meniscal transplantation

In an effort to restore normal knee anatomy and biomechanics, meniscal allografts can be used to replace the damaged meniscus. When surgical indications are adhered to, studies have shown excellent results in pain relief and improved function.[18] Surgical indications for meniscal allograft transplantation include prior meniscectomy, continued pain with intact articular cartilage, normal anatomic alignment, and joint stability.[18,38] Specific age limits are not available, but generally patients who are older than 50 to 55 years already have a degree of arthritis that would contraindicate the procedure. Other contraindications include inflammatory arthritis, obesity, and previous infection.[18]

Meniscus transplantation can be performed as either an open or arthroscopic technique. Other procedures that may be performed in conjunction with meniscal transplantation are high tibial osteotomy to provide improved alignment, or reconstruction of the ACL to increase joint stability. Success rates of meniscus allograft transplants vary depending on the criteria used to determine success. It has been shown that knees with advanced arthrosis have a greater risk for graft failure.[18]

Postoperative rehabilitation. In rehabilitation of allograft meniscal transplantation a conservative approach is recommended. Patients will present postoperatively as NWB and with ROM limitations of 0° to 90° flexion. Postoperative rehabilitation will vary widely, but should closely resemble the rehabilitation of a meniscal repair. Most surgeons will provide a program that allows running at 4 to 6 months and full activities at 6 to 9 months.[18]

ARTICULAR CARTILAGE LESIONS

Articular cartilage is known to protect the subchondral bone and to reduce friction of the joint.[62] It is suggested that isolated chondral lesions may progress to symptomatic degeneration of the knee, and therefore surgical intervention may be warranted to provide pain relief and restore normal joint congruity.[18,60] Surgical options include arthroscopic débridement, microfracture, osteochondral grafting, and autologous chondrocyte implantation (ACI).

Operative Management

The microfracture procedure involves several holes being punctured into the subchondral bone, which creates a bleeding response of marrow into the area of the chondral lesion.[87] The marrow formulates into a fibrocartilaginous clot to protect the underlying subchondral bone.[55,80,87] Osteochondral grafting is a procedure in which cylindrical osteochondral grafts are harvested from the NWB surface of the femoral condyles and strategically placed within the area of the chondral lesion.[41] ACI involves two surgical procedures. The first procedure is an arthroscopic evaluation of the chondral lesion as well as a chondrocyte biopsy from the articular cartilage from a small section of a femoral condyle. Those chondrocytes are then cultured for a approximately 3 weeks and then injected back into the area of the chondral lesion (see Fig. 10-6). The injected chondrocytes are held in place by either a periosteal patch from the patient's tibia or a synthetic collagen patch.[19,33,62] Variables such as patient age, weight, activity level, chondral lesion size, and other concomitant knee pathology dictate which procedure is best for each patient.

Postoperative Rehabilitation

Rehabilitation progression for microfracture, osteochondral grafting, and ACI procedures are quite similar. Most authors agree to minimize weight bearing if the resurfacing technique was performed on the weight-bearing surface of the tibia or femur. The patient may be NWB for 2 to 8 weeks after surgery.[33,39,56,80,87] If the surgery was for the patellofemoral joint, the patient may start weight bearing soon after surgery with their knee immobilized or in a hinged brace allowing up to 20° of flexion.[39,87] A CPM machine may be prescribed because this has been shown to be beneficial for tissue repair.[39] Primary goals throughout this time are to protect the healing tissue, initiate patella mobilization, minimize joint swelling, restore ROM, and to begin isometric exercises as discussed previously.[33,39] Cardiovascular fitness should be promoted with the use of a stationary bike with minimal resistance, or the use of an upper body ergometer (UBE).

At 8 to 10 weeks after surgery, the patient should be FWB and relatively limp-free. At this point, the patient may begin CKC exercises that progressively increase the amount of ROM and joint load throughout the tibiofemoral or patellofemoral joint, depending on which joint was injured. Exercises should also progress from bilateral to unilateral in nature. From 2 to 6 months after surgery, the patient should have normal gait mechanics, full ROM, and should be within 90% of their strength of the contralateral limb. Cardiovascular fitness activities progress from stationary biking to rowing, swimming, level walking, and then stair climbing throughout this phase of rehab. As exercises apply more load through the repair, continued use of modalities to treat and prevent inflammation is encouraged.

Authors seem to agree that returning to sport should happen between 6 and 12 months after surgery.[33,39,56] Low-impact activities such as skating and cycling may begin by 6 months after surgery. Basic agility work as well as pool running may also begin at this time. Roughly 8 months after surgery, the patient should start an interval running program on land as well as a plyometric exercise progression. High impact sports such as tennis and basketball should not start until close to 12 months out from surgery.[33]

PATELLOFEMORAL PATHOLOGIC CONDITIONS

A careful review of the anatomy and kinesiology of the patellofemoral joint and extensor mechanism is encouraged before discussing the examination and treatment of patellofemoral dysfunction. It is important for the PTA to understand the integrative functional role the hip, foot, and ankle play in providing optimal alignment for proper patellofemoral tracking. This section outlines the more commonly encountered problems affecting the patellofemoral joint, focusing on the fundamental rehabilitation concepts for conservative management as well as rehabilitation programs related to proximal and distal surgical realignment procedures.

Etiology

Pathology of the patellofemoral joint is one of the most common disabilities of the knee joint in orthopedic and sports medicine.[94] Several authors have speculated differences in flexibility, strength, and neuromuscular control to be causes of patellofemoral pain (PFP). What seems to be consistent is that people with PFP have decreased gastrocnemius and soleus flexibility[78] and decreased hip external rotation and abduction strength[78,89]; they also tend to demonstrate increased hip internal rotation with CKC activities such as running.[89] Most patients with PFP will complain of anterior knee pain with prolonged sitting (theater sign), stair ambulation, and squatting motions.

Physical Examination

The physical examination of a patient with PFP should include examining the posture of the patella relative to the femur, the lower extremity muscle stiffness and strength, and the overall lower extremity static and dynamic alignment and how these may cause the patella to track poorly in the trochlear groove of the femur.

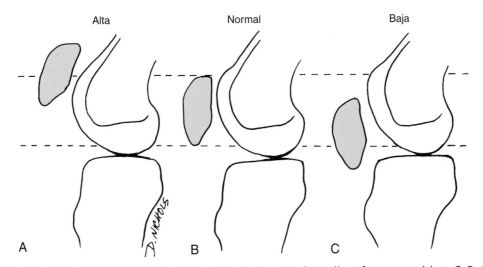

Fig. 18-21 Patella reference positions. **A,** Patella alta. **B,** Normal patella reference position. **C,** Patella baja.

In general, the patella is referenced to the femur in three positions (Fig. 18-21). A patellar posture that is more superior than normal is referred to as *patella alta*[50,67,96] and is associated with greater patellar instability.[67] Excessive hamstring tightness can increase patellofemoral compression because patellar excursion through knee extension is resisted by hamstrings, requiring more quadriceps force and causing increased compression forces of the patella into the femur (Fig. 18-22).[50] Testing for rectus femoris and iliotibial band (ITB) inflexibility should also be performed, because these structures have been linked to decreased PFP if flexibility is restored to normal.[94]

In addition to patellar posture and muscle stiffness, the **quadriceps angle (Q angle)** is a clinical assessment that relates to patellar tracking deviations and variations in the line or angle of pull of the quadriceps on the patella.[67] The Q angle refers to a line drawn from the anterior superior iliac spine (ASIS) through the center or axis of the patella and distally to the insertion of the patellar tendon on the tibial tubercle (Fig. 18-23, *A*). The Q angle can be increased by proximal tibial external rotation or distal tibia varus.[50,96] Figure 18-23, *B*, shows the various angles of muscular pull on the patella and how an increased Q angle can affect the tracking mechanisms of the patella during flexion and extension. Miserable malalignment syndrome (Fig. 18-24) is assessed with the patient in the standing position and provides objective data for the physician and PT about the entire lower extremity kinetic chain, patellar tracking dysfunction, and pain.[50,67,96] This syndrome is characterized by femoral anteversion (internal femoral rotation), "squinting" patellae (patellae facing toward each other), proximal external tibial torsion (which results in what is called the *bayonet sign*), and foot pronation.[9,96] Miserable malalignment syndrome results in an increased Q angle and can result in lateral tracking of the patella. It has been suggested that the Q angle is not just a valuable

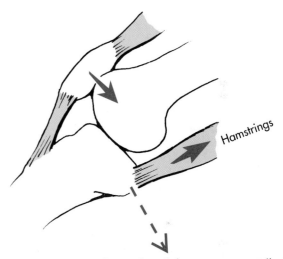

Fig. 18-22 Excessive hamstring tightness can contribute to increased patellofemoral compression.

tool as a static measurement; it should also be observed during CKC activity, such as a single leg squat.[79]

In light of this information concerning patellar posture, muscle inflexibility and weakness, Q angle, and lower extremity malalignment, the PTA must recognize that the result of these abnormalities is pain and dysfunction related to femoral and retropatellar articular (hyaline) cartilage degeneration from excessive loading of the patellofemoral joint.

Nonoperative Rehabilitation of Anterior Knee Pain

The initial course of treatment focuses primarily on controlling pain and swelling while modifying provocative activity. Activities that cause pain such as running and cycling must be temporarily reduced in order to decrease inflammation. Additionally, ice and nonsteroidal anti-inflammatory drugs (NSAIDs) are important modalities in the acute phase to reduce inflammation.

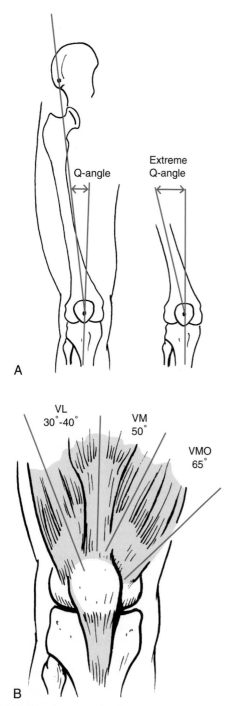

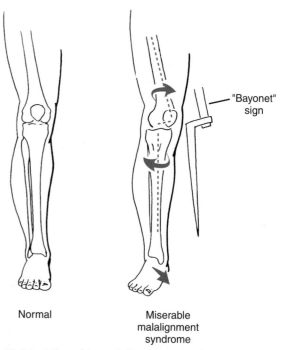

Fig. 18-24   Miserable malalignment syndrome. Anatomic alignment is assessed in the standing position. The miserable malalignment syndrome is characterized by combined femoral anteversion, "squinting" patellae, external tibial torsion, and foot pronation.

Fig. 18-23   A, The quadriceps angle is measured from the anterior superior iliac spine, through the axis of the patella, and distally to the insertion of the patellar tendon on the tibial tubercle. **B,** Angles of muscular pull on the patella. Patellar reference positions and the quadriceps angle can affect mechanical tracking of the patella because of muscular angles of pull. *VL,* Vastus lateralis; *VM,* vastus medialis; *VMO,* vastus medialis oblique.

Strengthening of the quadriceps muscle group is initiated by introducing isometric sets that do not produce pain. In some instances, submaximal isometric quadriceps sets are necessary at the beginning of the program to accommodate pain. The vastus medialis oblique

(VMO) is the focus of attention when addressing the quadriceps strengthening because of its ability to stabilize the patella superiorly and more importantly, medially.[9] The superior-medial pull of the vastus medialis muscle directly counteracts lateral tracking syndromes. Equally important, is to perform isolated strengthening exercises of the hip abductors, external rotators, and extensors.

In conjunction with quadriceps and hip strengthening, tight lateral structures that act to pull the patella laterally must be treated manually and with appropriate stretching. Stretching the hamstrings and ITB (Fig. 18-25, *A*) and performing manual patellar-stretching exercises (Fig. 18-25, *B*) are essential to counteract anterior knee pain that results for a lateral tracking patella.[94,95] Also, quadriceps, gastrocnemius, and soleus inflexibility should be addressed in the initial phase of rehabilitation.

Once acute inflammation has subsided, CKC strengthening exercises are introduced to promote higher level functional strengthening. Multiplane hip strengthening, leg press, squats, walls squats, and step-ups are all appropriate progressions. ROM, resistance, and step height may all need to be modified to allow the patient to perform without pain. It is important to understand that significant increases of patellofemoral joint stress are shown to happen between 0° and 30° of knee flexion with open-chain exercises, and between 60° and 90° with closed-chain exercises.[88]

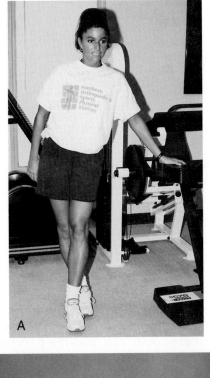

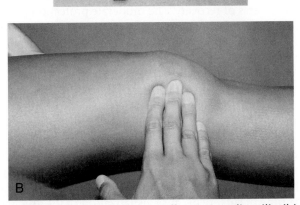

Fig. 18-25 Stretching the patella. **A,** Standing iliotibial band stretching. Stretching the lateral structures of the hip and knee can aid in minimizing lateral tracking of the patella and lateral compressive forces. **B,** Manual lateral patella stretching. The patient is instructed in autostretching of the patella. If the lateral retinaculum of the knee is tight and is causing the patella to track laterally, the patient can gently stretch the patella medially to stretch tight lateral structures.

Biofeedback units used on the VMO during CKC is an excellent way to emphasize proper muscular activation. CKC exercises should be progressed from bilateral to unilateral as pain and strength allow. Emphasis should be placed on alignment as the exercises progress. Encouraging joint stacking, where the patient controls hip adduction and internal rotation, will reduce valgus angulation across the knee and in turn will help reduce PFP.[64,99]

Supportive devices can help dynamically stabilize the patella and promote normal tracking throughout this phase of rehabilitation. Commercially available patellar stabilizing sleeves provide a lateral buttress support to the patella to minimize lateral tracking. Various taping methods can be incorporated for dynamic stability as well. The use of foot orthotics in patients with increased pronation has shown to be useful in decreasing pain by improving lower extremity alignment.[12] These devices may be necessary for the patient to progress through CKC strengthening without pain.

It is important to incorporate pain-free cardiovascular exercise to build muscular endurance and promote patellofemoral joint health. Elevated treadmill walking, both forward and backward, may be most beneficial for muscle activation while minimizing stress to the patellofemoral joint.[16,57] Swimming and using a stationary bike and elliptical trainer are all appropriate nonimpact cardiovascular modalities as long as they are pain free for the patient.

When considering return to sport and discharge criteria for patients with PFP it is important for the clinician to thoroughly evaluate lower extremity mechanics as it relates to alignment with running, jumping, and cutting activities. Lower extremity jumping mechanics appear to be consistently different among individuals with PFP.[99] Conservative treatment programs that include kinematic retraining may improve patient outcomes and prevent recurrence of this common orthopedic condition.[64,79,99]

Operative and Postoperative Management for Patellofemoral Pain

Surgical management of patellofemoral disorders can be classified as proximal realignment procedures, distal realignment procedures, and procedures to address articular cartilage abnormalities.[96]

Proximal Realignment

The basic goal of operative management for anterior knee pain related to lateral patellar tracking disorders is to reestablish appropriate extensor mechanism function and reduce patellofemoral contact forces.[35]

Proximal realignment procedures involve lateral retinacular release with or without VMO advancement.[93] Rehabilitation after proximal realignment procedures is essentially the same as for nonoperative treatment of anterior knee pain. However, pain and swelling after surgery, as well as specific tissue healing and time constraints, must be addressed carefully. Therefore the initial course of management after proximal realignment procedures is focused on the use of ice, lateral patellar compression, limb elevation, temporary immobilization, weight bearing as tolerated, and NSAIDs as prescribed by the physician. Control of pain and swelling is essential to reduce the quadriceps inhibition they produce.

Temporary immobilization is specifically related to management of the lateral retinacular release procedure. The rationale behind this procedure is to reduce the pull of the lateral structures contributing to the lateral retinaculum, including the vastus lateralis muscle. Therefore, in this specific procedure, early lateral retinacular stretching exercises and early knee flexion ROM exercises are needed to prevent the lateral structures that were released from scarring and counteracting the purpose of the surgery. In some cases the VMO is surgically cut and advanced distally to create a greater medial pull of the patella. Early flexion exercises may stretch the advancement of the VMO; therefore extreme caution is needed when encouraging motion after lateral retinacular release with advancement of the VMO. When the ROM has been advanced, early active quadriceps strengthening exercises must be delayed to allow for appropriate scarring and healing at the suture site.

Supine wall slides, stationary cycling, prone leg flexion and manual patellar stretching exercises are introduced as pain and swelling allow. Quadriceps strengthening is the foundation for a successful outcome after this surgical procedure. Open-chain remedial exercises (quadriceps sets and multiplane straight leg raises) give way to CKC functional exercises as soon as pain and tissue healing allow. Step-ups with biofeedback over the VMO, wall squats, leg presses, stair steppers, elliptical trainer and normalized gait mechanics are encouraged during the early stages of postoperative rehabilitation. Emphasizing proper knee alignment with CKC exercises is encouraged as discussed in the nonoperative care of PFP.

Distal Realignment

The goal behind distal realignment surgeries is to reduce severe patellofemoral compression loads and significant patellar subluxation by surgically removing the extensor mechanism's insertion (patellar tendon attachment on the tibial tubercle) and reattaching the tibial tubercle to a more mechanically advantageous site to improve the pull of the quadriceps (Fig. 18-26).[9]

Individual circumstances and surgical procedures dictate variations in this initial management plan. Significant modifications in rehabilitation are necessary with distal realignment procedures based on bone and soft-tissue healing and promotion of quadriceps strength. Generally, immobilization with a hinged range-limiting brace is used for 4 to 6 weeks.[9,96] Crutches are encouraged for about 6 weeks, with initial NWB progressing to toe-touch weight bearing and then to FWB over the full 6 weeks of immobilization.[9,96] Gradual progression of flexion ROM is advised; achieving approximately 100° of knee flexion for the first 2 weeks and progressing to 120° by 6 weeks.[9] Isometric quadriceps sets and straight-leg raises are encouraged once pain, swelling and tissue healing allow. With extensor mechanism repair, as well as radical distal realignment procedures, a few weeks' delay is necessary before initiating quadriceps sets and straight-leg raises so as not to endanger the

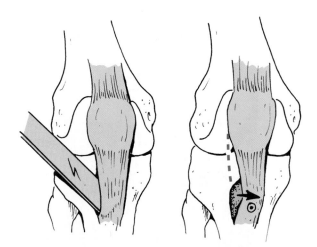

Fig. 18-26 Elmslie-Trillat distal realignment procedure for distal extensor mechanism.

surgical repair site. Many remedial quadriceps strengthening exercises can be performed in the brace during the early phases of recovery. The moderate protection phase after 6 weeks from surgery will be a similar progression of exercises as those mentioned with nonoperative rehabilitation.

Articular Cartilage Procedures

Arthroscopic procedures are used to directly address the condition of the articular cartilage on the undersurface of the patella and the femoral condyles in cases of anterior knee pain. The term chondromalacia describes retropatellar articular cartilage degeneration or softening. The diagnosis of chondromalacia only can be made at the time of surgery because visualization of the articular surface is necessary.[67,96]

Various surgical procedures are used to smooth rough articular surfaces and stimulate an inflammatory response to enhance healing. Perforation or abrasion of subchondral bone (chondroplasty, microfracture and abrasion arthroplasty) stimulate a communication between the damaged articular surface and vascular supply of subchondral bone.[9] Acute postoperative management includes ice, elevation, compression, NSAIDs, protected weight bearing and possible use of a CPM at home. The PTA must pay close attention to complaints of pain and objective signs of swelling with all exercise progressions. Progression of exercises has been discussed in the articular cartilage section of the chapter.

FRACTURES

This section briefly introduces management and rehabilitation programs associated with fractures of the patella, distal femur (supracondylar femur fractures), and proximal tibia (tibial plateau).

Patellar Fractures

Etiology

Fractures of the patella can occur with direct or indirect trauma.[96] The most common injury involves the patella making contact with a hard surface. Less frequently the patella can be fractured by a violent contraction of the quadriceps.[65,96] Avascular necrosis (AVN) can result if a transverse fracture occurs, because the vascular supply to the patella is reserved for the central portion of the distal pole, leaving the proximal segment of the transverse fracture prone to AVN.[65]

Nonoperative Rehabilitation

Rehabilitation management of nondisplaced patellar fractures treated with immobilization and limited weight bearing is primarily supportive throughout the literature. Nondisplaced patellar fractures are often treated conservatively with immobilization of the affected limb in full extension for 4 to 6 weeks.[59,65,96] The unaffected limb can maintain strength and flexibility using quadriceps strengthening exercises. Aerobic fitness can be enhanced with the use of single leg stationary cycling or an UBE. Ankle pumps are encouraged for the affected limb throughout immobilization. Quadriceps sets, short-arc knee extensions and straight leg raises are introduced gradually once sufficient bone healing has occurred. If quadriceps strengthening exercises and knee flexion exercises are initiated too soon, the force of muscle contraction and knee flexion stretching may separate and stress the fracture site, slowing the healing process and leading to fracture displacement.

Operative Management

Surgery for displaced patella fracture is indicated when the bone fragments exceed 3 to 4 mm in separation.[59] Stabilization of displaced patellar fractures is best accomplished with an open reduction with internal fixation (ORIF) procedure. Figure 18-27 portrays various patellar fracture patterns. The most common fixation devices are tension band wiring and cerclage wiring (Fig. 18-28). The tension band wire is a dynamic compression device that approximates and compresses the patellar fragments. The additional use of cerclage wiring adds to the stability of the repair and allows early joint motion without redisplacing the fracture fragments.[96]

Postoperative management for patella fracture

Generally, the knee is immobilized in 20° of knee flexion to support dynamic compression of the tension band wiring procedure. One week after surgery, active knee extension, submaximal quadriceps sets, and straight leg raises can be initiated. Flexion of the knee out of the immobilizer usually is limited to approximately 100° for at least 6 weeks to allow for proper bone healing. Weight bearing as tolerated (WBAT) with assistive devices is encouraged during the first few weeks after surgery. The patient should be progressed to FWB by the third week. The long progression of quadriceps strengthening exercises and the advancement of full knee flexion correlate with normal bone healing and individual tolerance. Care must be taken not to force aggressive knee extension strengthening exercises with heavy isotonic loads too early in the program. Normalizing gait and progression through CKC step-ups and squats replicates the sequencing outlined in the nonoperative section.

Supracondylar Femur Fractures

Operative Management

Distal femur fractures generally are classified as extraarticular, unicondylar, or bicondylar[65,67] (Fig. 18-29). These fractures are usually managed with an ORIF procedure. Figure 18-30 demonstrates fixation devices used for transverse supracondylar fractures, unicondylar fractures, and type C (T- and Y-pattern) fractures. The method of fixation focuses on fracture site stabilization and fragment apposition while minimizing the pull on the fracture site by the quadriceps, hamstrings, and calf muscles.[59,65]

Proximal Tibia Fractures (Tibial Plateau Fractures)

Operative Management

Displaced proximal tibial fractures are treated with an ORIF procedure. Figure 18-31 illustrates the different types of tibial plateau fractures. Various internal fixation devices used with different fracture patterns are illustrated in Figure 18-32. Postoperative management and rehabilitation of tibial plateau fractures follow the course of bone and soft-tissue healing. First, the patient is placed in a leg immobilizer or fracture brace in full extension. Active quadriceps sets are performed and the patient is generally NWB or partial weight bearing,

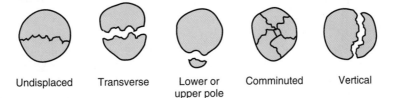

Undisplaced   Transverse   Lower or   Comminuted   Vertical
upper pole

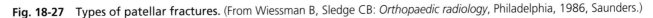

Fig. 18-27 Types of patellar fractures. (From Wiessman B, Sledge CB: *Orthopaedic radiology*, Philadelphia, 1986, Saunders.)

depending on the severity of the fracture. After initial surgical wound healing has occurred, knee flexion exercises can begin based on the patient's tolerance.

Nonoperative and Postoperative Management of Supracondylar and Tibial Plateau Fractures

Physicians usually treat nondisplaced distal femur and proximal tibial fractures nonoperatively with closed reduction of the fragments and tibial traction for approximately 8 to 12 weeks.[59] Physical therapy management of supracondylar and tibial plateau fractures is guided extensively by the healing process of bone and associated soft tissue. Generally, patients have limited weight bearing for 8 to 12 weeks. NWB is followed strictly until subsequent radiologic assessment determines secure bone healing. Arthrofibrosis and quadriceps adhesion to the bone are frequent problems, with significant bleeding and associated tissue damage in distal femur fractures. Therefore early postoperative management focuses on patellar mobility (within the confines of the knee brace or immobilizer), active quadriceps-strengthening exercises (quadriceps sets and straight-leg raises), and active knee flexion to minimize knee contractures. It is imperative to encourage strengthening and flexibility exercises for the uninvolved limb and instruct the patient in a general fitness program that does not compromise the healing of the injured limb.

Normalized gait mechanics and CKC strengthening are encouraged once it is determined that the fracture has healed enough to accept these compressive forces. CKC functional exercises (stair-steppers, short-arc step-ups, wall squats, and leg presses), and proprioception exercises (balance boards and minitrampoline) are added cautiously as the patient demonstrates improved quadriceps strength, increased knee ROM, and reduced pain and swelling, and as the necessary healing of bone and soft tissue occurs.

High Tibial Osteotomy

A tibial osteotomy procedure can be performed on patients who demonstrate advanced degenerative joint disease (DJD) of one compartment of the knee.[67] Most commonly, this is the medial compartment and is characterized by a varus (bow-legged) deformity that creates abnormal loads on the medial aspect of the tibiofemoral joint.[72] Less frequently, the lateral compartment is involved and creates a valgus deformity (knock-knees) (Fig. 18-33). This procedure is generally considered a temporary solution, approximately 10 years, before a total knee replacement (TKR) is considered.[67] Patients

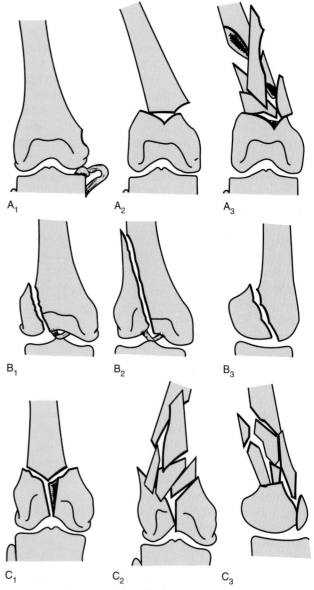

Fig. 18-29 Arbeitsgemeinschaft für Osteosynthesefragen/Association for the Study of Internal Fixation (AO/ASIF) classification of supracondylar fractures. (From Johnson KD: *Orthopaedic knowledge update III*, Rosemont, Ill, 1990, American Academy of Orthopaedic Surgeons.)

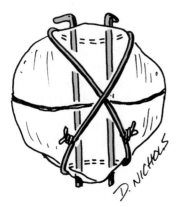

Fig. 18-28 Transverse fracture of the patella. Stabilization is achieved with tension band wiring and cerclage wiring.

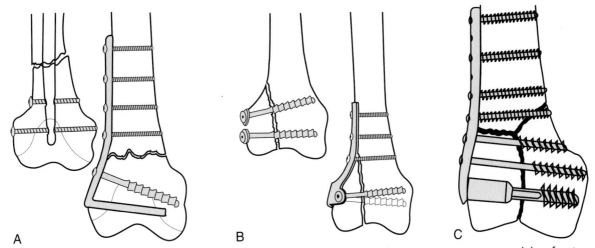

Fig. 18-30 Various methods of open reduction with internal fixation for transverse supracondylar fractures **(A)**, unicondylar fractures **(B)**, and T- and Y-condylar fractures **(C)**. (From McRae R: *Practical fracture treatment*, ed 3, New York, 1994, Churchill Livingstone.)

younger than 50 years of age with greater than 120° flexion have a higher probability of success with a high tibial osteotomy (HTO).[70]

HTO attempts to realign the tibiofemoral joint by surgically creating a wedge in the proximal tibia or distal femur, depending on varus or valgus deformity, and redistributing the forces and compressive loads more evenly across the joint (Fig. 18-34). In valgus deformity associated with lateral tibiofemoral compartment destruction, a distal femur (supracondylar) closing-wedge osteotomy is performed and is stabilized with a plate.[67,86] Depending on the wishes and training of the surgeon, some patients use CPM immediately postoperatively to facilitate early flexion motion.[86]

Postoperative Rehabilitation for High Tibial Osteotomy

Usually the knee is placed in an immobilizer in full extension with a suction drain inserted to help evacuate the excessive accumulation of blood. Initially, strengthening exercises (quadriceps sets, straight-leg raises in the splint, and gluteal sets) are performed and advanced from the first day postoperatively. Manual patellar stretching is encouraged once initial surgical wound healing has occurred, especially with distal femoral wedge osteotomy (preoperative valgus deformity caused by lateral joint compartment disease) because the procedure involves extensive invasion of the quadriceps.[86] If CPM is not used, the patient is allowed out of the immobilizer several times a day to perform active knee flexion exercises (Fig. 18-35). As patellar mobility (caudal-cephalic motion) improves, progressive knee flexion ROM exercises are added with the patient in a sitting position to allow gravity to influence the flexion range of the affected limb. Care must be taken to manually assist the affected limb from sudden flexion and encourage quadriceps relaxation.

Weight-bearing status after HTO is guided primarily by the time constraints of bone healing.[86] Usually touch-down weight bearing (TDWB) is allowed after surgery with the aid of crutches or a walker for up to 12 weeks.[86] Progressive resistive exercises for the quadriceps and hamstrings are initiated gradually within the first 3 to 4 weeks after surgery. Usually ankle weights, Thera-Band resistance, seated isotonic quadriceps and hamstring exercises, and cables and pulleys can be added cautiously during the moderate-protection phase of recovery (7 to 12 weeks).[91] Knee flexion ROM improvement is encouraged by using supine wall slides, seated knee flexion, prone knee flexion, and stationary cycling.

The initiation of functional CKC resistance exercises is deferred until the physician receives radiographic confirmation of secure bone union. Assistive devices for ambulation are discontinued once a minimum of 8 to 12 weeks has passed, fixation of the bone has occurred, and the patient demonstrates good quadriceps strength, improved knee flexion ROM, and confidence in a normalized gait pattern. CKC strengthening exercises can be progressed as discussed with previous sections. One must take caution with progressing CKC exercises as to not inflame an already arthritic knee.

Total Knee Replacement

Knee Arthroplasty

The indications for TKR are primarily to eliminate or reduce pain and improve functional activities in severely disabled patients.[34,36,67] Osteoarthritis (DJD) and rheumatoid arthritis contribute significantly to unicompartmental (medial or lateral), bicompartmental (both medial and lateral joint compartments), and

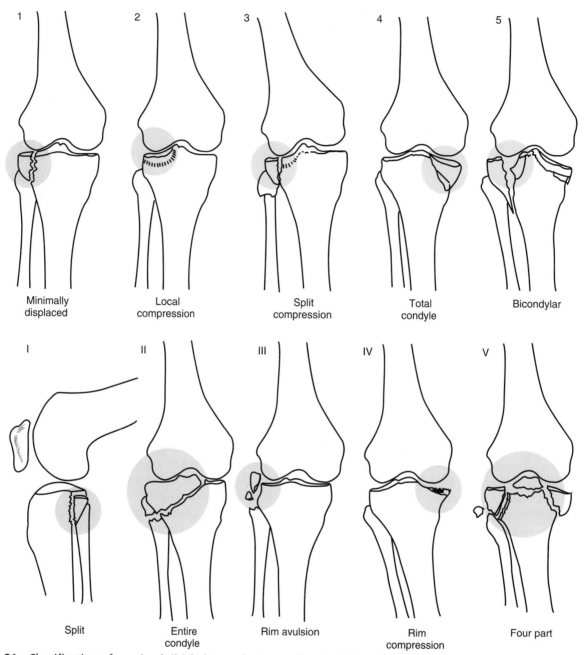

Fig. 18-31 Classification of proximal tibial plateau fractures. (From Loth T: *Orthopedic boards review*, St Louis, 1993, Mosby.)

tricompartmental (medial, lateral, and patellofemoral compartments) pain and dysfunction.[34,36,67,92]

Basic contraindications for TKR are active or recent septic arthritis, a "nonfunctioning extensor mechanism or severe neurologic dysfunction that prevents extension or control of the knee," and a neuropathic joint.[59,67]

TKR generally involves removing the degenerated articular surfaces of the tibia, femur, and patella, and replacing these structures with metal, plastic, or a combination of each. The goals are to relieve pain, uniformly transmit forces across the joint, create a horizontal joint in the stance phase of gait, restore anatomic and mechanical axes, provide adequate stability, and improve function.[34,36,67,92]

Prosthetic implants vary in their design by being constrained, nonconstrained, mobile-bearing, or fixed-bearing. Constrained, or conforming implants, sacrifice the cruciate ligaments (ACL, PCL, or both) and rely on the conformity between the components for stability. Nonconstrained (cruciate-sparing) implants retain the cruciate ligaments.[36,67,92] Fixed-bearing prostheses have a polyethylene (plastic) component fixated on the tibial tray. Mobile-bearing prostheses have a polyethylene platform which articulates between the metallic femoral prosthesis and tibial implant. The mobile polyethylene

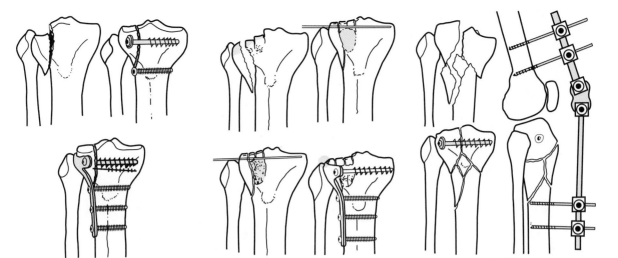

Fig. 18-32 Various methods of internal fixation of tibial plateau fractures. (From McRae R: *Practical fracture treatment*, ed 3, New York, 1994, Churchill Livingstone.)

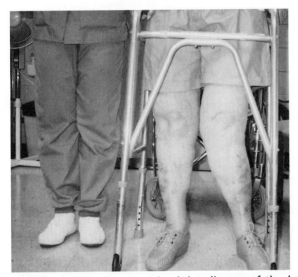

Fig. 18-33 Severe degenerative joint disease of the lateral compartment of the knee. Note the severe valgus deformity of the knee.

platform allows for better load-sharing throughout the polyethylene and theoretically reduces the wear of this implant.[13] Studies show similar outcomes with regard to ROM and function with these four implants,[11,46,82] however the prevalence of osteolysis was found to be slightly higher with the mobile-bearing implants.[46]

Prostheses can be secured with or without bone cement. The cementless prosthesis is porous-coated and allows the surrounding bone to grow into and adhere to the prosthesis, creating a direct biologic fixation.[36] Cemented implants have been shown to have better survival at 15 years than cementless implants.[5]

Although the most common approach used to perform a TKR is through an anterior medial parapatellar

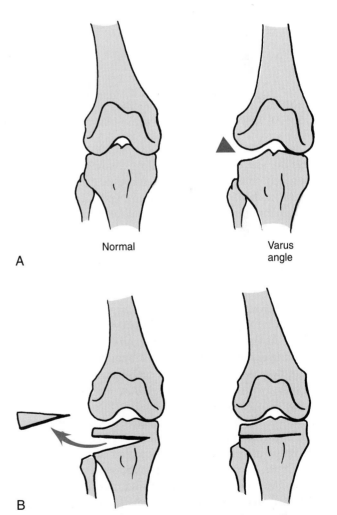

Fig. 18-34 High tibial osteotomy surgical procedure to redistribute compressive loads more evenly across the joint. **A,** Normal and abnormal varus angle. **B,** Wedge removed to change the angle of joint.

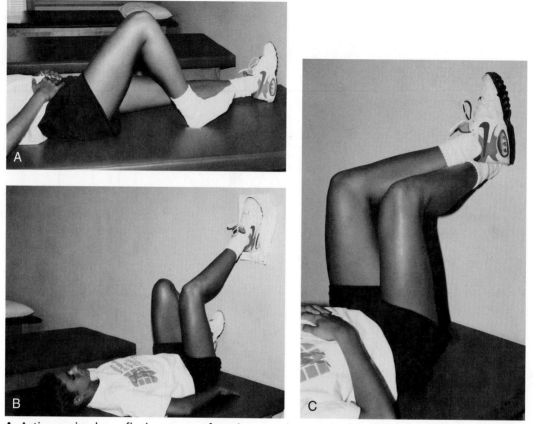

Fig. 18-35 **A,** Active supine knee flexion range-of-motion exercises are performed daily with the immobilizer removed. **B,** Supine wall slides. **C,** Supine active-assisted wall slides for gaining knee flexion.

incision, some surgeons are using a minimally invasive approach that spares cutting through the quadriceps. Several authors have shown improved function and a shorter inpatient stay[2,27,54] as well as decreased use of narcotics for pain management with the minimally invasive approach.[54]

Rehabilitation after Total Knee Joint Replacement

Weight bearing may be restricted longer in the noncemented group to allow for firm bone growth to the component.[36] Cemented components demonstrate a more secure fit earlier than the noncemented group, thus allowing earlier progression in weight bearing.

Immediate postoperative care uses a compression dressing with a knee immobilizer in full extension with the involved limb elevated 30° to 40° to minimize swelling and to prevent a knee flexion contracture. The maximum-protection phase of recovery focuses on reducing unwanted stresses that may loosen the prosthesis, while stimulating muscle strength, increasing ROM, and reducing pain and swelling. Remedial exercises that are initiated immediately after surgery include quadriceps, hamstring, and gluteal isometrics, ankle pumps, active assisted straight-leg raises, short-arc terminal knee extensions and knee flexion ROM exercises. Some authors report that CPM may be beneficial

in regaining knee flexion[34,36]; however, other studies suggest standard physical therapy exercises without the use of CPM result in the same quality of function and ROM after TKR.[8,23] The knee immobilizer can be removed to perform supine heel slides and supine hip and knee flexion exercises. Supine wall slides and active-assisted wall slides can be added as pain allows. As the midline surgical incision heals, the patella should be mobilized in a caudal-cephalic motion to reduce patellofemoral adhesions. The appropriate time to begin weight bearing depends on the fixation used, but generally the patient is instructed in a PWB gait with a walker or crutches within a day after surgery.[34] An ambulatory assistive device is retained for support until a normalized gait is achieved.

With the primary goal after TKR being to restore ROM, the secondary goal is to restore strength. Quadriceps strength is highly correlated with functional performance, and therefore should be a focus throughout rehabilitation.[69] Once the patient is able to start an outpatient rehabilitation program, continued efforts of progressing knee ROM and general lower extremity strengthening can be started, as summarized in Table 18-1.

It is common for the elderly population receiving TKR to demonstrate reduced cardiovascular fitness and strength; therefore a general conditioning program

Table 18-1	*Outpatient Rehabilitation Program after Total Knee Arthroplasty*
Impairment	**Intervention**
Range of motion	Exercise bike (10-15 min), started with forward and backward pedaling with no resistance until enough ROM for full revolution; progression: lower seat height to produce a stretch with each revolution
	Active assistive ROM for knee flexion, sitting or supine, using other leg to assist
	Knee extension stretch with manual pressure (in clinic) or weights (at home)
	Patellar mobilizations: 3 sets of 30 reps superior/inferior; medial/lateral as necessary
Strengthening	Quad sets, straight leg raises (with full knee extension), hip abduction (side lying), standing hamstring curls, seated knee extension, standing terminal knee extension from 45° to 0°, step-ups (5- to 15-cm block), wall slides to 45° knee flexion; 1-3 sets of 10 reps for all strengthening exercises
	Criteria for progression: exercises are to be progressed (e.g., weights, step height) once the patient can complete the exercise correctly and feels maximally fatigued at the end of each set
	Progression: 0.5- to 1.0-kg weights added to exercises, step-downs (5- to 15-cm block), front lunges, and wall slides toward 90° knee flexion
Pain and swelling control	Ice and compression as needed
Incision mobility	Soft tissue mobilization until incision moves freely over subcutaneous tissue
Functional activities	Ambulation training with assistive device as appropriate with emphasis on heel strike, push-off at toe-off, and normal knee joint excursions
	Emphasis on heel strike, push-off at toe-off, and normal knee joint excursions when able to walk without assistive device
	Stair ascending and descending step-over-step when patient has sufficient concentric and eccentric quadriceps strength
Monitoring vital signs	Blood pressure and heart rate are monitored at initial evaluation and as appropriate

ROM, Range of motion; *reps,* repetitions.
From Mizner RL, Petterson SC, Snyder-Mackler S: Quadriceps strength and the time course of functional recovery after total knee arthroplasty, *J Orthop Sports Phys Ther* 35:424-436, 2005.

should be started as soon as the patient can tolerate it. Early single-leg stationary cycling or UBE can be safely and effectively used to maintain or improve cardiovascular fitness. Because a TKR was performed to reduce pain and dysfunction related to osteoarthritis or rheumatoid arthritis, care must be taken to protect other affected joints during the initiation of a general conditioning program. In some cases, a swimming program may be more appropriate than either open- or closed-chain resistive exercises.

The PTA should expect the greatest amount of functional gain in the first 3 months of rehabilitation; however, improvements up to a year from surgery may be expected.[53] After TKR it is generally understood that participating in high-impact activities, such as jogging, basketball, football, and soccer, is not recommended.[43]

Summary

Throughout any rehabilitation process, whether the situation is treated nonoperatively, or postoperatively, understanding the principles of tissue healing and applying the appropriate loads (or no load) to the involved structure(s) is the foundation of physical therapy.

Prescribing a proper exercise program and using the appropriate tools to control inflammation throughout each phase of rehabilitation, will better allow patients to achieve their respective goals.

❖ GLOSSARY

Anterior drawer test: A clinical examination used to approximate the degree of anterior tibial translation relative to the fixed femur.

Closed kinetic chain (CKC) exercises: A system of interdependent articulated links in which motion at one joint produces motion at all other joints in the system in a predictable manner.

Hughston jerk test: Commonly used examination to sublux and reduce the tibia relative to the femur.

Lachman examination: The most common, specific, and clinically useful ligament stability test for the ACL.

Pivot shift test: Commonly used examination to sublux and reduce the tibia relative to the femur.

Quadriceps angle (Q angle): An imaginary line drawn from the anterior superior iliac spine through the center or axis of the patella and distally to the insertion of the patellar tendon on the tibial tubercle.

REFERENCES

1. Agel J, Arendt EA, Bershadsky B: Anterior cruciate ligament injury in national collegiate athletic association basketball and soccer: a 13-year review, *Am J Sports Med* 33:524–530, 2005.
2. Archibeck MJ, White RE Jr: What's new in adult reconstructive knee surgery, *J Bone Joint Surg Am* 88:1677–1686, 2006.
3. Arnoczky S, Adams M, DeHaven K, et al: Meniscus. In Woo SLY, Buckwalter JA, editors: *Injury and repair of the musculoskeletal soft tissues*, Park Ridge, Ill, 1988, American Academy of Orthopaedic Surgeons.
4. Baker LB, Liu SH: Collateral ligament injuries of the knee: operative and nonoperative approaches. In Fu F, Harner CD, Vince GV, editors: *Knee surgery*, Baltimore, 1994, Williams & Wilkins.
5. Baker PN, Khaw FM, Kirk LMG, et al: A randomised controlled trial of cemented versus cementless press-fit condylar total knee replacement, *J Bone Joint Surg Br* 89:1608–1614, 2007.
6. Barber FA: What is the terrible triad? *Arthroscopy* 8:19–22, 1992.
7. Barrack RL, Skinner H, Buckley SL: Proprioception in the anterior cruciate deficient knee, *Am J Sports Med* 17:1–6, 1989.
8. Beaupre LA, Davies DM, Jones CA, et al: Exercise combined with continuous passive motion or slider board therapy compared with exercise only: a randomized controlled trial of patients following total knee arthroplasty, *Phys Ther* 81:1029–1037, 2001.
9. Bennett JG: Rehabilitation of patellofemoral joint dysfunction. In Greenfield BH, editor: *Rehabilitation of the knee: a problem solving approach*, Philadelphia, 1994, FA Davis.
10. Beynnon BD, Fleming BC, Johnson RJ, et al: Anterior cruciate ligament strain behavior during rehabilitation exercises in vivo, *Am J Sports Med* 23:124–134, 1995.
11. Bhan S, Malhotra R, Kiran KE, et al: A comparison of fixed-bearing and mobile-bearing total knee arthroplasty at a minimum follow-up of 4.5 years, *J Bone Joint Surg Am* 87:2290–2296, 2005.
12. Bizzini M, Childs JD, Piva SR, et al: Systematic review of the quality of randomized controlled trials for patellofemoral pain syndrome, *J Orthop Sports Phys Ther* 33:4–20, 2003.
13. Callaghan JJ, Insall JN, Greenwald AS, et al: Mobile-bearing knee replacement: concepts and results, *J Bone Joint Surg Am* 82:1020–1041, 2000.
14. Cannon WD Jr, Vittori JM: The incidence of healing in arthroscopic meniscal repairs in anterior cruciate ligament-reconstructed knees versus stable knees, *Am J Sports Med* 20:176–181, 1992.
15. Carlson TJ: *The rationale behind meniscus repair, postgraduate advances in sports medicine*, Rosemont, Ill, 1987, Forum Medicus.
16. Cipriani DJ, Armstrong CW, Shannon G: Backward walking at three levels of treadmill inclination: an electromyographic and kinematic analysis, *J Orthop Sports Phys Ther* 22:95–102, 1995.
17. Clancy WG, Shelbourne DK, Zoellner GB: Treatment of knee joint instability secondary to rupture of the posterior cruciate ligament, *J Bone Joint Surg Am* 65:310–322, 1983.
18. Cole BJ, Carter TR, Rodeo SA: Allograft meniscal transplantation, *J Bone Joint Surg Am* 84:1236–1250, 2002.
19. Cole BJ, Pascual-Garrido C, Grumet RC: Surgical management of articular cartilage defects in the knee, *J Bone Joint Surg Am* 91:1778–1790, 2009.
20. Cooper DE, Deng XH, Burstein AL, et al: The strength of the central third patellar tendon graft, *Am J Sports Med* 21:818–824, 1993.
21. Daniel DM, Fritschy D: In DeLee JC, Drez D, editors: *Orthopaedic sports medicine: principles and practice, anterior cruciate ligament injuries*, vol 2, Philadelphia, 1994, Saunders.
22. DeLee JC, Bergfeld JA, Drez D, et al: In DeLee JC, Drez D, editors: *Orthopaedic sports medicine: principals and practice, the posterior cruciate ligament*, vol 2, Philadelphia, 1994, Saunders, 1994.
23. Denis M, Moffet H, Caron F, et al: Effectiveness of continuous passive motion and conventional physical therapy after total knee arthroplasty: a randomized clinical trial, *Phys Ther* 86:174–185, 2006.
24. Drez D, editor: *Knee braces: seminar report*, Rosemont, Ill, 1985, American Academy of Orthopaedic Surgeons.
25. Duncan JB, Hunter R, Purnell M, Freeman J: Meniscal injuries associated with acute anterior cruciate ligament tears in alpine skiers, *Am J Sports Med* 23:170–172, 1995.
26. Durselen L, Claes L, Kiefer H: The influence of muscle forces and external loads on cruciate ligament strain, *Am J Sports Med* 23:129–136, 1995.
27. Dutton AQ, Yeo SJ: Computer-assisted minimally invasive total knee arthroplasty compared with standard total knee arthroplasty, *J Bone Joint Surg Am* 91:116–130, 2009.
28. Einhorn AR, Sawyer M, Tovin B: Rehabilitation of intra-articular reconstructions. In Greenfield BH, editor: *Rehabilitation of the knee: a problem solving approach*, Philadelphia, 1993, FA Davis.
29. Engle RP, Meade TD, Canner GC: Rehabilitation of posterior cruciate ligament injuries. In Greenfield BH, editor: *Rehabilitation of the knee: a problem solving approach*, Philadelphia, 1993, FA Davis.
30. Fetto JF, Marshall JL: Medial collateral ligament injuries to the knee: a rationale for treatment, *Clin Orthop Relat Res* 132:206–217, 1978.
31. Frank C, Woo SL, Amiel D, et al: Medial collateral ligament healing: a multi-disciplinary assessment in rabbits, *Am J Sports Med* 11:379–389, 1983.
32. Fu FH, Baratz M: In DeLee JC, Drez D, editors: *Orthopaedic sports medicine: principles and practice, meniscal injuries*, vol 2, Philadelphia, 1994, Saunders.
33. Gillogly SD, Voight M, Blackburn T: Treatment of articular cartilage defects of the knee with autologous chondrocyte implantation, *J Orthop Sports Phys Ther* 28:241–251, 1998.
34. Goldstein TS: Geriatric orthopaedics, rehabilitative management of common problems. In Lewis CB, editor: *Aspen series in physical therapy*, Gaithersburg, Md, 1991, Aspen Publishers.
35. Grana WA, Kriegshauser LA: Scientific basis of extensor mechanism disorders, *Clin Sports Med* 4:247–257, 1985.
36. Greene B: Rehabilitation after total knee replacement. In Greenfield BH, editor: *Rehabilitation of the knee: a problem solving approach*, Philadelphia, 1993, FA Davis.
37. Greis PE, Bardana DD, Holmstrom MC, Burks RT: Meniscal injury: I. Basic science and evaluation, *J Am Acad Orthop Surg* 10:168–176, 2002.
38. Greis PE, Holmstrom MC, Bardana DD, Burks RT: Meniscal injury: II. Management, *J Am Acad Orthop Surg* 10:177–187, 2002.
39. Hambly K, Bobic V, Wondrasch B, et al: Autologous chondrocyte implantation postoperative care and rehabilitation, *Am J Sports Med* 34:1020–1038, 2006.
40. Hammesfahr R: Surgery of the knee. In Donatelli R, Wooden MJ, editors: *Orthopaedic physical therapy*, New York, 1989, Churchill Livingstone.
41. Hangody L, Fules P: Autologous osteochondral mosaicplasty for the treatment of full-thickness defects of weight-bearing joints: ten years of experimental and clinical experience, *J Bone Joint Surg Am* 85:25–32, 2003.
42. Hastings DE: The nonoperative treatment of collateral ligament injuries of the knee joint, *Clin Orthop Relat Res* 147:22–28, 1980.
43. Healy WL, Sharma S, Schwartz B, Iorio R: Athletic activity after total joint arthroplasty, *J Bone Joint Surg Am* 90:2245–2252, 2008.
44. Henning CE, Lynch MA: Current concepts of meniscal function and pathology, *Clin Sports Med* 4:259–265, 1985.
45. Hermann O, Weig TG, Plitz W: Arthrofibrosis following ACL reconstruction – reasons and outcome, *Arch Orthop Trauma Surg* 124:518–522, 2004.
46. Huang CH, Ma HM, Liau JJ, et al: Osteolysis in failed total knee arthroplasty: a comparison of mobile-bearing and fixed-bearing knees, *J Bone Joint Surg Am* 84:2224–2228, 2002.
47. Hughston J: *Knee ligaments: injury and repair*, St Louis, 1993, Mosby.

48. Hughston JC: Patellar subluxation in patellofemoral problem, *Clin Sports Med* 8:162–253, 1989.

49. Indelicato P: Non-operative treatment of the medial collateral ligament of the knee, *J Bone Joint Surg Am* 65:323–329, 1983.

50. Jacobson KE, Flandry FC: Diagnosis of anterior knee pain, *Clin Sports Med* 8:195–279, 1989.

51. Jensen JE: Systematic evaluation of acute knee injuries. In Larson RL, Singer KM, editors: *Clinical sports medicine*, Philadelphia, 1985, Saunders.

52. Karachalios T, Hantes M, Zibis AH, et al: Diagnostic accuracy of a new clinical test (the Thessaly test) for early detection of meniscal tears, *J Bone Joint Surg Am* 87:955–962, 2005.

53. Kennedy DM, Stratford PW, Riddle DL, et al: Assessing recovery and establishing prognosis following total knee arthroplasty, *Phys Ther* 88:22–32, 2008.

54. King J, Stamper DL, Schaad DC, Leopold SS: Minimally invasive total knee arthroplasty compared with traditional total knee arthroplasty, *J Bone Joint Surg Am* 89:1497–1503, 2007.

55. Knutsen G, Engebretsen L, Ludvigsen TC, et al: Autologous chondrocyte implantation compared with microfracture in the knee, *J Bone Joint Surg Am* 86:455–464, 2004.

56. Kon E, Gobbi A, Filardo G, et al: Arthroscopic second-generation autologous chondrocyte implantation compared with microfracture for chondral lesions of the knee, *Am J Sports Med* 37:33–41, 2009.

57. Lange GW, Hintermeister RA, Schlegel T, et al: Electromyographic and kinematic analysis of graded treadmill walking and the implications for knee rehabilitation, *J Orthop Sports Phys Ther* 23:294–301, 1996.

58. Linton RC, Indelicato PA: Medial ligament injuries. In DeLee JC, Drez D, editors: *Orthopaedic sports medicine* vol 2, Philadelphia, 1994, Saunders.

59. Loth TS: *Orthopaedic boards review*, St Louis, 1993, Mosby.

60. Maletius W, Messner K: The effect of partial meniscectomy on the long-term prognosis of knees with localized, severe chondral damage. A twelve-to-fifteen year followup, *Am J Sports Med* 24:258–262, 1996.

61. Malone T: Rehabilitation of the surgical knee: the therapist's view of surgery. In Davies G, editor: *Rehabilitation of the surgical knee*, Ronkonkoma, NY, 1984, Cybex.

62. Mandelbaum BR, Browne JE, Fu F, et al: Articular cartilage lesions of the knee, *Am J Sports Med* 26:853–861, 1998.

63. Markolf KL, O'Neill G, Jackson SR, McAllister DR: Effects of applied quadriceps and hamstrings muscle loads on forces in the anterior and posterior cruciate ligaments, *Am J Sports Med* 32:1144–1149, 2004.

64. Mascal CL, Landel R, Powers C: Management of patellofemoral pain targeting hip, pelvis and trunk muscle function: 2 case reports, *J Orthop Sports Phys Ther* 33:647–660, 2003.

65. McRae R: *Practical fracture treatment*, ed 3, Ronkonkoma, NY, 1994, Churchill Livingstone.

66. Metcalf RW, Burks RT, Metcalf MS, McGinty JB: Arthroscopic meniscectomy. In McGinty JB, Caspari RB, Jackson RW, Poehling GG, editors: *Operative arthroscopy*, ed 2, Philadelphia, 1996, Lippincott-Raven, pp 263–297.

67. Miller M: *Review of orthopaedics*, Philadelphia, 1992, Saunders.

68. Miller RH III: Knee injuries. In Canale ST, editor: ed 10, *Campbell's operative orthopaedics* vol 3, St Louis, 2003, Mosby, pp 2214–2235.

69. Mizner RL, Petterson SC, Snyder-Mackler L: Quadriceps strength and time course of functional recovery after total knee arthroplasty, *J Orthop Sports Phys Ther* 35:424–436, 2005.

70. Naudie D, Bourne RB, Rorabeck CH, et al: Survivorship of the high tibial valgus osteotomy. A 10- to 22- year followup study, *Clin Orthop Relat Res* 367:18–27, 1999.

71. Neumann DA: *Kinesiology of the musculoskeletal system*, St Louis, 2002, Mosby.

72. Noyes FR, Butler DL, Grood ES, et al: Biomechanical analysis of human ligament grafts used in knee ligament repairs and reconstruction, *J Bone Joint Surg* 66:344–352, 1984.

73. O'Donoghue D: Surgical treatment of fresh injuries to the major ligaments of the knee, *J Bone Joint Surg Am* 32:721–738, 1950.

74. Paletta GA, Levine DS, O'Brien SJ, et al: Patterns of meniscal injury associated with acute anterior cruciate ligament injury in skiers, *Am J Sports Med* 20:542–547, 1992.

75. Paulos LE, Noyes FR, Grood E, et al: Knee rehabilitation after anterior cruciate ligament reconstruction and repair, *Am J Sports Med* 9:140, 1981.

76. Paulos LE, Payne FC, Rosenburg TD: Rehabilitation after anterior cruciate ligament surgery. In Jackson DW, Drez D, editors: *The anterior cruciate deficient knee: new concepts in ligament repair*, St Louis, 1987, Mosby.

77. Piasecki DP, Spindler KP, Warren TA, et al: Intraarticular injuries associated with anterior cruciate ligament tear: findings at ligament reconstruction in high school and recreational athletes, *Am J Sports Med* 31:601–605, 2003.

78. Piva SR, Goodnite EA, Childs JD: Strength around the hip and flexibility of soft tissues in individuals with and without patellofemoral pain syndrome, *J Orthop Sports Phys Ther* 35:793–801, 2005.

79. Powers CM: The influence of altered lower-extremity kinematics on patellofemoral joint dysfunction: a theoretical perspective, *J Othop Sports Phys Ther* 33:639–646, 2003.

80. Saris DB, Vanlauwe J, Victor J, et al: Characterized chondrocyte implantation results in better structural repair when treating symptomatic cartilage defects of the knee in a randomized controlled trial versus microfracture, *Am J Sports Med* 36:235–246, 2008.

81. Sato N, Higuchi H, Terauchi M, et al: Quantitative evaluation of anterior tibial translation during isokinetic motion in knees with anterior cruciate ligament reconstruction using either patellar or hamstring tendon grafts, *Int Orthop* 29:385–389, 2005.

82. Seon JK, Park SJ, Lee KB, et al: Range of motion in total knee arthroplasty: a prospective comparison of high-flexion and standard cruciate-retaining designs, *J Bone Joint Surg Am* 91:672–679, 2009.

83. Seto JL, Brewster CE: Rehabilitation of meniscal injuries. In Greenfield BH, editor: *Rehabilitation of the knee: a problem solving approach*, Philadelphia, 1993, FA Davis.

84. Shelbourne KD, Nitz PA: The O'Donoghue triad revisited. Combined knee injuries involving anterior cruciate and medial collateral ligament tears, *Am J Sports Med* 19:474–477, 1991.

85. Shelbourne KD, Patel DV: Treatment of limited motion after anterior cruciate ligament reconstruction, *Knee Surg Sports Traumatol Arthrosc* 7:85–92, 1999.

86. Sisk TD: Knee realignment and replacement in the recreational athlete. In DeLee JC, Drez D, editors: *Orthopaedic sports medicine: principles and practice* vol 2, Philadelphia, 1994, Saunders.

87. Steadman JR, Briggs KK, Rodrigo JJ, et al: Outcomes of microfracture for traumatic chondral defects of the knee: average 11-year follow-up, *Arthroscopy* 19:477–484, 2003.

88. Steinkamp LA, Killingham MF, Makel MD, et al: Biomechanical considerations in patellofemoral joint rehabilitation, *Am J Sports Med* 21:438–444, 1993.

89. Souza RB, Powers CM: Differences in hip kinematics, muscle strength, and muscle activation between subjects with and without patellofemoral pain, *J Orthop Sports Phys Ther* 39:12–19, 2009.

90. Tenuta JJ, Arciero RA: Arthroscopic evaluation of meniscal repairs: factors that effect healing, *Am J Sports Med* 22:797–802, 1994.

91. Timm K: Knee. In Richardson JK, Iglarsh ZA, editors: *Clinical orthopaedic physical therapy*, Philadelphia, 1994, Saunders.

92. Tippett SR: Total knee arthroplasty: an overview, physical therapy implications and rehabilitation concerns, *Course Notes*, 1994.

93. Turba JE: Formal extensor mechanism reconstruction, *Clin Sports Med* 8:297–317, 1989.

94. Tyler TF, Nicholas SJ, Mullaney MJ, et al: The role of hip muscle function in the treatment of patellofemoral pain syndrome, *Am J Sports Med* 34:630–636, 2006.

95. Van den Dolder PA, Roberts DL: Six sessions of manual therapy increase knee flexion and improve activity in people with anterior knee pain: a randomized controlled trial, *Am J Phys* 52:261–264, 2006.

96. Walsh WM: In DeLee JC, Drez D, editors: *Orthopaedic sports medicine: principles and practice, patellofemoral joint*, vol 2, Philadelphia, 1994, Saunders.

97. Warren RF, Marshall JL: Injuries of the anterior cruciate ligament and medial collateral ligaments of the knee, *Clin Orthop Relat Res* 136:191–197, 1978.

98. Wilk KE: Rehabilitation of medial capsular injuries. In Greenfield BH, editor: *Rehabilitation of the knee: a problem solving approach*, Philadelphia, 1993, FA Davis.

99. Wilson JD, Binder-Macleod S, Davis IS: Lower extremity jumping mechanics of female athletes with and without patellofemoral pain before and after exertion, *Am J Sports Med* 36:1587–1596, 2008.

100. Wind WM Jr, Bergeld JA, Parker RD: Evaluation and treatment of posterior cruciate ligaments, *Am J Sports Med* 32:1765–1775, 2004.

REVIEW QUESTIONS

Short Answer

1. Which injury does this figure represent?

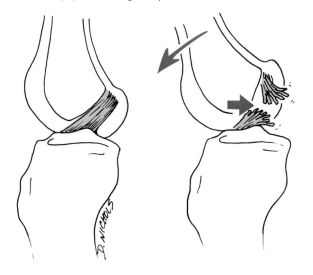

2. Identify the ligament and name the examination being performed in the following figure.

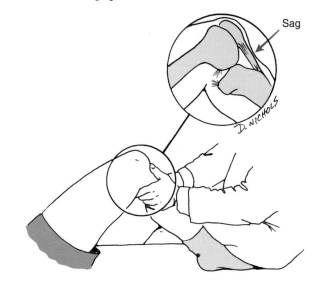

3. Name the mechanism of injury and identify the torn structure in this figure.

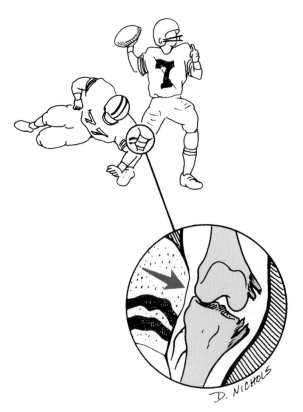

4. Match the names of meniscal lesions with the appropriate diagrams in the following figures. Select from these names:

_____Flap tear
_____Longitudinal tear
_____Parrot beak tear
_____Bucket handle
_____Radial tears

5. Match the following terms with the appropriate diagram:

_____Red-on-red zone
_____Red-on-white zone
_____White-on-white zone

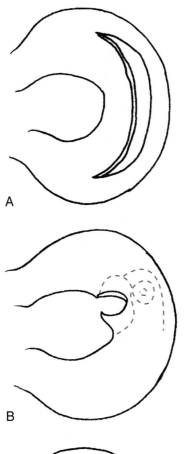

A

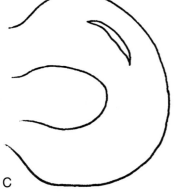

B

C

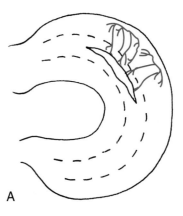

A

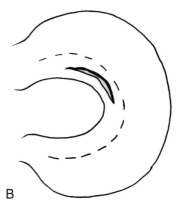

B

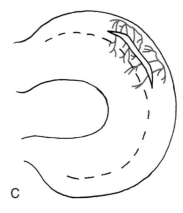

C

6. In the following figures, match the patellar reference description with the appropriate figure:

_____Patella baja

_____Patella alta

_____Normal

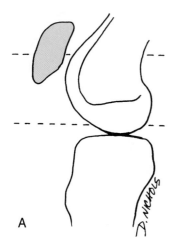

A

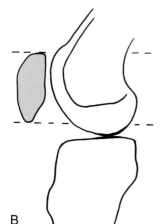

B

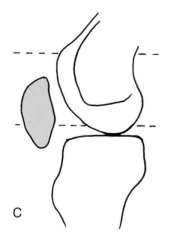

C

7. There is the frequent occurrence of significant bleeding and tissue damage with supracondylar fractures. List three early postoperative management techniques to prevent or minimize knee flexion contractures.

8. In the following figure, name the general type of fracture and pattern of injury, as well as identify the internal fixation devices used to secure the fracture fragments.

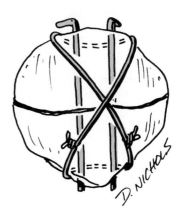

9. Name the four general types of implants used in a TKR.

True/False

10. Grade III MCL tears must always be treated surgically.

11. Patients should expect the majority of their gains after a TKR by 6 weeks postoperatively.

12. Normal gait mechanics should be restored by 2 weeks after an ACI procedure to the weight-bearing surface of the femoral condyle.

13. It is more common for male athletes to tear their ACL than female athletes of the same sport.

14. The Lachman test is a more specific clinical test than the anterior drawer test for examining ACL integrity.

15. Apley compression and distraction test is used to determine if the meniscus or ligament is injured.

19

Orthopedic Management of the Hip and Pelvis

Michael P. Reiman

LEARNING OBJECTIVES

1. Identify common hip fractures.
2. Outline and discuss common methods of management and rehabilitation of ordinary hip fractures.
3. Identify and describe common methods of management and rehabilitation after hip arthroplasty.
4. Identify and describe common soft-tissue injuries of the hip.
5. Outline and describe common methods of management and rehabilitation of soft-tissue injuries of the hip.
6. Identify common fractures of the pelvis and hip.
7. Discuss methods of management and rehabilitation for fractures of the pelvis and acetabulum.
8. Describe common mobilization techniques for the hip.

KEY TERMS

Comminuted fracture
Delayed union
Displaced fracture
Hip osteoarthritis

Malunion
Nonunion avascular
    necrosis
Osteitis pubis

Osteonecrosis
Pubalgia
Simple fracture

CHAPTER OUTLINE

The practicing physical therapist assistant (PTA) is exposed to many orthopedic problems involving the hip and pelvis. This chapter focuses attention on the more common classifications, management, and rehabilitation of hip fractures, joint reconstructive surgery (total hip arthroplasty), rehabilitation after hip replacement, and management of various pelvic fractures and soft-tissue injuries of the hip.

HIP FRACTURES

The clinical significance of hip fractures is reflected in the annual rate of fractures and the financial burden to the economy that hip fractures produce.[10,16] Goldstein[10] states that more than 300,000 fractures occur annually with an associated cost of $10 billion. Other authorities[4,16] report that 267,000 fractures occur annually, with a price tag of $33.8 billion.[4] Although fractures in general occur to all age groups, hip fractures are most common among elderly women.[4,16,17] Hip fractures in women can be attributed in part to the higher incidence of osteoporosis in this group[17]; with regard to age, hip fractures represent the most common acute orthopedic injury in the geriatric population.[16]

The classification of hip fractures is clinically significant for the PTA because the severity and location of the fracture profoundly affect surgical management and physical therapy interventions. The vascular supply to the femoral head and neck may be significantly compromised with certain fracture patterns and levels of severity (Fig. 19-1).[17] LeVeau[17] states, "The extent of the supply of blood to the head of the femur determines remodeling and healing after femoral neck fracture or hip dislocation."

Generally, hip fractures can be classified by location and described by severity (**simple** or **comminuted**).[9] Fractures of the hip can be located in the following areas:

- Extracapsular or intertrochanteric[9,10,21] (Fig. 19-2, *A*)
- Femoral neck or subcapital areas[11] (intracapsular) (Fig. 19-2, *B*)
- Proximal femoral shaft or subtrochanteric areas (Fig. 19-2, *C*)[11]

Secondary to the location and severity of hip fracture, the most significant complication is related to **osteonecrosis** and the loss of blood supply to the femoral head leading to avascular necrosis (AVN). Gross and associates[11] affirm, "any fracture of the neck (femoral) can disrupt this tenuous blood supply. As a result, there is an exceedingly high incidence of avascular necrosis of the femoral head after hip fractures." LeVeau[17] states, "avascular necrosis may occur after hip fracture in about 65% to 85% of the patients."

Three main clinical complications are noted with subtrochanteric fractures: **malunion, delayed union, and nonunion avascular necrosis.**[18] Two factors associated with malunion and nonunion of subtrochanteric hip fractures are:

- The subtrochanteric area of the proximal femur is cortical bone, which has a decreased blood supply.
- The subtrochanteric area is prone to large biomechanical stresses that can lead to loosening of various fixation devices.[18] This complication must be considered by the PTA when treating patients with this type of fracture.

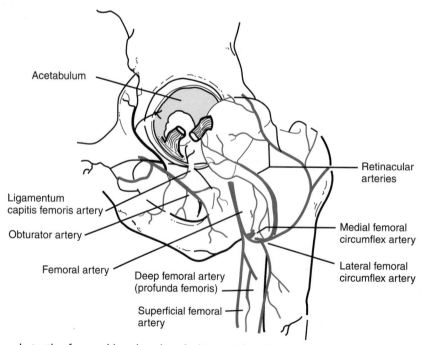

Fig. 19-1 Vascular supply to the femoral head and neck. (From Richardson JK, Iglarsch JK, editors: *Clinical orthopedic physical therapy*, Philadelphia, 1994, Saunders.)

Many options are available in treating hip fractures: The choice depends on the patient's age, location of the fracture, quality of bone, severity of the fracture (simple, **displaced**, or comminuted), activity level of the patient, associated soft-tissue injuries, and specific goals for the patient's return to activity. Generally, hip fractures are managed surgically with an open reduction with internal fixation (ORIF) procedure that secures the fracture fragments with various rods, nails, pins, screws, and plates.[9,10,16] Some hip fractures can be managed conservatively with bed rest, traction, and protected weight bearing.[18] For example, in a fractured greater trochanter where the displaced fracture fragment is less than 1 cm (as evaluated by the physician radiographically), the treatment could be bed rest for several days, range of motion (ROM) exercises, and limited weight bearing for 4 weeks.[18]

With an isolated lesser trochanteric fracture (most common in adolescents), the physician bases treatment on the amount of fragment displacement. If the fracture is displaced more than 2 cm, the physician could perform an ORIF procedure; if the fragments are in closer apposition, the physician may elect rest, protected weight bearing, and limited exercise for 3 to 4 weeks.[18] Figure 19-3 depicts common fixation devices used to secure fracture fragments using an ORIF procedure.

While treating patients with hip fractures, the PTA must be aware that venous thrombosis is a potentially critical complication after hip surgery. Without prophylactic medications to minimize thrombosis, statistics show that 40% to 90% of patients develop this condition after hip surgery.[18] Venous thrombosis is the most common complication after hip fracture in the elderly population of patients.[18]

Hip fractures and dislocations can occur in combination, as well as isolated events. Usually hip dislocations are either anterior or posterior (Fig. 19-4). Isolated hip dislocations generally are treated conservatively with bed rest, traction, and protected limited weight bearing for up to 12 weeks.[18] For example, with an anterior hip dislocation, bed rest with traction is prescribed, with specific precautions to strictly avoid extreme hip abduction and external rotation to prevent redislocation. Usually protected weight bearing is allowed when the patient can achieve painless hip ROM around 3 to 4 weeks after the incident.[18] Conversely an isolated posterior hip dislocation is treated with bed rest and traction in abduction with precautions to prevent hip abduction, flexion, and internal rotation to protect the joint from dislocation.[18]

Rehabilitation after Hip Fractures

The patient's overall preoperative physical and mental condition is a predictor of postoperative success. Patients with major cardiovascular or pulmonary disease processes, obesity, osteoporosis, dementia or poor upper body strength are at increased risk for postoperative complications. Overall mortality rates of 20% after 1 year, 50% at 3 years, 60% at 6 years, and 77% after 10 years have been reported.[7]

Although the overall goal of rehabilitation is to restore patients to preinjury level, this may not be realistic. Only 20% to 35% of patients regain their preinjury

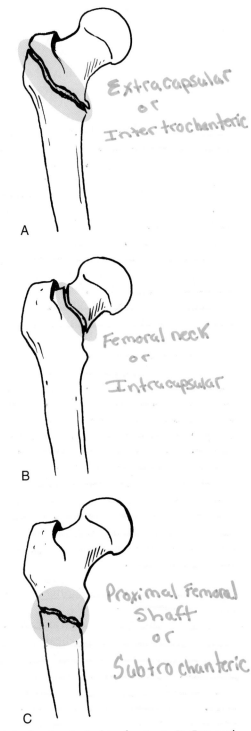

Fig. 19-2   A, Intertrochanteric hip fracture. **B,** Femoral neck fracture. **C,** Subtrochanteric hip fracture.

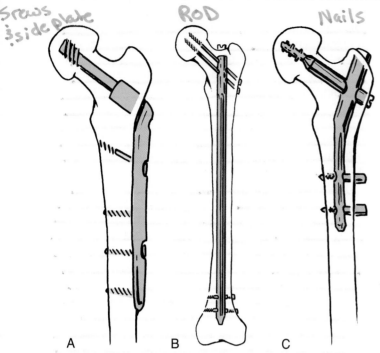

Handwritten annotations: "Screws 3side plate" (over A), "ROD" (over B), "Nails" (over C)

Fig. 19-3 Various methods of internal fixation for hip fractures. **A,** Screws and sideplate. **B,** Rod. **C,** Nails.

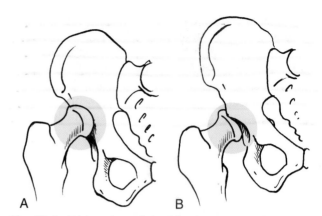

Fig. 19-4 Dislocation of the hip. **A,** Anterior dislocation. **B,** Posterior dislocation.

level of independence. As many as 15% to 40% require institutionalized care for more than 1 year after surgery. Many (50% to 83%) require devices to assist with ambulation.[14]

Any rehabilitation program used to treat hip fractures is highly individualized. The nature of the fracture type, classification, location, and method of internal fixation (if any) are considered, and the treatment program is adjusted to the patient's ability to cope with specific identified criteria. These criteria are established by the physical therapist (PT) and carried out by the PTA.

The progression from maximum to minimum protection closely follows the rate of bone healing. However, other factors are considered in safely and effectively providing an environment for the return to functional activities. In the maximum-protection phase of recovery (phase 1 to 21 days postoperatively, as described by Goldstein[9]), the fracture site is protected; pain and swelling are reduced; and isometric exercises, gentle protected ROM, and limited weight bearing begin.[9,17]

The general goals of recovery are to increase muscular strength specific to the surgery, improve overall conditioning, increase ROM of the affected hip, enhance aerobic fitness, increase local muscular endurance, reduce pain and swelling, reestablish normalized gait mechanics, and protect the healing structures from internal and external forces that can impede healing.[9,17]

During the maximum-protection phase the exercises used include active ankle pumps for both lower extremities, isometric quadriceps sets, gluteal sets, heel slides, hip abduction and adduction, and supine internal and external hip rotation. These exercises must be done at submaximal levels at first, and then progressively made more difficult according to the patient's tolerance.

Goldstein[9] identified a few major complications that occur, particularly during the maximum-protection phase of recovery. Generally, no combined diagonal or rotary forces are used in exercises during this phase. Hardware loosening and delayed healing may occur if increased torque is placed through the healing fracture site by excessive unwanted forces.[9] No active straight-leg raises or supine hip bridges should be performed during the first 6 to 8 weeks after surgery. Goldstein states, "The power generated by the massive hip muscles is so great during those exercises that there is a danger of displacing the fractured segments."[9]

In addition to rudimentary isometric quadriceps sets, gluteal sets, ankle pumps, and gentle hip-motion exercises, authorities advocate adding the exercises described in Figure 19-5 progressively during the first 3 weeks after surgery,[9] although exercises number 3 (forward bending of trunk) and 12 (hip extension in prone) are not advocated by the author of this chapter.

Early protected weight bearing is encouraged soon after surgery. Generally, touch down weight bearing (TDWB) or partial weight bearing (PWB) is allowed by the second day postoperatively. Weight-bearing status increases as dictated by the rate of bone healing (more than 8 to 12 weeks), which should be verified radiographically by the physician. Avoiding torque through the affected limb during standing minimizes loosening of the fixation device.

More demanding exercises are added as the bone and associated soft tissues heal. Closed-chain functional exercises are added as full weight bearing (FWB) is achieved. Partial wall squats and step-ups are usually initiated to regain concentric and eccentric muscle control of the quadriceps and hip extensors. A restorator or bike ergometer can be used during the early recovery phase if the patient can tolerate sitting, and depending on restrictions about hip flexion, ROM, and precautions.

Sitting

1. Knee extension (kicking)

   Slowly extend knee fully, hold for 1 second, and return slowly to flexed position under control.

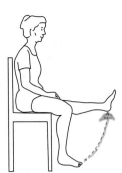

2. Hip flexion (marching)

   Lift alternate knees to chest, as if slowly marching in place while sitting.

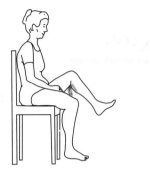

3. Forward bending of trunk

   Slowly reach hands down along the insides of the legs. Stop at the first pulling sensation. Return slowly to erect posture.

   Not Recommended

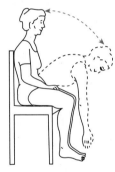

4. Armchair push-ups

   While seated, place hands on armrests (or push-up blocks) and extend both elbows, lifting torso from chair seat. Feet should be placed on floor for balance, support, and assist.

Supine Lying

5. Hip rotations

   With hips slightly abducted and knees extended, slowly roll legs in and out.

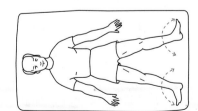

Fig. 19-5 Progressive hip exercises are employed during the first 3 to 4 weeks after surgery. (Modified from Goldstein T: *Geriatric orthopaedics,* Gaithersburg, Md, 1991, Aspen Publishers.)

6. Heel slides
   Slide heel along mat toward the buttocks and slowly return to original position.

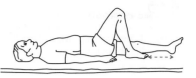

7. Knee to chest
   Flex hip, bringing knee toward the chest, and slowly return limb to extended position.

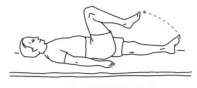

Supine

8. ~~Hip abduction/adduction~~
   Slowly spread legs apart and pull them together, keeping the knees extended and the toes pointed upward.

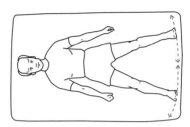

9. Terminal knee extension
   While supine with towel roll under knee, slowly contract the thigh muscles to bring knee into straightened position.

Prone Lying

10. Hip flexor stretch
    Lie prone for up to 20 minutes daily. Place pillow or bolster under ankles for comfort.

11. Knee flexion
    Flex knee and bring heel toward buttocks. Return to extended position.

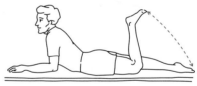

12. ~~Hip extension~~
    With knee flexed to 90°, lift knee slightly off mat without rotating pelvis and slowly lower knee to mat.

Not Recommended

Fig. 19-5, cont'd

The moderate-protection phase, defined as 3 to 6 weeks after surgery,[9] provides for more challenging exercises directed at regaining hip and knee motion, improving quadriceps and hamstring strength, and increasing strength to the hip extensors, abductors, and adductors. Standing four-position hip strengthening can be achieved initially without any resistance until a proper pattern of movement is achieved. Advancing this exercise can be accomplished using a cable system (Fig. 19-6), lower levels of Thera-Band, or ankle weights. The initiation of limited ROM leg presses can commence during this phase as well.

The late healing phase (after 6 to 8 weeks) is characterized by normalized gait mechanics and reduced use

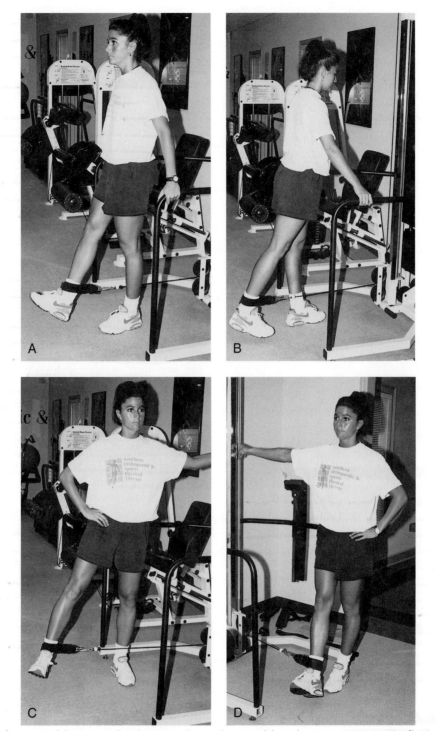

Fig. 19-6 Standing four-way hip strengthening exercises using a cable column system. **A,** Hip flexion straight-leg raise. **B,** Hip extension. **C,** Hip abduction. **D,** Hip adduction.

of assistive devices for ambulation. A treadmill can be used, with step cadence and stride length adjusted, to enhance gait and provide a stimulus for greater hip and quadriceps strength.

More advanced hip strengthening exercises can be added cautiously for more active patients. The stair-stepper stimulates hip extension strength and local muscular endurance, but extreme caution must be used when initiating various open- and closed-chain exercises after surgery for hip fractures. A fine line must be applied to avoid excessive forces (e.g., straight-leg raises or hip bridges), torque, and weight bearing while stimulating hip and knee motion and improving strength and function.

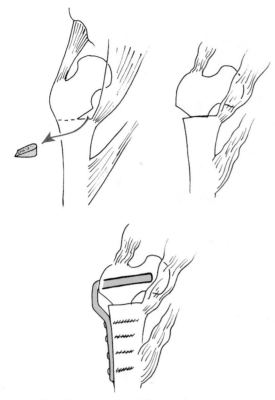

Fig. 19-7 Proximal femoral osteotomy.

PROXIMAL FEMORAL OSTEOTOMY

Intertrochanteric osteotomy may be performed when degenerative joint disease (DJD) is extensive and results in hip pain associated with subchondral bone erosion, articular cartilage fibrillation and fissuring, and hip joint incongruity.[15] The goal of this surgical procedure is to reduce pain and improve function related to advanced osteoarthritis by surgically changing the femoral neck-shaft angle so that healthy cartilage is exposed, thus "improving joint surface congruity."[15] Figure 19-7 illustrates this procedure and shows the changed neck-shaft angle relationship, reduced ligamentous and muscular tension, and improved joint articulation occurring after surgery.[15]

Rehabilitation after Proximal Femoral Intertrochanteric Osteotomy

Because a proximal femoral intertrochanteric osteotomy is performed to reduce symptoms related to advanced osteoarthritis (DJD) of the hip, the rehabilitation program must focus on joint protection principles (unloading forces through the hip) and postsurgical bone healing precautions. During the maximum-protection phase of recovery, avoiding unwanted forces, managing pain (with thermal agents or pain medication), using protected weight bearing (to unload the hip from repetitive articular cartilage destruction), restoring hip motion, and improving strength are stressed. Quadriceps-setting exercises, gluteal sets, ankle pumps, and gentle active hip ROM exercises are allowed from the first day after surgery.

Weight-bearing status is highly individualized but generally is progressed according to the rate and quality of bone healing. Typically, a walker or crutches reduces compressive loads through the hip during TDWB, PWB, and non–weight bearing (NWB) gait techniques. In most cases, protected weight bearing is strictly enforced for 8 to 12 weeks after this procedure.[15]

The contralateral hip, bilateral knee joints, and spine are targets of joint protection related to osteoarthritis. The PTA must fully recognize that the whole person—not just the affected joint—should be addressed during all phases of recovery. In keeping with joint protection, once the surgical incision has healed and the patient is allowed PWB status, an underwater treadmill, or unweighting device can be useful to enhance normalized gait mechanics in a protected weight-bearing environment. The buoyancy of the water allows reduced compressive loads through the hip.

Once radiographic evidence suggests secure bone healing, more challenging and intense strengthening exercises gradually are added. Isotonic knee extensions, leg curls, and standing hip abduction, adduction, flexion, and extension motions are strengthened through use of a cable system/wall pulleys, lighter Thera-Band resistances, and ankle weights. As with the rehabilitation post hip fracture, the PTA must recognize the advantages and disadvantages of these different therapeutic modalities. A major disadvantage of resistive bands or tubing is that the resistance increases as the range of the movement increases. This is a disadvantage to most muscle groups in the hip joint with these types of exercises since the length tension relationship of a muscle demonstrates maximal strength at approximately 80% to 120% of its resting length. At the very end range of these motions the hip musculature will potentially be actively insufficient and is required to resist the Thera-Band at its maximal resistance. The length–tension relationships between the resistance modality (resistive band/tubing) and the muscle do not match up in many cases. These same exercises can be performed in shortened ranges. The PTA must be cognizant as to the most favorable way to match up these length–tension relationships.

Extreme caution must be used with closed-chain strengthening exercises. Minimizing joint compressive loads, which may contribute to articular cartilage degeneration, is the cornerstone in the long-term care of severe osteoarthritis. Therefore functional weight-bearing exercises must be added judiciously and without increased pain.

A limited ROM leg-press exercise can be used as the first closed-chain activity. This may allow the PTA to systematically increase the resistance load while still using less load than the patient would encounter with FWB status. The compressive loads would therefore also be systematically increased. As healing progresses, mini step-ups, short-arc wall squats, and treadmill walking are added. A general conditioning program that encourages weight control, specifically using aerobic exercise (unloaded, upper body ergometer [UBE], or recumbent or semirecumbent stationary cycle ergometer), strengthening (while minimizing joint compressive loads and shearing joint motions), and flexibility should be implemented as soon as the patient can tolerate these activities.

HEMIARTHROPLASTY OF THE HIP

For femoral head osteonecrosis or severe femoral head fractures, hemiarthroplasty is used to eliminate pain and improve function. This procedure replaces the damaged femoral head with a bipolar prosthesis. Because hemiarthroplasty requires a normal acetabular surface,[15,22] it is rarely used for arthritis.[22] This is considered a conservative procedure[15] when compared with a total hip replacement. Hemiarthroplasty can be converted at a later date to total hip replacement if symptoms persist and the joint degenerates.[22] The term bipolar refers to two separate snap-fit components of one femoral prosthetic unit. A bipolar prosthesis is usually a large-diameter femoral head component that snap-fits snugly onto a smaller diameter femoral head, which is part of the total prosthetic unit.[9,15] A unipolar femoral prosthesis is a self-contained femoral head and shaft without additional components. The bipolar prosthesis usually produces less wear caused by friction and reduced impact loading of the acetabulum.[20]

FIXATION OF PROSTHETIC HIP COMPONENTS

As discussed in Chapter 9, the method of fixation of various prosthetic components directly affects the short- and long-term course of rehabilitation after hip arthroplasty. Both femoral and acetabular components usually can be secured to the bone with a cement, polymethylmethacrylate (PMMA), which is not actually an adhesive, but rather provides a strong interference fit between the prosthesis and the bone.[20] Or the components can be secured with a noncemented biologic tissue ingrowth prosthesis. Miller[22] recommends that cemented femoral stems be used only for patients older than 65 years of age, and that noncemented prostheses be used for younger patients. Weight-bearing precautions are related to the specific type of fixation procedure used to secure the prosthesis. Weight bearing generally is deferred for longer periods of time with a noncemented biologic tissue fit prosthesis so that the bone can grow into the porous coated femoral stem. Weight bearing with cemented

devices can progress at a slightly faster rate. However, in either case, rotational forces (torque) must be strictly avoided to minimize the loosening of components.

TOTAL HIP REPLACEMENT

Total hip arthroplasty (total hip replacement, [THR]) involves replacing both the femoral head and the acetabulum, as contrasted with a hemiarthroplasty, which replaces only the femoral head. Indications for the use of THR include the following:
- Rheumatoid arthritis
- Osteoarthritis (both femoral head and acetabulum)
- Osteonecrosis
- Fractures
- Juvenile rheumatoid arthritis (the most common indication for THR in adolescents)[20]
- Pain
- Reduced ambulation
- Significant alterations in activities of daily living (ADLs)[22]

Before discussing rehabilitation procedures, this chapter reviews pertinent complications and component designs related to THR because these issues influence specific physical therapy interventions and precautions.

Surgeons must select a proper femoral head size for each patient. In theory, a large-diameter femoral head may provide for greater ROM and inherent stability.[20,22] This makes sense because greater forces are necessary to dislocate a large-diameter head from the acetabulum. In practice, large-diameter femoral head components do not reduce the incidence of dislocation after surgery. Therefore the most commonly used head size is moderate (26 to 28 mm) rather than overly large (32 mm).[20,22]

One of the most common complications related to THR, using a noncemented femoral stem component, is persistent thigh pain with an antalgic gait (painful limp-gait) pattern. This thigh pain may last for 1 or 2 years after surgery and is reported in approximately 20% of all patients with this fixation type.[20,22]

The most significant complication after THR, with the highest mortality, is thromboembolic disease.[20] The entire rehabilitation team (PT, PTA, physician, etc.) must be concerned with this complication and monitor for this continually. While many of the signs of thromboembolitic disease after THR are the same as with any other lower extremity injury or surgery, some specific signs post THR would be localized tenderness and swelling along the distribution of the deep venous system of the hip, specifically the femoral vein along the anterior thigh.

Because the method of fixation is directly related to the initiation and progression of weight bearing after surgery with uncemented components, some authorities recommend TDWB on the second day postoperatively, gradually progressing to FWB by 8 weeks

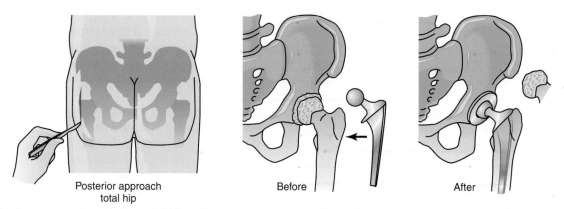

Posterior approach
total hip

Before

After

Fig. 19-8 Posterior approach for total hip arthroplasty procedure. (From Cameron MH, Monroe LG: *Physical rehabilitation: evidence-based examination, evaluation, and intervention,* St Louis, 2007, Saunders.)

postoperatively.[9] With a cemented (PMMA) prosthesis, Goldstein[9] suggests TDWB 2 days after surgery, progressing to FWB by the third week postoperatively. These timetables for weight bearing are directed by the biologic rate of bone healing and the wishes of the physician and are applied under the direction of the PT. A cemented component generally allows earlier motion and weight bearing than an uncemented prosthesis.

Loosening of the components has been estimated at 10% to 40% by 10 years postoperatively.[22] Loosening is more common among younger, more active patients, obese patients, patients with rheumatoid arthritis, and patients with previous hip surgery.[22] The PTA must be acutely aware of these factors when treating THR patients and recognize the increased potential for component loosening.

Postoperative dislocation of the hip after THR is another clinically significant complication occurring at rates between 1% and 4%.[22] These dislocations are multifactorial, requiring an awareness of the basic concepts of hardware design, fixation procedures, and surgical approaches and patient compliance with specific total hip precautions to avoid dislocation. The most immediate concern during the recovery from THR is teaching and reinforcing precautions to the patient, nursing staff, family, and other caregivers.

The PTA also should be familiar with the surgical approach used to gain exposure to the hip. Universal total hip precautions are intended to avoid the exact position the surgeon used to expose and dislocate the hip to carry out the procedure. Usually these precautions are as follows:

- Avoid hip adduction. This is usually accomplished by using an abduction wedge or pillow.
- Avoid hip internal rotation. The affected limb can be supported medially with pillows or a wedge to maintain the limb in neutral or slight external rotation.
- Avoid hip flexion greater than 90°.
- Avoid the combination (simultaneous performance) of hip flexion, internal rotation, and adduction for up to 4 months after surgery.[9]

The preceding precautions apply when a posterior (Fig. 19-8), posterolateral, or lateral approach is used. If an anterior surgical approach is used, combined hip extension and external rotation should be avoided.[9] Again, this variation is needed because the surgeon had to extend and externally rotate the limb to dislocate the hip and gain exposure for replacement.

Rehabilitation after Total Hip Replacement

Recovery from the significant trauma of THR requires extensive bone and soft-tissue healing. Following THR precautions, recovery may take up to 4 months or longer in some cases.

The rehabilitation program can be divided into maximum-, moderate-, and minimum-protection phases of recovery. The time frames associated with each phase depend on the individual patient's ability to achieve certain criteria of improved motion (being careful not to compromise THR precautions), increased strength, weight bearing status (taking into account whether the replacement has been secured with cement or a porous coated biologic ingrowth component), reduced pain, compliance with THR precautions, bed mobility, transfers, and improved confidence.

In the maximum-protection phase of recovery, the patient is instructed in bilateral ankle pumps, isometric quadriceps sets, gluteal isometrics, and active knee flexion (being careful to avoid excessive hip flexion) exercises. The contralateral limb can be exercised with active straight-leg raises, quadriceps sets, hamstring sets, ankle pumps, and full knee and hip mobility exercises. To ensure primary healing, all universal hip precautions must be enforced. (Avoid hip flexion, adduction, and internal rotation with a posterior, posterolateral or lateral surgical approach, and avoid hip extension and external rotation with an anterior approach.) In addition, the patient should be strongly cautioned to avoid the following positions and actions (Fig. 19-9), as outlined by LeVeau[17]:

- Do not sit in low chairs.
- Do not cross your legs.

No!   **Yes**

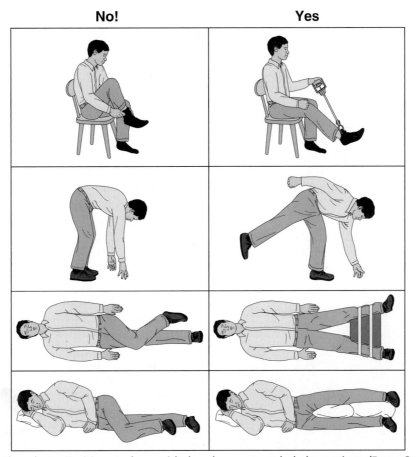

Fig. 19-9 Total hip arthroplasty: Positions to be avoided and recommended alternatives. (From Cameron MH, Monroe LG: *Physical rehabilitation: evidence-based examination, evaluation, and intervention,* St Louis, 2007, Saunders.)

■ Do not sleep on your side.

■ Do not bend forward at your hip (causes excessive hip flexion).

■ Do not squat.

Transfer training and bed mobility must be addressed immediately after surgery. The affected limb should be maintained in a stable, secure position during all transfers from bed to commode or wheelchair. A raised toilet seat is a basic requirement during the early phase of recovery. In addition, a raised and rigid (although padded) seat cushion is necessary to eliminate the sling effect of the wheelchair seat, which places the hip in an internally rotated position.[9]

The use of crutches or a walker is advocated for TDWB or PWB, depending on how the prosthesis is secured. A cemented prosthesis requires TDWB on the second day after surgery, with the patient gradually progressing to FWB by 3 weeks. An uncemented THR can begin with PWB; then the patient can progress to FWB up to 8 weeks after surgery.

The moderate-protection phase can begin when the patient has demonstrated improved quadriceps control, active knee flexion, reduced pain, compliance with all precautions and exercises, independent bed mobility and transfers, and improved gait (with necessary weight-bearing precautions). Moderate protection does not imply reduced THR precautions in any way. During this phase, more challenging exercises are added to more closely approximate functional activities. Light resistance exercises for quadriceps strengthening in a semi-recumbent position and elastic tubing (Thera-Band) also can be used to strengthen the hamstrings and hip extensors in a semirecumbent or seat-elevated position (Fig. 19-10). Standing exercises stress active hip motion (straight-plane motions, no combined rotational forces, THR precautions strictly enforced) and strengthening.

To enhance aerobic fitness, a recumbent bucket-seat bicycle ergometer or a UBE can be used. Increases in weight bearing are added as determined by component fixation, tissue healing constraints, and the wishes of the physician. Closed-chain functional activities begin between 3 and 8 weeks postoperatively[10] for cemented prostheses, with increased weight bearing orders by the physician. These activities can include sit-to-stand exercises with an elevated seat, partial supported knee bends (for concentric and eccentric quadriceps control), weight-shifting exercises, treadmill walking, mini step-ups, and standing resisted hip and knee extension (Fig. 19-11). For an uncemented prosthesis, closed-chain functional activities are deferred for 2 or 3 weeks longer than for cemented prostheses. However, standing straight-plane resistance exercises (hip extension, adduction, abduction, and flexion) are allowed between 3 and 8 weeks postoperatively.

The minimum-protection phase of recovery is initiated 12 to 16 weeks after surgery. Depending on individual cases, the physician may elect to discontinue THR precautions during this phase. A great deal of soft-tissue and bone healing must take place and muscular strength must improve dynamic stability before THR precautions are relaxed.

The minimum-protection phase is classically characterized by a return to normalized gait patterns without assistive devices, and by instruction in balance, coordination, proprioception, and advanced closed-chain

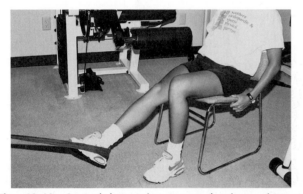

Fig. 19-10 Seated hamstring strengthening using an elastic band.

functional activities that duplicate the patient's specific ADLs. Most patients recover most of their hip motion during the first year after surgery.[20] Therefore at this phase of recovery (approximately 4 months after surgery) the patient may still demonstrate decreased motion, but must be reassured that more time is needed before assessing the ultimate degree of hip motion attainable.

While addressing proprioception, coordination, and balance after either knee or hip replacement (single-leg standing, eyes open and eyes closed, single-leg standing on a minitrampoline or balance board), the PTA must recognize that certain afferent neural input mechanoreceptors (type I, Ruffini; type II, pacinian; types III and IV, free nerve endings) will be lost because of the removal of the articulating joint surfaces. However, the joint capsule surrounding the joint replacement remains essentially intact and well supplied with mechanoreceptor feedback organs, which can be retrained and enhanced via appropriately applied weight shifting activities, balance board exercises, and closed-chain functional strengthening exercises.

Returning to higher level activities, including sport activity, should be a team approach discussion with the physician, PT, PTA and patient. Multiple factors should be considered, not the least of which would be presurgical activity level, experience in the activity/sport the patient wants to return to, strength, balance, proprioception, mobility status, and so on. A list of recommendations of activities and their level of recommendation is given in Box 19-1.

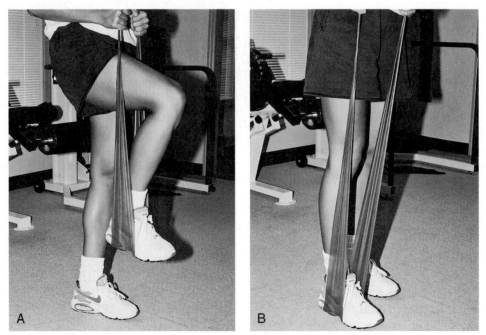

Fig. 19-11 Standing hip and knee extension press-down using an elastic band. **A,** Starting position. **B,** Finish.

BOX 19-1

Activity after Total Hip Arthroplasty

RECOMMENDED/ ALLOWED	ALLOWED WITH EXPERIENCE	NOT RECOMMENDED	NO CONCLUSION
■ Stationary biking	■ Low-impact aerobics	■ High-impact aerobics	■ Jazz dancing
■ Croquet	■ Road biking	■ Baseball/softball	■ Square dancing
■ Ballroom dancing	■ Bowling	■ Basketball	■ Fencing
■ Golf	■ Canoeing	■ Football	■ Ice skating
■ Horseshoes	■ Hiking	■ Gymnastics	■ Roller or inline skating
■ Shooting	■ Horseback riding	■ Handball	■ Rowing
■ Shuffleboard	■ Cross-country skiing	■ Hockey	■ Speed walking
■ Swimming		■ Jogging	■ Downhill skiing
■ Doubles tennis		■ Lacrosse	■ Stationary skiing machine
■ Walking		■ Racquetball	■ Weight lifting
		■ Squash	■ Weight machines
		■ Rock climbing	
		■ Soccer	
		■ Singles tennis	
		■ Volleyball	

From Healy WL, Iorio R, Lemos M: Athletic activity after total joint replacement, *Am J Sports Med* 29:377–388, 2001.

HIP OSTEOARTHRITIS

Hip osteoarthritis (OA) is defined as the focal loss of articular cartilage with variable subchondral bone reaction. The prevalence of OA ranges from 7% to 25% in adults aged 55 years and older in the white European population.[24] Although specific characteristics of hip OA have not always correlated with radiographic features, joint pain and functional impairment seem consistent.

Intervention goals for hip OA include relieving symptoms, minimizing disability, and reducing the risk of disease progression. Additional goals are education, modification of activities, maintenance of ROM if possible, instruction on proper diet and weight control, proper footwear, and the use of an assistive device if appropriate.

Conservative interventions that have demonstrated success in those patients with hip OA include gait and balance training, manual therapy techniques, and systematically progressed therapeutic strengthening.[2]

Functional, gait, and balance training is recommended to address impairments of proprioception, balance, and strength, which are all commonly found in individuals with lower extremity arthritis. The use of assistive devices, such as canes, crutches, and walkers, can be used in patients with hip OA to improve function associated with weight-bearing activities.

Regarding the use of manual therapy techniques, it was recommended that clinicians should consider the use of manual therapy procedures to provide short-term pain relief and improve hip mobility and function in patients with mild hip OA. Distractive techniques are particularly helpful to the patient with hip OA. Manual therapy techniques were also found to be superior in terms of relief of pain and improvement in function as compared with therapeutic exercise in all patients with hip OA, except those with highly limited function, high pain levels, and limited ROM.[13]

It was also recommended that clinicians should consider the use of flexibility, strengthening, and endurance exercises in patients with hip OA. The psoas muscle group should be assessed for lack of flexibility, and the gluteus medius should be assessed for weakness. Appropriately designed rehabilitation programs by the PT should be implemented. Strengthening of the weak gluteal muscles is addressed later in this chapter.

LEGG-CALVÉ-PERTHES DISEASE

In 1910, three researchers identified a hip condition that usually affects children between the ages of 4 and 8 years (the range is 2 to 12 years of age with the most common age being 6 years).[3] This condition, which is referred to as *Legg-Calvé-Perthes (LCP) disease* or *coxa plana*, is characterized as a noninflammatory, self-limiting (can heal spontaneously with or without specific treatment) syndrome in which the femoral head becomes flattened at the weight-bearing surface[11] as a result of disruption of the blood supply (AVN) to the femoral head in the growing child.[11,17] The long-term complications of the flattened femoral head lead to an incongruous joint surface and advanced DJD (Fig. 19-12).[11,17,19]

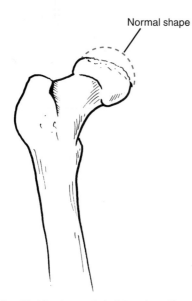

Normal shape

Fig. 19-12 Legg-Calvé-Perthes disease.

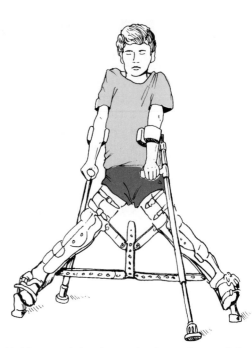

Fig. 19-13 An abduction orthosis can be used during the treatment of Legg-Calvé-Perthes disease to help maintain the femoral head seated within the acetabulum.

Throughout the management of this disease, the primary focus is on maintaining the femoral head within the confines of the acetabulum, regaining motion, and reducing pain and dysfunction.[11,17,19] In the acute or maximum-protection phase, reducing pain and dysfunction is generally accomplished using physician-prescribed nonsteroidal antiinflammatory drugs (NSAIDs), bed rest, and traction to take the load off the hip and restore motion in abduction.

Keeping the femoral head seated within the acetabulum can be accomplished using an abduction orthosis (Fig. 19-13).[11,17] To aid healing and reduce unwanted stress on the affected hip, the abduction orthosis can be worn as long as 2 years.[17] During this time, the brace can be removed for short periods each day to exercise the limb and attend to personal hygiene.[17] With the brace removed, the patient must maintain hip abduction during ROM exercises for the knee (flexion and extension), internal rotation of the hip, quadriceps strengthening, hip abduction, and hip extension strengthening exercises (gluteus medius and gluteus maximus).[17]

Surgical versus conservative intervention remains controversial as there is a lack of agreement on the benefit of surgical intervention versus conservative care. Patient prognosis is much improved if there is no collapse of femoral head.

PUBALGIA

Pubalgia is a collective term for all disorders causing chronic pain in region of pubic tubercle and inguinal region. Although typically resulting from athletic involvement, it can be present in other individuals. Pubalgia is often characterized by lower abdominal pain with exertion and minimal to no pain at rest. Unilateral presentation can be noted, although bilateral involvement is also possible. Identification of the contributing dysfunction is imperative in this wide-ranging condition. Arthrokinematic dysfunction of the pubic joint, sacroiliac joint dysfunction, muscle imbalances, among others, are all potential contributing factors to this dysfunction. Typically, stretching of traditionally tight muscle groups (psoas major and adductor muscle group) with strengthening of traditionally weaker muscles (gluteal muscles) is often indicated as long as it is pain free. Specific examples of gluteal strengthening exercises are given later in the chapter.

OSTEITIS PUBIS

Osteitis pubis is often part of the necessary differential diagnosis for pubalgia. These two dysfunctions are often confused. Osteitis pubis is characterized by pain and bony erosion of the symphysis pubis. The bony erosion is often a much later finding and therefore can complicate early diagnosis. These patients generally present with pain over the pubic area that radiates laterally across the anterior hip, which is usually aggravated by striding, kicking, or pivoting.

Examination findings include tenderness over the symphysis and proximal adductors, pain with adduction against resistance, and restricted hip rotation with pelvic obliquity and sacroiliac dysfunction.[8] A bone scan of the area may assist in differential diagnosis of this dysfunction versus pubalgia and athletic pubalgia (sports hernia).

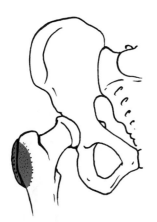

Fig. 19-14 Greater trochanteric bursitis.

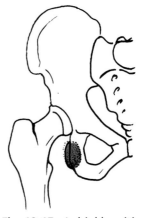

Fig. 19-15 Ischial bursitis.

Treatment is traditionally thought to be conservative, without any surgical intervention advantages. Treatment is aimed at addressing the primary dysfunction, whether it be muscle imbalance, joint mobility dysfunction, or some other cause. Similar to pubalgia, the treatment approach must be systematic and address the problem areas with consideration of progression principles.

SOFT-TISSUE INJURIES OF THE HIP

Bursitis

Trochanteric bursitis is a common soft-tissue injury affecting the hip in an active population of patients. The greater trochanter of the femur is most commonly affected. The trochanteric bursa may become irritated and inflamed because of excessive compression and repeated friction as the iliotibial band (ITB) snaps over the bursa while lying superior to the greater trochanter (Fig. 19-14).

Treatment for greater trochanteric bursitis is centered on relieving pain and inflammation while addressing the underlying cause of the condition. Rest, ice, and antiinflammatory medications are commonly used first to arrest the symptoms of pain and swelling. Any specific motions or activities (e.g., running) that may exacerbate the pain must be modified or eliminated. Intervention regarding this condition primarily consists of removal of the causative factors, stretching the soft tissues of the lateral thigh (especially the tensor fascia lata and iliotibial band); as well as focusing on the flexibility of the external rotators, quadriceps, and hip flexors. Strengthening of the hip abductors is essential, as is establishing a muscular balance between the hip abductors and adductors. Stretching is thought to be essential for reducing the compression and friction from the iliotibial band over the greater trochanter.

Specific strengthening exercises include quadriceps strengthening, hamstring curls, hip extension exercises (partial squats, leg press), and the previously

mentioned hip abduction exercises. Aerobic fitness can be maintained using a stationary cycle (although this is typically painful in this condition), UBE, treadmill, or stair-climber (if not painful). In any case, the ROM must be modified to limit hip and knee motion and avoid repeated snapping of the ITB over the trochanter. Ultrasound and hydrotherapy also may be useful during the acute phase of recovery.

Two other areas of bursitis commonly affecting the hip are ischial bursitis and iliopectineal bursitis. Ischial bursitis (Fig. 19-15) has also been termed *Weaver's bottom* and is characterized by pain over the ischial tuberosity underlying the gluteus maximus. It can be caused by direct contusion of the ischial tuberosity or extended periods of sitting.[11,23] Occasionally this condition can mimic a hamstring strain at the origin of the muscle at the ischial tuberosity.[11,23] This condition tends to affect thinner people and cyclists. Management is similar to other forms of bursitis: rest from the aggravating activity, ice packs, NSAIDs, and a judiciously applied program of stretching exercises that do not aggravate the symptoms. Generally, hamstring stretches are encouraged along with quadriceps-strengthening exercises. Somewhat unique to this particular bursitis is the use of a padded seat cushion as an intervention method because of the bursa location. Occasionally, conservative care fails and the physician may elect to inject the area with corticosteroids.[11]

Iliopectineal bursitis is characterized by either local tenderness over the iliopsoas muscle and tendon or diffuse radiating pain into the anterior thigh (Fig. 19-16).[23] Because the iliopectineal bursa lies deep to the tendon of the iliopsoas muscle, tightness of the iliopsoas alone and in conjunction with excessive hip extension can cause compression and frictional wear of the iliopectineal bursa. Pain may also be noted with passive hip flexion and adduction at the end range. Specific care centers on reducing pain and irritation using a program of rest, ice, antiinflammatory medications, and physical therapy interventions such as thermal agents, stretching, and strengthening exercises.

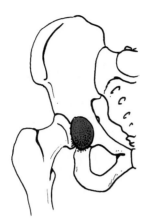

Fig. 19-16 Iliopectineal bursitis.

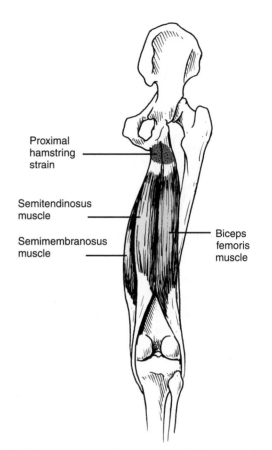

Fig. 19-17 Anatomy of posterior thigh musculature. Note proximal hamstring strain just inferior to the origin at the ischial tuberosity.

Unfortunately, in some cases of iliopectineal bursitis, stretching the tight iliopsoas muscle group increases pain over the bursa. Stretching of the psoas muscle perhaps should be deferred in cases where pain is exacerbated by such activity. The use of ice, hydrotherapy, ultrasound, and physician-prescribed NSAIDs can minimize the pain and allow for the initiation of quadriceps-strengthening exercises, hamstring stretches, ITB stretches, hip adductor stretches, and the beginning of an aerobic fitness program, as long as the symptoms do not increase. Specific stretching of the iliopsoas is indicated once initial healing has occurred and the acute inflammatory process is arrested.

Muscle Strains

Most acute injuries affecting the hip are musculotendinous strains of the hamstrings, iliopsoas, adductors, and rectus femoris.[11,23] Injuries to the hamstrings at the origin (ischial tuberosity) can be caused by sudden, forceful contraction of the hamstrings or by decelerating the lower leg against the concentric contraction of the quadriceps during running as the hamstrings contract eccentrically (Fig. 19-17).

Initial injury management involves the application of cold packs for 20 minutes, three to five times daily. Wrapping the affected limb with a compression bandage also can help relieve stress on the limb. Motions that produce pain and interfere with the healing process should be avoided. Two motions should not be attempted during the acute or maximum-protection phase of recovery: full knee extension combined with forward trunk flexion and full leg flexion.[3,4]

The use of crutches may be indicated during this phase to limit stress on the hamstrings. The PTA can significantly aid the patient in coping with a difficult problem during the early recovery phase. Sleeping may be extraordinarily painful. The PTA should counsel the patient to sleep supine with pillows under both knees to support the injured limb and to reduce passive nocturnal stretching by placing the hamstrings in a relaxed

position. As pain and swelling are reduced, active knee extension and leg flexion are encouraged (if the patient remains pain free) to help influence the direction of immature collagen fibers. The PTA must recall the intrinsic nature of muscle and tendon healing time constraints and avoid the temptation to encourage an aggressive stretching program for the hamstrings during the early maximum-protection phase of recovery. Sufficient time must be allowed for the torn tissue to scar and reorganize itself before subjecting the fragile immature collagen to excessive tensile loads that may impede healing. However, flexibility certainly must be addressed and is the focus of long-term recovery during the moderate- and minimum-protection phases of recovery, as defined by the significance of the injury; the patient's ability to achieve improved motion, strength, and pain-free gait; the physician's wishes; and the PT's direction.

Strength training proceeds according to the patient's individual situation and is strongly influenced by muscle and tendon healing constraints. Initially, isometric quadriceps sets and submaximal multiangle hamstring sets can be done as pain allows. Progressive strengthening can be achieved with prone manual resistive leg curls, ankle weights, or sitting Thera-Band leg curls. (This

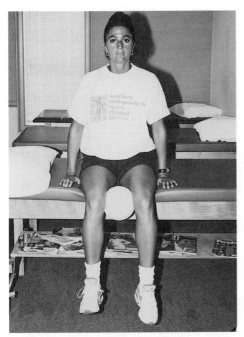

Fig. 19-18 Seated hip adduction isometrics.

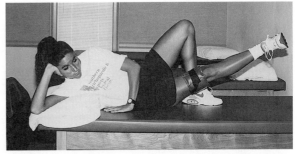

Fig. 19-19 Side-lying hip adduction concentric and eccentric contractions. Note the proximally placed resistance.

particular exercise strongly encourages slow eccentric hamstring muscle contractions.) An excellent, dynamic, and fun exercise to perform is scooting with a rolling adjustable-height stool. This exercise encourages knee flexion against resistance at various controllable speeds. Supine hip bridges can be added as function increases. Dependent on the patient's requirements, closed kinetic chain and higher functional demand exercises can be systematically implemented in order to allow individuals such as athletes a gradual return to their sport. The specific time frames for these different phases of the rehabilitation continuum must be determined with a team approach among the physician, PT, PTA, and patient.

An adductor muscle strain is termed a *groin pull*. A classic program of protection, ice, compression bandaging, crutches, and protected weight bearing during the acute or maximum-protection phase should be followed. As with other muscle and tendon strains, early aggressive stretching should be avoided. Once pain subsides, active hip flexion, gentle hip abduction and adduction motion, and knee ROM exercises should begin. Specific hip abduction stretching can be initiated, instructing the patient to perform the seated butterfly stretch, with a strong caution to proceed slowly without pain. Some authorities suggest waiting 3 to 6 weeks before instructing the patient in progressive resistance exercises.[11] However, resistance exercises can begin earlier, depending on the severity of the strain. To specifically strengthen the hip adductors, submaximal isometrics (Fig. 19-18) can give way to proximally placed resistance in various positions (Fig. 19-19).

Progression to more dynamic strengthening exercises depends on the specific goals established by the patient and PT. For example, in a young athletic population of patients eager to return to sports activities, a slide board can be an effective tool to introduce dynamic hip adduction and abduction motions (Fig. 19-20).

An iliopsoas muscle strain also is referred to as a *hip flexor pull*. This injury can occur from sudden, forceful extreme hip extension or by forced hip flexion against resistance.[23] A standard program of protection, rest, ice, and compression bandages with crutches and limited weight bearing is encouraged in the acute phase. Sleeping comfort can be enhanced by sleeping supine with pillows under the knees to reduce hip extension. Gentle, active hip flexion and extension exercises are begun once the initial healing phase has ended and the patient no longer complains of pain. A prolonged period of time may be needed to avoid hip extension (e.g., push-off during gait running or hip extension past neutral) and encourage healing. Gentle active stretching of the hip flexors can begin with the patient supine and the nonaffected knee and hip flexed. In addition, a hurdler's stretch can be initiated once the patient demonstrates improved hip extension motion without pain. The PTA should strongly encourage the patient to perform these stretches in a slow, static fashion without pain. Very close supervision is needed to guard against any ballistic, forceful, or violent motions that could impede healing and reinjure the affected limb.

Also, as previously mentioned with other conditions, correction of muscle imbalance and joint dysfunctions (as identified by the PT) need to be addressed. Antagonistic muscle group strengthening (gluteal muscles in this case) is necessary to maintain the newly gained flexibility achieved with stretching of the affected muscle. Some specific gluteal strengthening exercises with corresponding electromyographic percentage of maximal volitional contraction (values ± standard deviation) for the gluteus maximus and medius are as follows:

■ Side-lying hip abduction (gluteus medius: 42% ± 23%)[1]: patient lies on contralateral side with shoulder, hip and ipsilateral heel in contact with wall. Patient lifts ipsilateral lower extremity 6 to 12 inches in frontal plane, while keeping contact with wall

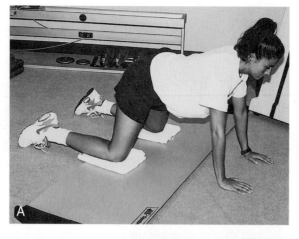

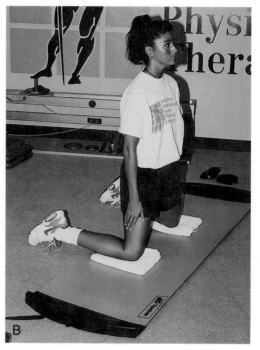

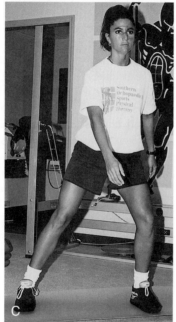

Fig. 19-20 Progressive slide board activities for dynamic closed-chain hip abduction and adduction. The series of exercises are begun. **A,** On hands and knees for support; the patient then slowly abducts and adducts both hips. **B,** Kneeling position is slightly more challenging. **C,** Standing position.

throughout the motion (Fig. 19-21, *A*). As the patient increases strength and requires less stabilization, he or she can move away from wall to perform this exercise as the PTA monitors compensation of abducting anterior to frontal plane.

■ Side bridge (gluteus medius: 74% ± 30%)[5]: patient lies on ipsilateral side with ipsilateral forearm directly below shoulder and lifts bilateral hips off table as demonstrated (Fig. 19-21, *B*).

■ Bilateral lower extremity bridge (gluteus medius: 28% ± 17%; gluteus maximus: 27% ± 13%; hamstrings: 35% ± 21%)[5,6]: patient lies supine with bilateral feet flat on table. Patient lifts bilateral hips off table to neutral spine position (Fig. 19-21, *C*).

■ Single lower extremity bridge (gluteus medius: 47% ± 24%)[5]: patient starting position as with bilateral bridge exercise. Patient lifts contralateral lower extremity with knee extended as patient lifts bilateral hips with ipsilateral lower extremity to neutral spine position (Fig. 19-21, *D*).

■ Standing hip abduction without weight (gluteus medius: 33% ± 23%)[1]: patient stands on contralateral lower extremity and abducts ipsilateral lower extremity 6 to 12 inches (Fig. 19-21, *E*).

Muscle Contusions

The most common contusion affecting the hip and pelvis involves the subcutaneous tissues of the iliac crest and is commonly termed a *hip pointer*.[12] Typically this injury can occur in one of two ways:

1. The iliac crest is contused by direct contact from an external force or falling on the exposed iliac crest.

2. There is a sudden forceful contraction or overstretching of the muscles attached to the iliac crest.[12]

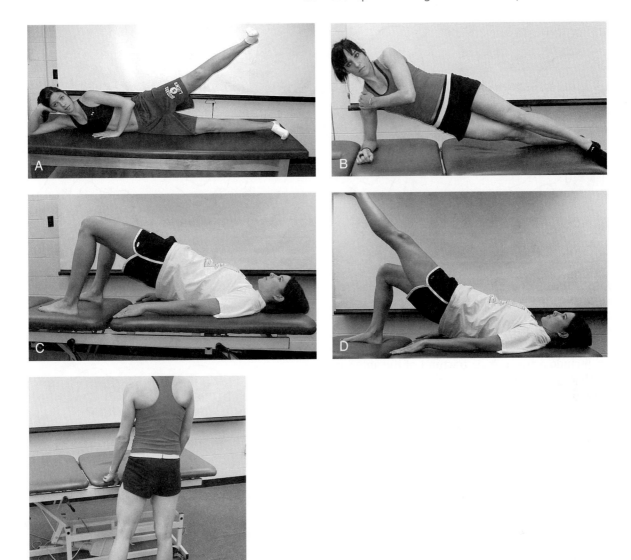

Fig. 19-21 **A,** Side-lying hip abduction. **B,** Side bridge. **C,** Bilateral lower extremity bridge. **D,** Single lower extremity bridge. **E,** Standing hip abduction.

This seemingly minor injury can be severe, causing extreme pain and dysfunction.

First, the patient is treated with protection, rest, ice, gentle compression wraps, crutches, and PWB. Initial soft-tissue healing must proceed without delay, so extreme caution is warranted to guard against unwanted forces or stress to the affected area. Stretching and strengthening of the affected hip commence once soft-tissue healing has progressed and pain is controlled. Usually in the moderate-protection phase, ultrasound, hydrotherapy, electrical stimulation, phonophoresis, or iontophoresis can be used at the discretion of the physician and PT to help control pain and swelling.

FRACTURES OF THE PELVIS AND ACETABULUM

General principles dealing with pelvic fractures and their classification with acetabular fractures dramatically show the PTA the extensive and potentially life-threatening nature of these injuries.[11,21,22] This discussion outlines the profound complications that may occur with pelvic fractures, giving the PTA a better understanding of the long-term rehabilitation needed in many cases of severe fractures.

The most basic classification of pelvic fractures refers to the injury as either stable or unstable.[11,21,22] Stable

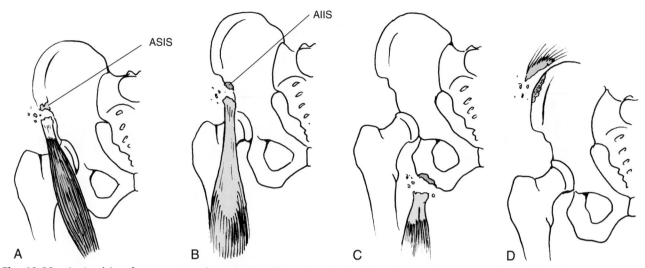

Fig. 19-22 A, Avulsion fracture anterior superior iliac spine. **B,** Avulsion fracture anterior inferior iliac spine. **C,** Avulsion fracture ischial tuberosity. **D,** Avulsion fracture iliac crest.

fractures include avulsion-type fractures of the anterior superior iliac spine, anterior inferior iliac spine, ischial tuberosity, and iliac crest (Fig. 19-22).[11,21] Avulsion fractures of the pelvis can be treated conservatively with rest, protected weight bearing, crutches, and avoidance of premature stretching and resistive exercises, which may delay bony union (usually within 6 weeks).[11]

McRae[21] advocates an ORIF procedure with avulsion fractures of the ischial tuberosity and fragment separation greater than 2 cm by saying, "Non-union is an appreciable risk, and if this occurs there may be problems with chronic pain and disability." Usually avulsion fractures of the ischial tuberosity can be treated with rest, keeping the hip extended and externally rotated to avoid continued stress on the healing bone, and enforcing protected weight bearing for approximately 6 weeks.[21] Once secure bone healing has been established, the PT may direct the assistant to carry out a gentle, progressive flexibility program to regain hip flexion. Strengthening exercises are added when the physician confirms radiographic evidence of secure union of the avulsion.

Other stable pelvic fractures include fractures of the superior pubic ramus, superior and inferior pubic rami on one side, and ilium (Fig. 19-23).[21] In general, stable fractures of the pelvis are treated nonsurgically with protection, bed rest (2 to 3 weeks),[21] and progressive motion and exercise once stable bone union has been confirmed.

Unstable pelvic fractures usually can be defined as either rotationally unstable but vertically stable, or rotationally and vertically unstable.[21] These severe injuries can be treated with an external fixator, ORIF procedure, or extended convalescence involving bed rest.[11,21,22] The PTA must be aware of complications after unstable pelvic fractures that can influence the time to begin

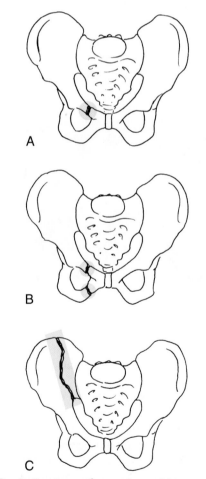

Fig. 19-23 A, Fracture of superior pubic ramus. **B,** Fracture of superior and inferior pubic ramus on one side. **C,** Fracture of the ilium.

rehabilitation procedures and can require protracted periods of recovery before physical therapy interventions. Box 19-2 outlines complications associated with these potentially life-threatening injuries.

The rehabilitation program employed after pelvic fractures is individualized and specific to the type and severity of fracture and the methods used to stabilize the fracture (ORIF, external fixator, and long-term convalescence). Because of the fragile hemodynamic nature of significant pelvic fractures, weight bearing of any kind is deferred for 8 weeks or longer.[21]

Initially the patient may be introduced to the vertical position using a tilt table. Pulse, respiration, and blood pressure are carefully monitored by the PTA as directed by the PT. Postural hypotension can be adequately addressed by gradually increasing the duration of elevation by small increments under the PT's direction. Maintenance of joint mobility is addressed early after surgery and during long periods of immobilization.

Active bilateral upper-extremity ROM begins as soon as the patient's condition is stable. Lower-extremity motion is limited to bilateral ankle pumps, gentle knee motion, and limited hip motion, depending on the nature of the fracture, fixation techniques used, stabilization of visceral damage (if any), and direction of the physician and PT. By far, the most significant clinical features associated with pelvic fractures are the potentially life-threatening complications, which can be acute or arise during early recovery or just after the acute phase of the injury. The PTA must closely supervise all vital signs before, during, and after all rehabilitation procedures. Once the physician has determined that the fracture site is stable and healed and the patient is medically stable, the PT may direct the PTA to follow a gradual program of general strength and fitness (a high priority with all patients requiring protracted periods of immobilization), quadriceps strengthening, hip motion, gait training, bed mobility, and transfer training.

The PTA must be aware that fractures of the pelvis also can involve the acetabulum. The acetabulum has an articular cartilage surface that allows for articulation between the femoral head and acetabulum. Care of this area is extremely important because the hip joint is a major weight-bearing structure.

The classification system used to identify specific patterns of acetabular fractures is defined by Loth[18] as the Letournel classification model (Fig. 19-24). Generally, these fractures are treated according to the severity of the fracture, usually with an ORIF procedure or, conservatively, with bed rest and traction to reduce compression of the joint.[21] Conservative management of acetabular fractures is reserved for severely fragmented acetabular floor fractures in which surgery cannot realign the fragments to anatomically reconstruct the articular surface.[21] An ORIF procedure is used to stabilize the fracture in all other cases.[18]

Protected weight bearing is encouraged for 8 to 10 weeks; in cases of nonsurgical management, weight bearing is permitted at 9 weeks. A lower-extremity strength program is initiated immediately after surgery and involves ankle motion, quadriceps sets, hamstring sets, gentle submaximal gluteal sets, and active knee and hip motion. As with all fractures, as bone healing progresses and the patient achieves individualized criteria (e.g., strength, motion, reduced pain, minimal swelling, increased weight bearing, and normalized gait), the rehabilitation program can be advanced, gradually incorporating more challenging functional exercises.

The PTA must remember the nature of specific acetabular fractures, since these fractures involve articular cartilage and bone. Therefore the initiation of closed-chain functional activities, which naturally require vertical loads, may be deferred for longer periods to allow for appropriate articular cartilage healing. If premature loads are directed through the weight-bearing surface of the affected articular cartilage of the acetabulum, delayed union may result.

COMMON MOBILIZATION TECHNIQUES FOR THE HIP

Reduced motion secondary to pain and fibrosis after fractures, soft-tissue injuries, and various hip arthroplasty techniques may warrant mobilization in conjunction with thermal agents, strengthening, stretching, and functional activities. The techniques presented here are identified by the PT as appropriate techniques to use based on pathology, the presence of pain, or defined limitations of movement. As with all mobilization techniques, the PT selects which techniques to use and the direction of force, amplitude, grades, velocity, and distractions (see Chapter 15).

Most important, patient comfort and compliance with relaxation before and throughout the treatment are of paramount concern. Before each treatment session, the patient should be placed in the most

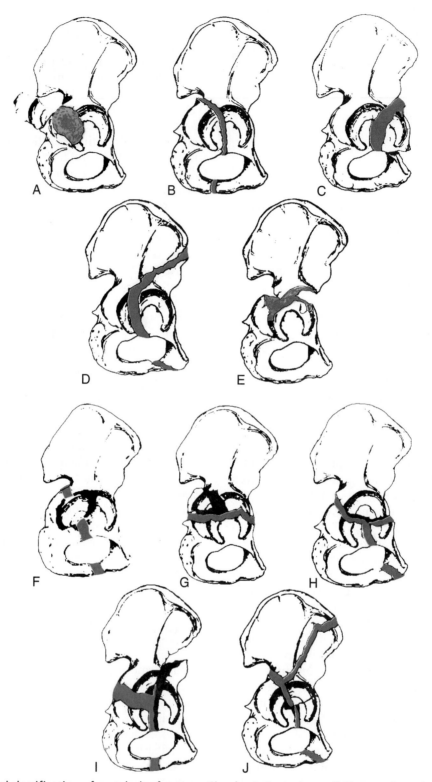

Fig. 19-24 Letournel classification of acetabular fractures. Simple: **A,** Posterior wall; **B,** posterior column; **C,** anterior wall; **D,** anterior column; **E,** transverse. Combined: **F,** Posterior column and posterior wall; **G,** transverse and posterior wall; **H,** T fracture; **I,** anterior column and posterior hemitransverse; **J,** both columns. (From Loth TS: Lower extremity. In *Orthopaedic boards review*, St Louis, 1993, Mosby.)

comfortable position with attention paid to supporting the affected limb. The application of thermal agents (e.g., hot packs or ultrasound) to the affected limb and surrounding structures may be helpful to compose and relax the patient before treatment. If the patient has physician-prescribed pain medications or muscle relaxants, it may be helpful to consult with the PT to suggest that the patient take these medications in a timely fashion before treatment to further enhance relaxation.

Other general rules of mobilization for the hip joint that should be implemented include:

- Warming of the tissues and body through exercise is advisable.
- Both the patient and the PTA must be in the correct position, relaxed and at ease.
- All techniques must be modified to suit both the PTA and the patient.
- Whenever possible, have the patient's body weight serve as a means of stabilization to prevent unwanted movement.
- Hand placement for mobilization should be as close to the joint as possible, with firm but comfortable grasp.
- Visualizing the joint surface, its direction, and contour will assist the PTA in correctly performing the technique.
- Whenever possible on hip joint mobilizations, the forearms should be positioned in line with the direction of the mobilization force to be applied.
- The PTA must use the minimum of force consistent with achieving the objective.
- Signs of overmobilization are:
  - Increase in pain
  - Increase in swelling
  - Decrease in mobility

Distraction

- Patient position: Supine with the leg positioned over the clinician's shoulder, hip in resting position.
- PTA position: Standing to side of the leg to be mobilized facing the patient's hip.
- Stabilization: The rest of the body on the table serves as stabilizing force. A belt may be wrapped around the patient's pelvis and the treatment table to help stabilize the pelvis.
- Mobilization: Position both hands on anterior and medial surfaces of the proximal thigh. Both hands move the femoral head away from the acetabulum at a 90° angle.
- Direction of force: Impart a caudal/inferior and lateral force to the hip joint by leaning back away from the patient (Fig. 19-25).
- Suggestions:
  - Maintain mobilizing and stabilizing hand as proximal to hip joint as possible.

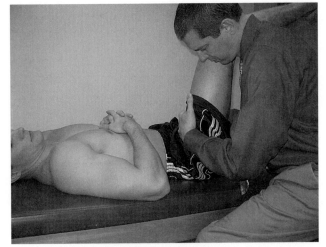

Fig. 19-25 Distraction.

- Hip joint is positioned in as close to the resting position as possible if conservative techniques are indicated. Approximating restricted ROM can be used if more aggressive techniques are indicated by PT.

Inferior Glide (Long Axis Distraction)

- Patient position: Supine on table, lumbar spine side-bent away from side to be mobilized.
- PTA position: Standing at the patient's foot facing the patient's hip.
- Stabilization: The rest of the body on the table serves as stabilizing force, especially with the lumbar spine side-bent away. A belt may be wrapped around the patient's pelvis and the treatment table to help stabilize the pelvis.
- Mobilization: Grab patient's leg proximal to the knee (supracondylar ridges of femur) with both hands. Distraction force in caudal direction imposed via both hands. PTA can lean back and use entire body for more aggressive mobilization if prescribed by PT.
- Direction of force: Directly inferior and along longitudinal axis from hip joint imparted via PTA body leaning back.
  - The result is distraction of the head of the femur away from the acetabulum (Fig. 19-26).

Posterior Glide

- Patient position: Supine with arms relaxed. Patient's dysfunctional side is flexed so that the foot is placed on the table just lateral to the noninvolved knee.
- PTA position: Standing on side opposite of dysfunction, directly facing the patient.
- Stabilization: Patient resting on table serves as stabilization. The dysfunctional lower extremity is placed in a position of flexion, adduction, and internal rotation such that the foot is placed on the table as stated above.
- Mobilization: PTA places bilateral hands on top of the knee on the dysfunctional side.

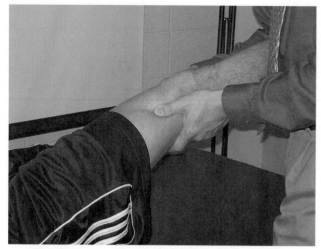

Fig. 19-26 Inferior glide (long axis distraction).

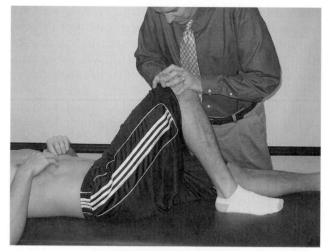

Fig. 19-27 Posterior glide.

■ Direction of force: Mobilization is imparted to the posterolateral hip and capsule through the long axis of the femur. Mobilization force is via PTA's body through his or her hands (Fig. 19-27).

■ Suggestions:
  ■ This technique can be progressed by adding more flexion, adduction, and/or internal rotation, eventually crossing mobilizing foot over other lower extremity.
  ■ Maintain good body mechanics to improve mobilization force.
  ■ Can use towel under ilium for greater posterior hip stretch.

Anterior Glide in Flexion, Abduction, and External Rotation

■ Patient position: Prone on table with dysfunctional hip in a position of flexion, abduction, and external rotation.

■ PTA position: Standing on side of dysfunction. Contact the proximal femur just distal the greater trochanter.

■ Stabilization: Patient's body resting on table serves as stabilizing force. A belt may be wrapped around the patient's pelvis and the treatment table to help stabilize the pelvis.

■ Mobilization: Mobilizing force is imparted to the hip through the proximal femur using passive accessory glides from posterior to anterior.

■ Direction of force: Passive accessory glides imparted from posterior to anterior (Fig. 19-28). Direction may also be imparted anterior-medial dependent on direction of restriction. Consider joint surface with mobilization.

■ Suggestions:
  ■ Maintain mobilizing and stabilizing hand as proximal to hip joint as possible.

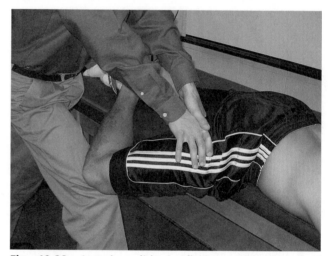

Fig. 19-28 Anterior glide in flexion, abduction, and external rotation.

  ■ Maintain mobilizing elbow in full extension to use entire body as mobilizing force in contrast to using only mobilizing upper extremity.

❖ GLOSSARY

Comminuted fracture: Any fracture with more than two fracture fragments.

Delayed union: Complication of subtrochanteric fractures characterized by any time that a fracture fails to unite in a normal time frame.

Displaced fracture: Any fracture in which there is loss of contact between surfaces.

Hip osteoarthritis: The focal loss of articular cartilage with variable subchondral bone reaction.

Malunion: Complication of subtrochanteric fractures characterized by a fracture in which successful union has occurred, but there is a degree of angular or rotatry deformity that exists.

Nonunion avascular necrosis: Complication of subtrochanteric fractures characterized by when blood supply to bone or segment of bone is compromised, leading to bone death.

Osteitis pubis: A disorder characterized by pain and bony erosion of the symphysis pubis.

Osteonecrosis: Subchondral bone necrosis secondary to vascular insufficiency.

Pubalgia: A term referring to all disorders causing chronic pain in region of pubic tubercle and inguinal region.

Simple fracture: A fracture in which the skin and soft tissues overlying skin are intact.

REFERENCES

1. Bolgla L, Uhl TL: Electromyographic analysis of hip rehabilitation exercises in a group of healthy subjects, *J Orthop Sport Phys Ther* 35(8):487–494, 2005.
2. Cibulka MT, White DM, Woehrle J: Hip pain and mobility deficits-hip osteoarthritis: clinical practice guidelines, *J Orthop Sports Phys Ther* 39(4):A1–A25, 2009.
3. Corrigan B, Maitland GD: The hip. *Practical orthopaedic medicine,* Newton, Mass, 1992, Butterworth-Heinemann.
4. Cummings SR, Nevitt MC: A hypothesis: the causes of hip fractures, *J Gerontol* 44:M107–M111, 1989.
5. Ekstrom R, Donatelli R, Carp K: Electromyographical analysis of core trunk, hip, and thigh muscles during 9 rehabilitation exercises, *J Orthop Sport Phys Ther* 37(12):754–762, 2007.
6. Ekstrom RA, Osborn RW, Hauer PL: Surface electromyographic analysis of the low back muscles during rehabilitation exercises, *J Orthop Sports Phys Ther* 38(12):736–745, 2008.
7. Elmerson S, Zetterberg C, Andersson G: Ten-year survival after fractures of the proximal end of the femur, *Gerontology* 34:186–191, 1988.
8. Fricker PA, Taunton JE, Ammann W: Osteitis pubis in athletes. Infection, inflammation or injury? *Sports Med* 12:266–279, 1991.
9. Goldstein TS: Treatment of common problems of the hip joint. In Goldstein TS, Lewis CB, editors: *Geriatric orthopaedics: rehabilitative management of common problems,* Gaithersburg, Md, 1991, Aspen Publishers.
10. Goldstein TS: The adult and geriatric hip. In *Continuing education course notes,* Boston, 1994, Quest Seminars.
11. Gross ML, Nasser S, Finnerman GAM: Hip and pelvis. In DeLee JC, Drez D, editors: *Orthopaedic sports medicine: principles and practice,* vol 2, Philadelphia, 1994, Saunders.
12. Henry JH: The hip. In Scott WN, Nisonson B, Nicholas JA, editors: *Principles of sports medicine,* Baltimore, 1984, Williams & Wilkins.
13. Hoeksma HL, Dekker J, Ronday HK, et al: Comparison of manual therapy and exercise therapy in osteoarthritis of the hip: a randomized clinical trial, *Arthritis Rheum* 51:722–729, 2004.
14. Jette AM, Harris BA, Cleary PD, Campion EW: Functional recovery after hip fractures, *Arch Phys Med Rehabil* 68:735–740, 1987.
15. Kozinn SC, Wilson PD: Adult hip disease and total hip replacement, *Clin Symp* 39(5):1–32, 1987.
16. Lewis CB, Bottomley JM: Orthopaedic treatment considerations. In *Geriatric physical therapy: a clinical approach,* New York, 1994, Appleton & Lange.
17. LeVeau B: Hip. In Richardson JK, Iglarsh ZA, editors: *Clinical orthopaedic physical therapy,* Philadelphia, 1994, Saunders.
18. Loth TS: Lower extremity. In *Orthopedic boards review,* St Louis, 1993, Mosby.
19. MacEwen GD, Bunnell WP, Ramsey PL: The hip. In Lovell WW, Winter RB, editors: *Pediatric orthopaedics,* Philadelphia, 1986, JB Lippincott.
20. McDonald D, et al: Total joint reconstruction. In *Orthopedic boards review,* St Louis, 1993, Mosby.
21. McRae R: *Practical fracture treatment,* ed 3, New York, 1994, Churchill Livingstone.
22. Miller M: Adult reconstruction and sports medicine. In *Review of orthopaedics,* Philadelphia, 1992, Saunders.
23. Saudek CE: The hip. In Gould JA, editor: *Orthopaedic and sports physical therapy,* ed 2, St Louis, 1990, Mosby.
24. Tepper S, Hochberg MC: Factors associated with hip osteoarthritis: data from the first National Health and Nutrition Examination Survey (NHANES-I), *Am J Epidemiol* 137:1081–1088, 1993.

REVIEW QUESTIONS

Short Answer

1. Name the type of injury in the following figure.

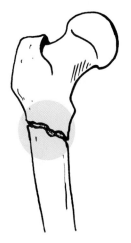

2. Name the type of injury in the following figure.

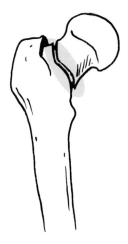

3. Name the type of injury in the following figure.

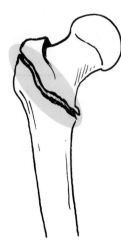

4. Name the soft-tissue injury in the following figure.

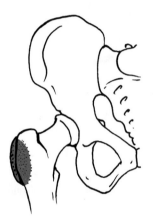

5. Name the soft-tissue injury in the following figure.

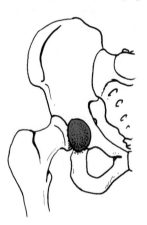

6. Name the soft-tissue injury in the following figure.

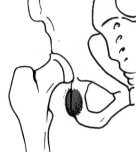

7. Label each muscle in the following figure.

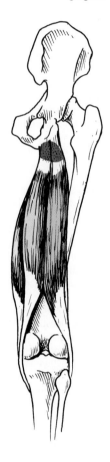

8. Identify the fracture type and location of injury in the following figure.

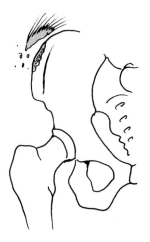

True/False

9. Hip fractures represent the most common acute orthopedic injury in the geriatric population.

10. The subtrochanteric area of the hip is prone to large biomechanical stresses, which can lead to loosening of various internal fixation devices.

11. The treatment of a fractured greater trochanter of the hip is always done with an ORIF procedure.

12. It is clinically significant that the simultaneous performance of hip flexion, internal rotation, and adduction be avoided for up to 4 months after THR surgery.

13. It is appropriate to actively encourage full knee extension after a hamstring strain during the first 3 weeks after injury.

14. Unstable pelvic fractures generally are defined as either rotationally unstable but vertically stable, or rotationally and vertically unstable.

15. Closed kinetic chain exercises are advocated during the early healing phases of recovery after acetabular fractures.

Orthopedic Management of the Lumbar, Thoracic, and Cervical Spine

Cheryl Sparks
Joseph Kelly
Gary A. Shankman

LEARNING OBJECTIVES

1. Outline and describe basic mechanics of the lumbar spine.
2. Discuss and apply the principles of fundamental mechanics of lifting.
3. Identify common sprains and strains of the lumbar spine.
4. Discuss common methods of management and rehabilitation of lumbar spine sprains and strains.
5. Identify and describe injuries to the lumbar intervertebral disc.
6. Define and describe methods of quantifying back strength.
7. Define and describe components of the back school model.
8. Define ergonomic and functional capacity evaluations.
9. Define spinal stenosis and describe methods of management and rehabilitation.
10. Define and contrast the terms spondylolysis and spondylolisthesis.
11. Describe methods of management and rehabilitation for spondylolysis and spondylolisthesis.
12. Identify common lumbar and thoracic spine fractures.
13. Define kyphosis, lordosis, and scoliosis.
14. Identify and describe methods of management and rehabilitation for kyphosis and scoliosis.
15. Identify and describe common cervical spine injuries, and discuss methods of management and rehabilitation.

KEY TERMS

Annulus
Directional preference
Disc
Disc protrusion
Extruded disc
Herniated nucleus pulposus (HNP)

Kyphosis
Lordosis
Nucleus pulposus
Radiculopathy
Scoliosis
Sequestrated disc

Spine stabilization
Thoracic inlet syndrome
Treatment-based classification (TBC)

CHAPTER OUTLINE

In an age when health care expenditures are a concern for many, back pain continues to cost billions of dollars in intervention and lost labor.[42,45] It is imperative that the physical therapist assistant (PTA) possess a sound understanding of the anatomy and appropriate management of patients with various spinal disorders. In this chapter the PTA is introduced to overall symptomatology and effective intervention strategies for some of the more prevalent diagnoses affecting the spine.

THE LUMBAR SPINE

Perhaps no other medical condition draws as much attention from researchers and clinicians as the identification and management of lumbar spine injuries. The primary cause of disability in the middle-aged working class adult is related to low back pain and accounts for approximately $50 billion in health care costs annually in the United States.[26,42,45] Lumbar spine injuries are also to blame for literally millions of lost work days per year in the United States and internationally. The rate of disability from injuries to the low back was estimated over a 10-year period to be a staggering 14 times greater than the rate of population growth for that same period.[1,15] Overall, lumbar spine injuries are the second leading cause of all physician visits in the United States and the prevalence of low back pain in the population is close to that of the common cold.[1,5,8,16,17,42]

Historically, absolute bed rest, medications, thermal agents (e.g., hot packs or ultrasound), and a series of rudimentary lumbar flexion exercises (e.g., pelvic tilts, single knee-to-chest, double knee-to-chest, and partial direct and oblique sit-ups) (Fig. 20-1) were the components of a typical protocol for lumbar sprains, strains, and disc-related pathologic conditions. It is now widely accepted that active rest and resumption of function has a significant impact on improving long-term outcomes.[20,24]

Basic Mechanics

The spine is made of 33 bones, which increase in size caudally. There are five regions including cervical, thoracic, lumbar, sacral, and coccyx. Components of the axial skeleton include osseous (bony) and nonosseous structures. Osseous structures include the vertebrae, and nonosseous structures are the intervertebral discs and the surrounding ligaments. Together these make up the normal spinal curves that define posture. These curves function to absorb shock and balance the center of gravity. The typical spinal vertebra has two portions: the body, which assists in weight bearing, and the vertebral arch, which protects the spinal cord. Also there are facet joints, or zygapophyseal joints, which guide range of motion (ROM) in the spine. These joints are plane joints, which glide relative to one another. The inferior aspect of the superior facet joint articulates with the superior aspect of the inferior facet joint. ROM is determined by the orientation of the facet joint. For example, in the cervical spine the facet joints are more horizontal in alignment, which allows for increased rotation. In the lumbar spine the joints have a vertical orientation, which allows for flexion and extension.

In the adult spine there are 23 intervertebral discs found in between the vertebral bodies (Fig. 20-2). The outer wall of the **disc** is called the *annulus* and comprises 12 to 18 concentrically arranged rings of fibroelastic cartilage.[30,56] Contained within the annulus is the **nucleus pulposus.** Nuclear material is a mucopolysaccharide gel[30] that transmits forces, equalizes stress, and promotes movement.[55] The annulus provides stability, enhanced movement between vertebral bodies, and minimal shock absorption. The greater portion of shock absorption comes from the vertebral body.[56,65]

The intervertebral disc is largely avascular and aneural. The vascular supply to the disc is provided by diffusion from the vertebral bodies above and below the disc.[14,30,49,56] The outer one third of the annulus is said to be innervated along with the facet joint capsule and exiting nerve roots.[14] When injured, without an intense vascular response, the disc has a limited capacity to heal and repair. In addition, degenerative changes also occur within the disc as a normal process of aging throughout the life span.

A popular theoretical model describes the fluid mechanics of the disc (nucleus pulposus) influenced by the motion of the lumbar vertebral segments.

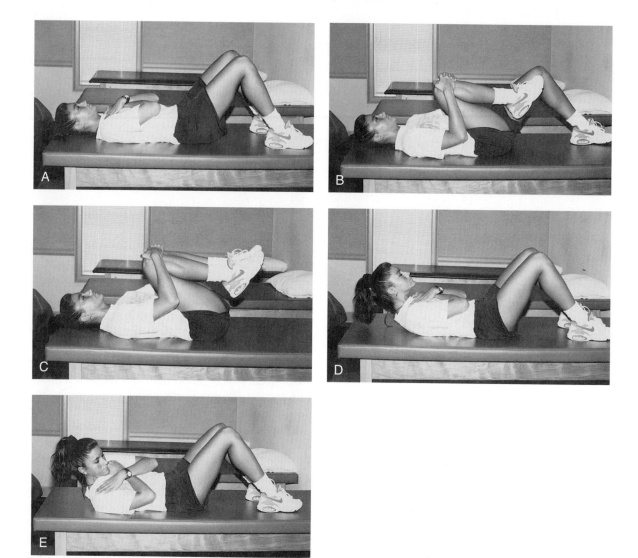

Fig. 20-1 Williams flexion exercises. **A,** Pelvic tilt. **B,** Single knee to chest. **C,** Double knee to chest. **D,** Partial direct sit-ups. **E,** Partial oblique sit-ups.

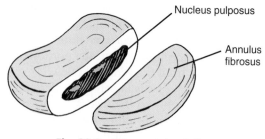

Fig. 20-2 Intervertebral disc.

McKenzie[49] describes flexion and extension motion of the spine as having clinically significant effects on the nucleus's direction of movement (Fig. 20-3, *A*). The theoretical model proposes when positional changes occur in the lumbar spine, from flexion to extension, the nucleus moves anteriorly (Fig. 20-3, *B*).[49] Conversely, when the spine moves from extension to full flexion,

the nucleus tends to displace or move posteriorly (Fig. 20-3, *C*). Thus it is necessary to fully understand the individual nature of each injury and avoid or enhance certain motions and postures as directed by the physical therapist (PT).

The amount of motion in the spine is primarily determined by the size of the vertebral body and the disc. Ligaments, fascia and musculature assist in restricting certain movements. The direction of motion is determined by the orientation of the facets. Spinal motions include flexion, extension, lateral flexion (side bending), and rotation.

The lumbar spine is composed of five anterior convex and posterior concave segments that produce the recognizable lordotic curve. Normal **lordosis** is increased with spinal extension and reduced with spinal flexion. The lumbar spine serves to support the weight of the upper body and dissipate compressive loads with

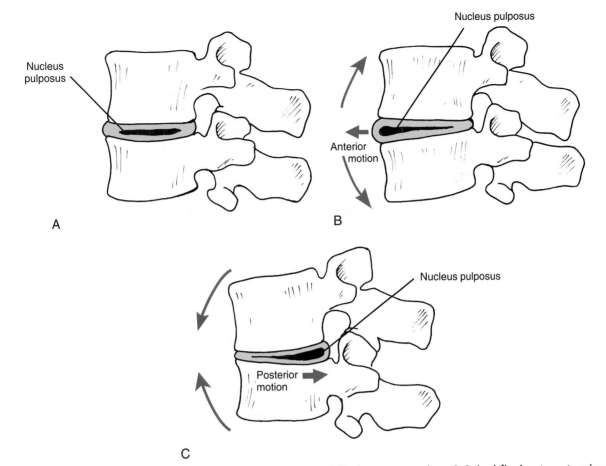

Fig. 20-3 Movement of the nucleus pulposus. **A,** Stasis. **B,** Spinal flexion to extension. **C,** Spinal flexion to extension.

minimal production of muscular torque. As a result significant forces are transmitted through the intervertebral disc during certain motions. Allman[1] describes lumbar motion and postural alterations as producing significant pressure within the disc (intradiscal pressure). The compressive forces that influence intradiscal pressure are as follows[1]:

■ Standing: Disc pressure is equal to 100% of body weight
■ Supine: Disc pressure is less than 25% of body weight
■ Side-lying: Disc pressure is less than 75% of body weight
■ Standing and bending forward: Disc pressure is approximately 150% of body weight
■ Supine with both knees flexed: Disc pressure is less than 35% of body weight
■ Seated in a flexed position: Disc pressure is approximately 85% of body weight
■ Bending forward in a flexed posture and lifting: Disc pressure is close to 275% of body weight

Intradiscal pressure also can be expressed in terms of pressure or load measured within the intervertebral lumbar disc. Cailliet[9] reports that isometric abdominal sets produce approximately 110 kg of pressure within the disc, whereas walking produces 85 kg; sitting, 100 kg; bilateral straight-leg raises in supine position, 120 kg; and lifting with a flexed torso and knees held straight, an astounding 340 kg of intradiscal pressure. This information may help clarify the rationale for protective postures, lifting protocols, and appropriate body mechanics, as well as prescribed exercises for specific lumbar spine conditions.

The PTA is strongly encouraged to thoroughly review the anatomic relationships among the lumbar vertebral bodies, discs, spinal canal, and nerve roots.

Muscle Strains

Spinal musculature includes the dorsally located superficial and deep paravertebral muscles. Deep paravertebral muscles include the semispinalis, splenius, multifidi, rotatores, interspinales, and intertransversarii. The more superficially located muscles include iliocostalis, longissimus, and spinalis. Anteriorly positioned are the rectus abdominis, the internal and external obliques, and the transversus abdominis. Injury to the muscles of the lumbar spine can be caused by sudden, violent contraction (e.g., attempting to lift a heavy object), rapid stretching, combined lumbar extension and rotation (torque), eccentric loading, and repetitive overuse resulting in microscopic damage to the muscle.

Although some authorities[27] point out that most low–back–related dysfunction results from soft-tissue injury, it is important to note that many other structures can potentially be involved (ligaments, disc, nerve tissue, and bone) and often the exact pathoanatomic cause of pain is elusive. The function however of the lumbar spine musculature is to contribute to dynamic stability.[55] Panjabi and co-workers[55] have identified the need for specific low back strengthening to reduce injury and "to stabilize the spine within its normal physiologic motions."

Muscle strains of the lumbar spine are common and general treatment goals are as follows[62]: reduce or eliminate inflammation (pain and swelling), restore muscle strength and control, restore flexibility, enhance cardiorespiratory fitness, restore function, and protect the affected area from further injury through education and supervised practice of proper lifting mechanics.

Ligament Sprains

Ligamentous support to the lumbar spine consists of the anterior longitudinal ligament (ALL), the posterior longitudinal ligament (PLL), the ligamentum flavum (LF), the interspinous ligament (ISL), and the supraspinous ligament (SSL). The ALL runs anteriorly along the vertebral body blending with the annulus of the disc to reinforce it anterolaterally. The PLL runs posteriorly along the vertebral body within the vertebral canal. It is more narrow and weaker than the ALL and offers little in terms of substantial support. The LF, lies within the vertebral canal and connects the lamina on the vertebral arch of adjacent vertebrae. The ISL lies between the spinous processes. It is well developed in the lumbar spine but weaker than the ALL, PLL, and LF. The supraspinous ligament attaches the tip of a spinous process to the next spinous process, traveling from the seventh cervical vertebra (C7) to the sacrum.

These spinal ligaments[69] can be injured by a sudden violent force or from repeated stress. The PT conducts a comprehensive examination of the patient to confirm or deny the presence of segmental instability (hypermobility resulting from ligament sprain) and evaluate the degree of pain with or without active or passive movement of the lumbar spine in general or in individual segments.[1,5] In addition to isolated ligament sprains, muscle strains can be superimposed, making the identification of specific single-ligament sprains exceedingly difficult. The management of lumbar ligament sprains essentially parallels the care of muscle strains. Each patient has specific, identified impairments and goals that must be addressed individually through the initial evaluation performed by the PT. The PTA, under the direction of the PT, must identify which specific

positions are contraindicated by carefully reviewing the initial evaluation data. Both the short- and the long-range goals for recovery from lumbar strains and sprains emphasize protecting the spine from unwanted forces and positions.

Radiculopathy

Radiculopathy is defined as mechanical compression or inflammation of a nerve root that causes neurologic symptoms in the lower extremities. This can be caused by encroachment on the spinal nerve root by osteophytes or a large disc herniation. Symptoms may include pain, numbness, tingling, weakness, burning, or paresthesias. This is frequently referred to as *sciatica* or a *pinched nerve.* However, a true radiculopathy consists of more than just pain and paresthesia; it often involves a change in reflexes, strength loss in a myotomal distribution, and sensory loss in a dermatomal distribution, which is identified by the PT during the initial examination.

Radiating pain into one or both lower extremities could signify nerve root compression from an adjacent herniated intervertebral disc. A sensitive test for nerve root compression or disc herniation requires the patient to be supine while the symptomatic leg is raised passively with the knee completely extended. This is called a *straight leg raise test.* When the uninvolved, or asymptomatic, lower extremity is tested in the same manner, this is called a *crossed straight leg raise test.* The crossed straight leg raise has been found to be highly specific for disc herniation. These tests are considered positive only if radicular pain is increased or reproduced.[21] Any positive findings noted during the initial examination performed by the PT should be confirmed or denied.[62]

Lumbar Intervertebral Disc Pathologies

Various terms are used to describe injuries to the disc. Although "slipped disc" is a common expression used to describe various ailments of the low back among the general population, a disc does not "slip" from within its confines between the vertebral bodies. Also incorrectly applied are the two terms, *disc bulge* and **herniated nucleus pulposus (HNP).** These are frequently used interchangeably. To clarify, a HNP can be defined by specific nomenclature to more precisely describe the injury. Miller[51] describes the three categories of HNP as protruded, extruded, and sequestrated. In a **disc protrusion,** the nucleus bulges against an intact annulus (Fig. 20-4, *A*). This would more closely resemble the layperson's disc bulge terminology. An **extruded disc** is characterized by the nucleus extending through the annulus, but the nuclear material remains confined by the posterior longitudinal ligament (Fig. 20-4, *B*). Finally, in a **sequestrated disc,** the nucleus is free within the canal (Fig. 20-4, *C*).

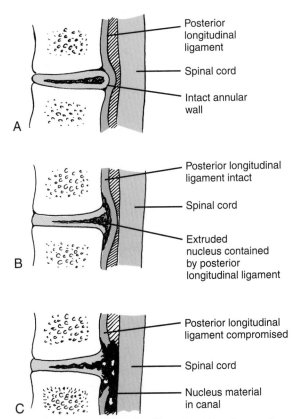

Fig. 20-4 Three categories of herniated nucleus pulposus. **A,** Disc protrusion. The nucleus bulges against an intact annulus. **B,** Extruded disc. The nucleus extends through the annulus; however, the nuclear material remains confined by the posterior longitudinal ligament. **C,** Sequestrated disc. The nucleus is free within the spinal canal.

Macnab[46] offers a variation of this classification model:

- Disc protrusion
  - Type I: Peripheral annular bulge
  - Type II: Localized annular bulge
- Disc herniation
  - Type I: Prolapsed intervertebral disc
  - Type II: Extruded intervertebral disc
  - Type III: Sequestrated intervertebral disc

Thus in a disc protrusion the annular fibers are intact, although the annulus bulges. A prolapsed disc has the nucleus contained only by the outer fibers of the bulging annulus.

Regardless of the exact nature of the injury, a HNP remains primarily a disease of young to middle-aged adults.[51] Common age-related degenerative changes that occur within the disc include decreased hydration, with a decreased water content from 70% to 88% by the third decade; biochemical changes in the glycosaminoglycans of the nucleus; and increases in collagen. As a result these changes make disc herniations rare in elderly people.[51,56]

When examining a patient who exhibits radicular signs, the PT confirms or denies the presence of peripheralization or centralization phenomena by observing a **directional preference.**[41,49] These conditions identified during the initial examination are defined by Kisner and Colby[41] as follows: "When repeating the forward-bending test, the symptoms increase or peripheralize. Peripheralization means the symptoms are experienced further down the leg." Centralization is defined by McKenzie[49] as, "the phenomenon whereby, as a result of the performance of certain repeated movements or the adoption of certain positions, radiating pain originating from the spine and referred distally, is made to move away from the periphery and toward the mid-line of the spine" (Fig. 20-5). The evaluation data obtained by the PT regarding the presence of a directional preference is essential in determining treatment.

Spondylolysis and Spondylolisthesis

Spondylolysis is a bony defect (stress fracture or fracture) in the pars interarticularis of the posterior elements of the spine (Fig. 20-6, *A*).[8,9,15,21,51,56,62] Spondylolisthesis, on the other hand, describes a forward slippage of one superior vertebra over an inferior vertebra (usually L4-L5 and L5-S1)[18,21] as a result of instability caused by the bilateral defect in the pars interarticularis (Fig. 20-6, *B*).[8,9,15,21,51,56,62] There are specific classification types, as well as degrees of slippage or "migration" of the vertebrae in the disease process of spondylolisthesis.[21] Five types, or classifications, have been identified, as follows[8,21,51]:

- Type I: Congenital or dysplastic. Results from a "congenital malformation of the sacrum or neural arch of L5, which allows forward slippage of L5 on the sacrum."[8] Most common in children.
- Type II: Isthmic spondylolisthesis. The most common type, affecting persons 5 to 50 years of age.[51] Usually a result of mechanical stress that causes a stress fracture at the pars interarticularis.[21,51]
- Type III: Degenerative spondylolisthesis. Most commonly affects the older population. Characterized by a loss of ligament integrity (or stability) that results in forward slippage of the vertebrae. Generally associated with the normal aging process.[8]
- Type IV: Traumatic spondylolisthesis. Caused by trauma that produces an acute fracture of the pars interarticularis. Casting is the most appropriate form of treatment.[8] Because of their generally high levels of physical activity, this type usually affects young patients.[51]
- Type V: Pathologic spondylolisthesis. Characterized by bone tumors that affect the pars interarticularis.

The degree or grade of slippage is determined radiographically by the examining physician and is defined as the amount of forward displacement of the superior vertebrae over the inferior vertebrae, as outlined in the following:[8,15,51]

- Grade I: 0 to 25%
- Grade II: 25% to 50%

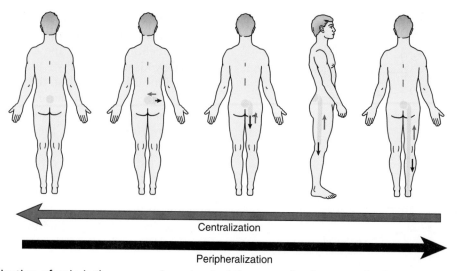

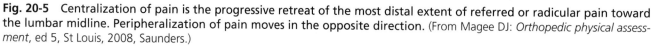

Centralization

Peripheralization

Fig. 20-5 Centralization of pain is the progressive retreat of the most distal extent of referred or radicular pain toward the lumbar midline. Peripheralization of pain moves in the opposite direction. (From Magee DJ: *Orthopedic physical assessment*, ed 5, St Louis, 2008, Saunders.)

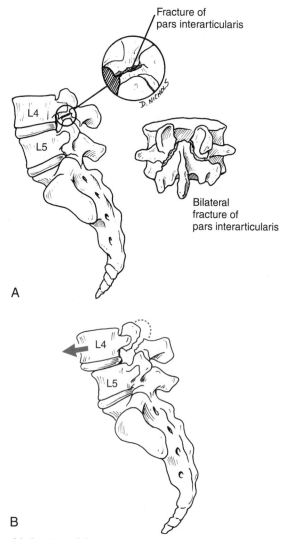

Fracture of pars interarticularis

Bilateral fracture of pars interarticularis

A

B

Fig. 20-6 Spondylolysis and spondylolisthesis. **A,** Spondylolysis. Fracture of pars interarticularis of the posterior elements of the spine. **B,** Spondylolisthesis. The resultant forward slippage of a superior vertebra over an inferior vertebra.

- Grade III: 50% to 75%
- Grade IV: 75% to 100%

The cause of the defect in the pars interarticularis is in part a congenital weakness in this area. In addition, the pars interarticularis is subjected to high levels of mechanical stress.[64,65] Authorities also suggest that the primary initial cause of the most common type of spondylolisthesis (isthmic) is fatigue fracture of the pars interarticularis.[65]

Patients primarily report pain with extremes of lumbar motion, especially extension. The pain generally follows the belt line.[37] During examination, the PT also may identify a palpable step-off between the affected lumbar vertebrae (usually L4-L5) because of the forward slippage.[15]

The management of spondylolisthesis is dictated by symptoms, as well as the degree of vertebral slippage (grades I to IV). For example, an adult with isthmic spondylolisthesis of radiographically determined grade I (0 to 25% slippage) may not experience significant symptoms with activity or extremes of lumbar extension. Thus treatment is aimed at preventing any progression to grade II (25% to 50% slippage). This usually is accomplished by instructing the patient to avoid ballistic lumbar extension, as well as vertical loading while seated or standing, so as to minimize anteriorly directed shearing forces on the spine. In addition, abdominal strengthening exercises, neutral **spine stabilization** exercises (controlled lumbar extension strengthening, isometrics, and rectus and oblique abdominal strengthening while in the neutral spine position), and stretching exercises for the trunk and lower extremities are encouraged.

The patient may require more specific attention when there is a greater degree of slippage with significant symptoms. Generally, pain and muscle spasm are addressed with physician-prescribed analgesics, muscle relaxants, nonsteroidal antiinflammatory drugs (NSAIDs), and agents (heat, ice, ultrasound, and electrical stimulation) to alleviate acute pain and swelling. If the pain is related to a fatigue fracture of the pars interarticularis, initial treatment focuses on managing stress to the fracture site using a lumbosacral corset or orthosis, which reduces anterior shearing forces through the fracture site and allows for bone healing.[21,37]

The cornerstone in the care of spondylolisthesis is application of abdominal and paravertebral muscle strengthening exercises to provide dynamic support for the spine during activity and avoidance of extreme lumbar extension. A young active patient must modify activities that directly influence the course of this disease. For example, weight lifting without proper precaution can contribute significantly to the occurrence of spondylolysis.[19]

Surgery is rare and usually is reserved for patients with radicular symptoms and high-grade slippage (grades III or IV), which compresses the nerve roots and causes neurologic signs.[8,51] The type of surgery advocated in these cases is a decompression laminectomy (to reduce compression of the nerve roots) with fusion to stabilize the vertebral segments.[8,51]

Rehabilitation after surgery for spondylolisthesis is deferred until solid bony union is determined radiographically. The patient is usually in a lumbosacral orthosis that does not permit lumbar extension. During immobilization, the patient can ambulate as tolerated and perform rudimentary ROM and strengthening exercises for the upper and lower extremities (ankle pumps, quadriceps sets, and knee ROM). Once bone healing is confirmed, a gradually progressive program of abdominal strengthening (from isometrics to concentric and eccentric abdominal contractions), lumbar ROM (avoiding dynamic, ballistic, and extreme lumbar extension), general conditioning, and a progressive return to function is advocated.[8,51]

Lumbar Spondylosis

Spondylosis is defined as osteoarthritis of the spine. X-ray findings may include bone spurs and osteophytes as well as fusing of adjacent levels in advanced stages. It is also referred to as *degenerative joint disease (DJD)*. Spondylosis is a degenerative process associated with aging. It can also be associated with decrease in disc height or degenerative disc disease. This degenerative process may lead to encroachment on the nerve roots and resultant neurologic symptoms.

Spinal Stenosis

Lumbar spinal stenosis is defined as a narrowing of the spinal canal, which constricts and compresses nerve roots (Fig. 20-7).[51] This gives rise to symptoms of neurogenic or spinal claudication, as follows:

1. Radicular ache into the thigh and less frequently into the calf[8]
2. Paresthesias into the lower extremity[29]
3. Disturbances in motor function[29]

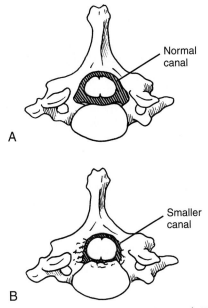

Fig. 20-7 Lumbar spinal stenosis. **A,** Normal. **B,** Stenotic spine. The narrow diameter of the spinal canal can lead to constriction and compression of nerve roots.

This condition occurs in males "twice as often as females"[51] and typically is observed during late middle age and older.[29,51]

Lumbar spinal stenosis is most commonly acquired as a result of degenerative arthritic changes that encroach on the diameter of the canal, producing nerve root compression.[51] The patient with stenosis frequently complains of pain and increased symptoms with lumbar extension. Extension of the lumbar spine in a patient with stenosis further compresses the spinal canal, thereby increasing pain and paresthesias.[15,29,51]

During ambulation and gait training, an elderly patient typically demonstrates a forward-flexed trunk posture when using a walker. Under careful observation and questioning, the patient may suggest that leaning forward feels better and reduces back and leg pain. The role of the PTA is to continually educate the patient, reinforcing appropriate postures, body mechanics, and lifting techniques. Sitting and sleeping changes, as well as a general physical conditioning and weight management programs are also addressed and have been identified as an important adjunct in the overall management of patients with spinal stenosis.[51] Whitman and colleagues[63] demonstrated that subjects with spinal stenosis experienced greater improvements in pain and recovery at 6 weeks with manual therapy, exercise, and walking than subjects who just performed routine flexion exercises and walking. The physical therapy team should work together to provide the appropriate manual intervention followed by specific exercise and a walking program for the best management of patients with spinal stenosis.

Lumbar Spine Fractures

Fractures of the lumbar vertebrae generally occur after a profound traumatic event and can be classified according to the forces that produce the fracture. For example, compression, flexion, extension, flexion-distraction, flexion-rotation, and lateral flexion are forces that produce fractures.[51] Lumbar spine fractures also can be described in terms that graphically depict a specific fracture deformity, including crush, wedge, burst, shear, slice, and teardrop fractures.[51]

Perhaps the most clinically relevant spine fracture for the PTA to consider is the vertebral compression fracture. Vertebral compression fractures are the most common osteoporosis-related spinal fracture with approximately 700,000 occurring per year, and the prevalence of vertebral compression fractures increases with age.[15,29,43]

Many benign activities can produce compression fractures in an elderly population of patients with osteoporosis.[8,43] Care must be taken to ensure that no rapid deceleration occurs when an elderly patient transfers to a bedside commode or any other hard surface. This seemingly trivial activity frequently causes multilevel compression fractures in patients with osteoporosis. Compression fractures produce symptoms ranging from acute local pain to essentially no signs at all.[43] Thus subtle complaints of pain caused by typical daily activities, such as bending, lifting, or rising from a chair, must be viewed with a high level of suspicion in elderly patients.[43]

Treatment of compression fractures focuses on relief of pain; authorities[29,43] advocate activity modification, physician-prescribed analgesics, NSAIDs, heat, ice, massage, and electrical stimulation to control pain, swelling, and associated muscle spasm. During the acute and subacute phases of recovery, the patient with compression fractures must avoid thoracic or lumbar flexion activities.[29] Repeated trunk flexion is contraindicated because it creates an anterior wedging of the vertebral bodies, producing greater stress and compression at the fracture site.[29] Appropriate exercise progression should target the muscles supporting or attached to the affected bone, and they will be determined by the PT. Exercises should be combined with postural correction, scapular stabilization, and improving weight-bearing patterns, strength, balance, and flexibility.

Compression fracture prevention education programs, especially in patients with osteoporosis, should focus on implementing an exercise program designed to increase strength, flexibility, and bone density, as well as improve balance, posture, and body mechanics to help maintain bone mass. Other preventative measures include identifying potential hazards in the home, selecting appropriate assistive devices, and general patient education.

Treatment-Based Classification

Rehabilitation of the lumbar spine is focused toward impairments rather than labeling pathoanatomic findings. As a result, when a patient experiences low back pain, the evaluating PT assimilates information from the patient history, examination, and current best evidence, and classifies the patient into the most appropriate category. The rehabilitation plan will include a multimodal approach that categorizes patients based on their overall symptomatology and response to a specific intervention. This system has been identified as **treatment-based classification (TBC)**.[6]

The TBC system consists of subgroupings through which the patient moves fluidly in and out of during the course of care. The interventions within these categories include manual therapy and exercise,[12,22] specific exercise for directional preference,[7,63] traction,[24,25] neuromuscular reeducation and stabilization exercise,[34,52,54] aerobic exercise, and recommendations to stay active. PTs will use their findings from the clinical examination to match the patient with the most appropriate intervention. Research has shown patients managed with this systematic approach experience significant decreases in pain and disability.[6,24] For the PTA it is important to be aware of the categories along with exercise and educational concerns within each.

Some patients with acute or chronic low back pain will benefit from first restoring mobility in the spine, and therefore these patients will initially be placed in the manual therapy and exercise category. The PT will address any segments that need to be mobilized before initiating an exercise program for the patient. Early exercises are chosen to enhance the restoration of normal movement in the lumbar spine and include pelvic rocking and abdominal bracing. Patients with short duration of symptoms (less than 2 or 3 weeks), no symptoms distal to the knee, and low fear-avoidance behaviors are expected to experience a 50% reduction in disability in 1 to 2 weeks on the Oswestry Disability Index (ODI) Questionnaire.[12,22] However the PT may choose to progress the patient gradually based on the presence of elevated fear avoidance beliefs noted on the Fear Avoidance Beliefs Questionnaire (FABQ).[28]

Patients with more chronic or recurring symptoms of low back pain are managed with neuromuscular reeducation and stabilization exercise. These patients often present with an average straight leg raise greater than 91° and the presence of aberrant motions. Exercises focus on recruitment and control of the multifidi, transversus abdominis, internal and external obliques, and the gluteal musculature. With this strategy, patients can also expected to achieve a 50% reduction in disability on the ODI in 8 weeks.[34]

In the presence of a directional preference, the patient experiences a centralization phenomenon where distal lower extremity symptoms and low back

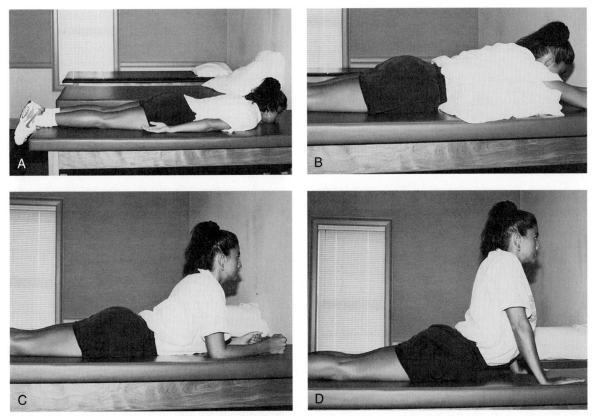

Fig. 20-8 Passive prone extension sequence. **A,** Patient lying prone without pillow for support. **B,** Patient prone with pillow under the chest for mild thoracic and lumbar extension. **C,** Patient propped up on elbows for improved extension. **D,** Patient prone with elbows extended for maximum extension.

pain are lessened with repeated movements into a particular direction. The symptoms become more centrally located with certain motions. An example of a repeated movement or prone progression is shown in Figure 20-8. Research has shown the adoption of the appropriate exercise program based on the patient's directional preference will allow for less pain and disability for up to 6 months.[7] Occasionally patients with distal lower extremity symptoms and neurologic signs will not demonstrate centralization with movement testing. In which case, the patient may benefit from mechanical traction in addition to specific exercises.[24]

The PTA should be extremely cognizant of any new reports of changes or worsening in patients' signs and symptoms and report these findings immediately to the evaluating PT. Some changes may include worsening or peripheralization of symptoms into the lower extremity, the presence of night pain, changes in bowel or bladder activity, or saddle anesthesia.

Invasive Management

When conservative physical therapy (including active rest, medications, exercise, and postural correction) fails to bring significant relief from symptoms, the physician may offer several invasive procedures. For some patients

whose persistent radicular pain (sciatica) cannot be controlled by conservative measures, the physician may prescribe an epidural steroid injection to relieve symptoms.[21,51] These injections are given only to relieve pain and reduce inflammation, and are not intended as a curative procedure to correct any neurologic deficits.

Patients may undergo surgery in the presence of a large disc herniation. As described by Miller[51] and Eismont and Kitchel,[21] the most common procedure is a laminotomy with a decompression discectomy. In this procedure the physician gains exposure to the herniated disc by cutting into the lamina and then removing all nonviable disc material, thereby decompressing the affected nerve root (Fig. 20-9). While some patients report good or excellent results with this particular surgical procedure, as many as 30% of these patients may have significant back pain at long-term follow-up.[18,51] Other invasive procedures exist, such as microsurgical discectomy and automated percutaneous discectomy.

Rehabilitation after any surgical procedure is highly patient-specific and directly related to the data obtained at the initial postoperative physical therapy evaluation. Generally, recovery closely parallels the criteria established with conservative management including neuromuscular re-education and stabilization exercise. However, extensive surgical exposure is necessary

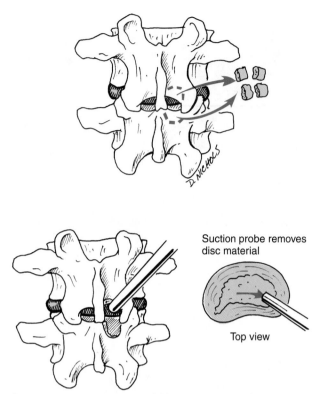

Suction probe removes disc material

Top view

Fig. 20-9 Laminotomy with decompression discectomy.

to perform a laminotomy with discectomy, and tissue-healing constraints influence recovery.

After surgery, the patient is taught bed mobility and transfer training using the log-roll technique to move from a supine to sitting position. Ambulation with a walker or crutches is generally allowed 1 day after surgery. Ambulation distance and endurance activities are increased according to each patient's ability. Rudimentary bed exercises can be performed the day after surgery and include active ankle pumps, gentle hip and knee flexion, and isometric exercises (quadriceps and gluteals). The PT guides the PTA concerning whether the postoperative patient will perform any isometric exercises. The PTA must instruct the patient in and reinforce proper breathing techniques if isometric exercises are done. The Valsalva maneuver is strictly avoided during all exercises.

For the first 3 days after surgery the patient is limited to sitting for no more than 1 hour at a time and must maintain proper spinal position with no flexion.[10] The PTA continually reinforces and encourages proper posture during the first week of recovery. The patient should be cautioned to avoid forward bending and trunk rotation.

More demanding and functionally relevant activities that do not stress the surgical site are added gradually. Transfers from supine to sitting and from sitting to standing must be demonstrated by the patient and observed by the clinician to be safe, efficient, and free from all unwanted stress. Throughout the first week, exercises can progress to include functional closed-chain activities while maintaining proper neutral spine positioning.

When initial wound healing is complete and pain is decreased, a more accelerated program of strengthening can begin. ROM is encouraged gradually as soon as the patient can tolerate these motions. Gentle active extension exercises and pelvic tilts (which promote pelvic motion, control, as well as limited-motion lumbar spine flexion and extension) begin early in the recovery phase.

The patient must achieve increased motion, controlled pain, improved endurance, and sufficient strength before beginning a general conditioning program after surgery. The longer recovery period is needed to allow for proper soft-tissue healing, bone healing, and control of inflammation and pain before subjecting the affected area to stress. From 3 to 5 weeks after surgery, the goals of recovery are identified as restored lumbar motion, normalized upper and lower extremity strength, improved aerobic fitness, and decreased pain and swelling.[10]

Progressive functional exercises can be added as the patient achieves these criteria. These include treadmill walking, balance activities, isotonic strengthening exercises, general flexibility exercises, and cardiovascular conditioning (via upper body ergometer, recumbent cycle ergometer, treadmill, stair-stepper, and cross-country ski machine).

Fundamental Mechanics of Lifting

Forces and stresses related to lifting, sitting, standing, walking, sleeping, and twisting are common to all activities of daily living (ADLs). O'Sullivan and colleagues[53] have identified a novel concept to instruct patients in proper lifting mechanics, listing the "five Ls" of lifting: load, lever, lordosis, legs, and lungs.

The load to be lifted is central to all concepts of lifting mechanics. The amount of weight to be hoisted should be appropriate for the task and for the individual attempting to lift it. The lever refers to keeping the object as close to the body as is functionally possible throughout the lift. If the object is held away from the body, the increased force (both intradiscal pressure and muscle strain) may strain the lumbar spine. Lordosis refers to maintaining a normal anatomic lordotic curve while lifting any object. Teaching the patient (and the PTA) to lift with the legs is basic to all lifting procedures. The muscles of the legs should be conditioned to fully participate during the lifting of any object from the floor. If the legs are not used fully, the muscles of the back may be necessary to absorb increased stress. The lungs refer to the use of proper breathing techniques during lifting. The Valsalva maneuver (closed glottis during attempted expiration) should be avoided and instruction given on exhaling during the actual lift.

Kaiser and co-workers[40a] have identified a lumbar stabilization model comparing two lumbar spine

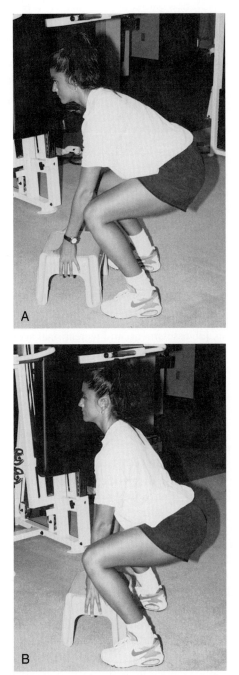

Fig. 20-10 Lifting postures. **A,** Flat back lifting position. **B,** Lifting with lumbar lordosis maintained.

postures during lifting. In the first posture (tested electromyographically) the starting position is characterized by a posterior pelvic tilt. The abdominal muscles are in a shortened position, the lumbar paravertebral muscles show no electromyographic activity, the posterior ligaments and posterior annular wall are stretched, the knees are in a position of decreased leverage, and the patient's center of gravity is posterior to the base of support (Fig. 20-10, *A*).[14] In the second posture, the patient's lumbar lordosis is maintained during the lift. The abdominal muscles are in their normal anatomic

length, the paravertebral muscles contracted, the posterior ligaments relaxed, the knees in an optimal leverage position, and the patient's center of gravity over the base of support (Fig. 20-10, *B*).

Prevention and Education for Back Dysfunction: The Back School Model

Although understanding and managing low back dysfunction is the focus of this section, prevention of lumbar spine injuries also is pertinent to this discussion, because the PTA is frequently directed to participate in and to carry out community-based back injury prevention programs under the supervision and direction of a PT. These education programs are commonly referred to as *back schools* and are designed to provide an understanding of anatomy, causes of back pain, lifting mechanics, posture, self-care for back pain, exercise, nutrition (weight management), ergonomics (which involves lifting, posture, general body mechanics, job modifications, and work site protection and redesign to minimize back injury), and stress reduction for high-risk patients and the population at large.

Often patients with a history of back pain are identified as ideal candidates to participate in these programs. Also, persons at risk (identified by job responsibilities, repetitive lifting, overweight condition, poor posture, poor body mechanics, relative weakness, and poor general physical conditioning) may be referred to these programs.

Many back schools involve a 1- or 2-hour class (consisting of lectures, slides, demonstration, and participation) each week for 4 to 6 weeks. Each session or class builds on the previous lecture to convey the principles seen in spinal anatomy, causes of back dysfunction, risk factors, posture, body mechanics, and treatment approaches.[1] Back schools can be based in outpatient physical therapy clinics, hospitals, industrial health clinics, wellness programs at work, or community fitness centers. In every case, the program should be under the direction and supervision of a PT, physician, or both.

Allman[1] has identified the outline in Table 20-1 as an appropriate general back school program. The curriculum clarifies the rudimentary concepts of education and prevention for a wide variety of back-related problems. The PTA who presents this information must be given specific information, evaluation data, indications, and contraindications for each patient participating in the back school program. In this way all phases of recovery and prevention can be individualized for each patient.

Most recently in a systematic review of completed research, Martimo and colleagues[48] concluded that the evidence to support back school programs is lacking. The effectiveness of a back school program in preventing pain, injury, and dysfunction is still under scrutiny. Despite this lack in evidence, there is still value in

Table 20-1	*Appropriate General Back School Program*
Education Topics	**Components of Education Topics**
Introduction to back dysfunction	The primary purpose is to increase the patient's awareness of back care, posture, and body mechanics.
Basic spinal anatomy and physiology: causes of back pain and dysfunction	1. Sprains and strains 2. Disc injuries (herniated nucleus pulposus) 3. Spinal stenosis 4. Spondylolisthesis
Risk factors associated with back injury	1. Poor general conditioning 2. Poor posture 3. Poor body mechanics and poor lifting style 4. Repetitive heavy lifting 5. Long-term sitting and driving 6. Stress (emotional)
Posture positioning and general body mechanics	1. Sitting 2. Sleeping 3. Standing 4. Lifting 5. Activities of daily living, job assessment, and recreational activities
Treatment approaches	1. Ice or heat 2. Stretching 3. Posture changes 4. Back support 5. Conditioning
General physical conditioning	1. Warm-up. Patients are introduced to the concept of a general warm-up preceding any physical activity. 2. Aerobic fitness. Patients are introduced to the methods, equipment, and implementation of general and specific endurance activities to improve cardiovascular fitness and control body weight. 3. Anaerobic power. Activities are outlined that develop intense physical effort of short duration. 4. Strength. Patients are instructed in methods to improve general body strength and specific lumbar extension strength exercises. 5. Flexibility. Patients are introduced to the philosophy, design, and implementation of daily, full-body stretching exercises with specific emphasis on the trunk and lower extremities. 6. Nutrition. Direct attention is focused on reducing the number of calories consumed by overweight individuals. Usually this education is conducted by a registered dietitian. 7. Relaxation techniques, stress reduction, and recreational activities are explored.

From Allman FL: Back school program. In *Introduction to back injuries*, Atlanta, 1990, The Atlanta Sports Medicine Clinic.

patient education by the PT and PTA. Future studies may provide evidence that back school programs prevent further injury.

Ergonomics and Functional Capacity Evaluations

In concert with back injury prevention through education and in accordance with the back school model is the concept of ergonomics and the implementation of functional capacity evaluations (FCEs), which are also referred to as *physical capacity assessments (PCAs)*, related to physical stress job analysis. The term ergonomics refers to a quantifiable system of job or ADL modification (or redesign) that allows for continued productivity while reducing work-related physical stress. As with the back school model, an FCE may require the PTA to prepare the evaluation area, set up all necessary testing equipment, and assist the PT with the collection, documentation, and storage of data. The implementation of an FCE is highly specific to the individual's job task. Its goal is to identify risk factors associated with a particular job or activity and then quantify the physical capacity of the individual being asked to perform the specific task to reduce the risk of back injury. In most cases an FCE is administered to a patient recovering from a back injury before returning to the job. An FCE also can be used as a screening tool to acquire data related to preemployment risk assessment and management of back injuries. Certain job or activity risk factors have been identified[33] that directly relate to the FCE. A few ergonomic risk factors are outlined by Hebert as follows[33]:

■ How much weight you lift
■ How often you lift
■ How low you bend to lift the load
■ How high you lift the load
■ How far you carry the load
■ How far you twist with the load
■ How far you reach with the load
■ How long you sit at your job
■ What the specific design of your seat is
■ If there is sustained or repeated bending, twisting, or reaching

Hundreds of factors may be related to job tasks. Each item to be tested in the FCE must be quantifiable and reproducible to enable the PT to make recommendations for reducing the risk of back injury. General testing parameters may be divided into categories that attempt to duplicate the requirements of the task to be performed while evaluating the patient's physiologic responses and assessing his or her physical abilities to carry out the task.

Table 20-2	*Testing Procedure that Identifies the Various Components of a Functional Capacity Evaluation*
Testing	**Procedure**
Musculoskeletal profile	1. Blood pressure
	2. Posture
	3. Gait
	4. Balance
	5. Range of motion
	6. Neurologic (reflexes)
	7. Sensory
	8. Muscle strength
Functional abilities screening	1. Push-pull
	2. Dynamic lifting
	3. Gross mobility
	4. Hand strength (grip dynamometer)
	5. Sitting and standing

From Work Site Partners, functional capacity evaluation system, industrial rehabilitation solutions. U.S. physical therapy system manual, Houston, 1994, USPT System Manual.

Authorities[60] advocate a multiphase testing procedure that identifies the various components of an FCE, as shown in Table 20-2. Within each FCE the aerobic end point (heart rate exceeds 85% of maximum heart rate) and biomechanical analysis of the patient's lifting-risk posture is assessed. In each section of the test, the parameters evaluated are performed directly as they relate to the specific job or task in question.

THE THORACIC SPINE

Thoracic Spine Muscle Injuries

Soft-tissue injuries of the thoracic spine usually involve some type of direct contact (contusion during athletic activities) or indirect overstretching or contraction of the thoracic muscles. Muscle contusions and strains of the thoracic spine occur primarily in younger active patients. The primary focus of management for these self-limiting injuries is the control of pain and swelling. Generally, ice is applied directly over the involved area during the acute stage of injury. Physician-prescribed analgesics, NSAIDs, moist heat applications, ultrasound, electrical stimulation, and massage are used judiciously to help control pain. Once pain has been effectively limited, the patient is allowed to participate in active ROM activities and strengthening exercises. The PTA may instruct the patient to perform seated, postural-awareness exercises that focus on thoracic extension and scapular retraction.

Prone thoracic and lumbar extension exercises are employed per patient tolerance. These involve a three-position progression from hands at the sides, to hands behind the head, and finally to arms fully extended while performing prone thoracic and lumbar extension. As pain is reduced and strength increases, the patient can begin isotonic strengthening exercises that focus on the scapular and thoracic spine muscles (Fig. 20-11).

Thoracic Disc Injuries

Thoracic disc herniations are rare (less than 0.3% of the population) and affect both men and women equally from the fourth through the sixth decades of life.[8] The most common segments affected are between the ninth and twelfth thoracic vertebrae.[8]

The type of treatment employed for thoracic disc herniations depends on whether the disc is herniated laterally or centrally.[8,21] A large central disc prolapse may produce symptoms of "spastic paraparesis, increased deep tendon reflexes, and a positive Babinski response."[21] However, lateral thoracic disc protrusions can produce signs more consistent with nerve root compression.

The PTA is exposed to both conservative care and postsurgical recovery after thoracic spine disc herniations. Less severe lateral disc herniations can be treated effectively with periods of active rest, analgesics, modalities to control pain and swelling, and epidural injections. More severe central disc herniations, involving progressive neurologic deficits, must be treated surgically to decompress the neurologic impingement.[8,21] Recovery after thoracic decompression closely follows the time necessary for healing of bone and soft tissue with extensive periods of supportive bracing to protect the affected spine from unwanted forces, and a progressive regimen of active motion, strengthening, and endurance activities, and a return to function with specific limitations delineated within the protocol developed by the surgeon and PT.

Kyphosis

Kyphosis is defined as an increase in the thoracic posterior convexity that is manifested by a rounded-back (and protracted scapulae) posture. Kyphosis can be subdivided into congenital, neuromuscular, and postural categories.[21] Osteoporosis, which can lead to multilevel thoracic compression fractures, causes anterior wedging of the involved segments and creates the kyphotic curvature.

The causes of pain associated with an increased thoracic convexity have been identified as stress originating from the posterior longitudinal ligaments, muscle fatigue resulting from stretched and weakened erector spinae and rhomboid muscle groups, and various postural and neurologic syndromes.[41]

The treatment of kyphosis depends on the degree of curvature, which is determined radiographically by the treating physician, any associated disc involvement, and the severity of symptoms.[5] In advanced cases of postural kyphosis with profound curvature and significant

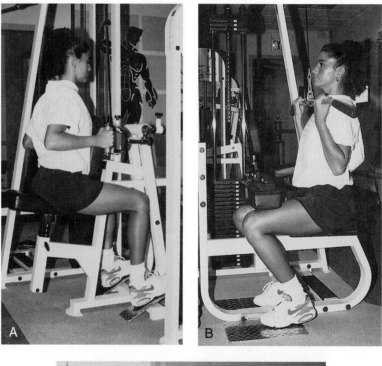

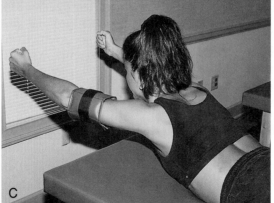

Fig. 20-11 Scapular and thoracic extension strengthening. **A,** Seated rowing machine to encourage scapular retraction. **B,** Latissimus bar pull-down in front. **C,** Prone lumbar and thoracic extension with scapular retraction using cuff weights. Notice the proximal placement of the resistance. As strength increases, the resistance can be moved to the patient's hands.

symptoms, the patient may require supportive bracing of the thorax to minimize the compression associated with anterior wedging of the vertebral bodies. With less severe kyphosis, the PTA plays a critical role in patient education, postural awareness, and the application of specific exercises to simultaneously stretch the anterior shoulder and pectorals and strengthen the thoracic extension muscles.

To effectively strengthen the scapular retractors, rhomboids, middle trapezius, and erector spinae of the thoracic region, a sufficient degree of freedom of movement in these areas is needed. Generally the anterior shoulder muscles and pectorals are shortened and relatively weak in response to the increased thoracic convexity. Therefore to provide the needed stimulus for full ROM strengthening, the anterior aspect of the thorax also must be addressed. Stretching the anterior shoulder muscles can be done both actively by the patient and passively, where the clinician provides the stretching. An effective active assisted stretch can be performed with the patient facing the corner of a room or standing in an open doorway. Both of the patient's hands are placed in a comfortable position on either side of the doorway. Then the patient slowly leans forward, providing a slow, static stretch to the pectorals and anterior shoulder. This position can be held for a prolonged stretch and usually is performed for multiple sets.

A passive stretch also can be employed with the patient in a seated position. With both of the patient's hands placed behind his or her head, the PTA stands behind the patient and grasps both elbows. The PTA delivers a slow posteriorly directed stretch to the pectorals and anterior shoulder muscles. To be effective, stretching must be performed consistently each day. Therefore the patient must perform stretches two or three times daily as part of a home exercise program. In addition to stretching the thorax, posterior thoracic strengthening must be addressed. The patient performs seated active scapular retraction exercises with an emphasis on maintaining an isometric contraction, or set, of the scapular muscles with each repetition.

As described, the patient does the three-progression prone thoracic extension exercises. In addition, the patient performs scapular adduction while lying prone with both arms held straight at 90°. Both arms are elevated while adducting the scapulae and holding the contracted position isometrically for 10 seconds.[41] This position can be modified slightly by having the patient hold weights while performing scapular adduction with both elbows flexed, creating more of a prone rowing motion.

The patient must perform both stretching and strengthening exercises daily as part of a home program. As the patient's motion improves and where posterior scapular strength increases, isotonic resistance exercises should be encouraged to a greater degree to provide increased stimulus for strengthening. In the home program, latex tubing or Thera-Band can be used in a seated rowing position to enhance scapular adduction. Commercially available isotonic rowing machines effectively provide greater resistance for the scapular muscles.

When treating postural kyphosis, the home exercise program must be carried out faithfully and the patient must develop an acute postural awareness at home and work. If the patient performs tasks at work that contribute to a rounded-shoulder position, modifications of these tasks is necessary. In many cases, the cause of poor thoracic posture is an inefficient work station arrangement in which the patient must maintain poor posture to perform tasks such as typing, writing, assembly work, or computer data entry. A simple adjustment in the height of the workstation so that it is closer to and centered midline with the patient encourages a more erect thoracic spine. Therefore the total care of the patient focuses on symptomatic pain relief using physician-prescribed analgesics, thermal agents, massage, and a comprehensive program of stretching, strengthening, education, and work site modifications.

Scoliosis

Scoliosis can be identified as any lateral curvature of the cervical, thoracic, or lumbar spine.[41] Scoliosis usually is idiopathic (cause unknown), but it also can result from neuromuscular causes or can be related to degenerative disease, osteoporosis, trauma, and postsurgical factors.[51] Kisner and Colby[41] identify the incidence of idiopathic scoliosis as being as high as 75% to 85% of all recognized types of scoliosis. Generally scoliosis can be recognized as either structural or nonstructural.[41]

Structural scoliosis is defined as an "irreversible lateral curve of the spine with fixed rotation of the vertebrae."[41] During the PT's initial evaluation of structural scoliosis, the clinician will observe whether the identified lateral curve decreases with forward trunk flexion. If not, structural idiopathic scoliosis is not corrected by changes in the patient's position or during active voluntary activities.[41] Nonstructural scoliosis is classified as reversible, wherein the lateral curve dissipates with positional changes. In either case, pain is the foremost presenting feature of scoliosis,[51] although cosmesis is a great concern. Other complaints involve decreased cardiopulmonary function (usually with thoracic curves greater than 65°) and neurologic symptoms associated with spinal stenosis.[51]

The nonoperative management of idiopathic scoliosis primarily involves the assistant in instructing the patient about therapeutic exercises outlined and prescribed by the PT. Scoliosis treatment involves both stretching and strengthening, much like kyphosis. Exercise by itself does not halt the progression or correct scoliosis.[41] The effective use of therapeutic exercise is intended primarily to improve spinal motion, increase muscle strength, and reduce back pain.[41]

In addition to exercises, bracing also has been advocated in the treatment of scoliosis.[41,51] However, bracing is intended to halt progression of the curve and not correct cosmetic deformity.[51] Perhaps the most commonly used brace for scoliosis is the Milwaukee brace.[41,51] Generally this brace is worn 23 or 24 hours a day.[41] However, Miller[51] suggests that part-time brace wearing is as effective as the traditional long-term application.

A fundamental principle in managing idiopathic scoliosis is stretching of the tight muscles on the concave side of the curve, while strengthening the muscles on the convex side of the curve. In addition, trunk axial elongation (stretching vertically) is important throughout exercise. As stated in the section on kyphosis, some freedom of motion must be available for strengthening exercises to be effective.

Stretching exercises directed toward the concavity must address all of the spinal muscles. Note that a right thoracic convexity results in a left lower thoracic concavity and associated right lumbar concavity with left lumbar convexity (Fig. 20-12). Strengthening exercises are performed for all of the muscles affected on the convex side of each lateral curve.

Various stretching exercises can be performed in prone, side-lying, or heel-sitting position.[41] While prone, the patient places both hands behind his or her head while tilting the thorax away from the concave side of the curve (Fig. 20-13, *A*). In another prone stretching exercise, the patient reaches overhead and extends the arm on the concave side, thereby effectively stretching the thoracic concavity (Fig. 20-13, *B*).

In the heel-sitting position, the patient places both hands forward and flat while emphasizing long-axis stretching. The lateral stretching component of this exercise is accomplished by having the patient slowly stretch both arms laterally away from the concave side of the curve (Fig. 20-14).

Static stretching also can be performed with the patient lying on his or her side. Place a small, soft rolled pillow or towel directly under the apex of the thoracic convex curve and support and stabilize the pelvis. For an advanced progression of side-lying stretching, the patient lies over the apex bolster toward the end of a treatment table (Fig. 20-15).

As alluded to in the preceding, trunk elongation (axial stretching) also is an effective stretching procedure used to treat scoliosis. Standing, the patient faces a wall and attempts to "walk up the wall" with both hands. The patient must reach as high as possible with both hands. A more progressive form of trunk

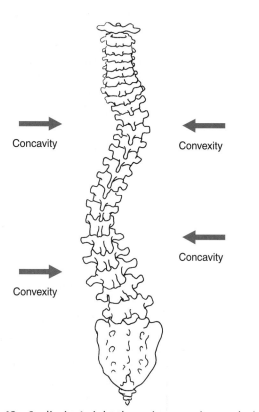

Fig. 20-12 Scoliosis. A right thoracic convexity results in a left lower thoracic concavity and an associated right lumbar concavity with left lumbar convexity.

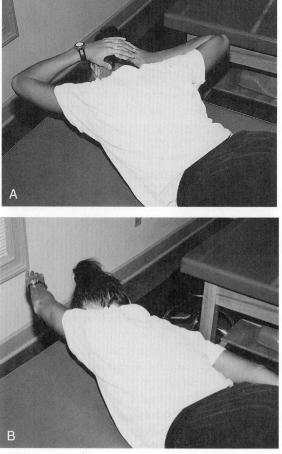

Fig. 20-13 Stretching exercises. **A,** Prone lateral trunk tilt. **B,** Prone lateral trunk tilt with arm stretch.

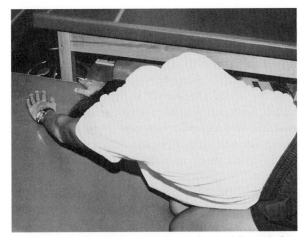

Fig. 20-14 Heel-sitting lateral trunk stretch with long-axis stretch and lateral stretch of both arms.

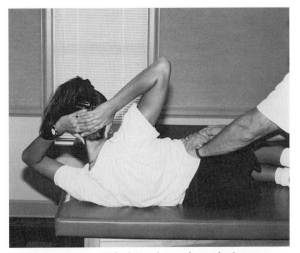

Fig. 20-16 Side-lying lateral trunk sit-up.

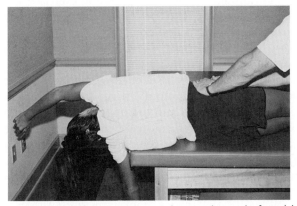

Fig. 20-15 Side-lying apex stretch over the end of a table.

elongation is to have the patient hang by both arms from an overhead bar.

Strengthening the thoracic and lumbar spine toward the convex side focuses on thoracic and lumbar extension strength and specific lateral strengthening maneuvers. Prone thoracic and lumbar spine active exercises were outlined and described in the preceding. These are effective when used early to enhance the strength of the thorax.

Specific lateral strengthening can proceed with the patient in a side-lying position on the concave side of the curve. The PTA should stabilize the trunk, then have the patient lift the trunk up toward the convex side of the curve (Fig. 20-16). This exercise can be viewed as a side-lying sit-up.

While this brief discussion has focused on a few rudimentary stretching and strengthening exercises for mild to moderate idiopathic scoliosis, an outline of surgical procedures to correct severe scoliosis is warranted. Surgery is reserved for severe symptomatic curves: those more than 50° to 60°.[51] With surgery, curves of this magnitude can be improved by approximately 50%.[41] The exact surgery performed depends on many factors.

However, a spinal fusion with or without Harrington rod instrumentation[41] is designed to elongate and stabilize the spine and thereby reduce pain and improve appearance.

Physical therapy after spine fusion for advanced, severe scoliosis requires extensive convalescence, the application of a postoperative brace, and limited activity for up to several weeks after surgery, depending upon the protocol designed by the collaborative efforts of the surgeon and PT.[41]

THE CERVICAL SPINE

Neck pain is thought to affect up to 66% of the population at least once in a individual's lifetime.[44] The economic burden of neck pain in the form of lost wages, cost of treatment, and workers compensation is high. This cost is second only to low back pain.[66] Individuals who experience an episode of neck pain may develop symptoms lasting more than 6 months.[4] Neck pain patients are frequently seen in outpatient physical therapy. Jette and associates[38] reported 25% of an outpatient physical therapy case load is represented by patients with neck pain. Women are also affected by neck pain more frequently than men.[66]

Without question, the most profound and catastrophic cervical spine injury is a fracture dislocation resulting in quadriplegia. The description of these spinal injuries is beyond the scope of this chapter. Once an evaluation is completed and a cervical spine fracture or spinal cord compression (myelopathy) is ruled out, patients with neck pain are often diagnosed with nerve root involvement or nonspecific mechanical neck pain. The pathoanatomic cause for neck pain is not identifiable for the majority of patients seen in physical therapy.[3] In a sample of healthy people without neck pain, up to 19% demonstrated abnormalities with imaging studies.[2] These abnormalities included disc protrusion or extrusion and impingement of the nerve root and spinal cord. The significant prevalence of abnormal findings with magnetic resonance imaging (MRI) in asymptomatic individuals can lead to medical misdiagnosis.

The evaluating PT will identify impairments in muscle, connective tissue, and nerves. As identified and explained in the section on the lumbar spine, rehabilitation of the cervical spine is focused towards impairments. This section identifies various soft-tissue and bony injuries of the cervical spine common to orthopedic physical therapy. General rehabilitation ideas are included with these pathoanatomic findings.

Whiplash Associated Disorder: Acute Sprains and Strains

Muscular strains of the cervical spine are common among young athletes and in association with motor vehicle accidents with flexion-extension, lateral flexion, and acceleration-deceleration "whiplash" type injuries.[59,67] Numerous impairments, stemming from bony and soft tissue injury, can be classified as whiplash associated disorder (WAD).[58] The U.S. annual cost associated with WAD is $29 billion.[66] The muscles that can be involved in cervical strains are the sternocleidomastoid, trapezius, scalenes, erectors, rhomboids, and levator scapulae.[67] The mechanism of injury producing cervical strains and sprains varies but includes hyperflexion, rotation, and lateral flexion of the head and cervical spine.[59]

Forces usually are great enough with automobile accidents that ligament injuries occur in conjunction with muscle strains. In fact, Stratton and Bryan's[59] experimental studies have demonstrated a wide range of tissue damage with hyperextension type automobile injuries:
1. Tearing of sternocleidomastoid muscle
2. Tearing of longissimus coli muscle
3. Pharyngeal edema
4. Tearing of anterior longitudinal ligament
5. Separation of cartilaginous end plate of the intervertebral disc

Similar types of injuries occur with hyperflexion injuries as a result of automobile accidents[59]:
1. Tears of the posterior cervical muscles
2. Tears of the ligamentum nuchae
3. Tears of the posterior longitudinal ligament
4. Intervertebral disc injury

The treatment of traumatic cervical spine sprains and strains is symptomatic during the acute stage of recovery. Patients may present with neck pain and referred upper extremity pain. The treating physician usually prescribes a course of analgesics, NSAIDs, or muscle relaxants; rest; and agents to control pain and swelling (heat, cold, ultrasound, and electrical stimulation). The healing constraints of muscle and ligament tissues differ; both must be addressed throughout recovery.

After the initial pain and swelling are controlled, the patient may be introduced to a series of active ROM exercises, cervical isometric strengthening exercises, and education in cervical posture mechanics. Initial ROM exercises must be approached cautiously to avoid reproducing the motion that caused the injury. As with all soft-tissue injuries, attention must be focused on protection of the affected area while striving to prevent further injury. If, for example, the mechanism of cervical sprain and strain was hyperflexion, care must be directed at avoiding the end range of head and neck flexion. Gentle active ROM exercises can proceed after moist heat application for 20 minutes to enhance muscle relaxation, relieve pain, and stimulate greater mobility.

Full recovery from acute sprains and strains of the cervical spine involves the elimination of pain and swelling initially, appropriate rest from any aggravating positions, protection from unwanted stress, the return of normal cervical spine ROM, enhanced muscle strength through isometric stabilization exercises, work site modifications, and postural-awareness activities (axial extension-retraction exercises).

Cervical Radiculopathy

Cervical radiculopathy is defined as mechanical compression or inflammation of a nerve root which causes neurologic symptoms into the upper extremities. Most common causes of radiculopathy are cervical disc herniation, spondylosis, and osteophytes.[61] The symptoms of peripheral pain, radicular signs, local cervical pain, and scapular pain are consistent with the symptoms of disc herniations observed in the lumbar spine.[59]

As with lumbar disc herniations, the initial goals are to relieve symptoms, reduce pain and swelling, control muscle spasm, and work toward centralizing the symptoms. Iglarsh and Snyder-Mackler[36] define improvement as "a decrease in the extent or intensity of the peripheral symptoms." The specific exercises for cervical disc herniation patients must be identified carefully by the physician and PT. Once the appropriate subgrouping of treatment is recognized, the PT organizes a comprehensive plan of pain relief, motion, strength, and postural education activities for the PTA to follow and apply.[11]

Cervical Spondylosis

In contrast to cervical disc herniations, cervical spondylosis involves chronic rather than acute degenerative disc, which results from "wear and tear on the weight-bearing structures of the cervical spine."[59] The symptoms are characteristic of spinal cord compression (myelopathy) or nerve root compression with radicular signs.[51] Cervical spondylosis is seen most often during the fourth and fifth decades of life and characteristically affects men more than women at the C5-C6 and C6-C7 segments.[51]

Sustained impact loading and repetitive microtrauma[59] are causative factors that can produce cervical cord impingement, nerve root impingement, osteophytes, bone sclerosis, loss of cervical lordosis, and central or posterolateral disc herniations.[51,59]

Initial physical therapy interventions focus on pain relief with the evaluation of thermal and electrical agents, physician-prescribed analgesics, and rest from aggravating positions. As with the evaluation of other disc conditions, the PT provides a comprehensive evaluation to accurately determine which motions cause pain and radicular symptoms and which relieve pain. From this detailed initial evaluation, the PT outlines and describes specific exercises consistent with these findings. In some cases, traction is an effective tool to minimize joint compressive loads and reduce cord compression or nerve root irritation.[51,57] The PT determines if mechanical traction or manual cervical traction is more appropriate. Isometric cervical spine stabilization exercises (four-way isometrics) and ROM exercises are initiated once pain has been reduced and the appropriateness of these activities is determined by the PT.

When cord compression (myelopathy) progresses and radicular pain persists, the physician can use various surgical interventions. Miller[51] describes an anterior cervical spine approach to accomplish a discectomy and fusion or a posterior approach for a foraminotomy or multilevel laminectomy to relieve cord or root compression.

Because cervical spondylosis is a chronic degenerative condition, long-term care involves protection from inappropriate and unwanted forces and instruction in cervical posture mechanics, flexibility exercises, and strengthening activities.

Cervical Facet Syndrome

The cervical facet joint is another possible source of neck pain.[50] Symptoms can include posterior neck stiffness, pain with cervical extension or rotation, cervicogenic headaches, and possible pain referral into the shoulder and scapula.[68] Degenerative changes to the cervical facet and surrounding soft tissue may cause this radiation. It is estimated that facet involvement affects 54% to 60% of chronic neck pain patients.[47] Appropriate interventions identified by the PT may include pain control, ROM, and exercise.

Thoracic Inlet Syndrome

Some texts cover thoracic inlet syndrome within the subject matter affecting the shoulder.[69] Because of the anatomic proximity of the structures involved, this condition is discussed within the context of the cervical spine. Authorities point out that the term *thoracic inlet syndrome* is a more precise and anatomically accurate term used to describe compression of vascular or neurologic tissues as they exit the "superior triangle opening of the thorax" (Fig. 20-17).[59,69] (This syndrome has been commonly called *outlet syndrome* in the past.) Specifically, proximal compression of the subclavian artery and vein, as well as the brachial plexus, are the

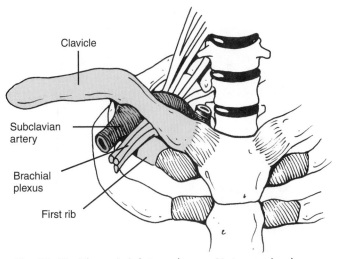

Fig. 20-17 Thoracic inlet syndrome. Note proximal compression of the subclavian artery and vein and the brachial plexus.

most probable neurovascular factors involved with thoracic inlet syndrome.[59] Many structures can cause compression of these tissues. Foremost is the presence of a cervical rib, a shortened or hypertrophied anterior scalene muscle, or malunion of the clavicle and subluxed first thoracic rib.[32,59,69] Symptoms of this condition include radicular signs of pain, numbness, tingling, weakness, and skin and temperature changes consistent with neurovascular tissue compression.[32,59,69]

Typically, physical therapy management addresses specifically defined limitations of movement and affected bony or soft tissues during the initial evaluation performed by the PT. An individualized comprehensive program of stretching, strengthening, and education can commence once the PT has determined which specific tissues are affected and identified any underlying causes of postural variations.

Soft-tissue stretching focuses on the anterior scalene muscles. The patient is instructed to laterally flex and extend the head to the opposite side of the shortened muscle (Fig. 20-18). Thoracic kyphosis tends to accentuate the symptoms of thoracic inlet syndrome, so pectoral stretching (facing an open doorway with hands on either side and leaning forward) and thoracic extension mobility and strengthening exercises are used to specifically address muscle weakness and soft-tissue restrictions. A host of clinically applicable thoracic extension mobility exercises can be used. Examples include seated scapular retraction, prone scapular and thoracic extension, and seated rowing activities with elastic tubing.

In addition to stretching and strengthening exercises, cervical posture correction is needed; poor cervical posture is a common problem in the workplace.[32] To address the forward head posture and tight anterior neck muscles, the patient can perform axial extension or cervical retraction stretching exercises, as described.

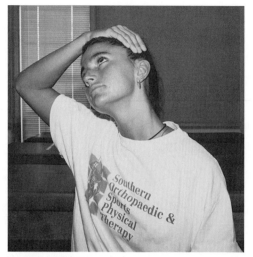

Fig. 20-18 Stretching of the anterior scalene muscles by laterally flexing and extending the head toward the opposite side of the shortened muscle. Note the gentle overpressure provided by the hand.

The effective management of thoracic inlet syndrome focuses on specific stretching of affected muscles, thoracic mobility, and extension strengthening, as well as education concerning proper cervical spine alignment and the performance of cervical retraction exercises.

Treatment Based Classification: Cervical Spine

Effective management of the cervical spine requires a multimodal treatment approach. The cervical spine TBC system assimilates information from the patient history and physical examination to classify the patient for the most appropriate treatment subgroup.[13,23] The five subgroups are labeled mobility, centralization, exercise and conditioning, pain control, and headache. As explained earlier, the patient moves fluidly in and out of these subgroupings during the duration of care. Preliminary research has identified that patients experienced improved outcomes when matched to interventions of their treatment subgroup.[23]

The cervical region is the most mobile region of the spine. Impairments in ROM in one vertebral level will change the motion in adjacent levels. The restoration of mobility in the cervical spine may be the first subgrouping chosen by the PT after the initial evaluation. Interventions may include mobilization, active ROM, passive ROM, and manipulation of the thoracic spine.[23] The PT will then initiate exercise in the form of ROM, strength, and conditioning with the PTA. Research suggests patients treated with manual therapy and exercise experience a clinically important reduction in pain.[31,35]

An important practical matter to consider when instructing patients to perform cervical ROM exercises is how to stabilize the trunk and shoulders. With both muscle and ligament damage, the long-term effect of healing is fibrous tissue contraction, which results in stiffness, restriction, and limitation of motion.[67] Therefore to effectively direct the stretch to the affected area, the surrounding structures must be supported and stabilized. For example, if a patient with a lateral flexion injury that results in muscle and ligament damage is instructed to gently stretch laterally away from the side of the injury, the opposite shoulder would elevate (because of the shortened tissues) if the shoulders are not stabilized, rendering the stretch ineffective. To stabilize the shoulder, the patient should perform the stretch while seated and use both hands to grasp under the seat. No shoulder elevation occurs when the patient attempts to stretch the head and neck laterally with the arms fully extended and secured under the seat.

Strengthening and conditioning exercise for the neck and upper quarter include the deep neck flexors. Prevailing theory suggests that stability of the cervical spine is dependent on deep neck flexor strength.[39] Jull and co-workers[40] reported retraining the deep cervical flexors in conjunction with manual therapy to the cervicothoracic spine can effectively decrease neck pain and headache with results being maintained at 1-year follow-up.[15] Precise instruction by the PTA for retraining deep neck flexor is very important for improved patient function.

Treatment of the deep neck flexors begins with the patient in the supine position. This exercise is designed to recruit the deep neck flexor muscles while avoiding co-contraction of superficial neck flexors. Instruction is given to the patient to keep his or her mouth closed, then to gently nod the head, performing a chin tuck. Hold this contraction for 10 seconds while observing for superficial muscle substitution (sternocleidomastoid). Progression of this contraction may occur once the patient is able to sufficiently contract without substitution. To increase intensity, instruct the patient to perform contraction then slightly raise his or her head off the supporting surface. Attention is once again focused on substitution of superficial muscles. Neutral spine position should be reinforced with cueing. The goal is to progress to an inclined position and then more functional positions with increasing control and strength.

Initial strengthening of the cervical spine may also include isometric stabilization exercises. Submaximal contractions and precise techniques are important and must be carefully explained and demonstrated to the patient. For isometric stabilization exercises, the patient performs a series of four-way isometrics in an anatomically neutral cervical spine position. The four-position isometric exercises are forward flexion, lateral flexion (right and left), and extension. In preparing to perform these exercises, the patient must demonstrate the ability to hold his or her head and neck in midline without excessive rotation, lateral flexion, forward flexion, or extension malalignment.

To begin, the patient should sit before a mirror to get visual feedback while maintaining proper head and neck alignment. The proper execution of the first isometric position of forward flexion should be explained and demonstrated. With one hand placed on the midline of the forehead (the patient must bring the hand into the described position and not rotate the head toward the hand), the patient should direct a posterior force to the forehead with the hand while resisting head and neck flexion, thereby stimulating isometric strengthening of the anterior cervical muscles. The patient should gradually and slowly build the resistance using the rule of 10s (gradually initiate isometrics with 2-second submaximal contraction, then hold for 6 seconds, then slowly reduce for 2 seconds) rather than suddenly applying maximal force (Fig. 20-19, *A*).

The patient should use both hands to support the occiput for the second position. The patient should maintain the head and neck in the anatomic midline position and not allow the head to flex forward. The patient should be encouraged to gradually apply an anteriorly directed force with both hands while resisting extension of the head. This position effectively strengthens the head and neck extensor group (Fig. 20-19, *B*).

The next position is lateral flexion. While the PTA observes proper head and neck alignment in the mirror, the patient should bring one hand to the side of the head but not allow the head to rotate or laterally flex to meet the hand. The patient should then apply lateral pressure while resisting this force. This position is

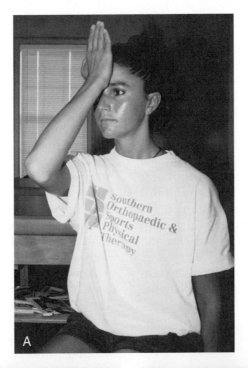

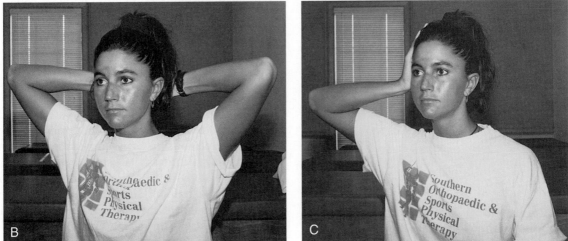

Fig. 20-19 Cervical isometrics. **A,** For forward flexion (notice the head must remain in midline and not be allowed to rotate). **B,** For head and neck extension. **C,** For lateral flexion

repeated on the opposite side. No head or neck motion must occur in each position. Usually the patient carries out a series of two to three sets of 10-second isometric exercises two to three times daily. As strength improves, the patient gradually increases the intensity, but avoids sudden or ballistic contractions (Fig. 20-19, C).

Educating the patient about cervical spine postural mechanics is as important as the actual management of any physical dysfunction. One of the most commonly recognized postural malalignment syndromes affecting the cervical spine is a forward head posture. Typically, this posture is characterized by a loss of flexion in the upper cervical spine region and a loss of extension in the lower cervical spine. The patient should perform axial extension or cervical retraction exercises. The PT determines which exercises are appropriate for each patient and identifies which patients are candidates for specific axial-extension exercises.

The PT may determine that the patient responds to repeated movements in a specific directional preference. A centralization phenomenon may occur where distal symptoms in the upper quarter decrease or abolish and symptoms increase or present near the central location of the cervical spine. The patient often responds to repeated retraction exercises in supine and sitting positions. Retraction exercises require the patient to be able to demonstrate a midline neutral position. The patient should sit in front of a mirror initially to perform this exercise correctly. Have the patient imagine that his or her head is resting on a conveyor belt. The patient must be able to align the ears with the shoulders and move the head straight back on the conveyor belt (Fig. 20-20). If done correctly, a "double chin" is produced as the patient moves the head back. If done incorrectly, the

head and neck move into extension. The patient should be encouraged to perform this exercise at home for multiple sets throughout the day or as prescribed by the PT.

The centralization subgroup includes repeated movements and also a co-treatment technique with the PT. The PT may request assistance of the PTA to perform a passive upper extremity movement on the patient while the PT mobilizes the cervical spine. The upper extremity movement follows the upper limb neurodynamic tension test for the median nerve. The PT will instruct the direction of the passive movement as well as the static position in order to mobilize the nervous system.

Upper Limb Neurodynamic Tension Test A: Median Nerve Bias

The upper limb tension test is assessed by placing the patient in the following positions:

■ Supine position
■ Scapular depression
■ Shoulder abduction
■ Forearm supination; wrist and finger extension
■ Shoulder lateral rotation
■ Elbow extension
■ Contralateral/ipsilateral cervical side-bending

Impairments in ROM and strength are frequently accompanied by pain. Pain control subgrouping will include those patients with high pain and disability scores noted on outcome measures. They may have been involved in a traumatic event or report very recent onset of symptoms. In many cases, these patients will present with poor tolerance to interventions and possibly elevated fear avoidance beliefs noted on the on the FABQ.[28]

Managing these patients requires patient reassurance. Gentle active ROM should be encouraged within the patient's pain tolerance. ROM for adjacent regions such as the shoulder and thoracic spine should also be included. The PT will address appropriate activity modification, which is then reinforced by the PTA. Often these patients will require more frequent collaboration with the PT for progression of interventions.

Mobilization of the Lumbar, Thoracic, and Cervical Spine

Although peripheral joint mobilization is covered in this text, axial skeleton mobilization techniques for the lumbar, thoracic, and cervical spine are not addressed. The extraordinarily complex arrangement and intimate anatomic relationship between vertebral segments and surrounding neurovascular structures require intense, exhaustive study and precise application of techniques after detailed training and clinical practice to be safe, effective, and efficient. The scope of the PTA's training is not consistent with the demanding working knowledge of neurovascular anatomy, biomechanics, and pathophysiology of the lumbar, thoracic, and cervical spine needed to provide mobilization techniques to these areas.

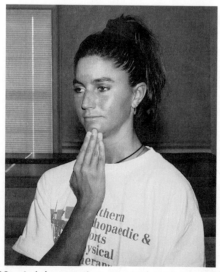

Fig. 20-20 Axial extension–cervical retraction. The head of the patient should move directly posterior. No head or cervical extension should occur. Attempt to produce a double chin without head or neck flexion.

❖ GLOSSARY

Annulus: The outer wall of a vertebral disc. It is composed of 12 to 18 concentrically arranged rings of fibroelastic cartilage.

Directional preference: During repetitive movements into either spinal flexion or extension, a patient's symptoms will either centralize or peripheralize. Those with a directional preference will have symptoms that centralize with a movement into their directional preference. It is thought that those with a directional preference have a more favorable prognosis than those who do not.

Disc protrusion: Condition in which nucleus bulges against an intact annulus.

Extruded disc: Condition characterizied by nucleus extending through the annulus, but nuclear material remains confined by the posterior longitudinal ligament.

Herniated nucleus pulposus (HNP): A specific type of disk bulge that is further subdivided into protusion, extrusion, and sequestration.

Kyphosis: An increase in the thoracic posterior convexity that is manifested by a rounded back (and protracted scapulae) posture.

Lordosis: The maintenance of a normal anatomic lordotic curve while lifting any object.

Nucleus pulposus: The [fiber/substance/gel] contained within the annulus.

Radiculopathy: Mechanical compression or inflammation of a nerve root that causes neurologic symptoms into the lower extremities. It can be caused by encroachment on the spinal nerve root by osteophytes or a large disc herniation. Symptoms may include pain, numbness, tingling, weakness, burning, or paresthesias.

Scoliosis: A disorder defined as any lateral curvature of the cervical, thoracic, or lumbar spine. It can be classified as either structural or nonstructural.[41]

Sequestrated disc: A condition in which the nucleus has breached the confines of the annulus and its free within the spinal canal.

Spine stabilization: Exercises performed to strengthen muscles in the trunk to provide a dynamic stabilization of the spinal segments.

Thoracic inlet syndrome: A term used to describe compression of vascular or neurologic tissues as they exit the superior triangle opening of the thorax. This syndrome has been commonly called *outlet syndrome* in the past.

Treatment-based classification (TBC): A multimodal rehabilitation plan that categorizes patients based on their overall symptomatology and response to a specific intervention.

REFERENCES

1. Allman FL: Back school program. *Introduction to back injuries*, Atlanta, 1990, The Atlanta Sports Medicine Clinic.
2. Boden SD, McCowin PR, Davis DO, et al: Abnormal magnetic resonance scans of the cervical spine in asymptomatic subjects. A prospective investigation, *J Bone Joint Surg Am* 72(8):1178–1184, 1990.
3. Borghouts JA, Koes BW, Bouter LM: The clinical course of prognostic factors of non-specific neck pain: a systematic review, *Pain* 77:1–13, 1998.
4. Bovim G, Schrader H, Sand T: Neck pain in the general population, *Spine* 19:1307–1309, 1994.
5. Brashear HR, Raney RB: *Affections of the spine and thorax, Handbook of orthopaedic surgery*, ed 10, St Louis, 1986, Mosby.
6. Brennan GP, Fritz JM, Hunter SJ, et al: Identifying subgroups of patients with acute/subacute "nonspecific" low back pain: results of a randomized clinical trial, *Spine* 31(6):623–631, 2006.
7. Browder DA, Childs JD, Cleland JA, et al: Effectiveness of an extension-oriented treatment approach in a subgroup of subjects with low back pain: a randomized clinical trial, *Phys Ther* 87(12):1608–1618, 2007.
8. Burkus JK: Spine. In Loth T, editor: *Orthopaedic boards review*, St Louis, 1993, Mosby.
9. Cailliet R: *Low back pain syndrome*, ed 3, Philadelphia, 1981, FA Davis.
10. Chappuis JL, Johnson GD, Gines AM: *A source guide for spine care*, Atlanta, GA, 1994, Greater Atlanta Spine Center.
11. Childs JD, Cleland JA, Elliott JM, et al: Neck pain: clinical practice guidelines linked to the International Classification of Functioning, Disability and Health from the Orthopedic section of the American Physical Therapy Association, *J Orthop Sports Phys Ther* 38(9):A1–A34, 2008.
12. Childs JD, Fritz JM, Flynn T, et al: Validation of a clinical prediction rule to identify patients with low back pain likely to benefit from spinal manipulation: a validation study, *Ann Intern Med* 141(12):920–928, 2004.
13. Childs JD, Fritz Piva SR, Whitman JM: Proposal of a classification system for patients with neck pain, *J Orthop Sports Phys Ther* 34(11):686–696, 2004.
14. Delitto RS, Rose SJ, Apts DW: An electromyographic analysis of two techniques for squat lifting, *Phys Ther* 67(9):1329–1334, 1987.
15. DeRosa C, Porterfield JA: Lumbar spine and pelvis. In Richardson JK, Iglarsh ZA, editors: *Clinical orthopaedic physical therapy*, Philadelphia, 1994, Saunders.
16. Deyo RA, Gray DT, Kreuter W, et al: United States trends in lumbar fusion surgery for degenerative conditions, *Spine* 30:1441–1445, 2005.
17. Deyo RA, Phillips WR: Low back pain: a primary care challenge, *Spine* 21:2826–2832, 1996.
18. Dietrich N, Kurowski P: The importance of mechanical factors in the etiology of spondylolysis: a model analysis of loads and stresses in the human lumbar spine, *Spine* 10:541–632, 1985.
19. Duda M: Elite lifters at risk of spondylolysis, *Phys Sports Med* 15:107–158, 1987.
20. Ehrmann-Feldman D, Rossignol M, Abenhaim L, et al: Physician referral to physical therapy in a cohort of workers compensated for low back pain, *Phys Ther* 76(2):150–156, 1996.
21. Eismont FJ, Kitchel SH: In DeLee JC, Drez D, editors: *Orthopaedic sports medicine: principles and practice, Thoracolumbar spine* vol. 2 Philadelphia, 1994, Saunders.
22. Flynn T, Fritz J, Whitman J, et al: A clinical prediction rule for classifying patients with low back pain who demonstrate short-term improvement with spinal manipulation, *Spine* 27(24): 2835–2843, 2002.
23. Fritz JM, Brennan GP: Preliminary classification of a proposed treatment based classification system for patients receiving physical therapy interventions for neck pain, *Phys Ther* 87(5):513–524, 2007.

24. Fritz J, Delitto A, Erhard RE: Comparison of classification-based physical therapy with therapy based on clinical practice guidelines for patients with acute low back pain: a randomized clinical trial, *Spine* 28(13):1363–1371, 2003.

25. Fritz JM, Lindsay W, Matheson JW, et al: Is there a subgroup of patients with low back pain likely to benefit from mechanical traction? Results of a randomized clinical trial and subgrouping analysis, *Spine* 32(26):E793–800, 2007.

26. Frymoyer JW: Predicting disability from low back pain, *Clin Orthop Relat Res* 279:101–109, 1992.

27. Fulton M: *Lower-back pain: a new solution for an old problem*, Rolling Meadows, IL, 1992, MedX.

28. George SZ, Fritz JM, Bialosky JE, et al: The effect of a fear-avoidance-based physical therapy intervention for patients with acute low back pain: results of a randomized clinical trial, *Spine* 28(23):2551–2560, 2003.

29. Goldstein TS: Treatment of common problems of the spine. In Lewis CB, editor: *Geriatric orthopaedics: rehabilitative management of common problems*, Gaithersburg, Md., 1991, Aspen.

30. Gould JA: The spine. In Gould JA, Davies G, editors: *Orthopedic and sports physical therapy*, ed 2, St Louis, 1990, Mosby.

31. Gross AR, Hoving JL, Haines TA, et al: A Cochrane review of manipulation and mobilization for mechanical neck disorders, *Spine* 29(14):1541–1548, 2004.

32. Hebert LA: *The neck-arm-hand book*, Greenville, Mass., 1989, IMPACC.

33. Hebert LA: *Your back for life*, Greenville, Mass., 1993, IMPACC.

34. Hicks GE, Fritz JM, Delitto A, et al: Preliminary development of a clinical prediction rule for determining which patients with low back pain will respond to a stabilization program, *Spine* 86: 1753–1762, 2005.

35. Hoving JL, Koes BW, de Vet HC, et al: Manual therapy, physical therapy or continued care by a general practitioner for patients with neck pain. A randomized controlled trial, *Ann Intern Med* 136(10):713–722, 2002.

36. Iglarsh ZA, Snyder-Mackler L: Temporomandibular joint and the cervical spine. In Richardson JK, Iglarsh ZA, editors: *Clinical orthopaedic physical therapy*, Philadelphia, 1994, Saunders.

37. Jackson DW: Low back pain in young athletes: evaluation of stress reaction and discogenic problems, *Am J Sports Med* 7:366–664, 1979.

38. Jette AM, Smith K, Haley SM, et al: Physical therapy episodes of care for patients with low back pain, *Phys Ther* 76:924–935, 1996.

39. Jull G: *Management of cervicogenic headaches. Physical therapy of the cervical and thoracic spine*, St Louis, 2002, Churchill Livingstone.

40. Jull G, Trott P, Potter H, et al: A randomized controlled trial of exercise and manipulative therapy for cervicogenic headache, *Spine* 27(17):1835–1843, 2002.

40a. Kaiser RK, Rose SJ, Apts DW: *An electromyographic analysis of two techniques for squat lifting*, Washington University School of Medicine, Applied Kinesiology Laboratory, Program in Physical Therapy.

41. Kisner C, Colby LA, editors: *Therapeutic exercise foundations and techniques*, ed 2, Philadelphia, 1989, FA Davis.

42. Knight M, Stewart-Brown S, Fletcher L: Estimating health needs: the impact of a check-list of conditions and quality of life measurement on health information derived from community surveys, *J Public Health Med* 23:179–186, 2001.

43. Lewis CB, Bottomley JM: *Orthopaedic treatment considerations, Geriatric physical therapy: a clinical approach*, New York, 1994, Appleton & Lange.

44. Linton SJ, Hellsing AL, Hallden K: A population based study of spinal pain among 35-45 year old individuals. Prevalence, sick leave and health care use, *Spine* 23(13):1457–1463, 1998.

45. Luo X, Pietrobon R, Sun SX, et al: Estimates and patterns of direct health care expenditures among individuals with back pain in the United States, *Spine* 29:79–86, 2004.

46. Macnab I: *Backache*, Baltimore, 1977, Williams & Wilkins.

47. Manchikanti L, Boswell MV, Singh V, et al: Prevalence of facet joint pain in chronic spinal pain of cervical, thoracic, and lumbar regions, *BMC Musculoskelet Disord* 5:15, 2004.

48. Martimo KP, Verbeek J, Karppinen J, et al: Effect of training and lifting equipment for preventing back pain in lifting and handling: a systematic review, *BMJ* 336(7641):429–431, 2008.

49. McKenzie RA: *The lumbar spine: mechanical diagnosis and therapy*, Waikanae, New Zealand, 1981, Orthopedic Physical Therapy Products.

50. McLain RF: Mechanoreceptor endings in human cervical facet joints, *Iowa Orthop J* 13:149–154, 1993.

51. Miller MD, editor: *Review of orthopaedics*, Philadelphia, 1992, Saunders.

52. Niemisto L, Lahtinen-Suopanki T, Rissanen P, et al: A randomized trial of combined manipulation, stabilizing exercises, and physician consultation compared to physician consultation alone for chronic low back pain,, *Spine* 28(19):2185–2191, 2003.

53. O'Sullivan JJ, Ellis JJ, Makofsky HW: The five "L's" of lifting, *Phys Ther Forum* 10(14):3–6, 1991.

54. O'Sullivan PB, Twomey LT, Allison GT: Evaluation of specific stabilizing exercise in the treatment of chronic low back pain with radiologic diagnosis of spondylolysis or spondylolisthesis, *Spine* 22:2959–2967, 1997.

55. Panjabi M, Abumi K, Duranceau J, et al: Spinal stability and intersegmental muscle forces. A biochemical model,, *Spine* 14(2): 194–200, 1989.

56. Paris SV: *The spine: etiology and treatment of dysfunction including joint manipulation*, Atlanta, Ga., 1979, Course Notes.

57. Raney NH, Petersen EJ, Smith TA, et al: Development of a clinical prediction rule to identify patients with neck pain likely to benefit from cervical traction and exercise, *Eur Spine J* 18(3):382–391, 2009.

58. Spitzer WO, Skovron ML, Salmi LR, et al: Scientific monograph of the Quebec Task Force on Whiplash-Associated Disorders: redefining "whiplash" and its management, *Spine* 20(Suppl 8): 1S–73S, 1995.

59. Stratton SA, Bryan JM: Dysfunction, evaluation and treatment of the cervical spine and thoracic inlet. In Donatelli R, Wooden MJ, editors: *Orthopaedic physical therapy*, New York, 1989, Churchill-Livingstone.

60. U.S. Physical Therapy: Work site partners, functional capacity evaluation system, industrial rehabilitation solutions, *Houston*, 1994:U.S.P.T. System Manual.

61. Wainner RS, Gill H: Diagnosis and nonoperative management of cervical radiculopathy, *J Orthop Sports Phys Ther* 30:728–744, 2000.

62. Watkins RG, Dillin WH: Lumbar spine injury in the athlete, *Clin Sports Med* 9:419–448, 1990.

63. Whitman JM, Flynn T, Fritz JM: Nonsurgical management of patients with lumbar spinal stenosis: a literature review and a case series of three patients managed with physical therapy, *Phys Med Rehabil Clin N Am* 15(1): 77–101, vi-vii, 2003 .

64. Wiltse LL: Spondylolisthesis in children, *Clin Orthop* 21:156–163, 1957.

65. Wiltse LL, Widell EH, Jackson DW: Fatigue fracture: the basic lesion in isthmic spondylolisthesis, *J Bone Joint Surg* 57A:17–22, 1975.

66. Wright A, Mayer TG, Gatchel RJ: Outcomes of disabling cervical spine disorders in compensation injuries. A prospective comparison to tertiary rehabilitation response for chronic lumbar spinal disorders, *Spine* 24(2):178–183, 1999.

67. Wroble RR, Albright JP: Neck and low back injuries in wrestling, *Clin Sports Med* 5(2):295–325, 1986.

68. Wyatt LH: Facet syndrome in the cervical spine, *J Amer Chiropr Assoc* 47(3):27–28, 2010.

69. Yahara ML: Shoulder. In Richardson JK, Iglarsh ZA, editors: *Clinical orthopaedic physical therapy*, Philadelphia, 1994, Saunders.

REVIEW QUESTIONS

Short Answer

1. Match the following list of percentages relating to intradiscal pressure with the appropriate and corresponding body position.

100%	Supine (knees flexed)
75%	Standing
35%	Bending forward
25%	Side-lying
275%	Supine

2. List the five Ls of lifting, as described by O'Sullivan, Ellis, and Makofsky.

True/False

3. The intervertebral lumbar disc is essentially avascular and aneural except for the periphery of the annulus, which is innervated.
4. Ligamentous sprains of the lumbar spine can occur from sudden violent force or repeated stress.
5. It is essential that all cases of HNP be treated with lumbar extension postures.
6. Manual muscle testing is the most effective way to quantify lumbar muscle strength and performance.
7. Lumbar extension exercises are advocated for spondylolisthesis.
8. Osteoporosis, which can lead to multilevel thoracic compression fractures, can cause anterior wedging of the segments, which in turn creates the kyphotic curve.
9. Scoliosis refers to a lateral curvature of the lumbar vertebrae.
10. Generally scoliosis can be categorized as structural or nonstructural.
11. With nonstructural scoliosis, positional changes result in a decrease in the curvature.
12. Therapeutic exercise (by itself) is intended to halt the progression of scoliosis and correct resultant deformity.
13. The use of bracing in the treatment of scoliosis is intended to halt the progression of the curve and is not identified as effective in correcting cosmetic deformity.
14. Axial stretching (trunk elongation) is not advocated for the treatment of scoliosis.
15. Cervical spondylosis is an acute cervical disc disorder.

21 Orthopedic Management of the Shoulder

Terry Trundle

LEARNING OBJECTIVES

1. Identify and describe methods, management, and rehabilitation for subacromial rotator cuff impingement.
2. Identify and describe methods of management and rehabilitation for tears of the rotator cuff.
3. Describe methods of management and rehabilitation for glenohumeral instability.
4. Discuss methods of management and rehabilitation for adhesive capsulitis.
5. Identify and describe common injuries of the acromioclavicular joint.
6. Describe common methods of management and rehabilitation for injuries of the acromioclavicular joint.
7. Identify and describe common fractures of the scapula, clavicle, and proximal humerus.
8. Outline and describe methods of management and rehabilitation of fractures around the shoulder.
9. Describe methods of management and rehabilitation after shoulder arthroplasty.
10. Describe common manual exercise techniques for the shoulder.

KEY TERMS

Bankart lesion   Glenohumeral joint   Hill-Sachs lesion

This chapter introduces common injuries, treatment, and rehabilitation procedures related to the **glenohumeral joint,** acromioclavicular (AC) joint, scapula, and proximal humerus. The shoulder is the most mobile of all joints with multiple planes of motion. This anatomical complex is made up of three main components, osteology, arthrology, and passive stabilizing structures. Osteology (bone) consists of the humerus, clavicle, and the scapula. Arthrology (joints) consists of glenohumeral, AC, sternoclavicular, and scapulothoracic articulation. Passive stabilizers are the labrum, superior glenohumeral ligament, middle glenohumeral ligament, inferior glenohumeral ligament, and capsule. Myology (muscle) provides dynamic support and stability and is made up of more than 18 major muscles that directly or indirectly provide mobility and stability of the entire shoulder complex.

Because of the complexity of the shoulder and surrounding tissues, the physical therapist assistant (PTA) is strongly encouraged to review pertinent anatomy and kinesiology of the glenohumeral, acromioclavicular, and scapulothoracic joints. Furthermore, the PTA should review the mechanisms of tissue healing because these principles clarify tissue-healing concepts and reinforce the need for early protected motion after injury, immobilization, and recovery of strength and function after injury to the shoulder complex. This section focuses on the recognition of certain orthopedic injuries and rehabilitation procedures used to reduce pain and swelling, improve motion, restore strength and endurance, and return the patient to normal function.

SUBACROMIAL ROTATOR CUFF IMPINGEMENT

A common cause of shoulder pain and dysfunction in laborers, athletes, and persons who do repetitive overhead lifting is subacromial rotator cuff impingement. In this disorder, the tendons of the rotator cuff are crowded, buttressed, or compressed under the coracoacromial arch, resulting in mechanical wear, stress, and friction.[15,20,23] Clinically, distinction must be made between primary and secondary impingement because there are important differences in treatment related to the specific cause of impingement.[15,20]

Primary shoulder impingement refers to mechanical compression of the rotator cuff tendons, primarily the supraspinatus tendon, as they pass under the coracoacromial ligament between the acromion and coracoid process.[15,32]

Secondary shoulder impingement is related to glenohumeral instability that creates a reduced subacromial space because the humeral head elevates and minimizes the area under the coracoacromial ligament.[20] This mechanical instability is the result of impairment of muscle coordination and weakness of the scapular stabilizers.

Age-related degenerative changes also can result in a decreased subacromial margin between the rotator cuff and coracoacromial arch. Bony osteophyte formation can occupy space under the anteroinferior surface of the acromion, which consequently reduces the available space. A reduction in available space in the shoulder is known as *anatomic crowding*. The supraspinatus tendon is the most common structure involved with rotator cuff impingement; the vascularity of the supraspinatus tendon is causative.[20,32] An area just proximal to the insertion on the greater tuberosity is hypovascular and is commonly referred to as a *watershed zone, critical zone,* or *critical portion*. This area of relative transient hypovascularity occurs with repeated arm motions from abduction to adduction, which compromises the blood supply to the area. The combination of reduced blood supply to the supraspinatus tendon and mechanical wear, stress, and friction as a result of repeated overhead motions can lead to primary impingement, supraspinatus tendinitis, and ultimately tears within the rotator cuff.[27,32]

The various stages of rotator cuff impingement are related to age and degenerative changes in the cuff itself. Neer[35] has identified three specific stages of impingement (tendinitis):

■ Stage I: Occurs in younger patients (usually younger than 25 years of age), but can occur at any age. Clinical features are edema and hemorrhage. Pain is worse with shoulder abduction greater than 90°.[2-5] It is essentially a reversible lesion that responds to conservative physical therapy interventions.[37]

■ Stage II: The fibrosis and tendinitis stage, which usually affects patients between the ages of 25 and 40 years.[1] It is classified as irreversible because of long-term repeated stress, wherein the supraspinatus tendon, biceps tendon, and subacromial bursa become fibrotic. Pain is the predominant feature and occurs with daily activities; it frequently causes the patient difficulty at night.

■ Stage III: Affects patients more than 40 years of age. It is characterized by tendon degeneration, rotator cuff tears, and rotator cuff ruptures. Usually associated with a long history of repeated shoulder pain and dysfunction, as well as significant muscle weakness and atrophy.

Various clinical tests can be used to identify the presence of pain related to specific maneuvers of the shoulder. During the initial evaluation performed by the physical therapist (PT), tests are used to elicit impingement signs. One of these is the Neer painful arc test, in which pain is reported while the shoulder goes through elevation with internal rotation. This test elicits impingement secondary to compression of the rotator cuff against the coracoacromial arch.[10] The Hawkins-Kennedy test is

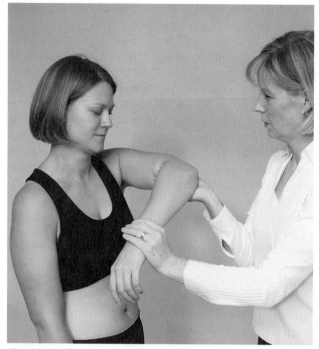

Fig. 21-1 The Hawkins-Kennedy impingement test demonstrates the impingement sign by forcibly medially rotating the proximal humerus when the arm is forward flexed to 90°. (From Magee DJ: *Orthopedic physical assessment*, ed 5, St Louis, 2008, Saunders.)

performed by elevating the shoulder to 90° in the scapular plane with internal rotation over pressure (Fig. 21-1). In most cases, elevation of more than 80° or 90° elicits pain. Therefore exercise and all activities that require the shoulder to elevate or abduct past 80° or 90° must be strictly avoided until all symptoms of pain have been eliminated.

Rehabilitation of Primary and Secondary Rotator Cuff Impingement

Kamkar and colleagues[20] have identified scapular weakness as leading to "function scapular instability," which affects scapular position during activities that cause a "relative decrease in the subacromial space." This secondary impingement requires the scapulothoracic muscles to be strengthened and stabilized before specific rotator cuff weakness can be addressed. Scapula thoracic articulation is known to many clinicians as the true core of the upper extremity. To effectively stabilize the humeral head so that it does not migrate superiorly, causing "winging" or "tipping," the scapular muscles (serratus anterior; upper, middle, and lower trapezius; levator scapulae; and rhomboid muscles) must be strengthened.[17,20,42] Thein[42] describes the clinical features of humeral head migration (secondary impingement) as possibly confusing the typical impingement picture. She reports, "If the supraspinatus is overworked trying to stabilize the humeral head, then it is unable

to effectively function to depress the humeral head. The resultant upward movement decreases the subacromial space and irritates the subacromial soft tissues, thus perpetuating the impingement process."

The initial evaluation performed by the PT is crucial in determining which exercises are to be performed to help stabilize the scapula and which should be avoided initially to reduce rotator cuff irritation with glenohumeral instability or superior migration of the humeral head.

Scapular stabilization exercises are only one component of a successful rehabilitation program.[9] In general a comprehensive rehabilitation program to address rotator cuff impingement, rotator cuff tendinitis (supraspinatus tendinitis), and degenerative tears of the rotator cuff tendons include modification of activities, local and systemic methods to control pain and swelling (nonsteroidal antiinflammatory drugs [NSAIDs], corticosteroid injections, ice, ultrasound, iontophoresis, phonophoresis), stretching and strengthening exercises, and a return to normal function after reevaluation by the PT and with continued maintenance of protective positions and general conditioning.[13,15]

The nonoperative treatment of impingement and symptomatic rotator cuff tears focuses on a three-phase, criterion-based rehabilitation program. The three phases of rehabilitation are as follows: (1) phase I, prefunctional; (2) phase II, return to function; and finally, (3) phase III, return to activity. Phase I, prefunctional, concentrates on relief of symptoms and initiating exercises to improve or maintain motion. Because impingement symptoms are usually made worse with overhead activities, the patient must modify activities of daily living (ADLs) and all other motions that may place the shoulder at or above 80° to 90° elevation. Home activities that require modification include cleaning hard-to-reach places and painting overhead. Work site tasks that must be adapted include heavy overhead lifting, manual labor, reaching, and climbing. Sporting activities such as tennis, golf, swimming, and baseball also must be modified to avoid impingement. The key to remember in each case is modification, not elimination, of compromising activities. For example, for a recreational tennis player, overhead serving should be avoided but all other ground strokes may be able to be maintained. For household activities and work site modifications, rearrangement and advanced planning of overhead tasks may be all that is needed to minimize the aggravating position of elevation past 80° or 90°. The PTA must constantly reinforce the concept of protective positioning and should encourage compliance throughout the course of rehabilitation.

In addition to activity modification, management of pain and swelling can be achieved with various physician-prescribed oral NSAIDs and physical therapy agents. Usually ice packs, ultrasound, some type of pharmacophoresis (iontophoresis and phonophoresis), and most recently, infrared laser application, are used to help control symptoms.

Throughout phase I, stretching exercises are performed to increase blood flow and contractility[15] and improve motion. The PTA must pay particular attention to performing all stretching activities, because many generalized shoulder stretches involve full forward shoulder elevation and abduction maneuvers. All phase I stretching should encourage nonballistic, slow, controlled, pain-free motion at less than 80° to 90° of elevation. Capsular mobility has been shown to be very helpful in increasing motion and preparing the surrounding muscles to assist in shoulder elevation in all planes of motion.[26,34] However, once symptoms are managed the patient can perform all stretches involving elevation and abduction if these stretches do not produce symptoms. Depending on the initial evaluation data gathered by the PT, the patient may be instructed in two specific stretches that authorities[15] suggest are effective in addressing posterior capsular tightness. Shoulder adduction across the chest (cross-body stretching) and internal shoulder rotation are used cautiously to improve posterior capsular tightness and overcome the limitations on motion of internal rotation of the shoulder. The effective use of the sleeper stretch to increase posterior capsular mobility has been reported. The concept of anterior capsular mobility has been presented as important for shoulder mobility to treat or prevent impingement while regaining horizontal abduction to prepare for tri-plane overhead motion.[25]

Initial strengthening activities that can begin during phase I generally include scapula stabilization exercises and light rotator cuff strengthening. The use of closed kinetic chain loading such as wall push-ups can be an effective pain-free low level muscle recruitment exercise. Closed kinetic chain (CKC) exercises will provide co-contraction and tri-plane stabilization with lower muscle contraction load than open kinetic (OKC) chain exercises.[5,46] Once the patient demonstrates improved motion and can do ADLs without pain, a progression through a series of OKC muscle strengthening can begin. Prone extension to the hip, side-lying external rotation, and scaption elevation without pain are some recommended exercises for rotator cuff recruitment toward strengthening (Fig. 21-2).[38] Specific rotator cuff strengthening exercises should focus on the supraspinatus muscle.[38] Studies demonstrate that the supraspinatus, infraspinatus, subscapularis, deltoid, latissimus dorsi, and pectoral muscles are effectively strengthened by arm elevation in the transverse plane, shoulder elevation with neutral rotation in the plane of the scapula (Fig. 21-3), prone horizontal shoulder abduction with external rotation (Fig. 21-4), and seated press-ups.[30]

Phase II, return to function, progresses with advanced scapular stabilization exercises that are encouraged as

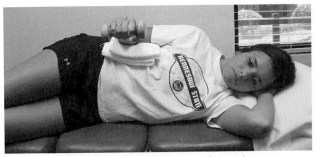

Fig. 21-2 Side-lying external rotation.

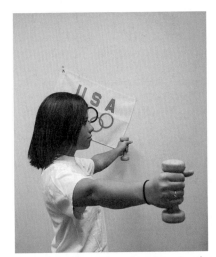

Fig. 21-3 Scaption. Shoulder elevation in the plane of the scapula.

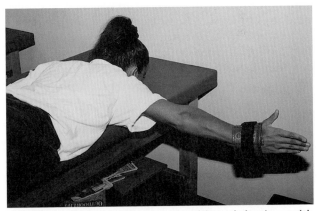

Fig. 21-4 Prone horizontal shoulder abduction with external rotation.

part of a comprehensive glenohumeral and scapulothoracic strengthening program. This phase of program uses progressive resistive strengthening via increased resistance while using OKC exercises. Electromyographic studies[33] have identified four basic scapular stabilization exercises that strengthen the upper, middle,

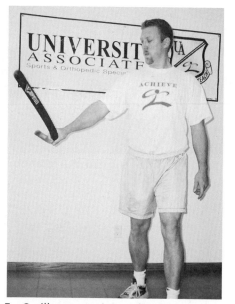

Fig. 21-5 Oscillatory training (Bodyblade, Hymanson, Playa del Rey, Calif.) for deltoid. (From Manske RC: *Postsurgical orthopedic sports rehabilitation: knee & shoulder*, St Louis, 2007, Mosby.)

and lower trapezius; the levator scapula; the rhomboid major; the pectoralis minor; and the middle and lower serratus anterior muscles.[8] The exercises are rowing, scapular plane elevation (scaption), press-ups, and push-ups followed by scapular protraction. As strength improves and when motion increases, a gradual return to normal function signifies the beginning of phase III, return to activity.[44]

The process of functional recovery is slow and must be done cautiously; overhead activities are introduced incrementally as the patient is able to demonstrate pain-free motion and the ability to perform strengthening activities. Some advanced return to activity phase exercises can include oscillatory training (Bodyblade) using tri-plane positioning (Fig. 21-5).[40]

Surgical Management of Shoulder Impingement and Rotator Cuff Tears

When physical therapy interventions fail to provide long-lasting relief and in cases of rotator cuff tears (Neer's stage III impingement, tendon degeneration, and cuff tears), various surgical procedures can be used to correct the underlying pathologic condition. With subacromial impingement not involving a specific rotator cuff tear, subacromial decompression (SAD) can be used to eliminate or diminish the abnormality causing the impingement between the humeral head and the undersurface of the acromion, allowing freer movement of the tendons without irritation. Acromioplasty includes beveling or reshaping of the acromion with detachment of the coracoacromial ligament. Distal clavicle excision (DCE) may

also be involved.[39] If there is an associated rotator cuff tear (small tear less than 1 cm, medium tear less than 3 cm, large tear greater than 5 cm), a SAD procedure is used in conjunction with direct repair of the rotator cuff defect. The SAD procedure can be performed as an open arthrotomy or as an arthroscopic procedure.[39]

Rehabilitation after SAD or rotator cuff repair closely parallels nonoperative rehabilitation of rotator cuff impingement. However, time must be allowed for healing of the soft tissues and bone after surgery. Some clearly identified differences exist between rehabilitation procedures used for decompression and small cuff tears (less than 1 cm) and repairs of medium (less than 2 to 3 cm) and large (greater than 4 to 5 cm) cuff tears with SAD.[39] With a small cuff tear repaired in conjunction with a decompression procedure, active motion and pain-free exercise can begin as soon as the patient can tolerate these activities.[39,44] However, if the rotator cuff tear is between 2 and 5 cm, tissue protection must be longer to allow for extensive soft-tissue healing. If full active range of motion (AROM) is allowed too early, healing of the rotator cuff may be compromised because of the stresses placed on the repaired tissues. The type of surgical procedure used, mini-open procedure or arthroscopic approach; the healing constraints must be considered for proper beginning of successful rehabilitation. Large cuff tears may require longer periods of time for recovery to achieve improved healing.[15]

Generally, recovery after SAD with or without rotator cuff repair follows a prescribed three-phase rehabilitation program.[42,44] Phase I, the prefunctional phase, lasts approximately 3 to 4 weeks[39,44] and focuses on control of pain and swelling with NSAIDs, oral analgesics, ice packs, ultrasound, phonophoresis (if needed), infrared therapy, and various degrees and durations of manual range of motion (ROM), depending on the extent of tissue injury. The concept of early protected manual motion applies depending on the precise nature of the injury and which surgical procedure is used. The prefunctional phase should include increasing ROM, scapula stabilization beginning with retraction, and adding protraction when the patient has pain-free arm control.

With small rotator cuff repairs (less than 1 cm), isometric submaximal muscle sets of the shoulder extensors, flexors, abductors, external rotators, and internal rotators can begin as early as pain allows. Active assisted ROM (AAROM) activities beginning with manual exercise must be performed pain free. Active biceps and triceps exercises are performed in the neutral humerus position beginning with isometrics then progress to light resistive exercises. ROM and strength gradually increase as pain and swelling are controlled.

At the end of this phase, the initial use of the upper body ergometer (UBE) may be introduced. The early

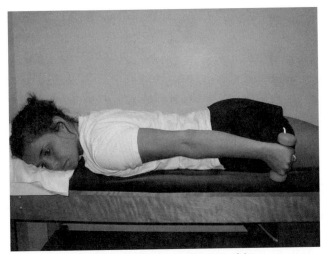

Fig. 21-6 Prone extension to hip.

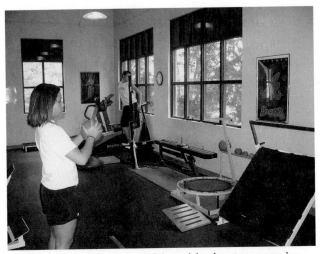

Fig. 21-7 Plyometric activity with plyo-toss exercise.

use of CKC activity with double-arm wall push-ups may be helpful for low level recruitment of shoulder muscles.[44,46] With increased arm control strength and motion, phase II, the return to function phase, can begin. It generally lasts from weeks 5 through 12 after surgery. During this phase, progressive motion can be used, although with caution for repetitive shoulder abduction and forward elevation above 90°. The use of Thera-Band strengthening of the rotator cuff should be performed in a short-arc pattern of motion, normally in the standing positions.[18,44] In addition, dumbbell isotonic concentric and eccentric exercises for recruitment of the humeral head decompression (rotator cuff) may begin using short-arc pain-free ROM. This program is known as *positional recruitment* for the purpose of low-level strengthening and progresses according to the tolerance of the patent and demonstration of arm control.[44] During phase II, progressive strengthening exercises for elevation in scaption are performed in allowing for what is known as *shoulder hike*. Prone positional exercise, such as prone extension to hip (Fig. 21-6) and short-arc prone scaption at 100°, and eccentric training of scaption has been very useful in treating shoulder hike.[30,38,44] Progressive resistive exercises (PREs) are a major part of the return to function phase. With some patients, based on good pain-free response to all rotator cuff exercise, advanced scapula stabilization and oscillatory training such as the Bodyblade may begin (see Fig. 21-5).

Phase III, the return to activity phase, can begin once the patient can demonstrate normal motion without symptoms and with improved strength. This phase lasts approximately from week 12 to beyond. Return to activity always includes the continuation of PREs. This aspect of rehabilitation is for the long haul.[44] Advanced CKC exercises such as single-arm wall push-ups on an uneven surface may be introduced. For the advanced patient,

plyometric activity with plyo-toss exercise may be used (Fig. 21-7).

During the return to activity phase the core rotator cuff strengthening exercises of forward elevation, scaption, prone horizontal abduction with external rotation, and press-ups, as well as scapular stabilization exercises of seated rows, prone scaption at 120° (Fig. 21-8), scaption, and press-ups for scapular protraction (push-ups with a plus)[20,33,38,44] form the foundation of improving strength that eventually leads to full functional recovery.

The prefunctional phases and periods of passive or manual control motion are extensive for rehabilitation after surgical repair of massive rotator cuff tears. Generally, no active shoulder motion or active concentric or eccentric strengthening is allowed for 2 to 3 months after surgery.[11] Extensive soft-tissue healing must proceed unabated to foster the recovery of functional motion and strength.

Initially the patient is placed in abduction pillow or shoulder immobilization after surgery to allow the repaired tissues of the rotator cuff and deltoid to be placed in a shortened position. Early active muscle strengthening and active motion are avoided to allow for appropriate healing. Generally, manual control passive ROM with full motion restriction is allowed during the first several weeks of recovery. AAROM activities, can begin 2 months after surgery.[11]

Submaximal isometrics and scapular stabilization exercises must be added cautiously 4 to 12 weeks after surgery.[11,44] Specific rotator cuff strengthening exercises[11] performed isotonically with dumbbells, Thera-Band, and similar devices are reserved until 3 months after surgery to accommodate the healing constraints of the tendons and muscles of the rotator cuff and deltoid. Full functional recovery of motion and strength may take up to several months after the repair of massive rotator cuff tears.[11,44]

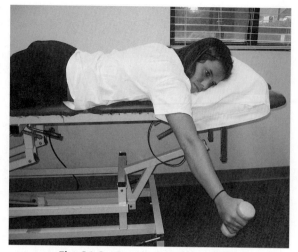

Fig. 21-8 Prone scaption at 120°.

GLENOHUMERAL JOINT INSTABILITY AND DISLOCATION

Dislocations and subluxations (partial dislocation) of the glenohumeral joint (the articulation between the humeral head and glenoid fossa of the scapula) frequently occur after indirect trauma with the arm abducted, elevated, and internally rotated (posterior dislocation).[16] The shoulder is the most commonly dislocated joint in the body,[16] and dislocation occurs in men more often than in women. Anterior dislocations occur more frequently than posterior dislocations.[16] Also, rotator cuff tears of various dimensions (small, less than 1 cm; medium, less than 3 cm; and large, greater than 5 cm) occur with relative frequency. Strege[41] reports that rotator cuff tears occur 30% of the time with acute anterior dislocations in patients older than 40 years of age and 80% of the time in patients older than 60 years of age.

Two associated injuries may occur as a result of acute glenohumeral dislocation and instability. Because the shoulder is the most mobile joint in the body, bony restrictions do not provide substantial restraint. Rather, the fibrocartilaginous glenoid labrum deepens the articulation between the humeral head and bony glenoid fossa. Injury to the labrum can occur if forces are great enough to dislocate the humerus from its confines within the glenoid. This injury is referred to as a *Bankart lesion*[3,36,41,42,44] and is defined as "an avulsion of the capsule and glenoid labrum off of the anterior rim of the glenoid resulting from traumatic anterior dislocation of the shoulder."[21,41]

The head of the humerus is subject to injury as a result of anterior shoulder instability. A **Hill-Sachs lesion** is a compression or "impaction fracture"[36] of the posterolateral aspect of the humeral head as a result of anterior shoulder instability.[3,36,41,42] This lesion results from instability and is not the essential cause of glenohumeral instability.[36,45]

As stated, anterior dislocations are more prevalent than posterior dislocations. However, shoulder instability can be defined as multidirectional, wherein the humeral head may sublux or dislocate anteriorly, inferiorly, and posteriorly.[36,41]

Nonoperative Management

The initial management of acute shoulder dislocations (anterior and posterior) calls for a period of protection lasting for up to 4 to 6 weeks.[16,36] All positions that may reproduce the mechanism of dislocation are avoided. In some cases immobilization is needed to promote healing.

Management of pain and swelling is addressed with physician-prescribed NSAIDs, analgesics, ice packs, electrical stimulation, or other physical agents such as ultrasound and infrared. During the protection period, the hand, wrist, and elbow of the affected shoulder must receive active motion and strengthening exercises that do not compromise the shoulder. Also, a general conditioning program of strength, flexibility, and endurance activities can begin. With an anterior shoulder subluxation (spontaneous reduction of the humeral head) or dislocation, the patient must avoid shoulder abduction and external rotation to allow proper capsular scarring and soft-tissue healing to occur. It is interesting to note that patients older than age 40 years who are not at significant risk of recurrent dislocation because of a relatively sedentary lifestyle may only need minimal protection for a couple of weeks before rehabilitation can begin and motion can be regained.[16,36]

The prefunctional phase of rehabilitation begins with manual control ROM, active assistive stretching for elevation, and assisted ROM exercises to help the patient regain lost motion if a relatively lengthy period of protection was warranted.

Initial strengthening begins with submaximal isometric exercises that can be safely started while the patient's shoulder is placed in the neutral humeral position. Isometric shoulder adduction and abduction, internal and external rotation, and elevation and extension can be performed at a pain-free level. Once the patient can demonstrate an increase from submaximal isometric contractions to near-maximal contractions, progressive internal and external rotation can begin with the affected shoulder in a minimal degree of abduction. When the symptoms of pain are reduced and the intensity and quality of muscle contractions are improved, the patient may increase ROM activities to forward elevation, extension, scapular mobility, and internal and external rotation and abduction. As the patient progresses to the return to function phase, combined shoulder abduction and external rotation are avoided. In fact, some authorities recommend avoiding extremes of shoulder abduction and external rotation for 3 months after removal of the sling.[16,36] The hallmark of the return to function phases of recovery after anterior shoulder dislocation or subluxation is progressive strengthening of the rotator cuff, anterior shoulder muscles, and scapular stabilizers, with particular attention given to eccentric strengthening of the posterior rotator cuff (infraspinatus and teres minor).[22,42,44] Thera-Band and handheld dumbbell weights are effective because of the wide variety of motions that can be addressed and can carry over to home exercises. Please refer to the previous section on rotator cuff exercises for a recommended home program.

Synchronous shoulder motion, or scapulohumeral rhythm, must be addressed before and throughout recovery from a shoulder dislocation. The 2:1 ratio of motion between the scapula and glenohumeral joint (meaning that for every 2° of glenohumeral flexion or abduction after the first 30° of shoulder motion, the scapula must rotate upwardly 1°)[24] must be addressed early to prevent the facilitation of abnormal motions between the scapula and glenohumeral joint during strengthening activities. This can be accomplished adequately by focusing on normalized scapular motion and stabilization exercises during the return to function phase as long as symptoms of pain and harmful glenohumeral joint positions are avoided.

Throughout each phase of recovery, various tissues that contain the humeral head in the glenoid fossa (glenoid labrum, capsule, and ligaments; superior, middle, and inferior glenohumeral ligaments; and musculotendinous rotator cuff) can be stressed or torn. By definition, glenohumeral instability identifies ligamentous and capsular restraints as being "attenuated"[27,28]; therefore the appropriate progressive application of strengthening activities for the rotator cuff and scapulothoracic muscles becomes central to the recovery of motion and function.

One way the PTA can address functional motions and stimulate the afferent neural input system is through CKC activities. CKC activities can enhance proprioception and promote dynamic joint stability.[16,28] Rhythmic stabilization through manual exercises and progression to other oscillation training such as the Bodyblade may be helpful.

Isotonic resistance exercises are quite challenging and stressful to the glenohumeral joint; consequently, many appropriate exercises must be modified to accommodate limitations of motion, pain, and the provocative positions of abduction and external rotation. The seated or supine chest press is an example of isotonic exercise that promotes anterior shoulder strength. However, this particular exercise can place the shoulder in a horizontally abducted position that stresses the anterior shoulder capsule, causing the head of the humerus to translate forward within the glenoid (Fig. 21-9). Progressive positional recruitment for strengthening using the PRE method is always continued throughout this phase of recovery.

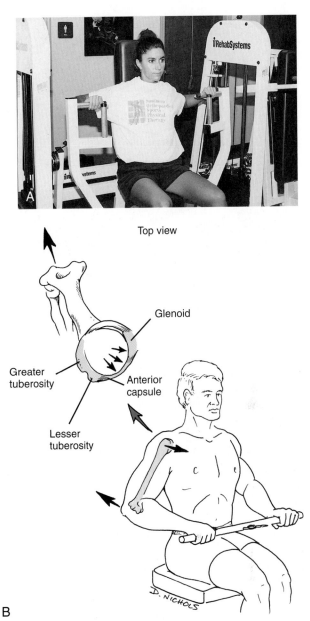

Fig. 21-9 **A,** Seated chest press. This initial position can place stress on the anterior shoulder capsule. **B,** In this figure, notice how the head of the humerus can rock forward within the glenoid, causing stress to the anterior shoulder capsule.

Local muscle endurance activities are done using an UBE, CKC exercise with the use of hands on the stairstepper (Fig. 21-10, A).[44] Weight-bearing closed-chain exercises such as wall push-ups (Fig. 21-10, B) for triplane strengthening can be introduced. These exercises provide proprioceptive stimulation to the mechanoreceptor system. Gradually, more challenging weight-bearing activities that demand progressive control of the glenohumeral joint in multiplane and diagonal motions are added (Fig. 21-11, A-C). A balance board also can help train the shoulder muscles to respond and fire quickly for sufficient stabilization (Fig. 21-11, D-E).

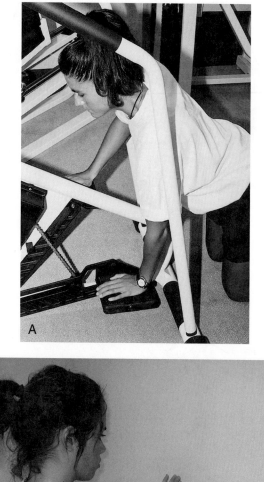

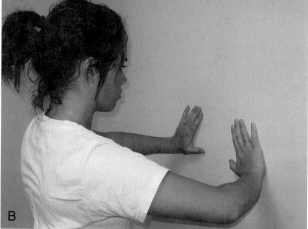

Fig. 21-10 Closed kinetic chain exercises. **A,** Stair-stepping activity. **B,** Wall push-up.

Cable systems offer various exercises and positions that duplicate functional activities. Cable systems are particularly useful in athletic patients, because sport-specific tasks can be reproduced with this equipment. In addition, a plyo-toss (plyometric) exercise for stabilization is part of the return to activity phase. Plyometric ball toss against a rebounder is an excellent exercise for advanced patterns (Fig. 21-12).[4]

The process of recovery after shoulder dislocation matches the degree of injury. Full functional recovery is not always possible. In some cases, minor stress causes the shoulder to dislocate again after acute traumatic dislocation. With repeated episodes of shoulder dislocation or subluxation, recurrent anterior instability can

result.[12,16] If patients fail to respond to an aggressive physical therapy program, the physician may choose one of several operative procedures to correct the instability. Patients with recurrent dislocations may receive an anterior capsulolabral reconstruction.[7] Patients with multidirectional instability may require a procedure known as a *capsular shift*.[23]

Operative Management and Rehabilitation

Because posterior shoulder dislocations account for only 2% to 4% of all shoulder dislocations,[36] this discussion focuses on repairs and rehabilitation procedures to enhance joint stability and promote function in patients with anterior glenohumeral instability. Surgical procedures for shoulder instability can be classified as open or arthroscopic techniques.[7,23,36]

The anterior capsulolabral reconstruction procedure essentially reattaches the capsule to the glenoid. Sometimes this is referred to as *corrective surgery for capsular redundancy*. All labral lesions are also repaired. A superior labrum, anterior to posterior (SLAP) repair, which is the repairing of the superior labral lesion, may also be involved.

Patients with anterior shoulder instability corrected via arthroscopy normally experience less postoperative pain and reduced soft-tissue damage.[44] Rehabilitation after open or arthroscopic stabilization for anterior glenohumeral instability requires a prefunctional phase of rehabilitation that emphasizes protected ROM. Slow and protective external rotation is performed up to 12 weeks postoperative to ensure healing of all soft tissue. A recommended external rotation incrimination is as follows:

■ 0° to 30° for 3 weeks
■ 30° to 45° for 6 weeks
■ 45° to 75° for 9 weeks
■ 75° to 90° for 12 weeks

Initial postoperative care begins with a period of immobilization in a shoulder immobilizer to allow for appropriate soft-tissue healing.[7] During this period, medications for pain and swelling may be prescribed by the physician. Frequently, ice packs are applied to the shoulder for 20 minutes, three to five times daily, as part of the home program to control postoperative pain and swelling. Also the patient can actively perform finger, hand, wrist, and elbow mobility exercises. In addition, submaximal isometric exercises can be initiated while the arm is still in the immobilizer. These must be performed pain free.

The degree and direction of shoulder motion allowed are specific to the surgical procedure, the wishes of the physician, and the direction of the PT. Generally, scapular protraction and retraction, manual control ROM, and assisted ROM exercises are performed to increase motion. The initiation of motion exercises is important because faulty scapulothoracic and glenohumeral

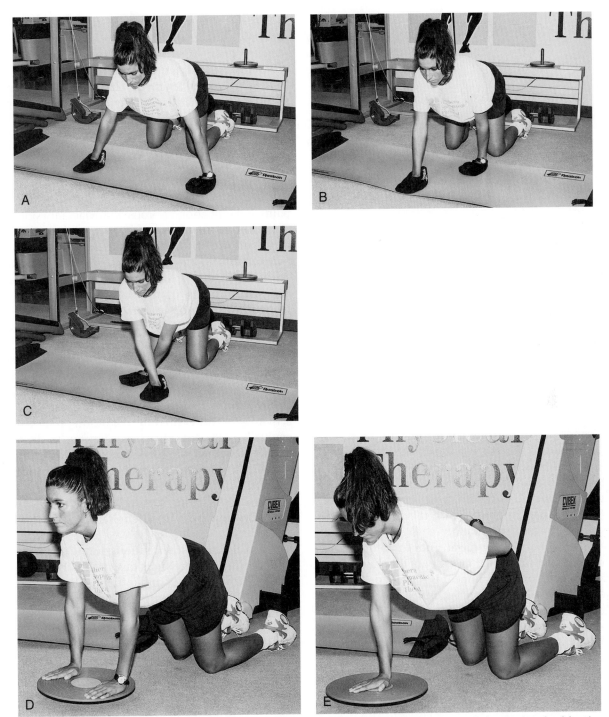

Fig. 21-11 Multiplane and diagonal closed-chain weight-bearing activities. **A,** Shoulder abduction and adduction on a slide board in a kneeling position. Extreme caution must be taken to ensure that a limited range of abduction be allowed when initiating this activity. **B,** Shoulder flexion and extension in a kneeling position. When beginning all slide board activities the patient must be able to eccentrically and concentrically control the affected shoulder globally. **C,** Diagonal patterns on the slide board. **D,** Closed kinetic chain wobble board activity for stimulating shoulder stability. Initially, both arms are used when introducing this exercise. **E,** When strength, control, and confidence improve, the patient can progress to one arm.

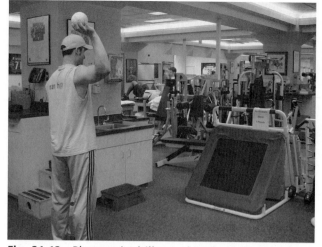

Fig. 21-12 Plyometric drill: one-hand standing baseball throw. (From Manske RC: *Postsurgical orthopedic sports rehabilitation: knee and shoulder*, St Louis, 2007, Mosby.)

mobility can be affected early. Care must be taken to encourage scapular motion, as well as glenohumeral mobility, and to identify any limitations affecting normal scapulohumeral rhythm. Progressive elevation and scapula control is recommended early in this phase of rehabilitation. Elevation is normally progressed to 135° to tolerance after 6 weeks postoperative. Slow progression of abduction is recommended. Therefore the PTA must be aware of the exact rationale behind limiting early active or passive shoulder abduction and external rotation.[44]

Progressive motion and strengthening exercises are allowed as the patient progresses to the return to function phase. Progressive shoulder strengthening must address both the glenohumeral and scapulothoracic joints. To recover functional mobility of the shoulder, a program of positional recruitment is suggested. Because the scapula forms the base of support for glenohumeral motion, stabilization exercises must be advanced. As the patient demonstrates improved mobility without complaints of pain, the quality of muscle contraction (from submaximal to maximal) must be encouraged gradually. PREs using a Thera-Band, dumbbells, or both within an active, pain-free ROM can begin, along with more challenging flexibility exercises, between 6 and 8 weeks after surgery.[7]

The eccentric contraction phase of each exercise must be encouraged. Applying this concept during the return to function phase involves emphasizing the eccentric loading phase of all internal rotation, abduction, external rotation, adduction, and shoulder elevation exercises.[4] Local muscle endurance also must be considered once the patient has achieved improved motion and strength. Usually an UBE or some other form of low-intensity, high-repetition shoulder-specific activity is appropriate. Functional activities, proprioception, and CKC exercises, are necessary for functional recovery.

During the return to activity phases of recovery, in order to stimulate the mechanoreceptor system, a complete program of advanced CKC exercises, plyo-toss (plyometrics) and sports specific training is designed. Generally the total length of rehabilitation after surgical stabilization of the glenohumeral joint ranges from 3 to 5 months.[7]

ADHESIVE CAPSULITIS

Adhesive capsulitis, which is also referred to as *frozen shoulder*, is characterized by decreased shoulder ROM, pain, inflammation, fibrous synovial adhesions, and reduction of the joint cavity.[1,3,6] Adhesive capsulitis occurs more commonly in females and affects patients between 40 and 60 years of age.[6] The two distinct classifications of frozen shoulder are primary and secondary adhesive capsulitis. Primary idiopathic frozen shoulder is the most common lesion and occurs spontaneously from unknown causes. Secondary adhesive capsulitis generally occurs after trauma or immobilization.[6,52]

Among older patients, secondary adhesive capsulitis can develop because of limited immobilization for as little as 1 or 2 days.[5,14] In the early stages of this disabling condition, pain occurs both at rest and during activity.[5,6,14] However, as the condition progresses, pain gradually subsides, then spontaneously disappears. Severely restricted motion and profound loss of function remain.[5,6,14] During the acute painful phase, treatment is focused on controlling inflammation and symptoms of pain. Physician-prescribed analgesics, NSAIDs, and intraarticular steroid injections can provide some pain relief.[6]

Physical therapy interventions during this acute painful stage include the judicious use of ice, heat, ultrasound, phonophoresis, and infrared. Also central to this initial management phase is the stimulation of pain-free motion and relaxation of muscle guarding of the glenohumeral joint, cervical area, and scapulothoracic muscles.[19] Passive, active, and active assisted motion exercise must occur within a pain-free ROM to stimulate removal of metabolic waste, increase local blood flow, and assist in the reduction of edema in the local tissues. Both wand and rope and pulley systems can be used early if they are performed in a slow, controlled, pain-free ROM. For severely restricted glenohumeral motion, the PT may prescribe the application of specific joint mobilization techniques to help modulate pain and reduce muscle guarding.[1,3,5,14,19,44] As addressed, grades I and II low-amplitude physiologic and accessory oscillations can help encourage relaxation while reducing pain.[19,44]

If the scapula is not stable and free from restriction while the patient attempts to regain shoulder motion and function, normal scapulohumeral rhythm cannot be obtained. Therefore early scapular stabilization exercises[3,37,44] can be employed as long as pain does not inhibit the correct performance of the exercise. Normalized motion must precede specific strengthening activities to avoid developing faulty shoulder mechanics.

The complete restoration of glenohumeral joint mobility is the goal of treatment for the late stage of adhesive capsulitis. The PT must identify the appropriate application of increased joint mobilization techniques to address specific capsular restrictions and initiate more challenging progressive resistance exercises.[48] When the patient demonstrates improved glenohumeral motion and appropriate scapulohumeral rhythm, strengthening exercises can begin for the deltoid, scapular muscles, rotator cuff, and upper-arm muscles.[9,44]

Although control of pain and inflammation is the primary feature of early physical therapy management, submaximal isometric exercise can be used to initiate strengthening if pain is not increased with exercise. Progressing from submaximal isometrics to maximal isometrics usually precedes the use of a Thera-Band or dumbbells for concentric and eccentric exercises. A comprehensive series of rotator cuff exercises[38,43] and scapular stabilization exercises[3] can be encouraged as early as pain and motion allow. To address normalized function, the patient does closed-chain resistance exercises and overhead loading along with proprioception exercises (e.g., balance board, slide board, and Plyoball) in a sequential, orderly fashion once sufficient strength, improved motion, and scapulohumeral rhythm have been established. Local muscle endurance activities focus on purposeful, functional movements that duplicate ADLs.

Again, pain control, restoration of motion, and improved function must be reinforced continually to encourage compliance with a home exercise program and the avoidance of positions that may exacerbate pain and muscle guarding.

ACROMIOCLAVICULAR SPRAINS AND DISLOCATIONS

Ligamentous sprains of the AC joint usually result from a fall on the acromion (direct force) or when force is transmitted from a fall on an outstretched arm proximally to the AC joint (indirect force).[50] AC joint sprains and dislocations are graded according to the degree of injury to specific ligamentous structures (AC and coracoclavicular ligaments), as well as the position of the clavicle in complete rupture of both the AC and coracoclavicular ligaments, as follows[50]:

■ First-degree, grade I AC joint sprain: Characterized by partial tearing of the AC ligaments, with resultant joint tenderness over the AC joint, no joint instability or laxity of the ligament, and minimal loss of function.[31]

■ Second-degree, grade II AC sprain: Complete rupture of the AC ligaments with partial tearing of the coracoacromial ligaments.[31,50] The patient has moderate pain, some dysfunction (reduction in shoulder abduction and adduction), and a palpable gap between the acromion and the clavicle.[1,30,31]

■ Third-degree, grade III AC ligament injury: Dislocation between the acromion and clavicle where both the AC and coracoclavicular ligaments are ruptured and the distal clavicle becomes displaced superiorly. Patients demonstrate marked pain and severe limitation of shoulder motion. Three additional classifications have been proposed that describe the degree of vertical, posterior, and inferior separation of the clavicle in grade III AC dislocation.[31]

Rehabilitation and management of grade I AC sprains focus on symptomatic relief. Typically, pain is controlled with the use of ice packs, NSAIDs, analgesics, and rest. Because the AC ligaments have been partially torn, the AC joint must be protected from further direct or indirect forces that may stress the AC ligaments. The patient may be allowed to resume activities within 2 weeks and usually does not require a rehabilitation program of significant duration.[1,31]

Grade II AC sprains require more direct attention to approximate the torn AC ligaments and allow for secure ligament healing. Usually this injury is managed nonoperatively using a shoulder immobilizer as needed for the short-term, and early ROM and stabilization exercises begin.[31] Again, modalities of choice may be used as needed.

As noted, there is usually a palpable step-off between the acromion process and distal clavicle with grade II AC sprains. This deformity represents a permanent loss of joint continuity because of lost ligamentous support between acromion and clavicle.[31]

The rehabilitation program continues with the prefunctional phase for a grade II AC sprain; active assisted to active exercises are allowed through pain-free ROM. Submaximal isometrics can be performed for all muscles of the shoulder girdle. However, care must be taken to avoid contractions that stress the AC joint; then isometric strengthening may be progressed for return to function. During this phase of rehabilitation inappropriate stress to the ligament should be avoided around the AC joint.

The return to function phase continues, using OKC and CKC advanced strengthening of the entire shoulder complex. Scapula stabilization continues to be vital for overall control of the upper extremity. PREs continue in the return to activity phase, including advanced scapula-cuff strengthening. Deltoid strengthening is advanced as tolerated. Thera-Band and dumbbells are effective and versatile tools for compliance and carryover to a prescribed home exercise program. The performance of scapular and humerus elevation exercises helps approximate the torn ligaments and provides dynamic muscular support to the torn structures. It is recommended that eccentric training progress slower, whereas plyometric with plyo-toss exercises and advanced rhythmic stabilization exercises are helpful for the more athletic patient. Rotator cuff strengthening is always recommended throughout all the advance phases of rehabilitation. In addition, a general conditioning program is warranted to improve or maintain aerobic fitness, strength, and flexibility.

The treatment of grade III AC sprains (dislocation of the distal clavicle and acromion process) may include surgical intervention. Although many surgeons advocate open surgical repair, others favor closed reduction, immobilization, and progressive rehabilitation. The nonoperative treatment of grade III AC sprains is centered on reducing the dislocation and maintaining the reduction.[31] The goals of the initial course of treatment in physical therapy is to minimize pain and swelling, with the modalities of choice, physician-prescribed NSAIDs, analgesics, and protection of the AC joint from unwanted stress, To ensure proper healing of the ligaments, the rehabilitation team must continuously reinforce compliance using the immobilizer for the recommended period prescribed by the treating physician.

While the patient is immobilized, submaximal isometric exercises can be initiated for the shoulder and scapula if no stress is applied to the healing ligaments. As with grade II AC sprains, the hand, wrist, and elbow of the affected arm can be safely and effectively strengthened during immobilization. Generally the nonoperative treatment of grade III sprains parallels the treatment plan for grade II sprains. The primary differences are the longer duration of immobilization and the more cautious and delayed application of motion and resistance exercises, so as not to adversely affect ligament healing. In some cases, nonoperative treatment is ineffective and surgical correction must be addressed.

The surgeon may elect to do open reduction with internal fixation (ORIF) to the AC joint to stabilize and approximate the joint. Another procedure calls for the surgeon to perform a modified reconstruction known as the *coracoacromial ligament transfer* and *clavicular reduction*. Most recently an autogenous tendon graft material has been used to reconstruct the AC joint.

Active motion and light resistance exercises for the hand, wrist, and elbow of the affected limb are encouraged in the early pre-function phase, normally lasting 4 to 6 weeks. Isometric exercises focus on the shoulder and scapular muscles once the AC joint is stabilized and protected from unwanted forces. Progressive active and active-assisted shoulder motion is allowed as pain and soft-tissue healing progress. After this period of protection to support the surgical reconstruction, the return to function phase begins the progressive strengthening. Return to function closely follows the patient's level of

motion and strength. As stated, heavy, intense resistance exercises must be based on the patient's tolerance. Advanced strengthening of the scapula, rotator cuff, and deltoids are included in the return to activity phase.

SCAPULAR FRACTURES

Most scapular fractures result from direct, severe trauma.[29,50] Therefore there is a high incidence of significant associated injuries, including other fractures, glenohumeral dislocations, pneumothorax, and neurovascular injuries.[29,41,50] Interestingly, fractures of the scapular body are the most common (49% to 89%)[50] and demonstrate the highest incidence of associated injuries (35% to 98%).[41] However, the treatment of fractures to the scapular body is conservative if associated injuries have not occurred, using ice and shoulder immobilization for 2 to 3 weeks.[29,41,50] During the immobilization period, hand, wrist, and elbow exercises can be initiated for the affected arm along with a general conditioning program. Early manual control ROM exercises for the shoulder begin as the pain and swelling subside.

Isometric exercises performed submaximally also can be initiated early if the patient remains pain free. As pain and swelling subside, strengthening exercises can be added within a pain-free ROM. Nonunion and malunion of this fracture are rare and usually are not associated with a loss of function or clinical symptoms.[41,50]

The second most common scapular fracture occurs to the glenoid neck. Williams and Rockwood[50] suggest that if the fracture is extraarticular, healing can occur at 6 weeks and that management involves conservative symptomatic care. Glenoid fractures also can be intraarticular, where the fracture extends through the glenoid fossa. The treatment of these fractures depends on whether there is associated glenohumeral instability. If no instability is present, these fractures are treated with shoulder immobilization and a return to motion and strength.[50] However, if there is glenohumeral instability associated with an intraarticular glenoid fracture, then surgical repair is needed to stabilize the fragments.[50] Usually an internal fixation device is inserted into the fracture fragments; therefore immobilization is needed to minimize stress at the fracture site. Manual control exercises can be initiated soon after surgery to minimize postoperative joint stiffness. Although gentle manual control shoulder elevation and external rotation are initiated 2 to 3 weeks postoperatively, active stretching and resistance exercises must be deferred for up to 6 to 8 weeks to allow for secure bone healing.[50]

CLAVICLE FRACTURES

Fractures of the clavicle occur as a result of direct or indirect trauma. These injuries are common and primarily affect men younger than 25 years of age.[52] Care is focused on achieving reduction of the fracture fragments, maintaining the reduction, and minimizing the immobilization of the glenohumeral joint of the affected arm.[52] Usually the patient is placed in a commercially available figure-of-eight bandage to maintain proper alignment of the area. The duration of immobilization varies, but authorities suggest that healing takes 4 to 6 weeks or longer.[52]

During the initial period of immobilization, with the figure-of-eight bandage, the hand, wrist, and elbow of the affected arm are exercised with active motion and resistance exercises. Unwanted stress to the fracture site is avoided during this period. In addition, the patient may perform submaximal isometrics for the shoulder and scapula once pain has been controlled. Manual exercises to the scapula is recommended before beginning OKC strengthening.[44]

Active shoulder elevation must not be greater than 50° to 70° until after 4 weeks (although patients may be encouraged to perform gentle active shoulder motion no greater than 60° when pain free).[50] As the healing process continues and when bone healing is confirmed radiographically (approximately 4 to 6 weeks), greater degrees of shoulder motion are allowed, with PREs added as tolerated.

If the fracture is located at the distal end of the clavicle, ORIF may be more appropriate, because these fractures tend to be unstable and do not maintain proper alignment with a figure-of-eight bandage.[41] The fragments of a displaced distal clavicle fracture usually are secured with an intramedullary fixation pin.[41]

PROXIMAL HUMERUS FRACTURES

Proximal humerus fractures usually are classified according to a four-part classification.[29,41] The four parts are the humeral head, lesser tuberosity, greater tuberosity, and humeral shaft.[41]

Physical therapy management of humerus fractures depends on the severity and complexity of the fracture, as well as the means used to secure fixation of the fracture site. Generally with nondisplaced one-part fractures (the most common type), the affected arm is placed in a immobilizer for a period of time and the patient is given analgesics and encouraged to apply ice liberally to minimize pain and swelling. Within the first 2 weeks, gentle active motion is allowed, as well as active motion of the elbow, wrist, and hand of the affected arm.[29] In fact, the patient may be allowed to remove the immobilizer for active motion exercises a few times each day.[29]

Submaximal shoulder isometrics are initiated as early as pain allows. Perhaps the most salient aspect of physical therapy care in proximal humerus fracture is the functional restoration of glenohumeral motion and strength after protracted periods of immobility to allow for appropriate bone healing. Early scapular motion

exercises minimize the restriction of scapular mobility. Submaximal scapular stabilization exercises[44] also can be encouraged early, as pain allows, to provide a stable base for glenohumeral motion exercises. Manual glides for mobility of the scapula maybe helpful. Manual glides to the glenohumeral joint may be needed if hypomobility is a side effect of prolonged immobilization. Progressive motion and resistance exercises for the deltoid, rotator cuff, and upper arm muscles closely parallel bone healing and the patient's ability to demonstrate improved motion without pain.

Other more complex fractures can require ORIF with screws and a plate, as well as prolonged periods of immobilization. As with all fractures, during immobility the patient can participate in a total body-conditioning program that does not compromise the healing of the fracture. In addition, the hand, wrist, and elbow of the affected limb must be exercised without stressing the fracture site.

The ultimate task after the healing of humerus fractures is regaining purposeful, functional strength and motion of the glenohumeral joint. Indeed, the time necessary to heal significant fractures may cause serious glenohumeral and scapular restrictions. The long-term healing restraints of bone form the primary guide for the physician and PT in deciding when to employ progressive motion activities and when to initiate strengthening tasks without compromising the fracture site.

Avascular necrosis (AVN) may be a risk with some significant fractures (displaced fractures of the anatomic neck).[29] For example, in an older population of patients with advancing osteoporosis who have four-part proximal humerus fracture, internal fixation may be poor because of the osteopenic bone. A prosthetic humeral head, known as *hemiarthroplasty*, may be more appropriate in this case.[41]

As the fracture begins to stabilize, and under the direction and supervision of the PT, some patients begin CKC exercises to stimulate the mechanoreceptor system (afferent neural input system) of the elbow, shoulder, and wrist and to effect proper bone healing (Wolff's law) by providing submaximal intermittent stress to the healing bone.

The PTA participates in the rehabilitation process of proximal humerus fractures by following and supervising a comprehensive program of early protected limited ROM, submaximal isometrics for the scapular stabilizers, rotator cuff, and upper arm muscles, and by providing continued protection for the injured site. As pain, motion, and bone healing progress, the PTA must carefully observe the scapulothoracic and glenohumeral motion. If scapulohumeral rhythm is adversely affected, specific attention must be addressed to regain a stable scapula and proper glenohumeral mobilization. In many cases if a restriction is noted, the PT may use scapular and glenohumeral mobilization techniques to modulate pain and encourage improved motion. However, the fracture site must be secure and stable, with radiographic confirmation of this, and the physician must order this protocol before mobilization can commence.

Functional shoulder activities and resistance exercises are added gradually as bone healing advances and the patient demonstrates greater confidence, motion, and strength without pain. Proprioception and CKC activities also may be added during the return to function phase of recovery in preparation for normalized purposeful motion and strength of the involved limb.

Total Shoulder Arthroplasty

With severe four-part fractures of the proximal humerus, AVN of the humeral head, osteoporosis, rheumatoid arthritis, and advanced osteoarthritis, the proximal humerus may be replaced with a prosthesis, or a total shoulder arthroplasty may be indicated.[14,41] The condition of the rotator cuff is a significant feature in patients receiving a hemiarthroplasty or total shoulder arthroplasty. Goldstein[14] reports that in patients suffering from rheumatoid arthritis, as many as 38% have a torn rotator cuff. If a rotator cuff tear is repaired in addition to the arthroplasty, postoperative immobilization may be as long as 4 to 6 weeks, with the affected arm held in an abduction splint to allow for healing of the repaired cuff.[2,14,47] When a patient has a massive rotator cuff tear or has had a revision of failed arthroplasty with rotator cuff tear a reverse prosthesis procedure may be needed. This procedure requires the surgeon to place the humeral component in the glenoid socket and the glenoid component into the proximal humerus. The rehabilitation objectives are usually the same as a regular arthroplasty,[6] but in some cases the progress will be slower.[47]

Thus a rotator cuff repair added to shoulder arthroplasty guides the course of rehabilitation and dictates the need for protective of limited motion, which leads to a longer program of rehabilitation.[5] In terms of restoration of shoulder motion, if the rotator cuff is not repaired, progressive range of motion though goal setting of the PT is carefully guided to regain functional motion.[49]

The prefunctional phase of rehabilitation after shoulder arthroplasty usually allows for early manual control assisted ROM and isometric exercises. Slow return toward external rotation is used to protect the healing of the subscapularis.[44] Isometric exercise may depend on soft-tissue healing and patient tolerance. Usually during the first postoperative week, the patient is allowed active exercise of the wrist, hand, and elbow of the affected shoulder. The postoperative immobilizer also is frequently removed for hygiene and exercises.[14] By the end of the first week, the immobilization device may be removed and manual control exercises initiated and AAROM exercises are continued. At the end of the second postoperative week, the patient is introduced to scapular motion and stabilization exercises while the quantity and quality of isometric exercises and motion exercises are progressed.[14] The assistant must encourage compliance with a comprehensive home exercise program of motion and strength. Wand-assisted exercises and pulley systems can be used as part of the home ROM program. Return to function phase will include light resistive strengthening, and more advanced scapula stabilization Thera-Band exercises are useful for the home exercise program. This usually begins between 4 and 6 weeks. Because the subscapularis has been taken down as part of this procedure, precaution is taken to protect against a return of external rotation that is too rapid. Additionally, early strengthening of the subscapularis is avoided to allow adequate heading of this muscle.[44]

If the patient has received a rotator cuff repair or neural prosthesis, the sequence of care and initiation of resistance exercise and active shoulder motion may be delayed. Functional use of the affected arm can be expected around 4 months postoperatively. However, Goldstein[14] suggests that for optimal results, the patient should participate in an active home exercise program long after discharge of rehabilitation.

MOBILIZATION OF THE SHOULDER

The precise application of specific peripheral joint mobilization techniques is extremely effective for pain reduction and restoration of normalized joint motion. In addition to various soft-tissue injuries and fractures, immobilization frequently causes limitations in scapulothoracic and glenohumeral mobility. For a normalized scapulohumeral rhythm to be restored, any limitations in motion must be identified early in the rehabilitation period.

During the initial immobilization, the PT documents all limitations of specific joint motion. Each limitation is addressed as part of the rehabilitation program. However, if the PTA recognizes delayed restoration of motion, reduced motion, or increased pain during the rehabilitation program, then he or she immediately must communicate this to the PT.

The following scapular and glenohumeral mobilization techniques represent only a few of the many techniques available. The PT decides which specific technique is to be used, when to apply the technique, in which direction, and with what amplitude, grade, or oscillation.

Before the PTA uses any mobilization technique, the position and comfort of the patient must be assessed. The use of oral physician-prescribed analgesics, thermal agents (e.g., heat, ultrasound, and ice), and proper body limb positioning enhance relaxation and compliance during treatment.

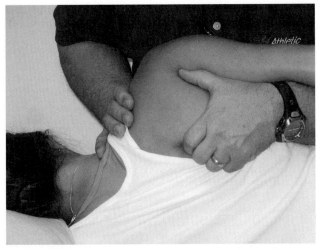

Fig. 21-13 Vertebral border scapular distraction.

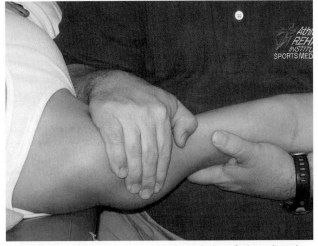

Fig. 21-14 Inferior and posterior glide of the glenohumeral joint.

Mobilization of the Scapulothoracic Joint

While the patient is in a side-lying position on the unaffected side, the scapula can be effectively mobilized in a superior and inferior direction, as well as distracted from the thorax. To distract the scapula, the PTA should stand facing the patient. The PTA should firmly grasp the medial or vertebral border of the affected scapula and purposefully distract the scapula away from the thorax (Fig. 21-13). To glide the scapula superiorly and inferiorly, the PTA should assume the same position and support the inferior border of the scapula. The PTA should use the hand on the inferior border to direct a force to glide the scapula in a superior direction, then use the hand on the superior border to direct a force to glide the scapula in an inferior direction.[21,44] In the same position the PTA can perform a lateral scapula glide. This technique is helpful to loosen subscapular soft tissue that may have become hypomobile during the postoperative or prefunctional phase of rehabilitation.

Mobilization of the Glenohumeral Joint

Anteroposterior glide of the glenohumeral joint can be accomplished with the patient supine. The PTA should sit near the affected shoulder. Wooden[51] recommends putting towels under the elbow of the affected shoulder in this position, to place the humerus in a more horizontal position. The humeral head should be grasped firmly with the thumb and fingers of one hand while the scapula is actively stabilized with the other hand. If the glenohumeral joint is stiff and motion is applied to the joint without stabilizing the scapula, the glenohumeral joint and scapula will move as a single unit. While stabilizing the humerus with one hand, the other hand is used on the humeral head to provide an inferiorly or posteriorly directed force. This procedure is also known as "over-the-top inferior glide." The over-the-top hand placement to the proximal humeral head provides a mild inferior directed shift (Fig. 21-14).

Lateral distraction of the humeral head can also be achieved while the patient is supine. The PTA should

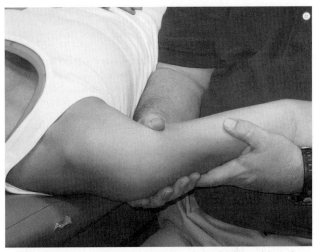

Fig. 21-15 Lateral distraction of the humeral head.

sit near the affected shoulder, then abduct the affected shoulder to 45° and the arm is supported by the PTA's hands. The PTA can use one or both hands to grasp the proximal humerus and direct a straight lateral force, effectively translating the humeral head from the glenoid (Fig. 21-15). Mild inferior glides of the glenohumeral joint may be helpful in regaining motion due to superior migration of the head of humerus.[44]

❖ GLOSSARY

Bankart lesion: Dislocation of glenohumeral joint or repetitive subluxation may lead to fractures of the anteroinferior aspect of the glenoid rim.

Glenohumeral joint: Greatest range of motion and least stable of any joint. Center core of motion.

Hill-Sachs lesion: Glenohumeral joint dislocation or repetitive subluxation, may lead to bone defect on posterolateral aspect of humeral head. Hill-Sachs lesion is also called *impression fracture.*

REFERENCES

1. Boissonnault WG, Janos SC: Dysfunction, evaluation and treatment of the shoulder. In Donatelli R, Wooden MJ, editors: *Orthopaedic physical therapy*, ed 3, St Louis, 2009, Churchill Livingstone.
2. Boudreau S, Boudreau E, Higgins L, et al: Rehabilitation following reverse total shoulder arthroplasty, *J Orthop Sports Phys Ther* 36(12):734–743, 2007.
3. Brumitt J: Scapular-stabilization exercises: early-intervention prescription, *Athl Ther Today* 11:15–18, 2006.
4. Davies GJ, Krauschar DR, Brinks KF, et al: Neuromuscular static and dynamic stability of the shoulder: the key to functional performance. In Manske RC, editor: *Postsurgical orthopedic sports rehabilitation: knee & shoulder*, St Louis, 2006, Saunders.
5. Dillman C, Murray T, Hintermeister R: Biomechanical differences of open and closed chain exercises with respect to the shoulder, *J Sport Rehabil* 3:228–238, 1994.
6. Duralde XA, Pollock RG, Flatow EL, et al: Frozen shoulder: prevention, diagnosis and management, *J Musculoskel Med* 10(9):64–72, 1993.
7. Durall CJ, Giangarra C, Humphrey CS: Anterior capsulolabral reconstruction. In Manske R, editor: *Postsurgical orthopedic sports rehabilitation: knee & shoulder*, St Louis, 2006, Saunders.
8. Ekstrom RA, BiFuleo KM, Lopau CJ, et al: Comparing the function of the upper and lower parts of the serratus anterior muscle using surface electromyography, *J Orthop Sports Phys Ther* 34(5):235–243, 2004.
9. Ellen MI, Rogers DP, Gilhool JJ: Practitioner flexibility strengthens shoulder rehabilitation protocol, *Biomechanics* January:45–52, 2000.
10. Ellenbecker TS: *Clinical examination of the shoulder*, St Louis, 2004, Saunders.
11. Ellenbecker TS, Baile DS, Kibler WB: Rehabilitation after mini-open and arthroscopic repair of the rotator cuff. In Manske RC, editor: *Postsurgical orthopedic sports rehabilitation: knee & shoulder*, St Louis, 2006, Saunders.
12. Ghodadra NS, Provencher MT, Verma NN, et al: Open, mini-open and all-arthroscopic rotator cuff repair surgery: indications and implications for rehabilitation, *J Orthop Sports Phys Ther* 39(2):81–89, 2009.
13. Gitterman G: Shouldering pain, *Adv Dir Rehabil* July:25–28, 2003.
14. Goldstein TS, editor: Treatment of common problems of the shoulder complex. In *Geriatric orthopaedics: rehabilitative management of common problems*, Gaithersburg, Md, 1991, Aspen.
15. Hawkins RJ, Mohtadi N: Rotator cuff problems in athletes. In DeLee JC, Drez D, editors: *Orthopaedic sports medicine: principles and practice*, vol 1, Philadelphia, 1994, Saunders.
16. Hayes K, Callanan M, Walton J, et al: Shoulder instability: management and rehabilitation, *J Orthop Sports Phys Ther* 32:497–509, 2002.
17. Hill Z, Sibilia K, Stone J, et al: Secondary impingement of the shoulder: examination and treatment techniques used by physical therapist, *Orthop Phys Ther Pract* 20:14–20, 2008.
18. Hughes CJ, McBride A: The use of surface electromyography to determine muscle activation during isotonic and elastic resistance exercises from shoulder rehabilitation, *Orthop Phys Ther Pract* 2:18–23, 2005.
19. Jewell DV, Riddle DL, Thacker LR: Interventions associated with an increased or decreased likelihood of pain reduction and improved function in patients with adhesive capsulitis: a retrospective cohort study, *Phys Ther* 89:419–429, 2009.
20. Kamkar A, Irrgang J, Whitney SL: Nonoperative management of secondary shoulder impingement syndrome, *J Orthop Sports Phys Ther* 17:212–224, 1993.
21. Kolstad K, Tyler T, Nicholas S: Rehabilitation of the shoulder. In Kumbhare DA, Basmajian JV, editors: *Decision making and outcomes in sports rehabilitation*, Philadelphia, 2000, Churchill Livingstone.
22. Laudner KG, Sipes RC, Wilson JT: The acute effects of sleeper stretches on shoulder range of motion, *J Athl Train* 43(4):359–363, 2008.
23. Levinson M, Altchek D: Capsular shift procedures: Neer and multidirectional instabilities. In Manske R, editor: *Postsurgical orthopedic sports rehabilitation: knee & shoulder*, St Louis, 2006, Elsevier.
24. Lippert L: Shoulder girdle. *Clinical kinesiology for the physical therapist assistant*, ed 2, Philadelphia, 1994, FA Davis.
25. McClure P, Balacuis J, Heilland D, et al: A randomized controlled comparison to stretching procedures for posterior shoulder tightness, *J Orthop Sports Phys Ther* 37(3):108–114, 2007.
26. McClure PW, Bialker J, Neff N, et al: Shoulder function and 3-dimensional kinematics in people with shoulder impingement syndrome before and after a 6-week exercise program, *Phys Ther* 84:832–848, 2004.
27. McClure PW, Michener LA, Karduna AR: Shoulder function and 3-dimensional scapular kinematics in people with and without shoulder impingement syndrome, *Phys Ther* 86:1075–1090, 2006.
28. McCluskey GM, Getz BA: Pathophysiology of anterior shoulder instability, *J Athl Train* 35(3):268–272, 2000.
29. McRae R: *Practical fracture treatment*, ed 3, New York, 1994, Churchill Livingstone.
30. Macrina L, Reinhold M: Arm forces, *Training and Conditioning* 18:48–51, 2008.
31. Matheson JW, Price CR: Rehabilitation after conservative and operative treatment of acromioclavicular joint injuries. In Manske R, editor: *Postsurgical orthopedic sports rehabilitation: knee & shoulder*, St Louis, 2006, Elsevier.
32. Matsen FA, Arntz CT, Lippitt SB: Rotator cuff. In Rockwood CA, Matsen FA, editors: *The shoulder*, ed 2, Philadelphia, 1998, Saunders, pp 755–840.
33. Mosely JB Jr, Jobe FW, Pink M, et al: EMG analysis of the scapular muscles during a shoulder rehabilitation program, *Am J Sports Med* 20(2):128–134, 1992.
34. Myers JB, Laudner KG, Pasquale MR, et al: Glenohumeral range of motion deficits and posterior shoulder tightness in throwers with pathologic internal impingement, *Am J Sports Med* 34:385–391, 2006.
35. Neer CS: Impingement lesions, *Clin Orthop* 173:70–77, 1983.
36. Pagnani MJ, Galinat BJ, Warren RF: Glenohumeral instability. In DeLee JC, Drez D, editors: *Orthopaedic sports medicine: principles and practice*, vol 1, Philadelphia, 1994, Saunders.
37. Porterfield JA, DeRosa C: *Mechanical shoulder disorders: perspectives in functional anatomy*, Philadelphia, 2004, Saunders, pp 129-159.
38. Reinold MM, Macrina LC, Wilk KE, et al: Electromyographic analysis of the supraspinatus and deltoid muscles during 3 command rehabilitation exercises, *J Athl Train* 42(4):464–469, 2007.
39. Schultz RA, Leetun DT, Warner CD: Subacromial impingement, acromioplasty and subacromial decompression. In Manske RC, editor: *Postsurgical orthopedic sports rehabilitation: knee & shoulder*, St Louis, 2006, Elsevier.
40. Schultz RA, Warner C: Oscillatory devices accelerate proprioception training, *Biomechanics* May:85–90, 2001.
41. Strege D: Upper extremity. In Loth T, editor: *Orthopaedic boards review*, St Louis, 1993, Mosby.
42. Thein LA: Rehabilitation of shoulder injuries. In Prentice WE, editor: *Rehabilitation techniques in sports medicine*, ed 2, St Louis, 1994, Mosby.
43. Townsend H, Jobe FW, Pink M, Perry J: Electromyographic analysis of the glenohumeral muscles during a baseball rehabilitation program, *Am J Sports Med* 19:264–272, 1991.
44. Trundle TL: *Rotator cuff syndrome: from impingement to post operative rehab*, Course Notes, Brentwood, Tenn., 2009.
45. Tyler TF, Nicholas SS, Seneviratne AN: The Bankart lesion. In Manske RC, editor: *Postsurgical orthopedic sports rehabilitation: knee & shoulder*, St Louis, 2006, Elsevier.

46. Uhl TL, Carver TJ, Mattacola CG, et al: Shoulder musculature activation during upper extremity weight-bearing exercise, *J Orthop Sports Phys Ther* 33:109–117, 2003.

47. Unverzagt C, Omar L, Hughes C: Case report: rehabilitation and outcomes for a patient following and implant of Reverse Delta III Shoulder Prosthesis, *Orthop Pract* 18(2):32–37, 2006.

48. Vermeulen HM, Rozing PM, Obermann WR, et al: Comparison of high-grade and low-grade mobilization techniques in the management of adhesive capsulitis of the shoulder: randomized controlled trial, *Phys Ther* 86:355–368, 2006.

49. Wilcox R, Arslanian L, Millett P: Rehabilitation following total shoulder arthroplasty, *J Orthop Sports Phys Ther* 35:821–836, 2005.

50. Williams GR, Rockwood CA: Fractures of the scapula In DeLee JC, Drez D, editors: *Orthopaedic sports medicine: principles and practice,* vol 1, Philadelphia, 1994, Saunders.

51. Wooden MJ: Mobilization of the upper extremity. In Donatelli R, Wooden MJ, editors: *Orthopaedic physical therapy,* New York, 1989, Churchill Livingstone.

52. Yahara ML: Shoulder. In Richardson JK, Iglarsh ZA, editors: *Clinical orthopaedic physical therapy,* Philadelphia, 1994, Saunders.

REVIEW QUESTIONS

True/False

1. Secondary subacromial impingement is related to glenohumeral instability, which creates a reduced subacromial space, because the humeral head migrates upward and maximizes the area under the coracoacromial ligament.
2. Age-related arthritic changes and bony osteophyte formation have no effect on subacromial impingement of the shoulder.
3. Posterior shoulder dislocations occur more often than anterior dislocations.
4. It is not uncommon for rotator cuff tears to occur with shoulder dislocation.
5. During immobilization for anterior glenohumeral dislocations, it is necessary to provide ROM and strengthening exercises for the hand, wrist, and elbow, as well as of the affected shoulder.
6. Secondary adhesive capsulitis generally occurs after trauma or immobilization.
7. Scapular fractures occur from indirect and insignificant trauma.
8. Active muscle contractions of the deltoid are contraindicated during the prefunctional phase following rotator cuff repair.

22 Orthopedic Management of the Elbow

Leonard C. Macrina

LEARNING OBJECTIVES

1. Identify and describe the principles for common overuse and soft-tissue injuries of the elbow.
2. Discuss common methods of management and rehabilitation of overuse, soft-tissue injuries of the elbow.
3. Identify and describe intercondylar fractures, radial head fractures, olecranon fractures, and fracture-dislocations of the elbow.
4. Describe methods of management and rehabilitation of various fractures and fracture-dislocations of the elbow.
5. Describe techniques to improve range of motion of a stiff elbow including common joint mobilization techniques.

KEY TERMS

Epicondylitis
Lateral epicondylitis

Ligament stability
Medial epicondylitis

Medial valgus stress
overload

CHAPTER OUTLINE

This chapter introduces the physical therapist assistant (PTA) to common soft-tissue injuries and fractures of the distal humerus and elbow. Specific attention is directed at identifying treatment programs used to control pain and swelling, improve motion, strength, and function of the elbow after injury, surgery, or immobilization.

SOFT-TISSUE INJURIES OF THE ELBOW

Lateral Epicondylitis

Commonly referred to as *tennis elbow,* **lateral epicondylitis** affects the common wrist extensor origin of the extensor carpi radialis longus, extensor carpi radialis brevis, extensor digitorum, and extensor digiti minimi.[8,29] The repetitive overuse of this area leads to tendinitis of the origin of the extensor carpi radialis brevis tendon (Fig. 22-1).[9,29]

Interestingly, lateral **epicondylitis** can affect anyone involved with repetitive activities of the wrist extensors.[28] Thus persons involved with the use of hand tools (e.g., hammer, screwdriver, or pliers) and various activities involving wrist rotation, pulling, extending, and hand grasping can be affected by lateral epicondylitis.[28]

Generally the patient suffering from lateral epicondylitis has pain with palpation of the lateral epicondyle, with active or resisted wrist extension, and occasionally with grasping of the affected hand.[8,23,28] Because this is a chronic overuse tendinitis, the intense inflammatory response in the affected area of the lateral epicondyle is "an attempt to increase the rate of tissue production to compensate for the increased rate of tissue microdamage."[28]

Management of Lateral Epicondylitis

Initial acute management focuses on resolving pain and swelling with the judicious use of ice massage directly over the affected area, phonophoresis or iontophoresis, physician-prescribed analgesics and nonsteroidal anti-inflammatory drugs (NSAIDs), rest, and protection of the area from unwanted stress to allow for healing.[8,23,28]

Relative rest rather than strict immobilization is used. A wrist cock-up splint can be used in severe cases to minimize stress on the inflamed wrist extensor tendons. The patient is allowed to remove the splint as needed to participate in controlled motion exercises that do not produce pain. Long-term, rigid immobilization is not indicated, because treatment goals are to not only reduce pain and swelling but also to encourage proper collagen alignment and scar tissue maturation.[23] Without early protected motion, excessive tissue scarring and random collagen fiber alignment would severely limit normalized motion and function of the elbow and wrist.

During the initial healing stage, the PTA must encourage the patient to avoid any and all motions that may adversely affect healing. Short-term modifications in activities of daily living (ADLs), sports, and job-related activities must be addressed to provide a pain-free environment for healing. When this initial program fails to bring significant relief of symptoms, some physicians elect to inject the area with a steroid to reduce the inflammation.[20,23]

In addition, active gentle static stretching is advised for the wrist extensors to produce normalized, pain-free wrist flexion and extension (Fig. 22-2). Although specifically addressing treatment for the elbow, active motion and resistance exercises for the elbow and shoulder can be initiated if no wrist motion occurs to increase symptoms.

The PTA can enhance the effectiveness of low-load, long-duration static stretching by applying moist heat

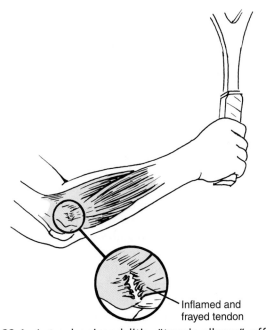

Fig. 22-1 Lateral epicondylitis, "tennis elbow," affects the common wrist-extensor origin.

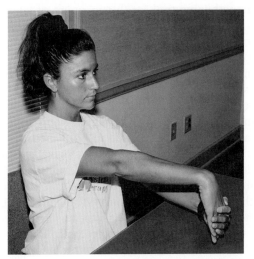

Fig. 22-2 Stretching of the wrist extensors.

packs (provided the acute inflammatory process has ended) or ultrasound to the lateral epicondyle to stimulate local circulation and relieve congestion caused by metabolic waste products and relax soft tissues in preparation for stretching.

Resistance exercise can begin as pain is reduced with active motion exercises. Generally, submaximal isometrics are used for wrist extension, flexion, forearm pronation and supination, and radial and ulnar deviation.

The PTA must carefully instruct the patient to perform all exercises within a pain-free range of motion (ROM). Throughout all phases of recovery, the patient must avoid stressful, pain-producing activities to prevent the exacerbation of the inflammatory condition. Progressive motion exercises and increased resistance exercise are the foundation for a return to functional activities. Concentric and eccentric muscle contractions are added once the patient can demonstrate increased quality of multiangle isometric contractions. Care must be taken when initiating both concentric and eccentric resistance exercises because frequently these contractions produce symptoms. Light resistance is advocated when having patients perform these exercises for the first time. An important component for all resistance exercises used with lateral epicondylitis is the performance of slow, controlled eccentric contractions. Eccentric muscle contractions produce greater tension than either concentric or isometric exercise. In addition, energy use involving adenosine triphosphate (ATP) is less for eccentric exercise than for either concentric or isometric exercise. Eccentric muscle contractions are, in fact, advocated by Curwin and Stanish[8] for the treatment of tennis elbow, and the rationale for the performance of eccentric exercise is described by Reid and Kushner[24] as, "Exercising the muscle eccentrically allows it to withstand greater resistance and prevent injury, which occurs by eccentrically loading an inflexible muscle."[24]

Resistive exercises emphasizing the eccentric phase are described in Figure 22-3, *A-B*. A hammer is an effective strengthening tool for the treatment of lateral epicondylitis. However, when instructing the patient to perform pronation and supination of the forearm for the first time, the PTA should have the patient hold the hammer close to its head (Fig. 22-3, *C*). As the patient gains strength and can control the resistance of the hammer eccentrically, the patient should gradually hold the hammer at the midshaft. As strength improves further, the patient should be allowed to hold the hammer at the end of the shaft, which requires greater eccentric muscle control, strength, and torque. In the same manner, strength can be gained for radial and ulnar deviation through use of the hammer. With a gradual return to functional activities, some physicians and therapists advocate the use of a counterforce brace to help dissipate the "overload forces" on the common origin of the wrist extensors (Fig. 22-3, *D*).[8,20,28]

Surgery is rarely necessary for this condition because physical therapy management frequently is effective. In rare instances when conservative means fail to reduce pain and improve function, the surgeon may elect to surgically excise the "angiofibroblastic tissue at the origin of the extensor carpi radialis brevis muscle."[29]

Medial Epicondylitis

Medial epicondylitis, an overuse condition, affects the origin of the pronator teres, flexor carpi radialis, flexor digitorum sublimis, and flexor carpi ulnaris at the medial epicondyle of the elbow.[23] Although it occurs less often than lateral epicondylitis (the ratio of lateral epicondylitis to medial epicondylitis is 7:1),[28] it is no less incapacitating to the patient. Again the dominant feature is pain with palpation over the medial epicondyle, active motion, and particularly with resisted wrist flexion and full passive wrist extension (Fig. 22-4).[23,24]

Management of Medial Epicondylitis

The acute management phase of this inflammatory overuse condition, also referred to as *golfer's elbow,* concentrates on the management of pain and swelling. Usually the physician prescribes NSAIDs, ice (protect the ulnar nerve), phonophoresis or iontophoresis, relative active rest (not immobilization), protection, and gentle active motion exercises. The criteria-based treatment plan parallels that for lateral epicondylitis, although it obviously focuses on the wrist flexors. Static low-load, long-duration stretching[3,4] can proceed as pain allows. The PTA must encourage the patient to avoid repetitive flexing of the wrist and pronating of the forearm if these motions produce pain. Modifications in lifting, twisting, pulling, or turning of the wrist and forearm must accompany each phase of recovery to avoid stress on the medial structures. Moist heat and ultrasound can be applied to the medial epicondyle before stretching once motion has improved without pain. Resistance training can then begin with submaximal isometrics, progressing to higher-quality isometric multiangle contractions, and ultimately to concentric and eccentric isotonic and isokinetic resistance exercises. The patient is instructed in the active use of the shoulder of the affected limb and strongly encouraged to follow a conditioning program to maintain or enhance cardiovascular fitness, strength, and flexibility throughout the rehabilitation process.

Although the resolution of pain and swelling is paramount for active use of the wrist and forearm, regaining lost motion caused by pain and muscular dysfunction is critical for function and a return to normal daily activities. The normal elbow ROM is 0° to approximately 145° of flexion.[29] However, most daily activities can be carried out within a functional ROM of 30° to 130° of flexion.[24,29] In addition, normal pronation of 75° and supination of 85° exceeds the functional arc of motion of 50° needed to carry out most ADLs. Therefore the PTA must

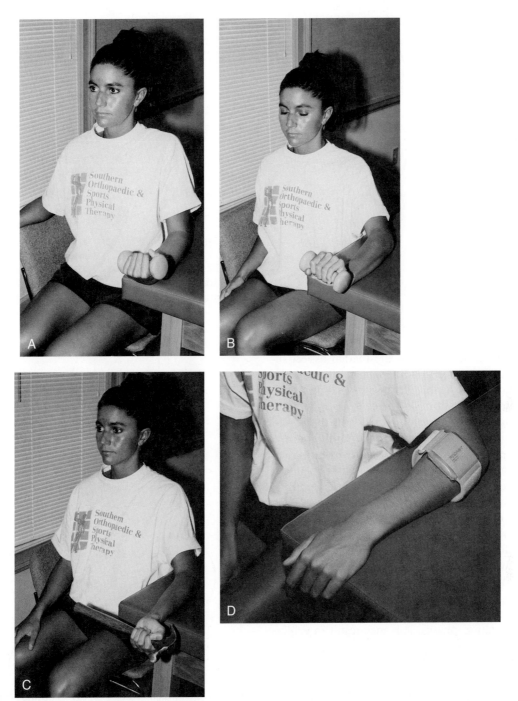

Fig. 22-3 Common wrist and forearm strengthening exercises. **A,** Wrist flexion. **B,** Wrist extension. Encourage slow, controlled, nonballistic concentric and eccentric contractions. **C,** Pronation exercise with a hammer. Notice that the grip is held close to the head of the hammer when first introducing this exercise. **D,** Counterforce brace may help spread or dissipate overload force on the common wrist extensor origin.

encourage pain-free early protected motion to facilitate the collagen fiber alignment needed for both functional scar maturation and purposeful motion to perform ADLs.

Medial Valgus Stress Overload

Injuries to the elbow often occur in the overhead athlete. The repetitive overhead motion involved in throwing is responsible for unique and sport-specific patterns of injuries to the elbow. These are caused by chronic stress overload or repetitive micro-traumatic stress observed during the overhead pitching motion as the elbow extends at over 2300°/s, producing a medial shear force of 300 N and lateral compressive force of 900 N.[11,32] In addition, the valgus stress applied to the elbow during the acceleration phase of throwing is 64 N·m,[11,32] which exceeds the ultimate tensile strength of the

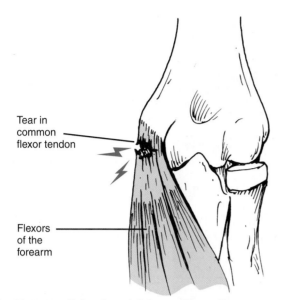

Fig. 22-4 Medial epicondylitis, "golfer's elbow." Repetitive overuse injury.

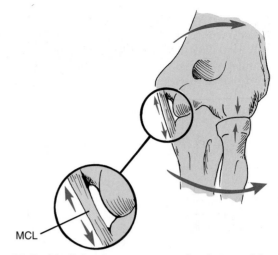

Fig. 22-5 Medial valgus stress overload. Repetitive valgus stress to the elbow may stress the capsuloligamentous structures of the elbow. *MCL,* Medial collateral ligament.

ulnar collateral ligament.[10] Thus the medial aspect of the elbow undergoes tremendous tensile (distraction) forces and the lateral aspect is forcefully compressed during the throwing motion.

Medial valgus stress overload, also known as *valgus extension overload* (VEO) occurs commonly among patients who participate in repetitive throwing and racquet sports such as javelin throwing, baseball, racquetball, and tennis.[9,21,23] The overhead athlete is susceptible to these specific elbow injuries. A number of forces act on the elbow during the act of throwing,[11,32] including valgus stress with tension across the medial aspect of the elbow. These forces are maximal during the acceleration phase of throwing. Compression forces are also applied to the lateral aspect of the elbow during the throwing motion. The posterior compartment is subject to tensile, compressive, and torsional forces during acceleration and deceleration phases. This may result in valgus extension overload within the posterior compartment, leading to osteophyte formation, stress fractures of the olecranon, or physeal injury.[1,35] These stresses approach the ultimate failure load of the ligament with each throw. The repetitive nature of overhead throwing activities such as baseball pitching, javelin throwing, and football passing further increase the susceptibility of medial elbow injuries including ulnar collateral ligament (UCL) injuries, by exposing the ligament to repetitive microtraumatic forces. Clinical differences exist between medial valgus stress overload and medial epicondylitis. Although medial epicondylitis represents a chronic overuse syndrome affecting the soft-tissue musculotendinous origin of the wrist flexors and pronators, medial valgus stress overload occurs to the capsuloligamentous structures (medial [ulnar] collateral ligament) as a result of repetitive valgus stress to the elbow (Fig. 22-5).[9,21,23]

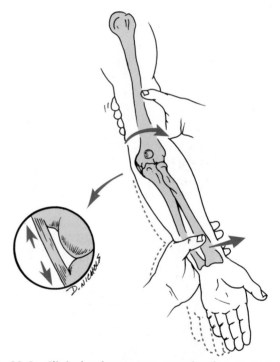

Fig. 22-6 Clinical valgus stress examination to test the stability of the medial (ulnar) collateral ligament.

Patients usually complain of pain over the medial aspect of the elbow and the posterior aspect of the olecranon.[21,23] During the physical therapist's (PT) initial evaluation, the PTA may observe the performance of **ligament stability** tests to confirm the presence of UCL laxity. The affected arm is held in 20° to 30° of flexion while the humerus is held in full external rotation to unlock the olecranon process from the olecranon fossa. A medial or valgus stress then is applied to the elbow to assess the stability of the UCL (Fig. 22-6).[21,23]

Management of Medial Valgus Stress Overload

Management of valgus stress injuries must take into account the healing constraints of ligaments. The patient may receive physician-prescribed NSAIDs, analgesics, ice massage, phonophoresis, or iontophoresis to reduce pain and swelling. Rest and protection of the injured medial ligamentous structures, while avoiding valgus stress, are the hallmarks of management. Because most of these injuries occur to active sports enthusiasts, the patient must omit activities that produce medial valgus stress. To ensure compliance, it may be necessary to suggest short-term rest from the activity, during which the patient should participate in running, cycling, and strength training and should perform flexibility exercises as long as no valgus load is applied to the elbow joint. In addition, the wrist, hand, and shoulder of the affected limb must be exercised during each phase of recovery.

The elbow is predisposed to flexion contractures due to the intimate congruency of the joint articulations, the tightness of the joint capsule, and the tendency of the anterior capsule to develop adhesions following injury.[33] The brachialis muscle also attaches to the capsule and crosses the elbow joint before becoming a tendinous structure. Injury to the elbow may cause excessive scar tissue formation of the brachialis muscle as well as functional splinting of the elbow.[33] Gentle low-load static stretching begins as soon as pain allows. Therefore the stretching regimen focuses on all wrist motions, forearm pronation and supination, and elbow flexion and extension as long as no symptoms of pain occur with these activities. If the patient continues to have difficulty achieving full extension using ROM and mobilization techniques, a low-load, long duration (LLLD) stretch may be performed to produce a deformation (creep) of the collagen tissue, resulting in tissue elongation.[12,27,30,31] This technique is extremely beneficial for regaining full elbow extension. The patient lies supine with a towel roll or foam placed under the distal brachium to act as a cushion and fulcrum. Light resistance exercise tubing is applied to the wrist of the patient and secured to the table or a dumbbell on the ground (Fig. 22-7). The patient is instructed to relax as much as possible for 10 to 15 minutes per treatment. The amount of resistance applied should be of low magnitude to enable the patient to perform the stretch for the entire duration without pain or muscle spasm. This technique should impart a LLLD over a prolonged period of time to achieve maximal benefits. Patients are instructed to perform this stretch technique several times per day, equaling 60 minutes of total end range time. Patients may perform a 15 minute stretch, 4 times per day.[16] This program has been extremely beneficial for patients with a stiff elbow.

The strengthening component of recovery must be modified to prevent any valgus stress or pain at end

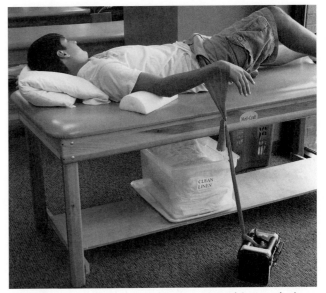

Fig. 22-7 Low-load, long duration stretching technique to gain elbow extension range of motion.

range extension. This ensures that the healing ligament is not receiving any additional tensile forces that may affect the healing capacity. Full ROM (flexion-extension) concentric and eccentric resistance exercise is allowed with light weights as motion and pain dictate. Wrist and hand exercises are encouraged early and pose no threat to the healing ligament. In addition, forearm pronation and supination with use of a hammer (as outlined) is employed as the patient is able to demonstrate improved motion without pain.

With time, the PT reassesses the stability of the medial collateral ligaments. If these structures demonstrate improved stability without pain, a gradual return to throwing can begin.

Surgery is considered if conservative treatment fails to restore function and eliminate pain. Degenerative changes, which are usually present in the adult, must be addressed surgically.[21,24] In general, an osteotomy is performed to remove osteophytes (bone spurs) and fibrotic, degenerated tissue.[21,24]

Acute rupture (grade III ligament rupture) of the medial (ulnar) collateral ligament can occur in skeletally mature adults if valgus stress is applied suddenly with sufficient force (Fig. 22-8).

First, these patients are managed conservatively with ice, NSAIDs, analgesics, and, most important, rest and protection. The progression from the acute, maximum-protection phase to return-to-normal function parallels treatment outlined for valgus stress injuries. However, because the ligament has been ruptured, a longer period of recovery is needed and rest and joint protection from valgus stress will last longer. Normal elbow function, which means flexion, extension, pronation, and supination, should be encouraged as early as pain and motion allow.

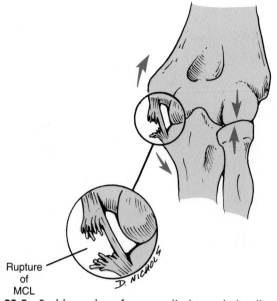

Rupture of MCL

D. NICHOLS

Fig 22-8 Sudden valgus force applied to a skeletally mature adult may result in rupture of the medial collateral ligament.

If early active protected joint motion and progressive resistance exercise have been used, authorities suggest that the injured patient can resume throwing activities approximately 3 months after injury.[21] However, surgery may be necessary to stabilize the joint if the patient does not demonstrate improved valgus stability and continues to have dysfunction.

Generally if the ulnar collateral ligament is ruptured midsubstance, a direct repair is carried out and a reconstructive procedure is performed. The palmaris longus or gracilis graft source is taken and passed in a figure-of-eight pattern through drill holes in the sublime tubercle of the ulna and the medial epicondyle.[2] A subcutaneous ulnar nerve transposition is performed at the time of reconstruction. Some surgeons are presently performing UCL reconstruction utilizing the docking procedure, as described by Rohrbough and colleagues.[26]

Postoperative rehabilitation begins immediately, with the patient's affected limb immobilized in a brace to protect against valgus stress. Instructions are given to perform hand, wrist, and shoulder exercises to maintain motion. Usually by the third week postoperatively, ROM should approach at least 20° of extension while slowly progressing to 110° of elbow flexion.[9] The continuous use of ice and therapeutic agents (e.g., ultrasound, transcutaneous electrical nerve stimulation, and galvanic stimulation)[24] are prescribed as necessary. Progressive resistance concentric and eccentric contractions are used for the wrist of the involved limb, whereas submaximal isometrics can begin for elbow flexion and extension.

Shoulder strengthening and flexibility exercises also can begin during the third week of recovery.[9] However,

care must be taken to avoid external shoulder rotation exercises because this motion produces valgus stress on the elbow.[9]

Usually by 4 to 6 weeks after surgery, ROM should be 0° to 130°.[9] In addition, concentric and eccentric resistance exercises for elbow flexion and extension are added progressively as tolerated. Gentle forearm pronation and supination exercises also can be made more challenging. From 2 to 4 months after surgery, functional training can begin with an emphasis on shoulder, elbow, and wrist strengthening, motion exercises, and plyometrics. Plyometric drills can be an extremely beneficial form of functional exercise for training the elbow in overhead athletes.[33,34] Plyometric exercises are performed using a weighted medicine ball during the latter stages of this phase to train the shoulder and elbow to develop and withstand high levels of stress (Fig. 22-9). Plyometric exercises are initially performed with two hands performing a chest pass, a side-to-side throw, and an overhead soccer throw. These may be progressed to include one hand activities such as 90/90 throws, and wall dribbles. For patients returning to sports that involve the upper extremity, such as golf, tennis, javelin, baseball, and softball, these patients are placed on an interval sport program as described by Reinold and colleagues.[25] Ultimately, it takes 10 to 12 months after elbow reconstruction and rehabilitation for valgus instability before a functional return to overhead, competitive sports is allowed.[21]

Lateral Collateral Ligament Injury

Stability of the elbow occurs mainly through the osseous configuration but secondarily through the medial and lateral collateral ligaments (LCLs). In particular, the lateral ligament complex prevents rotational instability between the distal humerus and the proximal radius and ulna. However, disrupting the soft-tissue constraints through a traumatic onset often results in subluxation or dislocation. The elbow is the second most commonly dislocated large joint after the shoulder.[14,15] In children younger than the age of 10 years, elbows are the most commonly dislocated joint.

In general, there are two main mechanisms of dislocation that have been suggested. Elbow dislocations are thought to result from hyperextension, in which the olecranon process is forced into the olecranon fossa and the trochlea is then levered over the coronoid process. Most elbow dislocations occur in a directly posterior or posterolateral direction. Very rarely will an anterior dislocation occur (~1% to 2%). Another proposed mechanism of injury is posterolateral rotation, in which combined forces of axial compression, elbow flexion, valgus stress, and forearm supination create a rotational displacement of the ulna on the distal humerus.

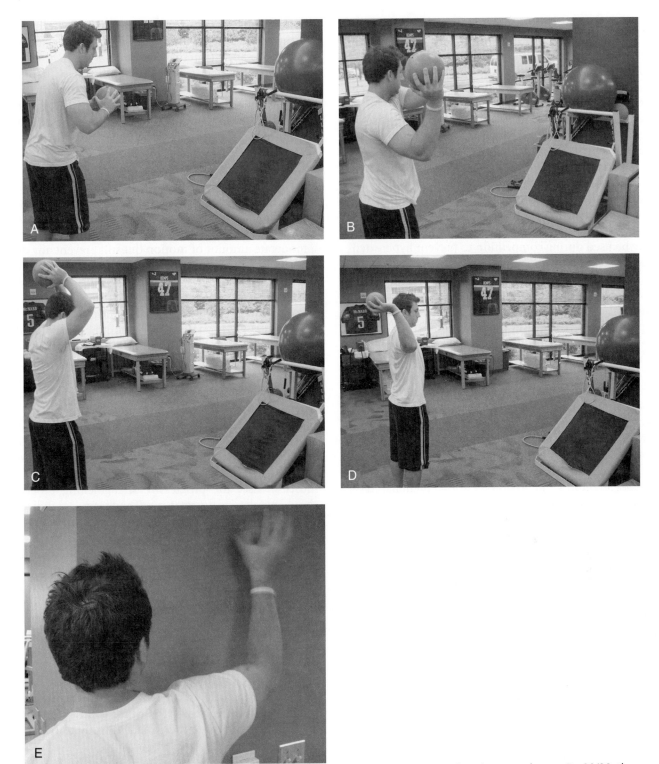

Fig. 22-9 **A,** Two hands performing a chest pass. **B,** Side-to-side throw. **C,** Overhead soccer throw. **D,** 90/90 throws. **E,** Wall dribbles.

Management of Lateral Collateral Ligament Injury
Nonoperative management

Nonoperative rehabilitation should commence immediately following the traumatic event. The focus of the rehabilitation is to restore ROM within the limits of elbow stability while slowly applying progressive stresses

to the healing structures. Modalities to control pain and swelling, such as cryotherapy and a compressive sleeve, may be used. Additionally, a hinged elbow brace with the forearm in a neutral or slightly pronated position is used to protect against excessive valgus and varus forces. The brace should restrict ROM to approximately

30° to 90° initially, then be progressively increased until full ROM is achieved without pain. A slow ROM progression for forearm supination and elbow extension will protect the healing LCL structures.

Strengthening activities may be initiated early on to prevent atrophy due to immobilization. Multiangle isometrics may begin during the initial phase of 1 to 10 days postinjury. Progressive resistance exercises for the elbow begin during the intermediate phase (days 10 to 14 postinjury). During the advanced phase, weeks 2 through 8 postinjury, functional progressions and sport specific activities are initiated. The athlete may be allowed to return to sports participation once sufficient strength, power, and endurance are obtained. A brace may be used during competition to prevent hyperextension and varus/valgus stresses.

Operative management

The reconstruction technique is intended to recreate the ulnar aspect of the LCL complex. O'Driscoll[22] recommends first repairing the avulsed origin of the lateral ligament complex to its isometric origin on the lateral epicondyle if possible. This is typically followed by augmentation of the repair with graft choices ranging from the palmaris longus, lateral triceps tendon, semitendonosus allograft or autograft, or even a plantaris allograft. The physician's preference will often dictate which graft is used during the reconstruction.

The rehabilitation program is designed to protect the healing structures and progressively load them based on healing constraints, degree of soft-tissue involvement and the ultimate functional goal of the patient. The following will briefly describe the rehabilitation program for this specific surgical procedure.

The rehabilitation program is initiated immediately following the surgical procedure to ensure adequate healing and protection. We have attempted to outline the postoperative protocol in three distinct phases to maximize functional outcomes: the immediate postoperative phase, the intermediate phase, and the advanced phase. The rehabilitation specialist should make every attempt to follow these guidelines, however the progression rate may differ among patients depending on the exact surgical procedure, physician preference, and the patient's individual characteristics.

During the immediate postoperative phase (weeks 0 to 3), the patient is placed in a 90° posterior elbow splint with full forearm pronation. This is used for the first 3 weeks to allow adequate soft-tissue healing of the graft within the bone tunnels. No elbow ROM activities are permitted during this time, particularly supination, which is generally limited for the first 4 to 6 weeks. Wrist and shoulder passive range of motion (PROM) and active range of motion (AROM) activities may be performed as long as there are no pain symptoms along the lateral elbow.

The patient may also begin gentle gripping exercises for the hand along with shoulder isometric activities. Shoulder rotation (internal and external) isometric exercises may not be performed during this phase, because of the varus and valgus moments at the elbow joint that may stress the healing soft-tissue structures. By the end of the third postoperative week, the patient may initiate AROM activities for the shoulder musculature, including the full can exercise, lateral raises, and internal/external rotation with tubing.

During the intermediate phase (weeks 4 to 7), the patient may gradually increase elbow PROM and progress strengthening activities. The elbow joint is protected by a hinged brace set from 30° to 100°. This will allow a moderate amount of motion but still prevent any deleterious end range stresses. The patient may unlock the brace by 10° per week and may discontinue using the brace by the end of the sixth week. The rehabilitation specialist may begin elbow PROM with the forearm in neutral or slight pronation. Care should be taken to not push the elbow into end range flexion or extension at this time. Full PROM may be expected by 8 to 10 weeks postoperative. If full ROM has not been achieved, then the LLLD guidelines mentioned earlier in the chapter may assist in obtaining the remaining ROM.

During the intermediate phase, the strengthening activities should focus on dynamic stability of the medial and lateral musculature. The patient may begin light isotonic strengthening for the wrist, forearm, and elbow muscles. Also, the progressive strengthening program should emphasize the rotator cuff and scapula stabilizers.

By week 8, the patient may progress to the advanced strengthening phase. The goals of this phase are to increase strength, power, and endurance while maintaining full elbow ROM. Aggressive strengthening exercises involving eccentric and plyometric contractions are also included, usually at 10 weeks postoperative. These sport-specific activities are progressed through increasing the number of repetitions, increasing the weight of the medicine ball or increasing the timed bouts of the activity to improve endurance. Beyond week 16, the patient is reassessed to determine strength levels before progressing to an interval sports program. Sufficient strength, generally within 15% of the contralateral side, and full ROM indicate the patient is ready to begin an interval program.[25]

FRACTURES OF THE ELBOW

Fractures of the Distal Humerus (Supracondylar Fractures)

By definition a supracondylar fracture is a transverse fracture of the distal third of the humerus.[17] These frequent injuries usually occur in children.[17,21,28] Supracondylar fractures generally are of two types.[7,17,29] Type

I is the most common and refers to an injury that occurs as a result of a fall on an extended, outstretched arm in which the distal humerus fragment is displaced posteriorly and is maintained in that position because of the strong pull of the triceps (Fig. 22-10, A).[7,29] Type II is considered a flexion injury and occurs after direct trauma to the posterior aspect of the elbow in which the distal humeral fragment lies anterior to the humerus (Fig. 22-10, B).[7,29]

The most common treatment of these fractures is by closed reduction and immobilization for 4 to 6 weeks. The affected arm is held in a flexed position to allow the triceps to help maintain the fracture in a stable position.[17,29]

As with all other fractures, the initial phase of recovery focuses on motion and strengthening exercises for the contralateral limb, general body conditioning, and active motion of the hand, wrist, and shoulder of the injured limb, as long as no undue stress is directed at the fracture site.

Physical therapy treatment after immobilization focuses on gentle active motion exercises, which can be preceded by the use of moist heat or a warm whirlpool to encourage relaxation, removal of wastes, and improved local circulation. In most cases, progressive active motion of the elbow and resistance exercises proceed as radiographic evidence confirms solid union, a minimum of 6 weeks has elapsed since surgery (consistent with the healing constraints of bone tissue), and the patient demonstrates improved motion without pain.

Complications arising from supracondylar fractures[18] include nonunion, malunion, and joint contracture. Perhaps the most disastrous complication results from vascular compromise.[7,17,18,29] As the fracture fragments are displaced, hemorrhage beneath the deep fascia produces an ischemic injury that creates an arterial and venous obstruction (usually affecting the brachial artery), leading to a Volkmann ischemic contracture (Fig. 22-11).[7,18,28] What is most important is that the clinical signs and symptoms of ischemic obstruction may not be noticed until the end of immobilization.[7] The symptoms of Volkmann ischemic contracture can occur throughout each phase of recovery after a supracondylar fracture.

Stralka and Brasel[28] outline six symptoms authorities define as indicating vascular obstruction:

■ Severe pain in the forearm muscles
■ Limited and extremely painful finger movement
■ Purple discoloration of the hand with prominent veins
■ Initial paresthesia followed by loss of sensation
■ Loss of radial pulse and later loss of capillary return
■ Pallor, anesthesia, and paralysis

Restoration of elbow function after supracondylar fractures initially focuses on motion exercises that do not stress the fracture site. Therefore passive stretching is

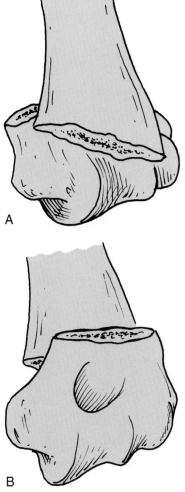

Fig. 22-10 **A,** Supracondylar fracture type I or extension-type fracture in which the distal humeral fragment is displaced posteriorly. **B,** Supracondylar fracture type II, or flexion-type in which the distal humeral fragment is displaced anteriorly.

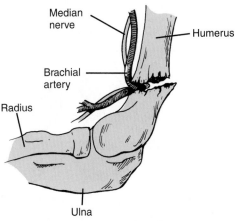

Fig. 22-11 Volkmann ischemic contracture.

contraindicated during the early healing phase.[17] Gentle active exercises for the upper arm, wrist, and shoulder, of course, should be performed to the patient's tolerance. Resistance exercises consisting of submaximal isometrics and progressing to concentric and eccentric muscle contractions are allowed, pending confirmation of secure union of the fracture fragments.

Intercondylar T or Y Fractures

In addition to nondisplaced or displaced transverse supracondylar fractures, potentially more significant fracture patterns can occur with falls or direct trauma to the elbow. Intercondylar fractures describe injuries that extend between the condyles of the distal humerus and involve the articular surfaces of the elbow joint.[7,17,18,29] According to Strege[29] and Miller,[18] there are four classifications of intercondylar fractures that display a T or Y configuration[7,17,21]:

■ Type I: A nondisplaced fracture that extends between the two condyles (Fig. 22-12, *A*)
■ Type II: A displaced fracture without rotation of the fracture fragments (Fig. 22-12, *B*)

■ Type III: A displaced fracture with a rotational deformity (Fig. 22-12, *C*)
■ Type IV: A severely comminuted fracture with significant separation between the two condyles (Fig. 22-12, *D*)

The type of fracture dictates a course of treatment that parallels the significance of the injury. With a type I nondisplaced fracture, treatment can be immobilization for approximately 3 weeks, followed by progressive, gentle active motion. Resistance exercises are deferred until secure bone union has been confirmed radiographically. With types II and III displaced fractures, the treatment is open reduction with internal fixation (ORIF) with the use of Kirschner wires, side plates, and lag screws to secure and stabilize the displaced fracture fragments (Fig. 22-13).[17,18,29] Type IV comminuted intercondylar fractures are treated differently for adults and elderly patients with poor bone quality (osteoporosis).[18,29] Adult patients are usually treated with an ORIF procedure to stabilize the fragments. However, in elderly patients with generally poor bone quality (osteopenic bone), a treatment procedure referred to as the *bag of*

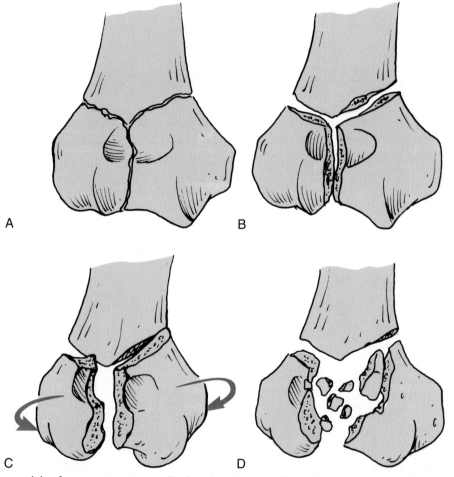

Fig. 22-12 **A,** Intercondylar fracture, type I, nondisplaced. **B,** Intercondylar fracture, type II, displaced without rotation. **C,** Intercondylar fracture, type III, displaced with rotation of fragments. **D,** Severely comminuted type IV intercondylar fracture with significant displacement.

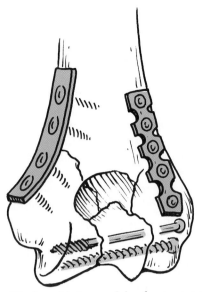

Fig. 22-13 Displaced intercondylar fracture open reduction with internal fixation.

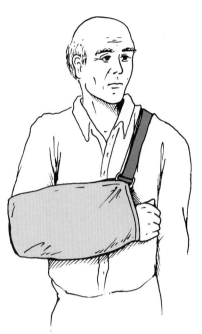

Fig. 22-14 In cases where elderly patients with osteoporosis suffer a severely comminuted intercondylar fracture, a treatment referred to as the *bag of bones technique* is used.

bones technique is used.[17,18,29] This technique calls for the use of a "collar and cuff" sling, with the affected elbow flexed as far as the limits of swelling and circulatory compromise allow.[29] With the elbow flexed and able to hang freely within the sling, gravity is used to help obtain possible reduction of the fracture fragments (Fig. 22-14).[18,29]

With intercondylar fractures of the elbow, the patient is instructed in a general conditioning program during immobilization while close attention is paid to avoiding all stress to the affected arm. In addition, the wrist, hand, and shoulder of the affected limb may be exercised with active motion if prescribed by the physician and PT. With intercondylar fractures, the anatomic relationship of the elbow (being extremely compact, with significant bony stability) dictates that the restoration of purposeful, functional motion becomes paramount during recovery. Soft-tissue scarring and bone callus formation can lead to early joint stiffness, arthrosis, and contractures.

During the early postimmobilization period, no passive manipulation or passive stretching can be performed.[29] Strege[29] reports an appreciable risk of joint ankylosis when passive stretching and manipulation are performed during early postinjury elbow rehabilitation.

Once wound closure has occurred after an ORIF procedure, the use of a whirlpool bath may aid local circulation, removal of waste, reduction in soft-tissue congestion, and enhancement of soft-tissue relaxation in preparation for protected active motion. Elbow flexion and extension, as well as forearm pronation and supination, are encouraged as prescribed by the physician and directed by the PT. Stable union of the fracture signifies more active involvement with progressive motion exercises and the initiation of resistance exercise

training to regain strength. If the patient demonstrates loss of motion, the physician and PT may decide to perform specific joint mobilization techniques once bone union is secure. This does not conflict with the mentioned contraindication for passive manipulation and stretching immediately after immobilization. Some patients ultimately may have residual loss of motion. However, functional activities can be performed with flexion and extension of 30° to 130° and pronation and supination of 50°.[29]

Radial Head Fractures

Another common fracture that occurs as a result of a fall on an outstretched arm is a radial head fracture. These fractures represent approximately one third of all elbow fractures and nearly 20% of all elbow trauma.[13]

The definition of the "carrying angle" of the elbow and the difference noted between men and women are important in understanding radial head fractures. The carrying angle is formed between the intersection of the long axis of the humerus and the axis of the ulna, with the elbow joint in full extension.[29] A normal carrying angle for men is 10° of valgus; in women, it is 13° of valgus (Fig. 22-15).[29] The clinical relevance is that a fractured radial head can lead to an increased valgus deformity and the varus elbow malalignment called a *gunstock deformity.*[13]

Radial head fractures generally are classified into four types, as follows (Fig. 22-16):
■ Type I: A nondisplaced fracture
■ Type II: A marginal fracture with displacement

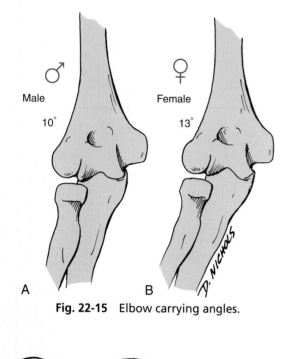

Fig. 22-15 Elbow carrying angles.

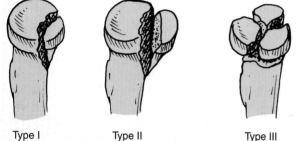

Fig. 22-16 Radial head fractures: type I, nondisplaced; type II, displaced; and type III, comminuted.

■ Type III: A comminuted fracture of the entire radial head

■ Type IV: Any radial head fracture with elbow dislocation[29]

Treatment options parallel the significance of the injury and dictate the course of rehabilitation. Patients with type I nondisplaced radial head fractures usually need a period of immobilization ranging from 5 to 7 days up to 3 to 4 weeks.[17,29] Usually, early active motion is allowed as soon as pain subsides. Because these fractures generally are stable (nondisplaced), healing occurs with very good results.[17] Terminal elbow extension may be recovered many months after type I radial head fractures.[17]

With a type II displaced fracture, the radial head can be excised or stabilized with an ORIF procedure. With a type III comminuted radial head fracture, the fractured area is excised.[13,17,18,29]

Rehabilitation after an ORIF or radial head excision usually calls for immobilization in a hinged splint to protect the healing bone and surrounding soft tissues. As noted, excision of the radial head can lead to increased varus or valgus deformity. In either case, migration of the radial shaft may occur after excision and place stress on the distal ligamentous radioulnar articulation.[13,17,18] Therefore any discomfort expressed by the patient at the distal radioulnar joint after excision of the radial head usually results from added stress on this area created by the disrupted proximal radial segment.[13,17,18] When the patient is immobilized, the hand, wrist, and shoulder of the affected limb are exercised as tolerated. The patient also is encouraged to participate in a general conditioning program of aerobic exercise, strength training, and flexibility exercises. Pain and swelling usually are managed satisfactorily by placing ice packs directly over the painful area. Early active ROM exercises are advocated 3 to 5 days postoperatively by some or deferred for up to 3 weeks by others.[13,29] Restoration of motion is the cornerstone for recovery after radial head fractures. As noted, joint restrictions secondary to arthrofibrosis and contractures can occur, with pronation and supination most commonly affected after radial head fractures.

The PT may elect to perform specific joint mobilization techniques to enhance pronation and supination if secure fixation has occurred after an ORIF procedure. Once wound closure has occurred, a whirlpool bath can be an effective adjunct preceding motion exercises. After excision of the radial head, resistance exercises of elbow flexion and extension and forearm pronation and supination can begin as soon as pain and motion allow. These exercises may be deferred for longer periods if an ORIF procedure was used so that stable bone union and soft-tissue healing can occur.

Olecranon Fractures

Olecranon fractures commonly result after a fall on the point of the elbow (olecranon process) or indirectly from forceful contraction of the triceps.[17] Generally, they are classified as either nondisplaced or displaced fractures. Displaced fractures of the olecranon have four subclassifications[18]:

■ Avulsion fracture, displaced

■ Oblique or transverse fracture

■ Comminuted fracture

■ Fracture-dislocation

The treatment for nondisplaced olecranon fractures requires immobilization for 6 to 8 weeks,[7,17] although as little as 3 weeks or less is used in some cases (particularly in older patients).[18,29] The position in which nondisplaced olecranon fractures are immobilized is somewhat controversial, in that some authorities advocate placing the affected arm in extension or slight flexion,[5,7,13,17] whereas others recommend placing the affected arm in 45° to 90° of flexion.[18,29] The rationale for placing the elbow in 45° of flexion is the likelihood of the loss of flexion after immobilization.[29] In addition,

Strege[29] suggests that immobilization should not exceed 45° because of the risk of displacing fracture fragments.

Usually, nondisplaced olecranon fractures are allowed gentle active ROM exercises after 3 weeks of immobilization. Flexion of the affected arm should not exceed 90° for the first 6 to 8 weeks after injury so that fracture fragments can heal.[13,29]

Displaced or comminuted fractures of the olecranon can be treated with an ORIF procedure to secure the fragments. With severely comminuted fractures, excision of as much as 80% of the olecranon can occur without loss of joint stability.[18,29]

Physical therapy can begin during the initial stages of immobilization. Active motion of the hand, wrist, forearm (pronation and supination), and shoulder can commence once acute pain has subsided. A general physical conditioning program is allowed as soon as tolerated by the patient. Active elbow flexion must not exceed 90° for the first 2 months after injury. Active resistance exercises for elbow extension must be minimized because the forceful contraction of the triceps can displace the fracture fragments before secure bone healing at 8 weeks. Resistance exercises for elbow flexion can begin earlier if motion is limited and the muscle contractions are submaximal. Submaximal isometric triceps extensions can proceed once bony union has been verified. Progressive concentric and eccentric loading is added as motion increases and secure fixation of the fragments has occurred.

Progressive flexion and extension movements must proceed cautiously and slowly to prevent displacement of the fragments. In addition, the patient must be carefully instructed to initially perform resistance exercises well within the limits of pain and motion restrictions to allow for proper bone healing. The strong contractions of the biceps during flexion and the triceps during extension activities are effective to gradually overcome most motion limitations observed early after injury or surgery. Full recovery after olecranon fractures may take 6 months to 1 year.[13]

Fracture-Dislocations

A fall on an extended outreaching arm causes isolated elbow dislocations and combined fracture-dislocations (Fig. 22-17).[9,17,19,24,28] Conwell[7] reports that "with the exception of the shoulder, the elbow is the most frequently dislocated joint in the body." This injury occurs most often in men, with the nondominant arm representing about 60% of these injuries.[19]

Posterior elbow dislocations are the most common, whereas anterior dislocations represent 1% to 2% of all elbow dislocations.[19] Associated fractures of the radial head occur in approximately 10% of elbow dislocations.[19,28] In addition, associated neurovascular injuries can occur with either isolated elbow dislocations or with fracture-dislocations.[17,19,28,29] Injuries involve the

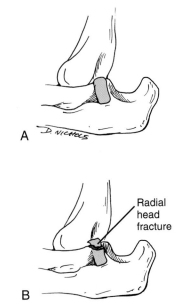

Fig. 22-17 A, Posterior elbow dislocation without radial head fracture. **B,** Posterior elbow dislocation with radial head fracture.

median, radial, and ulnar nerves, as well as the brachial artery with elbow dislocations.[19,29]

Isolated posterior elbow dislocations are managed with closed reduction and immobilization.[7,9,17-19,28] The elbow is placed in 90° of flexion in a splint for 3 to 6 weeks.[7,17,29] During this period, hand and shoulder motion is allowed if no offensive stress is applied to the elbow. Early active ROM exercises can begin during the first week after reduction.[29] However, no passive ROM or stretching is allowed because of the risk of myositis ossificans,[17,28] which results from aggressive passive stretching and mobilization. Active motion is not believed to cause this condition.[28] Therefore gentle active flexion and extension exercises are added as pain, swelling, and soft-tissue healing dictate. Because this injury represents a hyperextension trauma that significantly affects the joint capsule, muscle, tendon, and frequently ligamentous restraints, extensive soft-tissue healing is necessary for a stable, functional joint. The joint capsule of the elbow may require 8 to 10 weeks to heal satisfactorily.[9] Restoration of elbow extension therefore must proceed cautiously because the mechanism of injury is usually elbow hyperextension. Resistance exercises can begin as soft-tissue healing progresses. Eccentric and concentric resistance exercises for the biceps can be emphasized to reduce hyperextension forces.[9] Resistance-type exercises are deferred for at least 3 weeks to allow for acute symptoms to subside. However, aggressive elbow extension must be prevented until 8 to 10 weeks have elapsed.[9,19]

The most common complication after elbow dislocation is loss of extension.[19,28,29] Ten weeks after dislocation, a 30° flexion contracture is common, and a 10° flexion contracture is typically observed 2 years after injury.[19]

However unacceptable this loss of motion may be, it does not represent an "overwhelming functional deficit."[29]

The treatment of fracture-dislocations centers on the appropriate management of the fracture (most commonly the radial head) and reduction of the elbow. In most cases, radial head excision is performed to minimize the development of myositis ossificans.[28] Therefore with radial head excision, proximal migration of the radius can result in stress and pain to the distal radioulnar ligamentous articulation.[17,18,29]

Rehabilitation after fracture-dislocation of the elbow focuses on early protected active motion. Passive stretching again is strictly avoided during the early recovery phases of healing. With radial head excision, a loss of 25° to 30° of pronation and supination can be expected if postoperative immobilization lasts longer than 4 weeks.[28] As with isolated dislocation, loss of full elbow extension is not uncommon.

MOBILIZATION OF THE ELBOW

The rationale for specific joint mobilization is to avoid joint restrictions or hypomobility, which can limit the normal joint arthrokinematics.[6] In many instances, arthrofibrosis occurs as a result of immobilization and internal fixation methods used to stabilize fracture fragments.

The PT determines if mobilization is indicated after injury, surgery, or immobilization based on tissue healing constraints, the nature of the joint restriction (hypomobility of noncontractile tissue or articular surface dysfunction),[6] and whether passive motion is indicated for the treatment of joint limitations. The PT must clearly define the specific indications for mobilization with reference to the exact technique to be employed, rate of movement, amplitude of force, and direction of the force applied to the elbow. To obtain relaxation, the PTA must place the patient in a comfortable position, with specific attention paid to the support and stability of the shoulder, elbow, and arm of the patient. Before joint mobilization is applied, thermal agents are employed to reduce tissue congestion, aid in the removal of wastes, improve tissue extensibility, and enhance relaxation of the patient and the affected joint.

Injuries to the elbow that require mobilization should increase in flexion, extension, or both. Wooden[36] outlines three techniques used to enhance general motion, flexion, and extension of the elbow.

To enhance general mobility of the elbow, the patient should be supine with the affected elbow flexed to 90°. The shoulder of the affected limb is held at the patient's side or in an abducted position. The PTA places both hands at the proximal aspect of the forearm, and directs a straight lateral distraction force that directs the forearm away from the humerus (Fig. 22-18).

Humeral-ulnar abduction is employed to promote elbow extension.[36] The patient should be supine with

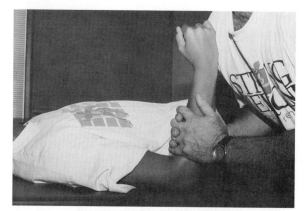

Fig 22-18 Elbow distraction.

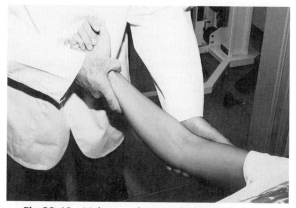

Fig 22-19 Valgus or humeral-ulna abduction.

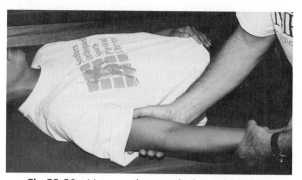

Fig 22-20 Varus or humeral-ulna adduction.

the affected arm abducted and the elbow slightly flexed. The PT sits to the patient's affected side with one hand stabilizing the distal lateral humerus and the other hand firmly grasping the ulnar aspect of the distal forearm. In this position, the PT directs a valgus or abduction force to the elbow (Fig. 22-19).[36]

An adduction technique is applied to increase elbow flexion.[36] The patient remains supine with the affected arm abducted. The PT sits to the patient's affected side and stabilizes the distal humerus on the medial aspect with one hand, while placing the opposite hand on the distal radial aspect of the forearm. In this position, the PT directs a varus or adduction force to the elbow (Fig. 22-20).

Although these few techniques are representative of the more common motions requiring mobilization, other positions and techniques can be used to enhance elbow motion.

❖ GLOSSARY

Epicondylitis: An inflammatory condition of the epicondyle of the medial or lateral elbow.

Lateral epicondylitis: A form of tendinitis commonly referred to as *tennis elbow*.

Ligament stability: Anterior band of the medial ulnar collateral ligament is the main ligamentous stabilizer.

Medial epicondylitis: An overuse condition also known as *golfer's elbow*.

Medial valgus stress overload: A condition that occurs commonly among patients who participate in repetitive throwing and racquet sports, it is also known as *valgus extension overload*.

REFERENCES

1. Andrews JR, Craven WM: Lesions of the posterior compartment of the elbow, *Clin Sports Med* 10(3):637–652, 1991.
2. Andrews JR, Jelsma RD, Joyse ME, et al: Open surgical procedures for injuries of the elbow in throwers, *Oper Tech Sports Med* 4(2):109–113, 1996.
3. Bandy WD, Irion JM: The effect of time on static stretch on the flexibility of the hamstring muscles, *Phys Ther* 74(9):845–850, 1994:Discussion, pp 850–842.
4. Bandy WD, Irion JM, Briggler M: The effect of static stretch and dynamic range of motion training on the flexibility of the hamstring muscles, *J Orthop Sports Phys Ther* 27(4):295–300, 1998.
5. Bennett JB, Tullos HS: Acute injuries to the elbow. In Nicholas JA, Hershman EB, editors: *The upper extremity in sports medicine*, St Louis, 1990, Mosby.
6. Bowling RW, Rockar PA: The elbow complex. In Gould JA, editor: *Orthopaedics and sports physical therapy*, ed 2, St Louis, 1990, Mosby.
7. Conwell HE: Injuries to the elbow, *Clin Symp* 21(2):35–62, 1969.
8. Curwin S, Stanish WD: *Tendinitis: its etiology and treatment*, Lexington, MA, 1984, DC Heath.
9. Dickoff-Hoffman S, Foster D: Rehabilitation of elbow injuries. In Prentice WE, editor: *Rehabilitation techniques in sports medicine*, St Louis, 1994, Mosby.
10. Dillman CJ, Smutz P, Werner S: Valgus extension overload in baseball pitching, *Med Sci Sports Exerc* 23:S135, 1991.
11. Fleisig GS, Escamilla RF: Biomechanics of the elbow in the throwing athlete, *Oper Tech Sports Med* 4(2):62–68, 1996.
12. Kottke FJ, Pauley DL, Ptak RA: The rationale for prolonged stretching for correction of shortening of connective tissue, *Arch Phys Med Rehabil* 47(6):345–352, 1966.
13. LaCroix E: Treatment of common problems of the elbow, forearm and wrist joints. In Goldstein TS, editor: *Geriatric orthopaedics: rehabilitative management of common problems*, Gaithersburg, MD, 1991, Aspen Publishers.
14. Linscheid RL, O'Driscoll SW: Elbow dislocation. In Morrey BF, editor: *The elbow and its disorders*, ed 2, Philadelphia, 1993, Saunders, pp 441–452.
15. Linscheid RL, Wheeler DK: Elbow dislocations, *JAMA* 194(11):1171–1176, 1965.
16. McClure PW, Blackburn LG, Dusold C: The use of splints in the treatment of joint stiffness: biologic rationale and an algorithm for making clinical decisions, *Phys Ther* 74(12):1101–1107, 1994.
17. McRae R: Practical fracture treatment. In McRae R, editor: *Injuries about the elbow*, New York, 1994, Churchill Livingstone.
18. Miller MD: *Review of orthopaedics*, Philadelphia, 1992, Saunders.
19. Morrey BF: In DeLee JC, Drez D, editors: *Orthopaedic sports medicine: principles and practices, elbow dislocation in the athlete*, vol. 1 Philadelphia, 1994, Saunders.
20. Morrey BF, Regan WD: In DeLee JC, Drez D, editors: *Orthopaedic sports medicine: principles and practice, tendinopathies about the elbow* vol. 1Philadelphia, 1994, Saunders.
21. Morrey BF, Regan WD: In DeLee JC, Drez D, editors: *Orthopaedic sports medicine: principles and practice, throwing injuries*, vol. 1 Philadelphia, 1994, Saunders.
22. O'Driscoll SW: Reconstruction of the lateral collateral ligament. In Yamaguchi K, King G, O'Driscoll SW, et al: *Advanced Reconstruction. Elbow*, Rosemont, Ill., 2007, American Academy of Orthopaedic Surgeons, pp 159–165.
23. Parks JC: Overuse injuries of the elbow. In Nicholas JA, Hershman EB, editors: *The upper extremity in sports medicine*, St Louis, 1990, Mosby.
24. Reid DC, Kushner S: The elbow region. In Donatelli R, Wooden MJ, editors: *Orthopaedic physical therapy*, New York, 1989, Churchill Livingstone.
25. Reinold MM, Wilk KE, Reed J, et al: Interval sport programs: guidelines for baseball, tennis, and golf, *J Orthop Sports Phys Ther* 32(6):293–298, 2002.
26. Rohrbough JT, Altchek DW, Hyman J, et al: Medial collateral ligament reconstruction of the elbow using the docking technique, *Am J Sports Med* 30(4):541–548, 2002.
27. Sapega AA, Quedenfeld TC, Moyer RA, et al: Biophysical factors in range-of-motion exercise, *Phys Sports Med* 9(12):57–65, 1981.
28. Stralka SW, Brasel JG: Elbow. In Richardson JK, Iglarsh ZA, editors: *Clinical orthopaedic physical therapy*, Philadelphia, 1994, Saunders.
29. Strege D: Upper extremity. In Loth TS, editor: *Orthopaedic boards review*, St Louis, 1993, Mosby.
30. Warren CG, Lehmann JF, Koblanski JN: Elongation of rat tail tendon: effect of load and temperature, *Arch Phys Med Rehabil* 52(10):465–474, 1971.
31. Warren CG, Lehmann JF, Koblanski JN: Heat and stretch procedures: an evaluation using rat tail tendon, *Arch Phys Med Rehabil* 57(3):122–126, 1976.
32. Werner SL, Fleisig GS, Dillman CJ, et al: Biomechanics of the elbow during baseball pitching, *J Orthop Sports Phys Ther* 17(6):274–278, 1993.
33. Wilk KE, Arrigo C, Andrews JR: Rehabilitation of the elbow in the throwing athlete, *J Orthop Sports Phys Ther* 17(6):305–317, 1993.
34. Wilk KE, Voight ML, Keirns MA, et al: Stretch-shortening drills for the upper extremities: theory and clinical application, *J Orthop Sports Phys Ther* 17(5):225–239, 1993.
35. Wilson FD, Andrews JR, Blackburn TA, et al: Valgus extension overload in the pitching elbow, *Am J Sports Med* 11(2):83–88, 1983.
36. Wooden MJ: Mobilization of the upper extremity. In Donatelli R, Wooden MJ, editors: *Orthopaedic physical therapy*, New York, 1989, Churchill Livingstone.

REVIEW QUESTIONS

Short Answer

1. In the following figure, identify the injury, mechanism of injury, and structure involved.

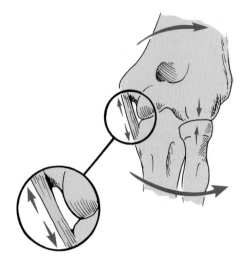

2. Name the most common type of supracondylar fracture.
3. In the following figure, identify the fracture type.

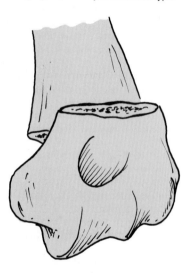

4. In the following figure, identify the general fracture, label the structure(s) that may be compromised, and identify the potential injury that may ensue.

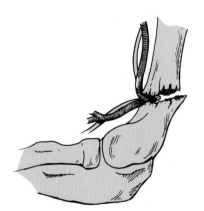

5. In the figure shown, identify the type and classification of fracture.

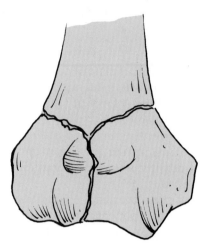

6. What is the most common direction of elbow dislocation?

True/False

7. In severe cases of "tennis elbow," the use of a wrist cock-up splint is advocated for the management of inflamed wrist extensor tendons.
8. During the subacute recovery phase of rehabilitation for lateral epicondylitis, initial instruction for patients to perform forearm pronation and supination must include the use of a hammer while holding the end of the shaft away from the head of the hammer.
9. Medial valgus stress overload is synonymous with medial epicondylitis.
10. The signs and symptoms of ischemic obstruction are always immediately evident after injury.
11. Passive stretching is advocated during the early recovery phase of healing after supracondylar fractures.
12. It is not uncommon for some patients to be left with some residual loss of ROM after intercondylar fractures.
13. After excision of the radial head in type IV comminuted fractures, the radial shaft may migrate and cause pain at the distal radioulnar joint.
14. Displaced or comminuted fractures of the olecranon can be treated with an ORIF procedure or, in cases of severely comminuted fractures, excision of as much as 80% of the olecranon.
15. With the exception of the shoulder, the elbow is the most frequently dislocated joint in the body.

23 Orthopedic Management of the Wrist and Hand

Marsha Lawrence

LEARNING OBJECTIVES

1. Identify and describe a common compression neuropathy of the wrist.
2. Discuss methods of management and rehabilitation of compression neuropathy of the wrist.
3. Identify and describe common ligament injuries of the wrist.
4. Describe and discuss methods of management and rehabilitation of ligament injuries of the wrist.
5. Describe methods of management and rehabilitation for distal radial and ulnar fractures.
6. Identify methods of management and rehabilitation for scaphoid fractures.
7. Identify and describe common metacarpal and phalanx fractures and methods of management and rehabilitation.
8. Describe methods of management and rehabilitation following surgery for Dupuytren's disease.
9. Identify and describe common extensor and flexor tendon injuries.
10. Discuss methods of management and rehabilitation of extensor tendon and flexor tendon injuries.
11. Identify methods of management and rehabilitation for complex regional pain syndrome.

KEY TERMS

Bennett fracture
Boxer's fracture
Carpal tunnel syndrome

Colles fracture
Compression neuropathy
Dinner fork deformity

Mallet finger
Nerve entrapment
Smith fracture

CHAPTER OUTLINE

This chapter introduces treatment of common orthopedic injuries and conditions of the wrist and hand. The focus is on interventions to control pain and swelling and improve range of motion (ROM), strength, and functional use of the wrist and hand while protecting surgical repairs. Patients often ignore their neck (especially if they are in a sling), shoulder, elbow, and forearm when the hand or wrist are injured so it is always important to include ROM and strengthening to the unaffected joints of the injured extremity. The referring physical therapist (PT) should be consulted before resuming general conditioning. Hand and wrist anatomy and kinesiology are complex so the physical therapist assistant (PTA) is strongly urged to review them before studying this chapter.

BONY INJURIES OF THE WRIST AND HAND

Fractures to the forearm, wrist, and digits are common. In general, their treatment and the timing of rehabilitation depend on the following:

1. The number of fragments in the fracture
2. The fragment orientation (displaced or in alignment)
3. The approach used to restore anatomic alignment (closed reduction or open reduction)
4. The method used to maintain the reduction (external fixation: casts, splints; internal fixation: pins, screws, or plates; or percutaneous fixation: pins that protrude through the skin into the bone)
5. Involvement of the articular surfaces

Before beginning any exercise program with these patients, it is important to know how stable the reduction is. Exercise can begin earlier and more aggressively with strong and stable fixation. It is also important to review any two-joint muscles that may cross involved and uninvolved joints because exercise to the proximal, uninvolved joint may jeopardize the fixation at the distal joint.

Distal Radial and Ulnar Fractures
Radius

The most common distal radius fractures are **Colles fractures**.[10] A Colles' fracture is defined as a radius fracture within 2.5 cm of the wrist in which the distal fragment is displaced in a dorsal direction.[10] This is also known as a **dinner fork deformity** due to the resemblance resulting from the shape of the wrist and hand following this fracture (Fig. 23-1). This injury is usually the result of a fall on the palm of an outstretched hand. Treatment of these common fractures is controversial and more than 85% require reduction.[10]

A **Smith fracture** is also referred to as a *reverse Colles fracture*.[10] The fracture usually occurs from a fall on the dorsum of the hand, with the resultant distal radial fragment displaced in a palmar direction (Fig. 23-2). The course of treatment is similar to the Colles fracture and the rehabilitation is the same.

Rehabilitation starts as soon as stable immobilization has been achieved. The goals are to reduce edema through positioning and retrograde massage and to maintain digit ROM through exercise. The distal edge of the cast or splint must be proximal to the distal palmar crease in order to allow full flexion of the metacarpal phalangeal (MP) joints. "Six-pack" exercises are taught and performed hourly while awake (Fig. 23-3).[6] These exercises maintain MP and interphalangeal (IP) ligament length and encourage differential gliding of the finger and wrist tendons. Passive assistance may be needed to achieve full range. Light gripping, pinching, and using the fingers is encouraged as long as there is no pain at the fracture site. Active forearm rotation within the limit of the cast should also be started. Shoulder pain should be evaluated further by the PT as proximal injuries can be overlooked in light of the distal radius fracture.

Some distal radius fractures require immobilization of the elbow to prevent forearm rotation for the first 3 weeks.[26] Once the cast is modified to free the elbow,

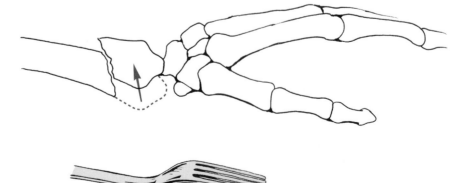

Fig. 23-1 Colles fracture with resultant dinner fork deformity.

active and passive exercise to the elbow can begin. The PT should be consulted before beginning resisted elbow flexion because of the attachment of the brachioradialis on the radial styloid. Strong contractions of this muscle may cause a loss of the fracture reduction.[26] Complications following distal radial fractures include: loss of reduction of the fracture fragments, nonunion (the break does not heal), malunion (partial healing or poor alignment), tendon adhesions, median nerve compression, instability, Volkmann ischemic contracture, and complex regional pain syndrome (CRPS).[10] The patient's pain, circulation and sensation should be monitored during each session and the exercises should be adjusted accordingly.

When the cast is discontinued, the patient may be placed in a soft splint between exercise sessions until the wrist muscles are stronger. Active and active assisted ROM to the wrist and forearm are initiated, making sure combinations of motion, such as flexion and ulnar deviation, are performed. Patients should be taught to isolate the wrist muscles from the finger muscles as they will have a tendency to lead wrist motion with the finger muscles. Encouraging the patient to hold a paper towel core while moving the wrist helps to accomplish this without adding resistance. Submaximal isometric exercises at various positions in the range are also started. Modalities to increase tissue extensibility or relieve pain are initiated as long as edema remains controlled. Strengthening is usually started 4 to 5 weeks after cast removal. The physician will order this only if the fracture site is no longer tender to palpation and evidence of bony union is seen. Closed-chain weight bearing is also gradually started at this time. Joint mobilization can be helpful in regaining full ROM. Patients generally return to work without restrictions about 10 weeks after cast removal.[26]

Patients with percutaneous fixation (sometimes called *external fixators*) can often follow the same exercise program outlined earlier (Fig. 23-4). The fixator stays in place until radiographs reveal evidence of bony healing, generally in 6 weeks.[6]

Distal Ulna Fractures

Fractures of the distal ulna usually occur in combination with distal radius fractures.[20] The medical management and rehabilitation follow the guidelines outlined above. Persistent pain with rotation or weight bearing suggests further evaluation of the triangular fibrocartilage complex is necessary to rule out tears (see later discussion).

Carpal Fractures

Fractures of the carpal bones are also usually caused by a fall on the outstretched hand. Scaphoid fractures are the most common, and trapezoid fractures, the least common.[1]

Scaphoid Fractures

A scaphoid fracture is often the result of a minor fall on the palm with the wrist hyperextended and radially deviated.[1] It is often dismissed as a sprain, delaying treatment. Pain and swelling in the area of the anatomic snuffbox that do not resolve over a few weeks, pain with wrist extension, and decreased grip strength are signs indicating further evaluation is needed.

The location of the fracture within the scaphoid determines the method of treatment. The blood supply to this bone enters distally, leaving the proximal portion without direct circulation when it is separated by a fracture (Fig. 23-5). Fractures in the proximal third of the bone have a high incidence of nonunion, and those that do heal take much longer, anywhere from 12 to 24 weeks of immobilization compared with 5 to 6 weeks for the distal portion.[1,4] Fractures that are not displaced or can easily be reduced are immobilized in a thumb spica cast. Nonreducible fractures require internal fixation with rigid immobilization. If nonunion and avascular necrosis (AVN) occur, bone grafts from the distal radius may be necessary.[4]

Rehabilitation should begin during immobilization as described under distal radial fractures. Edema reduction and ROM of the uninvolved distal joints are

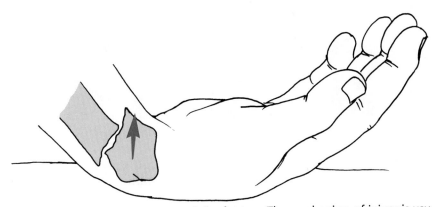

Fig. 23-2 Smith fracture, also referred to as a *reverse Colles fracture*. The mechanism of injury is usually a fall on the dorsum of the hand.

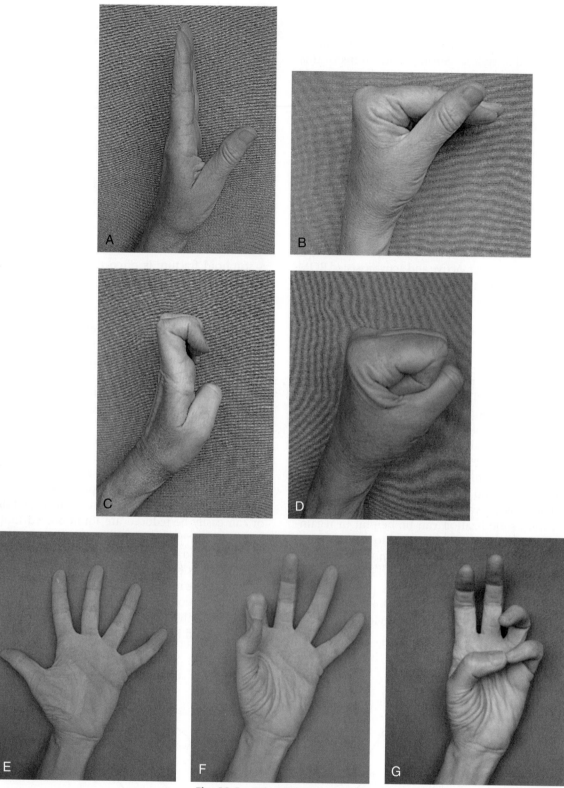

Fig. 23-3 "Six-pack" exercises.

the primary focus. Following cast removal, the patient usually wears a thumb spica splint between exercise sessions. Wrist exercises should focus on differential gliding of the wrist and finger muscles. Strengthening with exercise putty, sustained grip activities, and gradual closed-chain activities progress to tolerance. Patients usually return to full activity within 12 weeks after cast removal.[4] If the patient is having difficulty regaining motion, static progressive splinting, dynamic splinting, and joint mobilization can help restore full range.

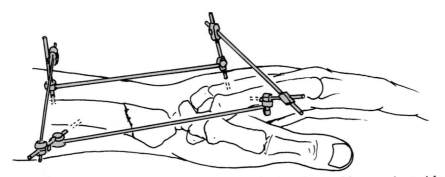

Fig. 23-4 External fixator for stabilization of severely displaced, unstable comminuted fractures.

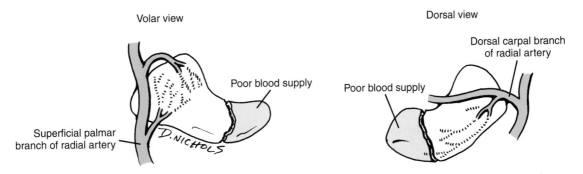

Fig. 23-5 Vascular anatomy of the scaphoid. The proximal pole of the scaphoid has a poor blood supply. If fractured in the proximal pole, there is the likelihood of avascular necrosis and resultant nonunion.

Metacarpal Fractures

Fractures of the metacarpals can occur in the base, shaft, neck, or head. These are due to falls, jammed fingers, or direct blows.[29] Fractures that are nondisplaced or minimally displaced are placed in a cast or splint for 3 to 4 weeks, usually including the joint above and the joint below the fracture.[30] The MP joint is placed in 45° to 60° of flexion to prevent collateral ligament shortening. Displaced fractures require surgical intervention and fixation by open or percutaneous techniques.

Fractures of the neck of the fourth or fifth metacarpal are called *boxer's fractures* (Fig. 23-6). These occur when the patient strikes a hard object with a clenched fist. Ironically, these are rarely seen in professional boxers.[30] These patients are immobilized with the wrist in slight extension and the MP joint flexed for 3 to 4 weeks.[29,30] The proximal interphalangeal (PIP) joints are free to flex and extend often within 24 hours. Edema control sometimes requires the use of an isotoner glove as well as massage and elevation.

Active range of motion (AROM) should emphasize isolated extensor digitorum communis motion, MP flexion, and composite flexion. Tendon adhesions to the fracture site or, in the case of open procedures, the skin, often limit gliding of the extensor tendons. A splint should be worn in between exercise sessions for an additional 2 weeks. At 6 weeks, passive ROM and resistance can be started emphasizing interossei strengthening in order to achieve full IP extension.[19] If the fixation is less

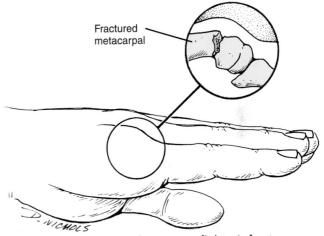

Fig. 23-6 Boxer's fracture, or fighter's fracture.

stable, ROM may be delayed until 3 to 4 weeks, then follow the course outlined previously. When the incision has healed, scar mobilization techniques should be started.

Bennett fracture is a fracture of the palmar base of the proximal first metacarpal.[30] The ligaments hold the fragment in place, but the remainder of the base is pulled radially and dorsally, resulting in a fracture-dislocation.[30] As with a boxer's fracture, treatment can be with closed reduction and rigid cast immobilization or with an open reduction with internal fixation (ORIF) procedure, depending on the severity of the fracture. There must be nondisplaced

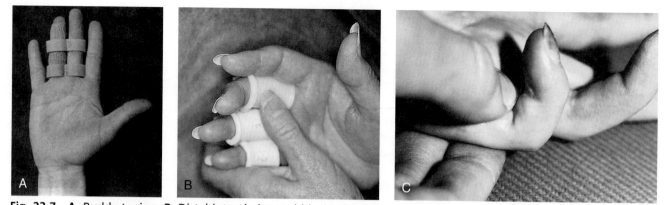

Fig. 23-7 A, Buddy taping. **B,** Distal interphalangeal blocking exercises with the metacarpal phalangeal in various positions. **C,** Manual blocking of the metacarpal phalangeal during active flexion of the proximal interphalangeal joint. (**A,** From Burke SL, Higgins JP, McClinton MA, et al: *Hand and upper extremity rehabilitation: a practical guide,* ed 3, St Louis, 2006, Churchill Livingstone. **B,** From Copper C: *Fundamentals of hand therapy: clinical reasoning and treatment guidelines for common diagnoses of the upper extremity,* St Louis, 2007, Mosby. **C,** From Early MB: *Physical dysfunction practice skills for the occupational therapy assistant,* ed 2, St Louis, 2007, Mosby.)

solid union at the fracture site before active motion can begin. If closed reduction is used, immobilization lasts 6 weeks to promote stable union.[30] If an ORIF procedure is used, immobilization is slightly shorter because of the rigid internal fixation. Rehabilitation closely parallels the treatment for a boxer's fracture with emphasis on regaining the thumb web space, opposition and composite flexion and extension. Resisted exercise, pinch, grip, and weight bearing on the palm with the thumb abducted can progress when stable fracture healing has occurred.

Phalanx Fractures

Phalanx fractures can occur at the neck, shaft, or base of the phalanx. Stable, closed, nondisplaced fractures are treated by buddy taping (Fig. 23-7, *A*) or with simple splints and immediate active ROM. More complex closed proximal and middle phalanx fractures should be placed in a hand-based splint for 3 to 4 weeks.[24] This splint should hold the MP joints in 50° to 70° flexion and the IP joints in 10° to 15° of flexion.[24] Once radiographic evidence of healing is confirmed, ROM can progress. The most common complication is loss of PIP joint extension.[9] Blocking exercises can help prevent the tendons from adhering to the fracture site (Fig. 23-7, *B, C*).

The distal phalanx is the most frequently fractured bone in the hand.[21] These fractures are usually splinted in extension using a small aluminum splint leaving the PIP joint free. Isolated PIP motion and MP motion can be started immediately. Often the nail bed is injured, leaving the finger hypersensitive and stiff. These patients are started on a program of desensitization, using touching, tapping, fluidotherapy, and vibration to overcome the hypersensitivity. Once movement can begin at the distal interphalangeal (DIP) joint, (usually at 3 weeks), the emphasis is on composite digit flexion and coordinated use of the digits. Patients often bypass the injured digit in functional

activities, so this is addressed in therapy with buddy taping, light grasping, and pinching exercises that isolate the thumb and the involved finger. If the terminal extensor tendon is disrupted (see "Mallet Finger" section), the DIP joint is splinted for 6 to 8 weeks. Aggressive passive flexion should be avoided because it may lead to an extensor lag.[21]

SOFT TISSUE INJURIES OF THE WRIST AND HAND

Ligament Injuries of the Wrist

Stability of the wrist depends primarily on intracapsular ligaments and not on intrinsic dynamic support from musculotendinous tissue.[34] Ligament sprains with varying degrees of carpal instability usually result from a fall with the wrist hyperextended (Fig. 23-8).[34]

Partial ligament injuries without carpal instability are immobilized in a short arm cast or splint for 3 to 4 weeks. Severe ligament injuries lead to carpal instability and reduction and maintenance of the alignment are more difficult. Options include rigid cast immobilization, closed reduction with percutaneous pinning, and ORIF (Fig. 23-9).[34] If cast immobilization is used to stabilize the joint, the patient is placed in the cast for 6 to 12 weeks, depending on the severity of the injury.[34] If closed reduction and internal fixation is required, the wrist is immobilized for about 2 months. After two months, the pins are removed, and the arm is placed in a cast for an additional 4 weeks.[34] With an ORIF procedure, the ligaments are directly repaired and the unstable carpal articulations are stabilized with wires or pins. The duration of immobilization is similar to that for closed reduction with percutaneous pinning.[34]

Regardless of the severity of the injury, the principles for rehabilitation are the same.[10] The initial goals are to

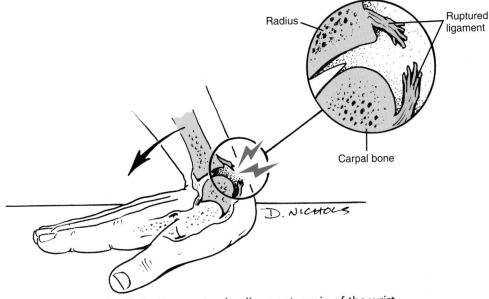

Fig. 23-8 Hyperextension ligament sprain of the wrist.

control pain and inflammation through the use of cold and electrical stimulation and to prevent edema through elevation, massage, light external compression wraps, and frequent digit active ROM within the limits of the immobilization. When the immobilization is removed, gentle, active, pain-free motion can begin in all planes. It is important to include forearm rotation and differential tendon glides between the wrist and fingers. As motion improves and pain subsides, submaximal isometric contractions can be used, progressing to resistance exercises and gradual closed-chain exercises. The last step is to gradually increase the speed of movement. Exercising with a metronome is helpful. Sustained gripping and concentric and eccentric exercises improve wrist strength. Protection of the wrist continues well into the final recovery stages of rehabilitation and the use of a wrist splint is encouraged in between exercise sessions.

Triangular Fibrocartilage Complex

Pain in the ulnar side of the wrist may indicate an injury to the triangular fibrocartilage complex (TFCC). The TFCC is formed by ligaments and an articular disk between the ulna and the ulnar carpal bones.[16] Injury to the TFCC can occur from an axial force applied to the ulnar side of the wrist during weight bearing and gripping (as in gymnastics) or a fall on the palm with the forearm pronated. The ulna is longer compared with the radius when the forearm is pronated.[16] This can lead to an ulnocarpal impaction syndrome that results in a torn articular disk and damage to the ulnar head and lunate. Distal radial fractures resulting in a loss of radial length can also leave the ulna longer than the radius. The central disc of the complex has poor blood supply so healing tears in it is difficult.[38] Treatment initially involves rest and splinting of the wrist and elbow to prevent

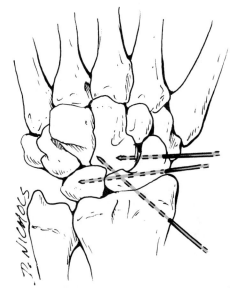

Fig. 23-9 Insertion of pins for stabilization after ligament sprain with carpal instability.

forearm rotation for 4 to 6 weeks, then a gradual program of ROM exercises and progressive strengthening.[38] Exercises should begin in supination, then progress to neutral, with pronated gripping and weight bearing being the final stage.[16] If the symptoms are not relieved by conservative methods, arthroscopic débridement or ulnar shortening are considered.[38]

Skier's Thumb

Skier's thumb is an acute sprain of the ulnar collateral ligament of the thumb. The mechanism of injury is a sudden valgus stress and hyperextension of the thumb, which results in either a partial ligament tear or a complete rupture (Fig. 23-10).[35]

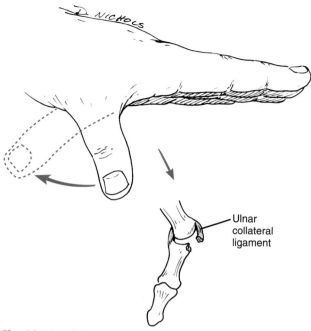

Fig. 23-10 Skier's thumb, also referred to as *gamekeeper's thumb.* Sudden valgus stress and hyperextension can result in partial or complete rupture of the ulnar collateral ligament of the thumb.

Partially torn ligaments can be treated nonsurgically with a thumb spica cast or rigid immobilization. The thumb carpal metacarpal (CMC) joint is abducted to 30° and the IP joint is left free for exercise. The splint is worn continuously for 3 to 4 weeks.[11,38] Edema reduction techniques are used as needed. At 3 to 4 weeks, the splint can be removed for active thumb MP and composite CMC, MP, and IP joint motion. Progressive strengthening can begin at 5 to 6 weeks and the protective splint is decreased except for heavy activities. Unrestricted use is delayed until 3 months postinjury.

Complete injuries may require surgery because they can be associated with a fracture of the proximal phalanx, or the distal end of the ligament may be displaced by the adductor muscle insertion preventing healing (Stener lesion).[11,38] A short arm thumb spica cast is applied for approximately 4 weeks.[35] The IP joint is left free and active flexion and extension is started immediately to prevent adherence of the extrinsic tendons. At 4 weeks, the cast is replaced by a splint and the program progresses as discussed earlier except strengthening, which should be cleared by the surgeon—usually at about 6 weeks. Scar massage and nightly application of silicon to the scar should help flexibility. The goal is a pain-free, stable thumb with pinch and grip values comparable to the uninjured hand. Unrestricted use is permitted around 3 month postsurgery.[1]

De Quervain Disease

De Quervain disease is a condition affecting the abductor pollicis longus and the extensor pollicis brevis tendons and sheaths (Fig. 23-11).[36] These tendons comprise

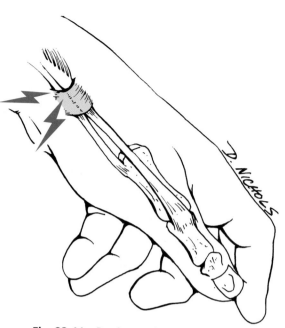

Fig. 23-11   De Quervain tenosynovitis.

the first dorsal extensor compartment and pass through a fibro-osseous tunnel lined with synovium between the distal radius and the extensor retinaculum. Repeated tension, such as that from simultaneous abduction and extension of the thumb and medial and lateral deviation and extension of the wrist, creates friction that can lead to swelling and thickening of the connective tissue and narrowing of the tunnel.[13,36] While many sources describe the process as a tendinitis, or an inflammation of the tendon, or tenosynovitis, an inflammation of the sheath, others dispute this finding and refer to it as a tendinosis or degeneration of the tendon cells and collagen.[2]

The disease presents as pain on the radial side of the wrist that is aggravated by use of the thumb. Swelling and, in some cases, nodules may be palpable. Pain is increased by ulnar deviation of the wrist when the thumb is clasped in the palm (Finkelstein test)[13,36] It is a cumulative trauma disorder frequently caused by overuse of the hand and wrist.[13]

Traditional conservative management includes activity modification aimed at avoiding the provocative motions and/or wrist and thumb immobilization. In addition, ice and high voltage, pulsed, galvanic electrical stimulation (HVPGS) may help symptoms. Iontophoresis is frequently ordered, but its effectiveness has not been established.[2] Passive motion in the pain-free range of the wrist and thumb should be done daily and progression to active motion can begin as tolerated. Strengthening can be initiated once active ROM is pain free and should emphasize eccentric as well as concentric motions of the wrist and thumb. All muscles of both thumbs should be strengthened because they have been shown to be weak compared with normal individuals.[8] The speed of ROM should gradually be increased as the final step in rehabilitation. Patients should be prepared for a recovery time of months rather than weeks.[2]

If conservative care fails to relieve symptoms, the physician may inject the first dorsal compartment with a corticosteroid to reduce pain and inflammation. Chronic cases of De Quervain disease require surgical release of the compartment. The affected wrist is immobilized for approximately 1 week with a compression bandage. The surgeon will indicate when exercises can begin as directed by the PT, with specific attention directed to tendon gliding, pain, and scar management once the sutures are removed. Resistance can progress as outlined under the conservative program.

Tendon Injuries

Tendon injuries are classified into zones according to the location of injury. There are different zones for extensor tendons as compared with flexor tendons. The management of tendon injuries is precise and is determined by the level of injury, the type of repair, and any associated injuries.

Extensor Tendon Injuries

Injuries to the extensor tendons are often treated as trivial, but they require careful management to maintain the dynamic balance of the fingers and wrist. Extensor muscles are weaker than the flexors so restoration of strength is important. On the back of the hand, these tendons are superficial and have a large surface area that makes them susceptible to injury and adhesions.[27] An in-depth discussion of all levels of injury and methods of repair is beyond the scope of this text, but two of the more common injuries are discussed below. The PTA should follow the PT's instructions precisely when working with an extensor tendon repair.

Mallet finger

Interruption of the extensor tendon mechanism over the DIP joint (zone 1) is referred to as a *mallet finger*. These injuries can be purely tendon or can include a fracture of the distal phalanx (Fig. 23-12). The imbalance that is created by the unopposed force of the flexor digitorum profundus muscle, positions the DIP joint in flexion and, with time, may lead to hyperextension of the PIP, resulting in a "swan neck deformity"[27] With either tendon rupture or avulsion fracture, the treatment is the same. The recommended treatment of a closed injury is continuous, uninterrupted splinting of the DIP joint for 6 weeks in hyperextension with the PIP joint free. The splint may require modification as swelling subsides, but care should be taken to not allow the DIP to change position during the adjustment. Active flexion and extension of the PIP joint begins immediately, but the adjacent finger DIP joints are not actively exercised. At 6 weeks, active flexion of the DIP joints begins. Initially, only 20° of flexion is allowed. The extension splint is reapplied at night for 4 more weeks. The patient is advised against

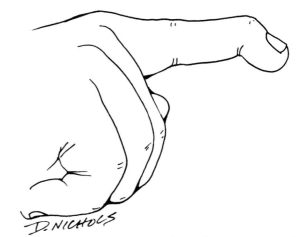

Fig. 23-12 Mallet finger. Avulsion fracture or tendon rupture results in distal interphalangeal joint flexion contracture.

using a strong muscle effort, and passive flexion is contraindicated. The flexion angle is increased each week as long as full extension is maintained. Full active flexion is delayed until at least 3 months postinjury. If an extension lag develops, full-time splinting is resumed.[5,27]

The patient should be informed that full motion may take 6 months. If the patient is noncompliant, a K-wire may be inserted to maintain the extended position. This is removed at 6 weeks and the program progresses as discussed earlier.

Boutonnière deformity

Interruption of the central tendon and triangular ligament at the PIP joint (zone III) allows the head of the proximal phalanx to herniate dorsally resulting in a boutonnière deformity (Fig. 23-13).[27] This displacement leads to imbalance between the intrinsic and extrinsic muscles of the finger. The resultant position of the finger is flexion of the PIP joint and hyperextension of the DIP. If the deformity can be corrected passively, the finger is held in full PIP extension for 6 weeks with the MP and DIP joints free. The goal is to approximate the ends of the tendon so they can heal together. The PTA should alert the PT if swelling decreases and the splint or cast is loose, requiring remolding. Active and passive DIP flexion is encouraged. After 6 weeks, active motion of the PIP is initiated but the digit is splinted in between sessions for 2 to 4 weeks. Just as with the mallet finger, the patient gradually increases active flexion of the PIP joint. The splint is gradually decreased as long as full PIP extension is maintained. The patient should be warned that treatment may be required for 6 to 9 months.[27]

If the deformity cannot be passively reduced or is associated with a fracture or other injury, surgical intervention is indicated. The postoperative course will depend on the structures repaired and the specific procedure performed.

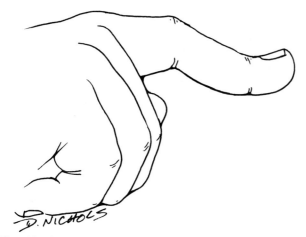

Fig. 23-13 Boutonnière deformity, proximal interphalangeal flexion with distal interphalangeal extension.

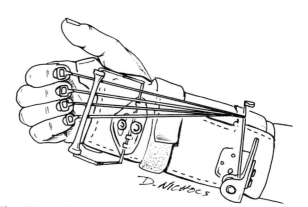

Fig. 23-14 Postoperative protective splint with rubber band traction after flexor tendon repair.

Flexor Tendon Injuries

The restoration of function following a flexor tendon injury requires careful balance between protecting the repair and gliding the tendon. The goal of surgery and therapy is a strong repair that glides freely. The flexor sheath and the pulley system in the digits provide a smooth gliding surface that is mechanically efficient. The level of the repair, the timing, the suture pattern and strength and any associated nerve or blood vessel injury all affect the timing of therapy. Even the most carefully applied program can result in stretching, gapping, or even rupture of the repair. Failure to glide the tendon will result in scarring within the pulley system and loss of active flexion. Ideally, these cases should be managed by a certified hand therapist (CHT) (either a physical or an occupational therapist with advanced training in hand rehabilitation) who is in close communication with the hand surgeon.

As with extensor tendons, the flexor tendons are classified into zones. The most difficult is zone 2, which extends from the level of the MP joints to the insertion of the flexor digitorum superficialis (FDS) just distal to the PIP joint. Injuries in this zone may involve both the FDS and the FDP tendons.[31]

There are presently three approaches to flexor tendon rehabilitation and the choice depends on the factors listed earlier as well as the patient's ability to comply.[31] In all of the methods, the flexor tendon is held on slack with wrist flexion, the MP joints flexed, and the IP joints allowed full extension.

1. Immobilization: Following repair, the wrist and hand are casted or splinted for 3 to 4 weeks before beginning active and passive exercise. This is generally reserved for children or adults who are unable to cooperate in their care.
2. Early passive mobilization: Passive flexion and active extension are allowed within the limits of the splint. Rubber band traction is sometimes used to pull the fingers passively into flexion (Fig. 23-14).
3. Early active mobilization: With these programs, the tendon is moved actively within 48 hours of repair and within carefully outlined limits set by the surgeon. These programs are only for the most compliant patient who can attend therapy frequently.

The splint is worn for about 4 weeks. After the initial 4 weeks, it may be modified to move the wrist into neutral and active motion is progressed. Specific progression to isolated joint motion or passive extension should be discussed in detail with the PT and surgeon.

Strengthening is initiated at about 8 weeks and the patient is generally informed that return to full, unrestricted use will take 3 months at a minimum.[31] If the tendon becomes adherent and cannot glide, surgery will be considered to free the tendon from the scar.

Dupuytren Disease

Dupuytren disease in the hand is first observed with the formation of pits and firm nodules that lie just below the skin of the palm (Fig. 23-15).[18] The nodules can be composed of overactive fibroblasts producing collagen or can be from "bunching" of the skin in response to a longitudinal contraction of the underlying fascia.[18] This tissue is not random, but appears along longitudinal tension lines in the palm or digits. The tissue undergoes contraction and maturation resembling that of normal wound healing. There is no known "trigger" but the tissue becomes thicker and eventually forms cords that become firm and tendon-like and the affected digits and thumb lose extension. The progression is variable and will be limited to nodules in some patients or progress to full flexion of the affected digits in others. Patients may report some tenderness with pressure on the nodules but pain is not a primary complaint. The greatest incidence is in white males of northern European descent, although it has been reported in all races and both sexes.[28] Initially, treatment is centered on patient reassurance and education. Reported conservative treatment includes the injection of steroids that may soften

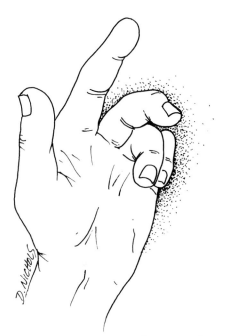

Fig. 23-15 Dupuytren contracture most commonly affects the ulnar digits, with flexion contracture of the ulnar metacarpal phalangeal joint.

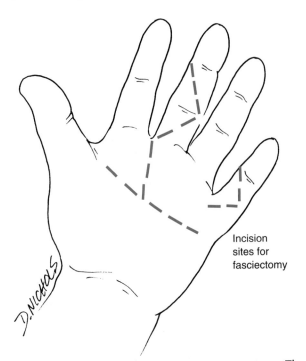

Incision sites for fasciectomy

Fig. 23-16 Fasciectomy for Dupuytren contracture. The dotted lines represent the surgical incision that is usually left open and not sutured together.

the nodules or collagenases, which are chemicals known to break down collagen.[3]

Once the disease interferes with function, a surgeon should be consulted. There is disagreement regarding the best surgical approach for treatment, but there are four main techniques currently in the literature.[17] They are:

1. Fasciotomy: cutting the contracted fascia blindly by inserting a small blade
2. Regional fasciectomy: removal of only the diseased fascia (Fig. 23-16)
3. Extensive fasciectomy: removal of the diseased tissue and any tissue with the potential of becoming diseased
4. Dermofasciectomy: removal of the skin overlying the diseased tissue as well as the diseased tissue. This is replaced by a full thickness skin graft or in some cases, left open to granulate in.

The goals of physical therapy postoperatively are to optimize the conditions for wound repair, minimize edema and pain, maintain the surgically achieved extension, gain full composite flexion and restore muscle balance around the affected joints.

Immediately after surgical release, the patient is fitted with a dorsal blocking splint that allows active flexion but limits full extension at the MP joints.[5,23] This splint is used for the first 2 to 3 weeks to avoid tension and vascular compromise in the healing incisions. Static, volar extension splints can be added at 10 days. After the incisions have closed, the dorsal splint is replaced by a hand-based volar splint that holds MPs as well as the IP joints in the full available extension. This splint is worn

an average of 3 months postoperatively at night and for short periods during the day, depending on the patient's ability to maintain the extension during wound and scar maturation. The CHT designs, fabricates, and adjusts the splints. The PTA should check the fit at each visit and alert the CHT when volume changes or improvements in the ROM necessitate splint adjustment. Wound care may include use of the whirlpool to loosen devitalized tissue, but care should be taken to avoid a completely dependent position because of edema concerns. Elevation, retrograde massage, and external compression can assist with edema reduction. If a skin graft was used, the donor site should also be monitored. The application of specific cross-fiber scar massage and silicon are appropriate once the wounds have healed. The PT should be consulted before massage is started on the skin graft margins. Active ROM emphasizing composite and isolated joint flexion and extension, abduction and adduction of the MP joints and opposition of the thumb should begin immediately postoperatively but care should be taken to avoid tension across the suture lines. Sensation should be monitored and protective techniques should be taught to those patients whose sensibility is compromised. Paresthesias often result from stretching the digital nerves and should resolve as healing progresses. The PTA should be aware of the early signs of CRPS. If this is suspected, it is important to inform the PT so the treatment program can be modified appropriately[23,25] (see later discussion). Passive ROM, gradual strengthening, and closed-chain weight bearing can begin as soon as wound healing permits.

Carpal tunnel syndrome

A **compression neuropathy** occurs when adjacent structures constrict a peripheral nerve, limiting its blood supply and resulting in impaired nerve conduction. Specific sites have been associated with compression of the radial, ulnar, and median nerves. If the adjacent tissue restricts gliding of the nerve, the nerve will be subjected to stretch that can also result in paresthesias and pain. This is referred to as a *nerve entrapment.* The most common compression neuropathy in the upper extremity is that of the median nerve at the wrist.[32]

Carpal tunnel syndrome (CTS) refers to the symptoms that occur when the median nerve is compressed or entrapped at the wrist. The carpal tunnel is formed by the carpal bones and the transverse carpal ligament and contains the median nerve and nine flexor tendons (Fig. 23-17). Increased friction and pressure within the tunnel constrict the nerve and produce sensory problems such as decreased sensation, pain, and tingling; and motor problems including loss of the thenar intrinsic muscles (flexor pollicis brevis [FPB], abductor pollicis brevis [ABPB] and opponens pollicis [OP], and loss of the first two lumbrical muscles.

There are many possible causes for CTS, including anatomic changes from arthritis, fractures, or cysts; systemic conditions such as diabetes, hypothyroidism, aging, pregnancy, or alcohol abuse; environmental factors such as solvent exposure or decreased temperatures; and occupational factors such as tasks requiring forceful, repeated motions in extreme postures (cumulative trauma), or vibration.[32]

The clinical symptoms of CTS include numbness of the thumb and radial digits, tingling, pain that is often worse at night, clumsiness in hand activity, weakness of grip and pinch, atrophy of the thenar muscles, and swelling in the hand and forearm.[12,22]

Conservative physical therapy management of carpal tunnel syndrome focuses on identifying and altering the factors that may produce symptoms. Extreme flexion or extension of the wrist compress the contents of the tunnel, so patient education should be directed to avoiding these positions. Anything that constricts the wrist such as tight sleeves, watchbands and bracelets or applies pressure over the median nerve when the pronated arm is resting against a desk can contribute to the problem. Custom splints that hold the wrist in 0° to 20° of extension should be worn day and night[22] for several weeks to keep the carpal tunnel open. Deep (1 MHz) pulsed ultrasound, nerve gliding exercises, carpal bone mobilization, and yoga have all been shown to be successful in reducing the symptoms.[22]

Medical management may include nonsteroidal antiinflammatory drugs (NSAIDs), or the physician may elect to inject the area with a corticosteroid to reduce

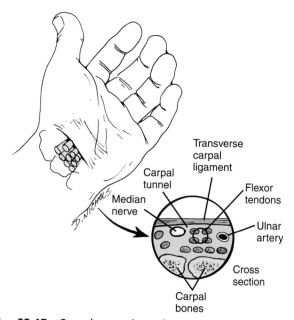

Fig. 23-17 Carpal tunnel syndrome. Compression neuropathy of the median nerve.

pain and swelling.[12] Failure of nonoperative treatment or the presence of thenar atrophy are indications for surgical intervention. In surgery, the transverse carpal ligament is divided and any inflammatory tissue removed. The wrist is immobilized for 1 to 2 weeks, but digit ROM can begin immediately. The patient is taught to avoid simultaneous wrist and finger flexion in order to avoid bowstringing of the flexor tendons. Nerve gliding and differential tendon gliding (Fig. 23-18) is emphasized to avoid adhesions.

When healing permits, scar massage is initiated and silicon can be used. Gradual, controlled, weight bearing on the palm is also helpful. The patient should be informed that full weight bearing may be painful for 6 months. Strengthening is started after suture removal and progressed as tolerated. Return to work should include patient education to avoid possible contributing factors as described earlier.

Complex Regional Pain Syndrome

One of the most difficult problems in hand rehabilitation is the treatment of CRPS. This term is used for clinical conditions in which the pain resulting from an injury is abnormally severe and/or prolonged compared with that of a normal postinjury response. This includes conditions such as reflex sympathetic dystrophy (RSD) and causalgia, but has replaced the use of these terms.[14,39] CRPS is further subdivided into type 1: without a nerve injury, and type 2: with a nerve injury. Both of these categories are further subdivided based on the presence or absence of sympathetic nerve involvement.[14]

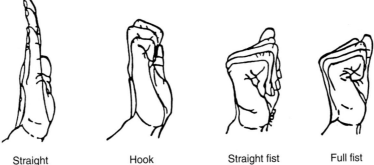

Straight   Hook   Straight fist   Full fist

Fig. 23-18 Nerve gliding and differential tendon gliding exercises. (From Hayes EP, Carney K, Wolf J, et al: Carpal tunnel syndrome. In Mackin E, Callahan AD, Skirven TM, et al: *Rehabilitation of the hand and upper extremity*, ed 5, St Louis, 2002, Mosby.)

Signs and symptoms

The presentation of this syndrome is variable, but there are four primary characteristics:

- Pain: This can range from localized pain to a delayed, abnormally painful reaction to light touch that extends beyond the actual location of the stimulus.[14,39] These patients often cannot tolerate any spontaneous touch; even air blowing on the extremity can produce extreme pain.
- Trophic changes: Atrophy results in differences in hair and nail growth, shiny, tight skin, loss of fat pads in the fingertips, and osteopenia.[14,15,39]
- Autonomic disturbances: This system controls microvascular perfusion and sweat gland activity. The patient may present with the affected fingers being warm or cool compared with the other side. There may be profuse sweating or extreme dryness of the skin. Edema usually is present. There may be dramatic color changes from pale and cyanotic, to mottled to red and warm, all within the same treatment session. Increased sympathetic nerve activity may also lead to increased pilomotor activity (goose bumps).[14,15,39]
- Functional impairment: The patient is reluctant to use the hand and/or entire extremity because of pain. Fine and gross coordination are disturbed. A typical, imbalanced hand posture is assumed with the MPs in extension and PIPs in either flexion or extension. The patient may have difficulty localizing tactile stimuli and may have an altered perception of his own hand, regarding it as foreign.[7]

Incidence

This condition is seen in both sexes, but is most prevalent in 30- to 55-year-old women. There is a higher incidence in smokers. The most common injury associated with CRPS is fracture of the distal radius and ulna.[14] Patients often report a tight cast as their first sign of discomfort. Other surgeries complicated by postoperative CRPS include carpal tunnel release, De Quervain release, distal ulna surgery, and dermofasciectomy for Dupuytren release.[14]

Diagnosis

The diagnosis is made based on clinical criteria, and early recognition and treatment are the best predictors of pain relief and functional recovery.[14] Bone scans, radiographs, cold stress tests, and microvascular perfusion tests contribute to the confirmation of the diagnosis.[14,39] PT evaluations of pain threshold, fine and gross coordination, grip strength, and ROM provide additional information.[14,15,39] The use of agents that interrupt the sympathetic nervous system differentiate types of CRPS and are used as part of the treatment when the sympathetic system is implicated.[14,15,38]

Treatment

A multidisciplinary approach including the surgeon, internist, pain specialist, PT, PTA, psychologist, and/or psychiatrist is recommended.[14,15,39] Pharmacological management falls into two categories: analgesics to relieve pain, and drugs that affect the sympathetic nerves, such as antidepressants and corticosteroids.[14,39] Surgery may be considered to correct the underlying source of pain, if it is identified. This can be a nerve entrapment, neuroma, or joint derangement.[14]

The PTA is in the optimum position to observe and report the patient's response to treatment and may be the first clinician to notice the onset of symptoms. Care should be taken to avoid increasing the symptoms. Pain control must be implemented before therapy can progress. Pain control may be helped by the use of heat or cold modalities, contrast baths in which extremes of temperature are avoided, transcutaneous electrical nerve stimulation, continuous passive motion (CPM), and hydrotherapy. Desensitization programs and sensory reeducation techniques can help. Edema should be treated through positioning, compression garments, and intermittent compression pumps, as the patient may not tolerate retrograde massage.

The entire limb should be treated with special attention to the shoulder because adhesive capsulitis is frequently present.[38] Maintenance of motion is a primary goal. Splints are used between exercise sessions to help prevent contractures and reduce pain. Active ROM with special attention to the MP and PIP joints, isometrics, and gentle, pain-free passive ROM can be used. Light, bimanual activities can help integrate the involved extremity and restore movement patterns. Aerobic activities to increase cardiac output may help stabilize the vasomotor system and assist the patient to feel some physical accomplishment. Joint mobilization is not indicated and can be detrimental. Positive results have been reported for stress loading programs. These programs use active distraction and compression of the extremity during which the patient alternates weight-bearing scrubbing with weighted carrying. This provides proprioceptive input to the extremity without joint motion.[33]

The treatment of these patients requires patience and creativity on the part of the PTA. Recovery is usually gradual and is dependent on the full, active participation of the patient.

MOBILIZATION OF THE WRIST AND HAND

The use of peripheral joint mobilization techniques can be quite effective to modulate pain and increase motion of the wrist and hand. The specific applications of these techniques are determined by the PT, and the appropriate direction and amplitude of force are dictated by the specific injury and degree of soft-tissue and bone healing.

Moist heat, electrical stimulation, and gentle active exercise can be used immediately before mobilization to encourage soft-tissue relaxation and evacuation of waste from the injured area. In addition, physician-prescribed analgesics, muscle relaxants and NSAIDs, may be effective before beginning mobilization techniques.

The position of the patient is a critical feature of effective mobilization. The injured extremity must be positioned to provide comfort, relaxation, and support while affording the clinician access to the extremity.

As with other joints, many different techniques are used. This discussion introduces only a few of the more common and easily performed techniques. The intricate and complex nature of the wrist and hand demands mastery of anatomy, kinesiology, pathomechanics of injury, and biomechanics to effectively perform the more difficult techniques described in orthopedic texts.[37]

Mobilization of the Wrist

Anterior, posterior, medial, and lateral glides of the wrist are performed with the patient either sitting with the affected arm supported or supine. The PTA uses one hand to stabilize the distal radius and ulna on the dorsal aspect while firmly grasping the proximal row of carpal bones with the other hand.[37] Using the hand supporting the carpal bones, the PTA directs an anterior and posterior force or a medial and lateral force to "glide" the carpal bones from the stabilized distal radius and ulna (Fig. 23-19).[37]

Distraction of the carpals is done with the patient either sitting or supine. The hand position is exactly the same as described in the preceding, but the direction of force is distal or longitudinal to the radius and ulna. This direction of force distracts or displaces the carpal bones from the stabilized radius and ulna (Fig. 23-20).[37]

Mobilization of the Hand

Anterior, posterior, medial, and lateral glides of the MP joint can be performed with the patient supine or sitting. The PTA uses one hand to stabilize the shaft of the affected metacarpal while firmly grasping the proximal phalanx with the other hand. With the metacarpal firmly stabilized, the PTA uses the hand contacting the phalanx to direct an anterior, posterior, or medial and lateral force that glides the MP joint (Fig. 23-21).[37]

Distraction of the MP joint occurs with the patient in the same position as described in the preceding. With the hand placement the same, the direction of force is applied to distract the phalanx from the stabilized metacarpal (Fig. 23-22).[37]

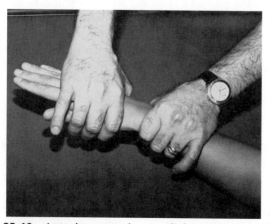

Fig. 23-19 Anterior-posterior, medial, and lateral glides of the wrist.

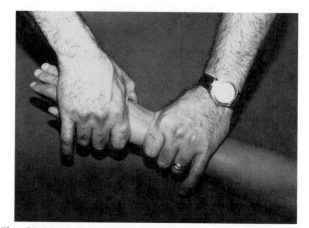

Fig. 23-20 Long axis or longitudinal distraction of the wrist.

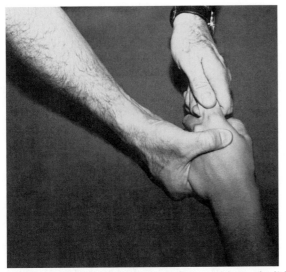

Fig. 23-21 Anterior-posterior, medial, and lateral glides of the metacarpal phalangeal joint.

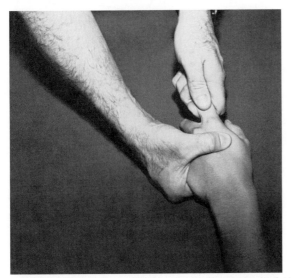

Fig. 23-22 Long axis or longitudinal distraction of the metacarpal phalangeal joint.

✤ GLOSSARY

Bennett fracture: Fracture of the palmar base of the proximal first metacarpal.

Boxer's fracture: Fractures of the neck of the fourth or fifth metacarpal caused by a strike to a hard object with a clenched fist.

Carpal tunnel syndrome: A group of symptoms that occur when the median nerve is compressed or entrapped at the wrist.

Colles fracture: A radius fracture within 2.5 cm of the wrist in which the distal fragment is displaced in a dorsal direction.

Compression neuropathy: Disorder that occurs when adjacent structures constrict a peripheral nerve, limiting its blood supply and resulting in impaired nerve conduction.

Dinner fork deformity: The deformity seen following a Colles fracture due to the position of the wrist and forearm resembling a dinner fork.

Mallet finger: Interruption of the extensor tendon mechanism over the DIP joint.

Nerve entrapment: Disorder that occurs when adjacent tissue restricts gliding of the nerve. The nerve will be subjected to stretch that can result in paresthesias and pain.

Smith fracture: A type of fracture also known as a *reverse Colles fracture* that occurs from a fall on the dorsum of the hand, with the resultant distal radial fragment displaced in a palmar direction.

REFERENCES

1. Amadio PC, Taleisnik J: Fractures of the carpal bones. In Green DP, Hotchkiss RN, Pederson WC, editors: *Green's operative hand surgery*, Philadelphia, 1999, Churchill Livingstone.
2. Ashe MC, McCauley T, Khan KM: Tendinopathies in the upper extremity: a paradigm shift, *J Hand Ther* 3:329–334, 2004.
3. Badalamente MA, Hurst LC: Efficacy and safety of injectable mixed collagenase subtypes in the treatment of Dupuytren's contracture, *J Hand Surg Am* 32:767–774, 2007.
4. Brach P, Goitz R: An update on the management of carpal fractures, *J Hand Ther* 16:152–160, 2003.
5. Evans RP, Dell PC, Fiolowski P: A clinical report of the effect of mechanical stress on functional results after fasciectomy for Dupuytren's contracture, *J Hand Ther* 15:331–339, 2002.
6. Fernandez DL, Palmer AK: Fractures of the distal radius. In Green DP, Hotchkiss RN, Pederson WC, editors: *Green's operative hand surgery*, Philadelphia, 1999, Churchill Livingstone.
7. Forderreuther S, Sailer U, Straube A: Impaired self-perception of the hand in complex regional pain syndrome, *Pain* 110:756–761, 2004.
8. Forget N, Piotte F, Bourbonnais D, et al: Thumb strength and mobility in de Quervain's disease, *J Hand Ther* 4:441–442, 2006.
9. Freedland A, Hardy M, Singletary S: Rehabilitation for proximal phalangeal fractures, *J Hand Ther* 16:129–142, 2003.
10. Frykman G, Kropp WE: Fractures and traumatic conditions of the wrist. In Hunter JM, Schneider LH, Mackin EJ, et al, editors: *Rehabilitation of the hand*, St Louis, 1995, Mosby.
11. Glickel SZ, Barron OA, Eaton R: Dislocations and ligament injuries in the digits. In Green DP, Hotchkiss RN, Pederson WC, editors: *Green's operative hand surgery*, Philadelphia, 1999, Churchill Livingstone.
12. Hunter JM, Davlin LB, Fedus LM: Major neuropathies of the upper extremity: the median nerve. In Hunter JM, Schneider LH, Mackin EJ, et al, editors: *Rehabilitation of the hand*, St Louis, 1995, Mosby.
13. Kirkpatrick WH, Lisser W: Soft tissue conditions: trigger fingers and Dequervains's disease. In Hunter JM, Schneider LH, Mackin EJ, et al, editors: *Rehabilitation of the hand*, St Louis, 1995, Mosby.
14. Koman AL, Poehling G, Smith TL: Complex regional pain syndrome: reflex sympathetic dystrophy and causalgia. In Green DP, Hotchkiss RN, Pederson WC, editors: *Green's operative hand surgery*, Philadelphia, 1999, Churchill Livingstone.
15. Lankford L: Reflex sympathetic dystrophy. In Hunter JM, Schneider LH, Mackin EJ, et al, editors: *Rehabilitation of the hand*, St Louis, 1995, Mosby.
16. La Stayo P, Lee MJ: The forearm complex: anatomy, biomechanics and clinical considerations, *J Hand Ther* 2:137–145, 2006.
17. McFarlane RM, MacDermid JC: Dupuytren's disease. In Hunter JM, Schneider LH, Mackin EJ, et al, editors: *Rehabilitation of the hand*, St Louis, 1995, Mosby.
18. McGrouther DA: Dupuytren's contracture. In Green DP, Hotchkiss RN, Pederson WC, editors: *Green's operative hand surgery*, Philadelphia, 1999, Churchill Livingstone.

19. McNemar T, Howell J, Chang E: Management of metacarpal fractures, *J Hand Ther* 16:143–151, 2003.
20. Melone CP: Fractures of the wrist. In Nicholas JA, Hershman EB, editors: *The upper extremity in sports medicine*, St Louis, 1990, Mosby.
21. Meyer FM, Wilson RL: Management of non-articular fractures of the hand. In Hunter JM, Schneider LH, Mackin EJ, et al, editors: *Rehabilitation of the hand*, St Louis, 1995, Mosby.
22. Muller M, Tsui D, Schnurr R, et al: Effectiveness of hand therapy interventions in primary management of carpal tunnel syndrome: a systematic review, *J Hand Ther* 2:210–228, 2004.
23. Mullins PA: Postsurgical rehabilitation of Dupuytren's disease, *Hand Clin* 1:167–174, 1999.
24. Page S, Stern P: Complications and range of motion following plate fixation of metacarpal and phalangeal fractures, *J Hand Surg Am* 23:827–832, 1998.
25. Prosser R, Conolly WB: Complications following surgical treatment for Dupuytren's contracture, *J Hand Ther* 9:344–348, 1996.
26. Reiss B: Therapists' management of distal radial fractures. In Hunter JM, Schneider LH, Mackin EJ, et al, editors: *Rehabilitation of the hand*, St Louis, 1995, Mosby.
27. Rosenthal E: The extensor tendons: anatomy and management. In Hunter JM, Schneider LH, Mackin EJ, et al, editors: *Rehabilitation of the hand*, St Louis, 1995, Mosby.
28. Ross DC: Epidemiology of Dupuytren's disease, *Hand Clin* 1: 53–62, 1999.
29. Singletary S, Freeland A, Jarrett C: Metacarpal fractures in athletes: treatment, rehabilitation and safe early return to play, *J Hand Ther* 6:171–179, 2003.
30. Stern P: Fractures of the metacarpals and phalanges. In Green DP, Hotchkiss RN, Pederson WC, editors: *Green's operative hand surgery*, Philadelphia, 1999, Churchill Livingstone.
31. Stewart KM, Van Strien G: Postoperative management of flexor tendon injuries. In Hunter JM, Schneider LH, Mackin EJ, et al, editors: *Rehabilitation of the hand*, St Louis, 1995, Mosby.
32. Szabo RM: Entrapment and compression neuropathies. In Green DP, Hotchkiss RN, Pederson WC, editors: *Green's operative hand surgery*, Philadelphia, 1999, Churchill Livingstone.
33. Watson HK, Carlson L: Treatment of reflex sympathetic dystrophy of the hand with an active "stress loading" program, *J Hand Surg* 12 (5Pt1):779–785, 1987.
34. Wilgis EFS, Yates AY: Wrist pain. In Nicholas JA, Hershman EB, editors: *The upper extremity in sports medicine*, St Louis, 1990, Mosby.
35. Wilson RL, Hazen J: Management of joint injuries and intraarticular fractures of the hand. In Hunter JM, Schneider LH, Mackin EJ, et al, editors: *Rehabilitation of the hand*, St Louis, 1995, Mosby.
36. Wolfe S: Tenosynovitis. In Green DP, Hotchkiss RN, Pederson WC, editors: *Green's operative hand surgery*, Philadelphia, 1999, Churchill Livingstone.
37. Wooden MJ: Mobilization of the upper extremity. In Donatelli R, Wooden MJ, editors: *Orthopaedic physical therapy*, ed 3, St Louis, 2009, Churchill Livingstone.
38. Wright HH, Rettig AC: Management of common sports injuries. In Hunter JM, Schneider LH, Mackin EJ, et al, editors: *Rehabilitation of the hand*, St Louis, 1995, Mosby.
39. Zhongyu L, Paterson Smith B, Smith TL, et al: Diagnosis and management of complex regional pain syndrome complicating upper extremity recovery, *J Hand Ther* 2:270–276, 2005.

REVIEW QUESTIONS

Short Answer

1. Name the most common compression neuropathy of the wrist.
2. A fracture-subluxation of the proximal first metacarpal describes what type of fracture?

3. Identify the injuries or deformities in the following figures.

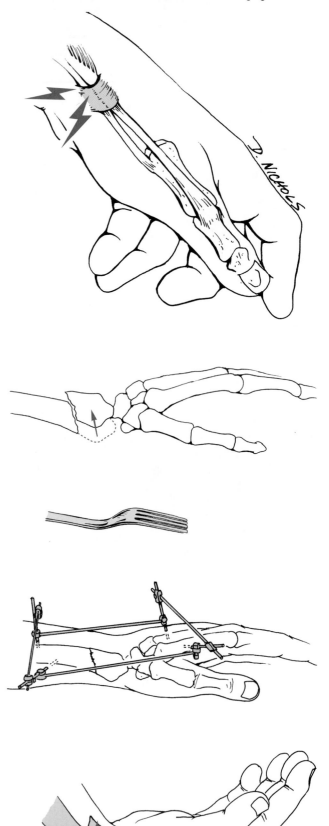

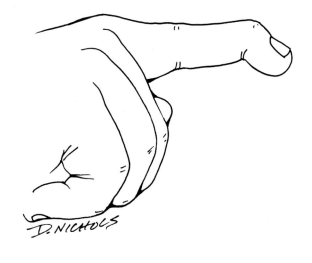

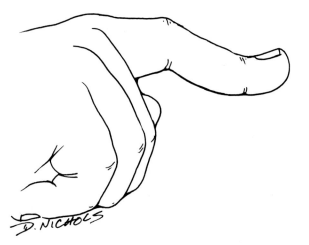

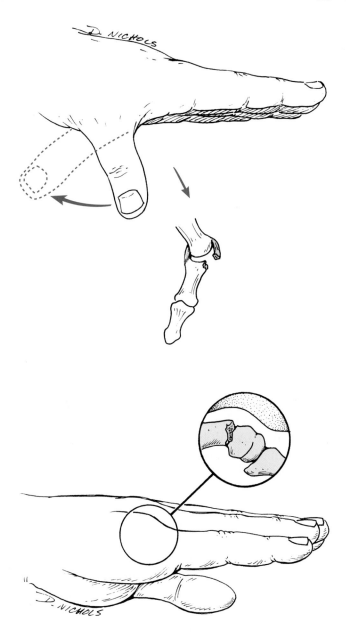

4. A rupture or avulsion fracture of the extensor tendon that results in a DIP joint flexion contracture is called _____ .

5. A rupture or stretch of the central extensor tendon at the PIP joint that creates PIP flexion with DIP extension is called a

_____ .

True/False

6. Generally, motions that produce repetitive ulnar deviations can create tenosynovitis at the first dorsal compartment of the wrist.

7. The stability of the wrist is primarily dependent on musculotendinous support and intracapsular ligaments.

8. A Colles fracture is the most common of all wrist fractures.

9. AROM of the fingers in a Colles fracture patient should start when the cast is removed.

10. Scaphoid fractures are considered the most common fractures that occur to the carpal bones.

11. Although occasionally tender nodules are present, Dupuytren disease is commonly not painful.

12. Surgery should be considered for a patient with Dupuytren disease if the loss of finger extension interferes with his function.

13. There is usually a direct relationship between the severity of injury and the degree of pain experienced by persons suffering from CRPS.

14. It is true that at no point in the course of recovery from RSD is aggressive active motion prescribed in the presence of pain.

PART VI

MANAGEMENT OF ORTHOPEDIC CONDITIONS BY AFFLICTION

In this section, the physical therapist assistant (PTA) is introduced to essential, common, and foundational principles of rheumatic diseases, pain management, and components of bracing, orthotics, and prosthetics. Within the daily provision of physical therapy practice, spanning most settings, the PTA will be exposed to and responsible for the delivery of services related to rheumatic disease, pain, and the application of bracing, orthotics, and prosthetics. The management of these critical conditions and services require knowledge of sound scientific principles of anatomy, physiology, and pathomechanics. Most importantly, however, is the sober and responsible application of treatment strategies delivered under the direction of the supervising physical therapist, which this section provides for the student and practicing clinician.

Consistent with the corpus of information in this text, the PTA is presented information related to foundations of disease processes and pathology of rheumatic diseases, as well as neuroanatomy and pathophysiology of pain management. The PTA is introduced to the materials, components, use, and application of various braces, orthotics and prosthetics. Foremost in this section is the relevant clinical application of therapeutic interventions in light of the basic science motif established and endorsed throughout the text.

In the study of this section, students and clinicians are strongly encouraged to carefully and thoroughly review Part II, "Review of Tissue Healing" (Chapters 7 through 12), Part IV, "Mobilization and Biomechanics" (Chapters 14 through 16), and Part V, "Management of Orthopedic Conditions by Region" (Chapters 17 through 23). Each of these sections provide the essential material on which to ground practical, functional, and purposeful interventions using established basic science knowledge of tissue healing, biomechanics, and orthopedic pathologic conditions.

24 Rheumatic Disorders

Steven Elliott

LEARNING OBJECTIVES

1. Identify causes of arthritis.
2. Discuss different types of arthritis.
3. Discuss similarities and differences for osteoarthritis and rheumatoid arthritis.
4. Discuss the effects and benefits of exercise with arthritis.
5. Discuss common methods of management and rehabilitation of arthritic conditions.
6. Discuss principles of joint protection.
7. Discuss general pharmacologic interventions for arthritic conditions.
8. Discuss the different surgical options for arthritic conditions.
9. Discuss pathophysiology and management of rheumatic disorders.

KEY TERMS

Atrophy

Closed-chain exercises

Connective tissue

Infection

Inflammation

Malaise

Open-chain exercises

Proteoglycan

CHAPTER OUTLINE

Arthritis affects the lives of 37 million Americans, and it is the leading cause of disability in American adults. The Centers for Disease Control and Prevention (CDC) estimate that by the year 2020 nearly 60 million people will be affected by rheumatic disease, a blanket term covering the more than 100 different conditions that may cause pain, stiffness, and sometimes swelling in or around joints.[2,15] Individuals affected with arthritis can suffer from pain, joint stiffness, swelling, and overall decrease in functional ability.[23] The causes of arthritis are not fully understood, but there are certain characteristics that can predispose an individual to developing arthritis, include obesity, inactivity, age, and gender.[15,23] Though the prevalence of arthritis increases with age, it is more commonly found in women than in men.[15,23]

ARTHRITIS

Osteoarthritis

Osteoarthritis (OA) is the most common form of arthritis and generally the most painful and disabling joint disorder.[2,15,19,26] There is no single cause of osteoarthritis; however, it may be a combination of biomechanical, metabolic, and genetic factors.[24,26] Prevalence of OA has been shown to increase with age and is more common in women older than 45 years of age. Risk factors associated with OA include obesity, trauma, **infection**, and repeated joint overuse.[2,15,19,26]

OA primarily affects the articular cartilage (which is composed of type II collagen, chondrocytes, and proteoglycans) that surrounds the subchondral bone (Fig. 24-1).[2,24] Patients with OA have decreased synthesis and increased catabolism of the cartilage matrix. OA initially damages the cartilage, causing it to become thinner and thereby decreasing **proteoglycan** synthesis. Initially chondrocytes can maintain the cartilaginous matrix (which consists of proteoglycans and collagen), but after time focal synovial membrane **inflammation** develops, releasing cytokines, which increase the release of metalloproteinases.[2] Metalloproteinase further breaks down cartilage collagen and proteoglycans.[2,15] Generally OA is not considered to have any inflammatory response, but new research shows signs of inflammation can exist.[2,15]

Osteoarthritis most commonly effects weight-bearing joints, such as the knee, hip, or spine.[2,15,23,24] Joints in the hands can also be affected: the first carpometacarpal joint, distal and proximal interphalangeal joints (DIP and PIP joints, respectively), and the first metatarsophalangeal joint are other common sites for OA.[24] In patients with OA of the hands, Bouchard and Heberden nodes, bony overgrowths at the PIP joints and the DIP joints, are often present (Fig. 24-2).[19,24,27] Pain associated with OA usually occurs with activity and is relieved with rest.[19,24] Other signs of OA include morning stiffness lasting 20 to 30 minutes, joint locking, a gel sensation in the joint, a bony appearance of the joint, crepitus, and effusion.[19,24] Radiographic imaging can show a progression of subchondral bone sclerosis and cysts, osteophytes, and joint space narrowing.[13,24] Carpal tunnel syndrome can even be caused by both osteoarthritis and rheumatoid arthritis (RA).[27]

Management of Osteoarthritis

Although there is no cure for OA, preventive measures can be taken to slow down the progression of the disease or better manage the symptoms. Obesity places extra stress on joints and is a key risk factor that can be prevented or remedied with proper diet and exercise.[19,24] The addition of vitamin D and calcium to a patient's diet can also reduce the occurrence and progression of OA.[19] Muscle weakness and repetitive motions or trauma contribute to the onset of OA.[24] Studies also have shown that immobilizing the joint for longer than 30 days can increase the risk of cartilage damage.[4] Given the positive and negative effects of changes in behavior it is imperative to educate the patient on joint protection, health behavior changes, and the importance of exercise to the management of arthritis.

Education is the most important component to the management of OA. Patients must be educated on the progression of the disease and management of pain with supportive devices, alteration in activities of daily living (ADLs), or thermal modalities. Exercise and weight control are key components to a patient's success with OA.[2,24]

Research has shown that every pound of body weight increases the forces in the knee by 2 to 3 pounds during single leg stance.[38] Exercise, specifically flexibility, and strength training, has been shown to decrease pain and improve function in individuals with OA.[24] Maintaining flexibility is an important first step because it helps decrease stiffness and allows for more comfortable movement.[2]

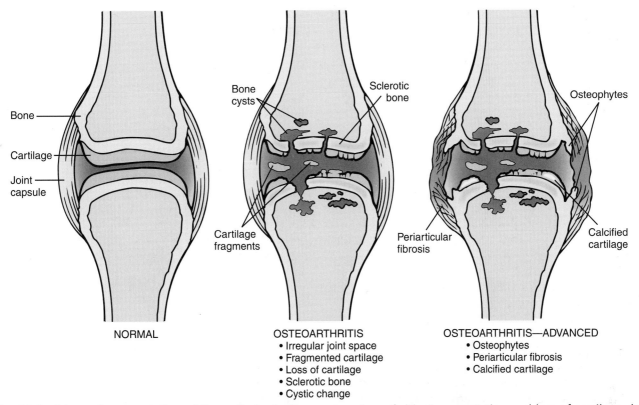

Bone

Cartilage

Joint capsule

Bone cysts

Sclerotic bone

Cartilage fragments

NORMAL

OSTEOARTHRITIS
- Irregular joint space
- Fragmented cartilage
- Loss of cartilage
- Sclerotic bone
- Cystic change

Osteophytes

Periarticular fibrosis

Calcified cartilage

OSTEOARTHRITIS—ADVANCED
- Osteophytes
- Periarticular fibrosis
- Calcified cartilage

Fig. 24-1 Schematic presentation of the pathologic changes in osteoarthritis. Fragmentation and loss of cartilage denude the subchondral bone, which undergoes sclerosis and cystic change. Osteophytes form on the lateral side and protrude into the adjacent soft tissues, causing irritation, inflammation, and fibrosis. (From Damjanov I: *Pathology for the health-related professions*, ed 3, Philadelphia, 2006, Saunders.)

Slow progression of the exercise program is important so as to not exacerbate symptoms. Patients should be progressed to 15 minutes of stretching without an increase in symptoms before initiating strength training.[2,24] Strength training improves the ability to absorb shock, support joints, and protect from injury.[2,26] When choosing an appropriate exercise it is important to keep in mind how much stress in being placed on the joint. **Closed-chain** weight-bearing exercises can create shear and compressive forces across the lower extremity joints and may be a contraindication pending severity of OA. **Open-chain exercises,** therefore, are encouraged in patients with OA.

Rheumatoid Arthritis

Rheumatoid arthritis is the second most common form of arthritis, and while it can be equally disabling as OA, it can also lead to increased mortality. This increased mortality has been shown in some research to have systemic causes.[12] The progression of RA also leads to difficulty with ADLs and disability. Along with most arthritic conditions, RA affects women more commonly than men and occurs at 20 to 40 years of age.[2,14,19] Both genetic and environmental factors have been linked as causes of RA.[14,19]

Although the exact etiology of RA is unknown, it is believed to start with a viral or bacterial infection that triggers an autoimmune response.[2,14] The immune response causes the body to attack its own tissue, leading to breakdown of joints.[2,14] RA affects the synovium lining, which then expands, damaging the extracellular matrix, cartilage, and bone.[2,14,26] This autoimmune response also activates T cells, which secrete cytokines, causing expansion of the synovial layer. Cytokines increase activation of fibroblast-like cells and macrophages leading to breakdown of cartilage and bone (Fig. 24-3).[2,14]

Early signs and symptoms associated with RA include fatigue, weight loss, fever, and musculoskeletal pain. Later signs or symptoms include pain, tenderness, swelling, redness, and stiffness in specific joints.[2,7,14,19] Unlike OA, RA morning stiffness can last hours and even all day. Fatigue in patients with RA may cause the patient to need to rest through the day.[2] Extraarticular manifestations can affect the lungs, heart, blood vessels, eyes, skin, and other organs.[2,7,19] It is important for the physical therapist assistant (PTA) to be able to distinguish the main differences between OA and RA (Table 24-1).

A unique feature of RA is the rheumatoid nodules, which occur on bony prominences, extensor surfaces, or pressure points.[2,19] There are several common physical changes that occur[36]:
- In the fingers and toes
  - Swelling of the joint
  - Hyperflexion and extension

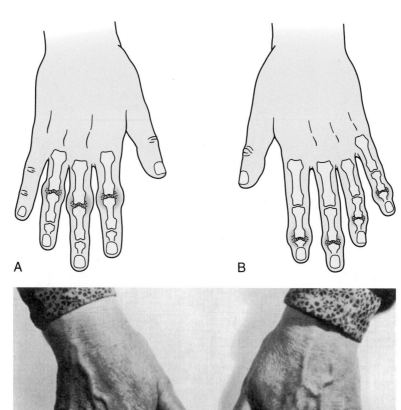

Fig. 24-2 Degenerative joint disease (osteoarthritis) of both hands. **A,** Bouchard nodes. **B,** Heberden nodes. **C,** Osteoarthritic enlargement of the distal interphalangeal joints (Heberden nodes) and the proximal interphalangeal joints (Bouchard nodes) is present. The metacarpal phalangeal joints are not affected. (**A** and **B,** From Magee DJ: *Orthopedic physical assessment,* ed 5, St Louis, 2008, Saunders. **C,** From Polley HF, Hunder GG: *Rheumatologic interviewing and physical examination of the joints,* Philadelphia, 1978, Saunders.)

- Volar subluxation
- Ulnar deviation
- Hallux valgus
- Hammer toes
- In the hand
  - Swan neck deformity (hyperextension of PIP and flexion of DIP)
  - Boutonnière deformity (flexion of PIP with hyperextension of DIP)
  - Ulnar deviation of fingers

Management of Rheumatoid Arthritis

When treating a patient with RA, education and prevention are vital. Some important objectives of physical therapy all have a common theme of prevention: prevent pain, deformities, loss of normal function, and loss of normal social, physical, and work capabilities. An exercise routine should start with stretching and range of motion (ROM) exercises in pain-free ranges,[2,14] and patients with RA should be informed not to overstretch an inflamed tissue to avoid any tears. To prevent contractures and muscular **atrophy** it is crucial to maintain full ROM of joints through a graded exercise routine.[14] Muscle conditioning is also a key component of management, and strength can be increased through isometric and dynamic exercise. Application of heat before exercise can result in better performance.[19] Generally during an acute exacerbation, isometric exercises are recommended. During subacute and chronic phases patients can implement dynamic exercise. Do note that

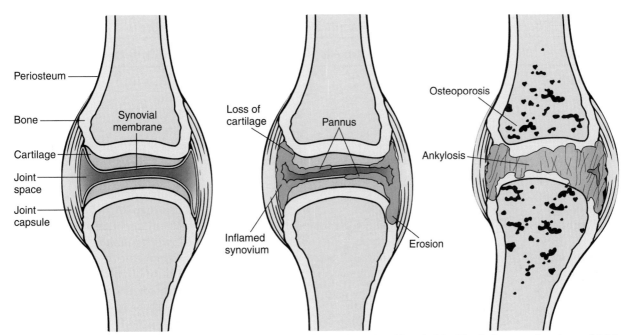

Fig. 24-3 Schematic presentation of the pathologic changes in rheumatoid arthritis. The inflammation (synovitis) leads to pannus formation, obliteration of the articular space, and finally ankylosis. The periarticular bone shows disuse atrophy in the form of osteoporosis. (From Damjanov I: *Pathology for the health professions*, ed 3, St Louis, 2006, Saunders.)

vigorous activity should be avoided during an exacerbation of symptoms. Any exercise that causes pain longer than 1 hour after exercise should be eliminated.[19]

The current management approach with medication is to start early with disease-modifying antirheumatic drugs (DMARDs) because they have been shown to slow RA progression. Nonsteroidal antiinflammatory drugs (NSAIDs) are the most commonly used drugs to decrease pain and swelling and increase ROM. Corticosteroids are also used for swelling, pain, and fatigue and tend to decrease symptoms faster. Biological response modifiers block cytokines, therefore decreasing the breakdown of cartilage and bone.[14] More in-depth explanation of the pathophysiology of these drugs will be explained later.

Reactive Arthritis

Reactive arthritis, or Reiter syndrome, is most commonly an abrupt onset of arthritis in young men presenting with the triad, conjunctivitis, urethritis, and oligoarticular arthritis.[7,18,19] Conjunctivitis is also known as *pinkeye*, which is inflammation of the conjunctiva (outermost layer of eye and inner surface of eyelid). Urethritis is inflammation of the urethra and presents as painful urination. Oligoarthritis is a form of arthritis with inflammation in two to four joints. Reiter syndrome usually presents within days or weeks of a dysenteric or sexually transmitted infection.[18,19] The arthritis is usually asymmetrical and involves the weight-bearing joints, such as the toes, ankles, and knees, then ascends to the axial skeleton and upper extremities.[7,18,19] Other symptoms present with Reiter syndrome are oral ulcers, penile lesions, keratoderma blennorrhagicum, and plantar

heel pain.[7,19] Approximately 80% of individuals with Reiter syndrome are positive for human leukocyte antigen B27 (HLA-B27).[7,19] The human leukocyte antigen system is the name of the major histocompatibility complex in humans. The major HLA antigens are essential elements in immune function. Sacroiliitis is observed in about 60% of patients with chronic Reiter syndrome. Management of Reiter syndrome includes NSAIDs and physical therapy similar to that used to treat ankylosing spondylitis.

Psoriatic Arthritis

Psoriatic arthritis is a seronegative inflammatory joint disease affecting a small percentage of people with psoriasis.[13,19] Psoriasis is an inherited chronic inflammatory skin disease that is characterized by silvery scales on a bright red plaque (Fig. 24-4).[5,13] In most cases the skin disease precedes the arthritis symptoms by several months to years.[9] Psoriatic arthritis closely resembles rheumatoid arthritis, but has differences such as DIP involvement, psoriasis or family history, nail pitting, and "sausage" appearance of digits.[7,14,19] Gender does not appear to predispose one to psoriatic arthritis, but it generally begins at ages 30 to 50 years.[9,13,18] Psoriatic arthritis is usually asymmetric and involves the small joints of hands and feet.[7,13,32] However, larger axial joints such as the sacroiliac joint can be affected in later phases of disease. Sacroiliitis usually occurs unilaterally, whereas ankylosing spondylitis is bilateral.[13,18] Imaging reveals a "pencil-in-cup" deformity caused by erosion and destruction of the phalanx bones that makes them look like a sharpened pencil at the end of the bone

Table 24-1	*Differential Diagnosis between Rheumatoid Arthritis and Osteoarthritis*	
Differential	**Rheumatoid Arthritis**	**Osteoarthritis**
Joints affected	Any joint	DIP > PIP
		Spine
		Hip
		Knee
Age	Any age	More common >40 years
	Most common ages 20-60 years	
Gender	More common in women	More common in men <45 years and women >45 years
Relative severity	More than OA	Less than RA
Disease pathogenesis	Autoimmune: Immune system attacks body	Condition of wear and tear with aging or injury
Joint involvement	Symmetric	Asymmetric
Joint destruction	Due to inflammation	Due to biomechanical stress
Deformities	Swan neck	Heberden nodes
	Ulnar deviation	Bouchard nodes
	Wrist subluxation	
	Boutonniere deformity	
Erythrocyte sedimentation rate	Markedly increased	Mild increase
Connective tissue flexibility	Increased	Decreased
Morning stiffness	>1 hour	<30 minutes
Rheumatoid factor	Positive in 70%	Negative
Imaging	Juxtaarticular osteoporosis, erosions	Osteophytes
		Eburnation
		Reduced joint space
Management	Physical therapy/occupational therapy	Paracetamol
	NSAIDs	Weight loss
	Gold	Joint replacement
	Penicillamine	Exercise
NSAID response	Usually some relief	Variable relief

(Fig. 24-5).[5,7,32] Furthermore, psoriatic arthritis can cause fingernail thickening, pitting, and separation from the nail bed.[9] Finally, periosteal reactions (formation of new bone) can be seen on x-rays.

Management for psoriatic arthritis is similar to that of rheumatoid arthritis.[7,18,32] Although there is no cure for psoriatic arthritis, NSAIDs can be used to treat inflammatory symptoms.[5,13] Most of the time the disease is mild and not destructive; therefore treatment consists of symptom management.[5,13]

Juvenile Rheumatoid Arthritis

Many rheumatic diseases in children exist, consisting of both acute and chronic conditions, with juvenile rheumatoid arthritis (JRA) being one of the most common.[44] JRA, a chronic inflammatory disease, actually covers three types of childhood arthritis: pauciarticular, polyarticular, and systemic.[7,13,32,44] The etiology of JRA is unknown, but is thought to be triggered by environmental factors or infection in children with genetic predisposition.[13,44] "JRA is similar to adult RA in the fact that the immune system mistakenly attacks the joints and organs, causing inflammation, destruction, fatigue, and other local and systemic effects."[13] JRA occurs before the age of 16 years and affects girls more commonly.[7,13,44] To confirm diagnosis the child must have the arthritis for at least 6 consecutive weeks.[44] Other symptoms of JRA are fever, rash, fatigue, anemia, loss of appetite, stiffness, irritability, altered mobility, and change in ADLs.[44]

Pauciarticular JRA is characterized by asymmetric synovitis of four or less joints.[7,13,44] There are usually no systemic features and it most commonly affects the knee, elbow, and ankle (Fig. 24-6).[13,44] Two subtypes of pauciarticular JRA exist: early onset and late onset.[7,13,44] Early onset pauciarticular JRA occurs before the age of 5 years and usually affects girls. Early onset pauciarticular JRA left untreated can result in iridocyclitis that can lead to visual impairments.[7,13,44] The second subtype, late onset pauciarticular JRA, occurs between the ages of 10 and 12 years and is more common in boys. This subtype affects large weight-bearing joints and entheses (insertion point of tendon into bone).[44] These children

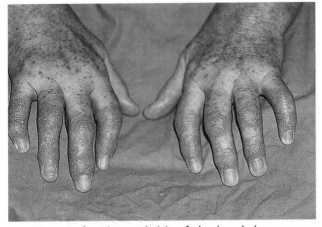

Fig. 24-4 Deforming arthritis of the hands in a person with psoriatic arthritis. (From Callen JP, Greer K, Paller A, et al: *Color atlas of dermatology*, ed 2, Philadelphia, 2000, Saunders.)

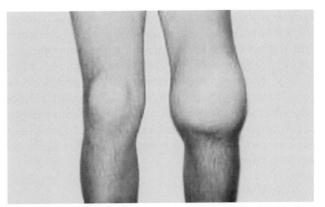

Fig. 24-6 An affected knee in a patient with pauciarticular juvenile rheumatoid arthritis. (From Kliegman RM: *Nelson essentials of pediatrics*, ed 5, St Louis, 2006, Saunders.)

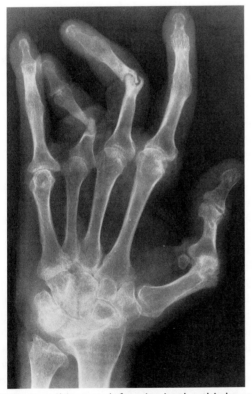

Fig. 24-5 Pencil-in-cup deformity in the third proximal interphalangeal joint and bony ankylosis involving the wrist and phalanges of second and fifth digits. (From Eisenberg RL: *Comprehensive radiographic pathology*, ed 4, St Louis, 2008, Mosby.)

often have spinal involvement that may develop into a spondyloarthropathy.[13,44]

Polyarticular JRA is synovitis in more than four joints and is more common in girls.[7,13,44] It usually manifests with symmetrical involvement of the small joints of the hands or feet, wrists, elbows, shoulders, knees, hips, ankles, cervical spine, and temporomandibular joints.[13,44] Bursitis and tendinitis can occur because they too are lined with synovial tissue. Unlike pauciarticular JRA, polyarticular JRA can have systemic features, including low grade fever, anemia, leukocytosis, mild hepatosplenomegaly, and lymphadenopathy.[44]

The last type of JRA is systemic JRA (Still disease) which can occur at any age and does not favor girls or boys.[13,44] Systemic JRA is characterized by a rash, synovitis in one or more joints, and an intermittent high grade fever.[7,13,44] The fever usually occurs in the afternoon and evenings and will return to normal with the child feeling better.[13,44] Because the fever can precede all other symptoms these children are often initially evaluated for fever of unknown origin.[44] The rash usually appears with the fever and is salmon pink, 2 to 5 mm in diameter, and has an erythematous perimeter.[44] Other signs and symptoms of systemic JRA include **malaise**, irritability, anemia, hepatitis, peptic ulcer disease, leukocytosis, thrombocytosis, lymphadenopathy, hepatomegaly, splenomegaly, pericarditis, and pleuritis.[13,44]

Management of Juvenile Rheumatoid Arthritis

Management for children with JRA is a combination of medication, physical therapy, and occupational therapy. Main objectives of therapy should be to control pain and inflammation, promote mobility, and improve function.[13,44] Control of pain and inflammation is usually done with NSAIDs, which have been shown to decrease stiffness, pain, and swelling in children with JRA. Other medications used with JRA are corticosteroids, DMARDs, infliximab, and immunosuppressants.[13,44] ROM is the strongest indicator of functional disability in children with systemic JRA.[13] Therefore, all joints should be stretched through the full ROM twice a day to maintain good mobility.[44] Heat can be used before stretching to help warm the muscles and decrease pain before stretching. Splinting and serial casting can also be used to help maintain or gain ROM.[44] Resistive exercise is also important and has been shown to change the immune response, with lower levels of cytokines and higher levels of antiinflammatory compounds.[13] Aquatic therapy is an appropriate management for JRA because the heat can help relax the muscles and decrease pain.[44] Even though the patient with JRA is only a child, education in joint protection and energy conservation is still important. Furthermore, always try to make the exercise program fun, interesting, and interactive to keep the child involved.[44]

Septic Arthritis

Septic arthritis is the invasion of a joint by an infectious agent causing arthritis. Septic arthritis usually occurs from a bacterial infection, but can be viral, mycobacterial, or fungal. Bacteria are introduced into the joint by the bloodstream from an infection elsewhere or from direct penetration after a wound, surgery, or local infection.[42] Two common types of septic arthritis are gonococcal and nongonococcal.[19,42]

Gonococcal Arthritis

Gonococcal arthritis usually occurs in healthy individuals and is two to three times more common in females.[19,42] Initially the patient will experience 1 to 4 days of noninflammatory joint pain in the wrist, ankle, knee, and elbow. Chronic arthritis or tendonitis are common symptoms preceding gonococcal arthritis.[42] Patients tend to have a characteristic asymptomatic skin lesions with 2 to 10 small necrotic pustules over the extremities, especially the palms and soles.[19]

Management of gonococcal arthritis

Gonococcal arthritis usually responds well to drug therapy in 24 to 48 hours, and therefore is not as destructive as nongonococcal bacterial infections.[19,42]

Nongonococcal Arthritis

Nongonococcal bacterial infections are primarily monoarticular and in large weight-bearing joints and wrists.[19,42] Previous joint damage from a disease like RA or intravenous drug users have increased risk of infection.[19,42] *Staphylococcus aureus* is the most common cause of nongonococcal septic arthritis.[19,42] Nongonococcal septic arthritis is marked by a sudden onset of acute arthritis with pain, swelling, and heat in one joint.[19] The hip, wrist, shoulder, and ankle can all be affected, but the knee is the most common. Chills and fever often accompany the symptoms of nongonococcal septic arthritis.[19]

Management of nongonococcal arthritis

Management should be initiated quickly with systemic antibiotics addressing the causative organism. If the specific organism cannot be determined then bacterial antibiotics are recommended.[19] Aspiration of the affected joint will keep the joint free of destructive exudates.[19,42]

Early intervention is important because ankylosis and articular damage can occur if management is delayed. Immobilization and heat can help decrease the joint pain.[19] Rest, elevation, and immobilization are used during the acute phase of the disease.

As stated before, early diagnosis and management are important because of the potential for harm if septic arthritis goes untreated.[42] Risk factors to keep in mind are infection elsewhere in the body, very old or young age, presence of other systemic diseases, recent joint aspiration or surgery, prosthetic joints, immunosuppression, and intravenous drug abuse.[13,42] An infected joint will be painful, tender, and have limited motion, but may not have redness, heat, and swelling, especially if treatment includes immunosuppressants.[42] Finally, remember that prevention is always a key component of physical therapy, so passive and then active ROM should be started as soon as possible to prevent contractures and loss of strength.[42]

Arthritic Conditions of the Spine

Arthritic conditions of the spine, otherwise known as *spondyloarthropathies*, have their main effect on the axial skeleton. Clinically the patient will have low back pain that increases with rest and improves with activity. Spondyloarthropathies have the following characteristics:

- They run in families.
- They are more common in men.
- Onset is before the age of 40 years.
- Patients generally have inflammatory arthritis of the spine or the large peripheral joints.
- Patients have an absence of autoantibodies in the serum.
- They are associated with the presence of HLA-B27.[19]

Ankylosing Spondylitis

Ankylosing spondylitis is a type of inflammation that affects the synovium of the spinal arthrodial joints as well as all the joint ligaments of the spine at their insertion points into the bone (enthesitis). It begins in the sacroiliac joints in nearly all patients and spreads superiorly up the spine.[18] As the disease progresses the spine becomes more rigid (ankylosed) and develops flexion deformities.[18] The disease also leads to formation of bony bridges called *syndesmophytes* between the vertebra. Structurally the patients will lose the lumbar curve, have reduced chest expansion, and have an increase in thoracic kyphosis.[18,22] Other changes noted in radiographic imaging are squaring of vertebrae and destruction of the sacroiliac joints[32] (Fig. 24-7).

Ankylosing spondylitis has a greater incidence in men and the age of onset is usually in the late teens to early 20s.[18] Hypomobility is likely to be seen in men between ages 40 and 50 years and in women older than 50 years.[27] Patients with ankylosing spondylitis usually will complain of alternating buttock pain that radiates down the thigh and that increases with rest

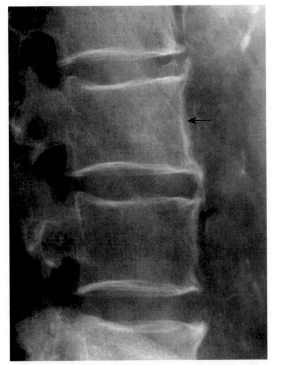

Fig. 24-7 Ankylosing spondylitis of the spine. There is vertebral body squaring resulting from mineralization of the anterior longitudinal ligament, which fills in the normal anterior concavity of the vertebral body *(arrow)*. (From Adam: A, Dixon AK, Grainger RG, et al: *Grainger & Allison's diagnostic radiology: a textbook of medical imaging*, ed 5, Philadelphia, 2008, Churchill Livingstone.)

but decreases with activity, a hot bath, or a shower.[18] Patients may show signs of peripheral arthritis such as swelling, redness, and tenderness. Constitutional symptoms include fever, fatigue, weight loss, and elevated erythrocyte sedimentation rate (ESR).[18] Ankylosing spondylitis can often be confused with sacroiliac arthritis, however there are several differences between these two diseases (Table 24-2).

Management of ankylosing spondylitis

Management for ankylosing spondylitis includes both physical therapy and drug therapy. Early rehabilitation of ankylosing spondylitis is crucial because it has been shown to significantly reduce the impact of disability.[18] Therapeutic exercise along with antiinflammatory drug therapy is important in managing ankylosing spondylitis. Benefits of exercise include improved mobility, posture, and function. Education is key to starting management of patients with ankylosing spondylitis. Patients should try to exercise when pain level is low and they are least tired. Starting an exercise session with heat application and light motion exercises can help loosen the joints and decrease pain for exercise.[18] Before starting the patient on a strengthening regimen, the therapist should always try to improve mobility of the spine, which can reduce pain and stiffness in the patient.[18] Physical therapy should focus on stretching the anterior flexor muscles and strengthening the extensors. Specifically, therapy should focus on strengthening

Table 24-2	Differential Diagnosis between Ankylosing Spondylitis and Sacroiliac Arthritis	
Differential	**Ankylosing Spondylitis**	**Sacroiliac Arthritis**
History	Bilateral sacroiliac pain that may refer to posterior thigh	Bilateral sacroiliac pain referring to gluteal area (S1-S2 dermatomes)
	Morning stiffness	Morning stiffness (prolonged)
	Male predominance	Coughing painful
Observation	Stiff, controlled movement of pelvis	Controlled movement of pelvis
Active movement	Decreased	Side flexion and extension full
		Slight limitation of flexion
Passive movement	Decreased	Normal
Resisted isometric movement	Pain and weakness, especially if sacroiliac joints are stressed	Pain, especially if sacroiliac joints are stressed
Special tests	Sacral stress tests probably positive	Sacral stress tests probably positive
Sensation and reflexes	Normal	Normal
Palpation	Tender over sacroiliac joints	Tender over sacroiliac joints
Diagnostic Imaging	X-rays diagnostic	X-rays diagnostic
Lab tests	Erythrocyte sedimentation rate increased	Normal
	HLA-B27 human leukocyte antigen present in 80%	

From Magee DJ: *Orthopedic physical assessment*, ed 5, St Louis, 2008, Saunders.

the postural muscles, back and neck extensors, shoulder retractors, and hip extensors and abductors.[18] A prone program is a good management option to stretch the anterior muscles.[18] Postural exercises are also beneficial, including standing against a wall with heels, buttocks, and shoulders touching the wall. Also, patients should try to sleep with as much extension as tolerable and lay prone at least 15 minutes a day.[18] Aquatic therapy is another management option that can help reduce discomfort and provide an avenue for relaxation, stretching, and strengthening.[18] Finally, breathing exercises are important because of the decreased chest expansion that occurs with ankylosing spondylitis.

Pharmacologic intervention is usually NSAIDs to help decrease pain and stiffness, allowing for normal ADLs and exercise. Indomethacin is the most effective NSAID used with ankylosing spondylitis for decreasing night pain and morning stiffness.[18,19] Sulfasalazine, which reduces the levels of acute phase reactants, may act as a "disease-modifying" agent. Sulfasalazine can decrease the peripheral symptoms associated with ankylosing spondylitis. Immunosuppressant drugs are reasonable for the severe cases when a patient cannot participate in physical therapy.[18,19]

NONARTHRITIC RHEUMATIC DISEASES

Gout

Gout is a metabolic disorder characterized by deposition of monosodium urate crystals in the joints, soft tissue, kidneys, and other connective tissue (Fig. 24-8).[7,13,19,42] Once urate crystals are present they can cause acute or chronic inflammation by stimulating inflammatory mediators.[7,13,19,32,42] The deposition of monosodium urate crystals is the outcome of hyperuricemia, which is the presence of high levels of uric acid in the blood. Hyperuricemia is due to the overproduction and/or underexcretion of uric acid.[7,13,19,32,42] Overproduction of uric acid is more common in individuals with a history of lymphoma, leukemia, or psoriasis.[13,19] Overproduction can also be due to enzyme abnormalities, hematologic malignancies, or other causes of rapid cell turnover.[42] Underexcretion of uric acid is more common with obesity, fasting, medication (such as diuretics or cyclosporin), renal insufficiency, hypertension, hypothyroidism, hyperparathyroidism, and acidosis.[13,19,42] Alcoholism increases risk of gout by both increasing production and decreasing the renal excretion of uric acid.[13,19,42]

Gout most commonly affects men older than the age of 30 years with occasional cases in postmenopausal women.[7,13,19,42] Acute monoarticular onset of inflammatory arthritis that is worst at night characterizes gout. Although the metatarsophalangeal joint of the great toe is the most common site of pain, the ankle, knee, wrist, elbow, and fingers can all be affected.[13,19,42] The involved joints usually become tender, swollen, warm, and red.[13,19,42] A fever often occurs along with the joint complaints.[13,19] The early initial episodes only last 3 to 10 days and then a patient can go months to years with no symptoms.[13,19,42] Severe gouty attacks suddenly return with more frequency affecting more joints and lasting longer.[13,19,42] The gout can become chronic with multiple joint damage leading to loss of function and disability.[13,19] Tophi, visible deposits of crystallized

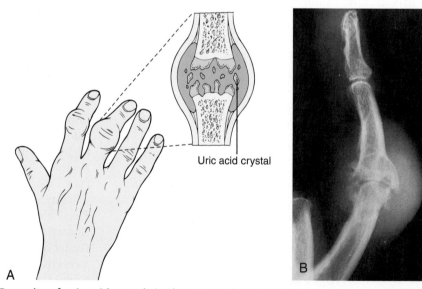

Fig. 24-8 Gout. **A,** Deposits of uric acid crystals in the connective tissue have a chemotactic effect and cause exudation of leukocytes into the joint. **B,** Severe joint effusion and periarticular swelling of proximal interphalangeal joint of finger. **(A,** From Frazier MS, Drzymkowski JW: *Essentials of human diseases and conditions,* ed 2, Philadelphia, 2000, Saunders; **B,** From Eisenberg RL: *Comprehensive radiographic pathology,* ed 4, St Louis, 2008, Mosby.)

monosodium urate, usually occur several years after the first episode of gout.

Management of Gout

Management of acute gout focuses on the arthritis and then addresses the hyperuricemia.[13,19] NSAIDs are the most common management for acute gout decreasing both inflammation and pain.[13,19,42] Corticosteroids are also used, but mainly when a patient has a contraindication for NSAIDs.[19] Another management option is to use drugs to inhibit tubular reabsorption of uric acid to promote urinary excretion.[39] Furthermore, rest, elevation, and joint protection are important during acute gout to further promote decreased inflammation.[13,42] Between or after the acute attacks hyperuricemia is addressed to help prevent future episodes.[13,19,42] Management when symptom free includes changes in diet, avoidance of hyperuricemic medications, colchicine, and reduction of serum uric acid. Dietary changes that can decrease the risk of gout are weight loss, moderation of alcohol, and avoidance of high purine foods.[13,19] Controlling the hyperuricemia is important to prevent gout from becoming chronic.[13]

Fibromyalgia

Fibromyalgia is a chronic widespread muscle pain syndrome.[8,13,19,21] By definition fibromyalgia is widespread pain lasting at least 3 months with physical findings of 11 to 18 tender points (Fig. 24-9).[8,13,21] Common characteristics of fibromyalgia are chronic widespread pain, aching, fatigue, and stiffness. Patients may also complain of headaches, sleep disorders, mood disorders, irritable bowel syndrome, and paresthesias.[28] Fibromyalgia is most common in women aged 20 to 50 years.[8,13,19] The exact etiology and pathogenesis of fibromyalgia is not fully understood, but is thought to be disturbances in different systems of the body. One common thought is that pain results from abnormalities of central sensory processing.[8] New research characterizes fibromyalgia as a biological disorder associated with neurohormonal dysfunction of the autonomic nervous system (ANS) because of the objective biochemical, endocrine, and physiologic abnormalities.[13] Furthermore, abnormalities in the hypothalamic–pituitary–adrenal axis, reproductive hormone axis, ANS, and immune system have been found in patients with fibromyalgia.[13] The onset

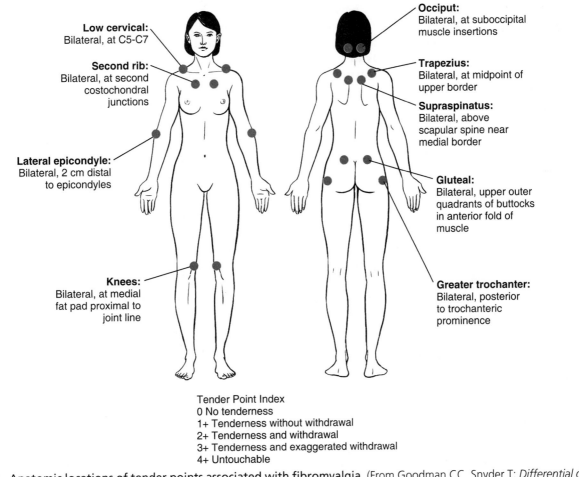

Low cervical:
Bilateral, at C5-C7

Second rib:
Bilateral, at second costochondral junctions

Lateral epicondyle:
Bilateral, 2 cm distal to epicondyles

Knees:
Bilateral, at medial fat pad proximal to joint line

Occiput:
Bilateral, at suboccipital muscle insertions

Trapezius:
Bilateral, at midpoint of upper border

Supraspinatus:
Bilateral, above scapular spine near medial border

Gluteal:
Bilateral, upper outer quadrants of buttocks in anterior fold of muscle

Greater trochanter:
Bilateral, posterior to trochanteric prominence

Tender Point Index
0 No tenderness
1+ Tenderness without withdrawal
2+ Tenderness and withdrawal
3+ Tenderness and exaggerated withdrawal
4+ Untouchable

Fig. 24-9 Anatomic locations of tender points associated with fibromyalgia. (From Goodman CC, Snyder T: *Differential diagnosis for physical therapists: screening for referral*, ed 4, Philadelphia, 2007, Saunders.)

of fibromyalgia may be due to prolonged stress or anxiety, trauma, rapid steroid withdrawal, hypothyroidism, and viral and nonviral infections.[8,13] Fibromyalgia may start as localized pain and after months or years become widespread.[8] The pain associated with fibromyalgia is often described as burning or aching, and sometimes tender, stiff, throbbing, and sore.[8,13] Even though fibromyalgia pain is widespread, patients will have one or two locations that are the worst, which are usually the neck, shoulders, and back.[8,19,21] Sleep disturbance is one of the other more common symptoms in fibromyalgia.[8,13,19] Patients will complain of exhaustion even after a night of sleep, which is because of the disordered non-rapid eye movement sleep.[35] Also, patients with fibromyalgia have increased motor activity and restlessness during sleep, which accounts for increased fatigue.[35] Other common symptoms are fatigue, subjective numbness, chronic headaches, dizziness, Raynaud phenomenon, and irritable bowel and bladder.[8,13,19,21] Symptoms tend to be exacerbated with noise, stress, tiredness, weather changes, trauma, noxious smells, and too much or too little exercise.[8,13,28]

Management of Fibromyalgia

The first step in treating a patient with fibromyalgia is to make sure the patient understands they have a diagnosed syndrome that is a legitimate disorder with real symptoms and there is an effective management.[8,19] The management for fibromyalgia needs to be multidisciplinary and address education, stress management, nutrition and lifestyle training, medication, muscle pain, and exercise.[13] Pharmacologic management focuses on managing the pain and sleep disturbances.[8] Antidepressants are commonly used with fibromyalgia because of their positive effects on pain, sleep, and fatigue.[8,21] The antidepressants work well with some patients because the chemicals in the body that control pain and sleep also control mood.[21] Other drugs used to treat fibromyalgia are muscle relaxants, antianxiety medications, and sleep aids.[9]

Exercise is an important aspect of fibromyalgia management and is shown to have numerous benefits.[8,13,19,21] The exercise program should not be progressed too fast and it is suggested to have the patient to start below a level they believe they can accomplish.[8] Modalities are useful in decreasing a patient's acute pain, therefore allowing them to start an exercise program.[13,21] Stretching can help improve flexibility and decrease pain. Stretching should be done in a pain-free range and can start with 10- to 15-second holds and then progress up to 1 minute. It is important to perform stretches at least once a day. Heat alone can help with muscle pain, but it is also beneficial to use heat before stretching.[8,21] Aerobic exercise has been shown to decrease pain and improve function in patients with fibromyalgia.[8,21] The exercise routine can be broken into

several shorter bouts throughout the day or one longer 30-minute session. Depending on the patient's fitness level, some may need to start with 5 minutes daily and work up to 30 minutes slowly. It is very important that the patient avoid overexertion because this can lead to increased symptoms.[8] Strengthening can help reduce the risk of muscle damage, but the patient should attempt to reduce eccentric muscle work.[8] Patients should pause for about 4 seconds between repetitions to allow for complete muscle relaxation. Lifting above the head and shoulders should be avoided to reduce risk of shoulder girdle injury or overuse. Furthermore water therapy or aerobics is a good alternative because the warmth and decreased pressures can lead to better relaxation.[8]

Systemic Lupus Erythematosus

Systemic lupus erythematosus (SLE) is a chronic inflammatory autoimmune disorder that may affect multiple organ systems.[7,13,19,37] SLE is most common in women during their childbearing years and is rarely found in older individuals.[7,13,19,37] In SLE the body produces antibodies against itself.[13] The antigen–antibody complexes in tissues suppress the body's immunity and damage tissues. The etiology of SLE is unknown, but environmental and genetic factors are believed to be the most related with evidence also supporting interrelated immunologic and hormonal factors.[13] Many risk factors exist for SLE with hereditary factors at the forefront, along with physical and mental stress, streptococcal or viral infections, exposure to sunlight or ultraviolet light, and abnormal estrogen metabolism.[13] Diagnosis for SLE is not difficult if the patient presents with common symptoms associated with SLE. The American Rheumatism Association has diagnosis criteria for SLE in which the patient needs to show 4 or more of the 11 symptoms. If the patient shows a few symptoms then diagnosis is made using clinical judgment along with supportive laboratory testing.[19,37]

The clinical symptoms of patients with SLE are variable and most will not present with exactly the same symptoms. The severity of SLE can vary drastically from a treatable rash or fatigue to a life-threatening illness.[19,37] The skin, joints, lungs, kidneys, blood, and other organs and tissues can be affected.[13,19,32,37] General signs of SLE include fever, fatigue, anorexia, weight loss, and myalgias.[19,37] Joint involvement is one of the earlier symptoms and occurs in more than 90% of patients.[19] Symmetrical polyarthritis is common in any joint, but is usually found in small joints of hands, wrists, and knees.[13,37] SLE presents like RA, but is not usually destructive or deforming.[13,19,32,37] When deformities are present, ulnar deviation, swan neck deformity, fixed subluxations of fingers, tenosynovitis, and tendon ruptures can occur.[13,37] Recurrent inflammation of tendons and other supportive structures of the joints can lead to ulnar deviation of the second to fifth fingers and subluxation of the metacarpophalangeal joints, which is referred to as *Jaccoud arthropathy*.[37,45] Jaccoud arthropathy is correctable with no radiographic signs of erosion.[37] Also, observe patients for signs of osteonecrosis or septic arthritis, which will present as persistent monoarthritis primarily in the shoulders, hips, or knees.[37]

Another common symptom in SLE is skin rashes over areas exposed to sunlight. Butterfly rash is an acute inflammatory rash over the nose and checks.[13,19,32,37] Discoid lupus is characterized by raised, red, scaly, and scarring rashes that can develop around the face, scalp, ears, and upper extremities (Fig. 24-10).[13,19,37] Other cutaneous manifestations include alopecia, oral ulcers, fingertip lesions, periungual erythema, nail fold infarcts, splinter hemorrhages, livedo reticularis, urticaria, panniculitis, and Raynaud phenomenon.[13,19,37] Other clinical findings in SLE are associated with the renal, hematologic, cardiopulmonary, immune, and central nervous systems.[13,19,37]

Management of Systemic Lupus Erythematosus

Systemic lupus erythematosus is marked by remissions and relapses and therefore management is focused on addressing symptoms quickly during an exacerbation.[19,37] Patient education is important for successful management of SLE. Relapses are less likely if activities are controlled and sometimes limited.[13] Also, after an exacerbation, return to activity should be slow and pain free.[13] Joint pain is managed similar to RA, with NSAIDs as the primary medication for minor symptoms.[19,37] Patients should be cautioned against prolonged sun exposure and should use sunscreen regularly. Topical corticosteroids are often used for rashes or skin lesions.[19,37] Because of the use of corticosteroids, patients will have a higher risk of osteoporosis, so weight-bearing exercises should be incorporated into the management plan.

OSTEOPOROSIS

It is not uncommon for patients with arthritic conditions to concomitantly have osteoporosis, a disease characterized by low bone mass and microarchitectural deterioration of bone tissue, which leads to enhanced bone fragility and a consequent increase in fracture risk (Fig. 24-11).[29] The decrease in bone mass is due to decreased osteoblast activity, which builds bone, and/or increased osteoclast activity, which reabsorbs bone.[43] Remodeling of bone, which maintains bone mass, is performed by osteoblasts and osteoclasts and occurs about every 120 days. However, between the ages of 30 and 40 years, bone resorption starts to exceed bone formation and density decreases.[25] The bone then becomes weaker because of the decreased quantity of bone, however, the quality of bone remaining has not been altered.[7,32]

There are many risk factors associated with osteoporosis, such as a sedentary lifestyle, white or Asian race, thin

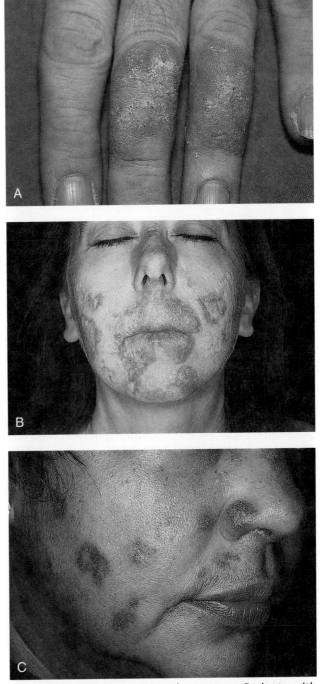

Fig. 24-10 Discoid lupus erythematosus. Patients with skin changes associated with discoid lupus erythematosus can present with a variety of signs. **A,** Hypertrophic discoid lupus erythematosus with prominent adherent scale. **B,** Round or oval cutaneous lesions can occur on the face or other parts of the body. **C,** Round or oval cutaneous lesions as they appear on a dark-skinned individual. (From Callen JP, Greer K, Paller A, Swinyer L: *Color atlas of dermatology*, ed 2, Philadelphia, 2000, Saunders.)

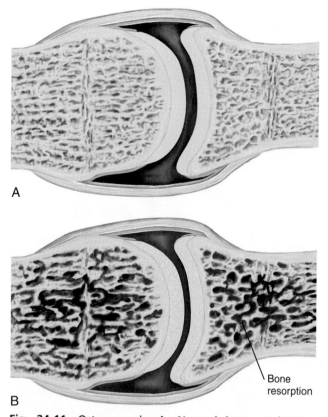

Fig. 24-11 Osteoporosis. **A,** Normal bone and joint. **B,** Osteoporotic changes shown with bone resorption greater than bone formation resulting in weakened trabeculae and increasing risk for fracture. (From Jarvis C: *Physical examination and health assessment*, ed 3, Philadelphia, 2000, Saunders.)

body frame, smoking, excessive alcohol intake, immobilization, early menopause, low calcium and vitamin D intake, and corticosteroid treatment.[25,32] Osteoporosis prevalence is more common in women and is directly associated with age. Peak bone mass is usually reached by age 20 to 25 years and then slowly declines, especially after menopause. The peak bone mass is generally higher and the decline in bone mass is less rapid in men.[29] For more on osteoporosis and bone healing.

The clinical features associated with osteoporosis are kyphosis, vertebral compression fractures, hip fracture, and distal radius fractures.[29] However, a true diagnosis is made by measuring bone mineral density. The most popular method to measure bone mineral density is dual energy x-ray absorptiometry (DEXA).

Preventive measures for osteoporosis include a proper diet with adequate calcium and vitamin D, weight-bearing exercises, and an estrogen therapy evaluation at menopause.[32] Prevention or management of osteoporosis needs to include weight-bearing activities and strength along with endurance exercise.[39] Management for osteoporosis should include a combination of medication (bisphosphonates, teriparatide, strontium ranelate), nutrition (calcium and vitamin D), and

exercise (aerobic, weight-bearing, and resistance exercise). Getting the correct amount of both vitamin D and calcium are important for healthy bones. Calcium alone will not lead to strong bones, because vitamin D is needed to transport the calcium into the bone.[9] Strength training exercises are important for postmenopausal women with osteoporosis, because they can increase or stabilize bone density of the hip and spine while also improving muscle mass, strength, and balance.[26] Furthermore, increasing the strength of the back extensors can help decrease symptoms of osteoporosis.[26]

TREATMENT IN RHEUMATIC DISEASE

The primary goal of management is to improve function of the patient, therefore allowing for a better quality of life. Secondary goals include:

■ Decreasing pain
■ Increasing ROM
■ Increasing strength.
■ Increasing joint stability
■ Decreasing biomechanical stress on joints
■ Increasing cardiovascular tolerance to activity (especially in RA)
■ Improving efficiency and safety of gait
■ Promoting independence with ADLs
■ Educating about joint protection, energy conservation techniques, functional abilities, and limitations

These goals can be achieved with an eclectic management program including modalities, stretching, strength and aerobic training, and education. Numerous studies have shown different modes of exercise to be beneficial in decreasing a patient's signs and symptoms of arthritis, so it is important for the patient to have a balanced exercise routine.[25]

Rehabilitative Management of Rheumatic Disorders

Modalities

Modalities are not a cure for disease, but application of both cold and heat can help decrease symptoms and allow for better function.

Cold

During an acute exacerbation of symptoms, patients should use cold to decrease inflammation, pain, and swelling.[9,17] Cold has been shown to have beneficial effects on pain, function, and stiffness.[17] Cold should be avoided in patients with inadequate thermoregulatory response.[17] Cold decreases pain by slowing or blocking nerve conduction, decreasing activity of the muscle spindle, and releasing endorphins. Veins in the tissues contract because of the coldness and decrease blood flow and capillary pressure, therefore decreasing swelling.[17] Histamine release is blocked by cold, which also decreases inflammation.

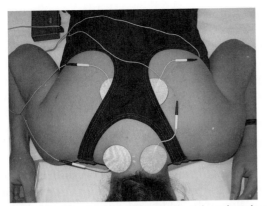

Fig. 24-12 Treatment of upper back and neck pain with electrical stimulation. (From Cameron MH: *Physical agents in rehabilitation: from research to practice*, ed 3, St Louis, 2009, Saunders.)

Heat

During subacute or chronic phases of rheumatic diseases, heat is more appropriate to decrease pain and increase ROM.[17] Heat should be avoided during an acute phase of inflammatory arthritis and in people who have decreased thermoregulatory response. Other contraindications include swelling, fever, infection, hemorrhage, or malignancy.[17] Heat can increase the pain threshold, increase blood flow, wash out pain-producing metabolites, and decrease muscle guarding.[9,17] Heat increases the extensibility of **connective tissue** and therefore should be combined with a low-stress prolonged stretch to increase flexibility.[17]

Electrical stimulation

Transcutaneous electrical nerve stimulation (TENS) is an effective management to decrease pain (Fig. 24-12).[17] A TENS units should never be placed close to the heart in a patient with a pacemaker.[11] TENS uses the gate theory to block pain by stimulating larger sensory fibers, which then block the smaller pain C fibers. C fibers innervate the synovium and joint capsule, so blocking pain perception in these fibers is beneficial to decreasing pain in patients suffering from arthritis.[17] One study has shown decreased inflammation, joint volume, and joint pressure from use of TENS.[17]

Stretching

Stretching is an important component of exercise in arthritis because it can relieve stiffness, increase joint mobility, and increase muscle length.[34] Intensity, duration, and frequency of stretching should take into consideration the phase of arthritis (Table 24-3).

In the acute phase patients should decrease activity and rest the inflamed joint.[34] Splinting also helps to reduce pain and inflammation by immobilizing or supporting the joint.[16] Reduced stress on the joint capsule and synovial lining through splinting reduces pain and

Table 24-3	*Joint-Specific Management Suggestions*
Joint	**Management Suggestion**
Hand	Encourage full finger flexion against minimum force
	Stress wrist extension
	Stress wrist ulnar deviation
	Maintain thumb web space
	Metacarpal-phalangeal
	• Avoid power grasp, lateral pinch, palmer pinch
	• Use palm over fingers
	• Two hands instead of one
	• Use forearm for lifting phalanges
	• Swan neck
	• Avoid intrinsic plus
	• Encourage PIP flexion with MP extension
	• Boutonnière
	• Avoid fingers flexed at rest
	• Daily DIP flexion with PIP extension ROM
	• Stress MTP extension with PIP and DIP flexion
Wrist	Avoid stirring with utensil diagonal in palm
	Avoid heavy lifting (hook grasp for bag)
Elbow	Avoid flexion contractures
	Avoid loss of supination/pronation
Shoulders	Not usually involved early
	Avoid decreased ROM all planes
	Tenderness inferior and lateral coracoid
	Be careful of GH subluxation
Spine	Core stabilization
Hip	Avoid sitting with legs crossed
	Avoid asymmetrical weight bearing
	Open seat ankle
	Avoid loss of abduction and rotation
	Avoid flexion contracture
Knees	Stand up with knees apart to prevent valgus
	Avoid hyperextension
Feet	Arch supports
	Hallux valgus
	Sit to stand with COG forward

COG, Center of gravity; *DIP*, distal interphalangeal; *GH*, glenohumeral; *MP*, metacarpal phalangeal; *MTP*, metatarsophalangeal; *PIP*, proximal interphalangeal; *ROM*, range of motion.

inflammation.[16] Rest is needed during the acute phase, but gentle ROM to maintain joint motion is still important. The goal of stretching in the acute phase is not to gain flexibility, but to maintain it, so do not overstretch the tissues. Tensile strength is decreased in inflamed tissues, therefore tears are more likely to occur. ROM exercise should be performed at least once a day to maintain proper flexibility.[34]

During the subacute or chronic phase of arthritis the goal is to increase flexibility, so a stretch at the end range of joint motion should be maintained. Intensity of the stretch should be gentle during subacute arthritis and aggressive during the chronic phase. Stretching should be performed two to three times a day with two to five repetitions performed on each joint.[34] If symptoms are subacute, five warm-ups with two to five more aggressive stretches can help improve motion. When joint symptoms are chronic, three to five warm ups with one to two maximum tolerated stretches are recommended. Each stretch should be held 10 to 30 seconds depending on the pain involved.[34] Pain should never last longer than 1 to 2 hours after exercise, but if pain persists longer than 2 hours, the intensity of exercise needs to be decreased.

Strengthening

There is an abundance of research supporting the benefits of exercise in rheumatic diseases. Muscle balance and conditioning are important aspects of physical activity because they provide joint stabilization and help the patient remain functional and independent with ADLs.[25] In OA, regular exercise has been shown to decrease joint pain and disability.[39] Exercise in patients with RA increases muscle strength and functional capacity without increased pain or medication.[39] Furthermore, resistive training can improve muscle disability, physical performance, and pain with no increase in arthritic symptoms[10]; strong muscles can help absorb shock through a joint whereas weak muscles cannot provide stability or control.[34] Strengthening is important, but is more effective when using the correct resistance for the phase of disease.

During an acute phase, resistive exercises need to be gentle with little pressure on the joints so that symptoms are not increased. Isometric exercises, those during which muscles are contacted without joint movement, are therefore recommended because of the minimal increase in joint pressure. Increased strength can also occur with isometric contractions held 6 seconds at 70% maximum effort and repeated 5 to 10 times a day.[34] Placing the joint at midrange during contractions allows for safer exercise. If symptoms increase, decrease intensity to avoid joint irritation, but if pain does not subside 1 to 2 hours after exercise, the exercises should be terminated until the patient is past the acute phase of an arthritis flare-up.

When a patient reaches the subacute phase, isotonic exercises, those during which the muscle contracts against a constant load resulting in joint movement, should be implemented.[34] The exercises should be performed through a pain-free ROM, but the American College of Sports Medicine states that 3 sets of 8 to 10 repetitions should be performed for each exercise.[1] If the patient is older than 50 years of age, however, 10 to 15 repetitions are recommended.[34] The appropriate amount of resistance is determined when the patient is able to perform all repetitions with no increase in symptoms but a minor feeling of fatigue at the end of each set. Once a patient can perform all repetitions easily, resistance should be increased slightly (1 to 2 pounds).[25] When working with larger muscle groups, such as the chest, back, or leg, an increase of 5 pounds should not aggravate symptoms. Even though the joint is not in an acute flare-up, precautions should be taken to avoid exacerbation of symptoms. Open-chain exercises are less stressful on the joint because the weight of the body is not sustained by the joint. All major muscle groups should be addressed during exercise, but focus should be placed on muscles crossing the joint or joints affected by arthritis.

Patients in the chronic phase of arthritis should be able to perform more vigorous activity without increasing joint symptoms. During this phase physical therapy should challenge the patient with increased intensity and repetitions. Exercises should again be performed through the full available ROM of each joint, and incorporating proprioceptive neuromuscular facilitation (PNF) patterns will allow for more muscles to be recruited for each motion and help prepare the patient for more functional movements. Balance activities should also be performed to decrease risk of falls and further train the body functionally. Strength training should be performed two to three times a week and not repeated two days in a row to allow for proper recovery. When performing any exercises, always position for optimal joint protection.

Aerobic Exercise

Aerobic activities are beneficial to all individuals for overall health and to decrease the risk of disease. Patients with arthritis often believe that rest is the only answer to decrease joint pain, but inactivity may actually exacerbate arthritic symptoms.[25] RA has many extraarticular manifestations, so aerobic exercise is an especially important part of management. Aerobic activity should be performed three to five times a week for 20 to 30 minutes continuously.[1] If the patient cannot tolerate 30 minutes of continuous exercise, the patient should be encouraged to perform several shorter activities throughout the day that add up to 30 minutes. As the patient's cardiovascular endurance improves, the amount of time spent in continuous exercise may increase. The intensity of exercise should be 70% to 85% of the patient's maximum heart rate (calculated as 220 minus age). The therapist should also explain that any hobby or activity that increases their heart rate can be considered exercise.

Aquatic Therapy

Water is an excellent medium to allow for an increase in pain-free movement while decreasing the stress on the joints. Aquatic exercise is unique because it can support, resist, or assist with exercises depending on the motion. Decreased joint compression, muscle relaxation, and sensory input from the pressure and temperature in the water help to decrease pain,[34] so aquatic therapy programs can increase strength, flexibility, and aerobic fitness in patients with knee or hip OA.[46] The resistance of water provides a means to strengthen muscles: the faster a patient moves through the water, the more resistance the patient experiences. Fins or water weights can be used to provide more resistance and progress strengthening (Fig. 24-13). The buoyancy of the water helps unload the body's weight-bearing joints, which can decrease stress and pain. As the patient's pain decreases and strength and endurance improve, the water level can be decreased to allow for more weight bearing. Recommendations from Minor[33] are as follows:

■ Select a pool with a water temperature of 84° F to 92° F (29° C to 33° C).
■ Exercise in sufficiently deep water to minimize joint compression (midchest to shoulder level).
■ Use nonslip, padded footwear to reduce foot discomfort.
■ Choose aquatic exercise programs specifically designed for people with arthritis.
■ Receive instruction in proper technique before starting a swimming or deep water running program.

Medical Management of Rheumatic Disorders

Drugs play an important role in rheumatic disorders by delaying the progression of the diseases and controlling the symptoms. Although the drugs are helpful in their own way to the specific diseases, there are side effects and risks, so careful consideration of the risk-to-benefit ratio needs to be taken when deciding drug use. As a PTA, it is important to know the effects of the different drugs to explain those effects to patients. It is important to educate patients on staying regular with their medication, because many drugs take months to start working and need to be taken regularly to get an appropriate amount in the bloodstream. There are numerous drugs to help rheumatic disorders, and they fall into the following categories: analgesics, NSAIDs, corticosteroids, biological response modifiers, and DMARDs.

Analgesics

The main role of an analgesic is to decrease pain, which is prevalent in patients with rheumatic disorders. Analgesics are primarily used with OA or in the early phases of RA, where inflammation is not as prevalent.[31] There are several analgesics available to patients with rheumatic disorders, most notably acetaminophen, oxycodone, propoxyphene, and tramadol. Acetaminophen is one of the safest and most cost-effective drugs available. Other pain reducers, such as propoxyphene, oxycodone, and tramadol, are often used but have more side effects and higher risk of dependence. Tramadol is the least likely to cause dependence and is therefore often used first; however, tramadol does contain opioids, which decrease the sensation of pain through the central nervous system. Opioids can cause sleepiness, dizziness, and constipation.[31] Education on the side effects is important so patients can report any side effects.

Nonsteroidal Antiinflammatory Drugs

NSAIDs have both analgesic and antiinflammatory effects but have no effect on arthritis progression.[13] There are many NSAIDs, including ibuprofen (Motrin), aspirin, naproxen, indomethacin, meloxicam (Mobic), choline, and magnesium salicylates.[9,31] NSAIDs inhibit cyclooxygenase (COX), which is an enzyme that converts arachidonic acid to prostaglandin, a molecule that has many roles including the promotion of inflammation and pain. COX has two different isomers: COX-1 and COX-2. COX-1 may be the main contributor in the adverse side effect of gastric bleeding and ulcers. COX-2 is mainly involved in inflammation of tissues; therefore,

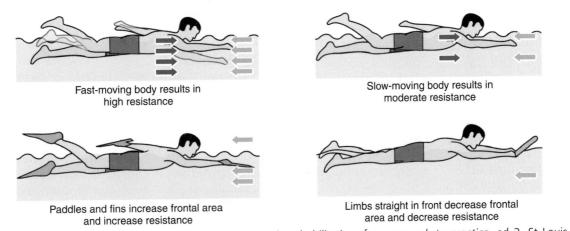

Fast-moving body results in high resistance

Slow-moving body results in moderate resistance

Paddles and fins increase frontal area and increase resistance

Limbs straight in front decrease frontal area and decrease resistance

Fig. 24-13 **Resistance.** (From Cameron MH: *Physical agents in rehabilitation: from research to practice*, ed 3, St Louis, 2009, Saunders.)

COX-2 inhibition may be the key factor in the use of NSAIDs.[19,31]

NSAIDs given at a lower dosage act more as an analgesic, but NSAIDS given at a higher dosage have more of an antiinflammatory effect. Low doses of NSAIDs may therefore be more appropriate with OA and early phase RA.[6] Late phase or severe RA may require a higher dosage. Educating the patient on the importance of regularly taking their NSAID to get proper dosage is important. Symptoms should decrease in the first 2 to 3 weeks of NSAID use, however some patients will respond better to different medications, so a different NSAID should be tried if the patient does not feel any improvement after 3 weeks.[19] Side effects to watch for include gastrointestinal bleeding and ulcers, dizziness, headaches, and drowsiness. Nausea and abdominal irritation are common and can be reduced by taking medication with food.[31]

Corticosteroids

Patients with inflammation as a primary symptom or who do not respond to NSAIDs are good candidates for corticosteroids.[6] Several corticosteroids are available including prednisone, dexamethasone, hydrocortisone, and betamethasone.[19,31] Corticosteroids are primarily used on a short-term basis to decrease symptoms and allow for other management methods to be used, such as physical therapy. Though corticosteroids usually provide the fastest and most effective antiinflammatory response long term usage has been shown to increase the risk of osteoporosis. Patients using corticosteroids should take precautions to make sure they get adequate calcium and vitamin D. Corticosteroids given by intraarticular injection should not be repeated more than three to four times in a year because of increased loss of blood supply to the bones. Oral and intravenous options are also available for giving corticosteroids. Most patients will feel a decrease in symptoms within 24 hours of dosage. Corticosteroids are often given along with NSAIDS or DMARDs.[13]

Disease-Modifying Antirheumatic Drugs

DMARDs are generally started as soon as a definite diagnosis of rheumatoid disease is made because they work in the early phases of the inflammatory process, can decrease arthritic symptoms, and possibly decrease the rate of damage to bone and cartilage.[13,19,31] DMARDs decrease this damage by suppressing the immune system, but generally take several weeks to months to produce effects.[9] DMARDs are primarily used with patients diagnosed with RA and systemic lupus erythematosus, but DMARDs may also used for psoriatic arthritis and ankylosing spondylitis.[9,31]

There are several types of DMARDs, including methotrexate, oral gold, penicillamine, sulfasalazine, and antimalarial drugs. Methotrexate is generally the first option for severe RA because of its long-term efficiency

and its antiinflammatory and immunosuppressant effects.[9,19,31] Methotrexate tends to produce results within 2 to 6 weeks, as opposed to other DMARDs that can take up to 6 months.[19,31] As stated earlier, it is important for the PTA to be cognitive of side effects for each drug. Methotrexate side effects include nausea, vomiting, diarrhea, mouth ulcers, decreased white blood cell count, megaloblastic anemia, and liver fibrosis or cirrhosis.[31]

Oral gold was one of the first DMARDs that showed improved symptoms in the majority of patients, but it has several side effects that start to negatively impact the risk-to-benefit ratio. Penicillamine was another DMARD used; it has many adverse side effects with about the same amount of beneficial results as oral gold. Sulfasalazine has been shown to be effective in treating spondyloarthropathies and juvenile RA.[9,31] Sulfasalazine has antibacterial, antiinflammatory, and immunomodulatory properties and has been shown to inhibit tumor necrosis factor-alpha which coordinates the autoimmune process.[31,41]

Biological Response Modifiers

The main purpose of biological agents is to inhibit the chemicals that are key factors in the inflammation and autoimmune processes. Unlike DMARDs, biological response modifiers target specific components of the immune system, thereby avoiding its widespread suppression.[9] Two chemicals that current RA drugs are addressing are tumor necrosis factor (TNF) and interleukin-1 (IL-1). TNF is a cytokine that activates lymphocytes and leukocytes, two inflammatory cell types that destroy the synovium of joints.[19,31] TNF inhibitors can be more effective than methotrexate in early phases of RA, but the two have been used in combination with favorable results.[19] Side effects are minimal with TNF inhibitors, but can include fever, chills, dyspnea, hypotension, and possibly higher chances of infection.[32] IL-1 receptor antagonist is designed to slow the rate of joint damage. This is done by blocking interleukin-1 alpha and beta, which play a role in immune and inflammatory responses in the body.

Supplements

Glucosamine and chondroitin sulfate are two safe supplements widely used for pain with arthritis.[31] Glucosamine is a natural substance that is a precursor in the synthesis of glycosaminoglycans, which are present in cartilage. Glucosamine therefore helps the body build and repair cartilage.[20] Chondroitin sulfate is a glycosaminoglycan and is thought to draw fluid into the cartilage, allowing for better joint function and protection from destructive enzymes.[20,31] There are no serious side effects documented with either of these supplements and they are readily available.[20,31,40] According to Richy and colleagues,[40] patients taking glucosamine and chondroitin reported improved scores on a visual analog scale for both pain and mobility. These two supplements have an excellent safety record and have been shown to be effective in managing the symptoms of arthritis in the knee and hip.[30]

Surgical Management of Rheumatic Disorders

Surgery should only be considered after conservative management, such as physical therapy, has shown to be ineffective in relieving symptoms or improving function. There are always risks when having a surgery, so encourage the patient to ask their medical doctor questions about the surgery being recommended. Most surgeries used to help patients with arthritis are effective in decreasing pain and improving movement of the affected joint. There are numerous surgical options, including:

■ Synovectomy
■ Osteotomy
■ Resection
■ Arthrodesis
■ Arthroscopy
■ Arthroplasty

Synovectomy

A synovectomy is the removal of synovium infected with inflammation. Removing the inflamed synovium can decrease symptoms and prevent or slow destruction of a joint.[9] Patients who continue to have inflammation after pharmacologic intervention are good candidates for this procedure; however, if the joint is degenerative without synovial inflammation then a synovectomy will not be beneficial. Synovium does grow back so the long-term benefits of a synovectomy are unknown.[19]

Osteotomy

An osteotomy is a procedure during which bone is cut to change the alignment of the joint to a better position (Fig. 24-14). Osteotomy can improve weight-bearing position of the lower extremities to aid in ambulation and is commonly used to correct coax vera, genu valgum, and genu varum.[9] Osteotomy is one option that can be used to delay the need for a total joint replacement. During the rehabilitation of a patient after an osteotomy the therapist needs to be careful to not cause trauma or torque on the extremity. Stretching and exercise should be done in a gentle manner, and pain in these activities should last no longer than 1 hour. Osteotomy may be used for a patient with a spondyloarthropathy disease who has severe deformities of the lumbar spine.[18]

Resection

Resection is a procedure during which part or all of a bone is removed from a stiff or immobile joint, creating a space between the bones (Fig. 24-15). The empty

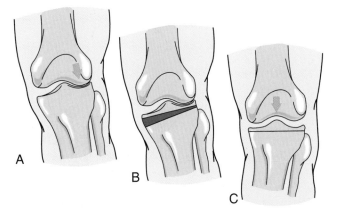

Fig. 24-14 Osteotomy of tibia for genu valgum (valgus deformity); anterior view of left knee. **A,** Weight-bearing force is concentrated on one compartment of knee. **B,** Wedge of bone is removed from tibia. Amount of bone removed is determined by how much correction in angulation is necessary. **C,** Distal portion of tibia is swung to proximal portion. Correction of angulation obtained allows weight-bearing forces to be more evenly distributed through both compartments of knee. (From Monahan FD: *Phipps' medical-surgical nursing: health and illness perspectives*, ed 8, St Louis, 2007, Mosby.)

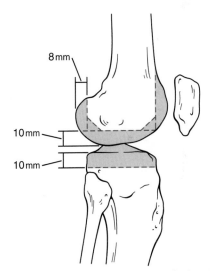

Fig. 24-15 In the measured resection technique, as much bone and/or cartilage is removed as will be replaced by the thickness of the arthroplasty components. This method attempts to restore the anatomical joint line level. (From Magee DJ: *Pathology and intervention in musculoskeletal rehabilitation*, St Louis, 2009, Mosby.)

space fills with scar tissue, which can be more flexible.[9] Patients with severe arthritis of the foot can have bone resection in the foot to improve walking and pain. Other common sites for resections are the wrist, thumb, and elbow. The main goal of the surgery is to improve function and decrease pain.

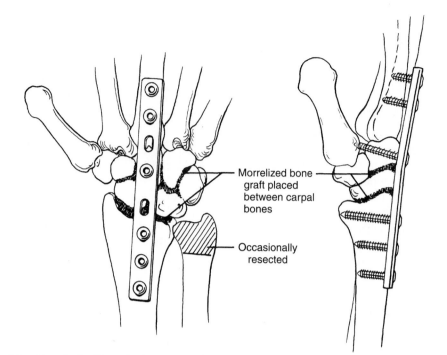

Morrelized bone graft placed between carpal bones

Occasionally resected

Fig. 24-16 **Total wrist arthrodesis.** (From Burke SL: *Hand and upper extremity rehabilitation: a practical guide*, ed 3, St Louis, 2006, Churchill Livingstone.)

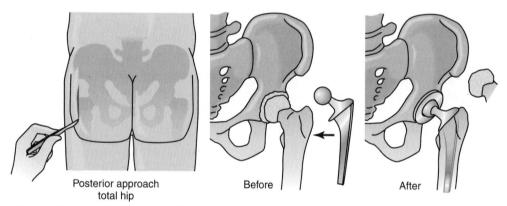

Posterior approach total hip

Before

After

Fig. 24-17 **Total hip arthroplasty procedure.** (From Cameron MH: *Physical rehabilitation: evidence-based examination, evaluation, and intervention*, St Louis, 2008, Saunders.)

Arthrodesis

Arthrodesis is the artificial ossification between two bones or a bone fusion (Fig. 24-16). By fusing, the joint pain is decreased and the joint can better sustain weight. The two bones lose flexibility but are pain-free and sturdy.[9] Common sites for arthrodesis are the ankles, wrists, fingers, and thumbs. Arthrodesis is used less commonly, but can be beneficial for a chronically infected and painful joint.[19]

Arthroplasty

Arthroplasty is a procedure for rebuilding joints that have been damaged, become painful, and are less functional (Fig. 24-17). Total joint replacement is a very successful method for decreasing pain and improving the functional ability of individuals, but generally the surgery is used in people older than the age of 65 years because the new joint only lasts about 10 to 15 years. The arthritic joint is replaced with metal, ceramic, and plastic parts. The two most common joint replacements are knee and hip, but shoulder, elbow, ankle, and knuckles also can be replaced.[19] In general, patients are expected to return to normal function, strength, mobility, and ROM after 6 months.[3] Hip and knee arthroplasties are common surgical interventions in patients with OA[24]; total hip arthroplasty is the most common procedure in patients with ankylosing spondylitis.[18]

Arthroscopy

Arthroscopy is not a procedure but rather a means of performing a procedure. The arthroscope is a thin tube with a light at the end connected to a screen. Arthroscopic surgery allows for exploration of a joint to determine what is wrong and to determine how extensive the damage is. Biopsies, cutting loose tissue, repairing cartilage, or smoothing rough surfaces can all be done arthroscopically. Arthroscopic surgery can have a faster recovery time than more invasive procedures, because only small incisions are required and minimal anesthesia is used. Surgeries commonly performed arthroscopically are meniscus repairs, rotator cuff repairs, cartilage damage repairs, and labral tear repair.

❖ GLOSSARY

Atrophy: A wasting; a decrease in size of an organ or tissue.

Closed-chain exercises: Distal end of extremity is fixed to the ground or to a device. For example, keeping your feet on the ground while bending knees.

Connective tissue: Tissue that supports and connects other tissues and parts of the body. Connective tissue has comparatively few cells. Its bulk consists of intercellular substance or matrix, whose nature gives each connective tissue its particular properties.

Infection: The presence and growth of a microorganism that produces tissue damage.

Inflammation: Nonspecific response that occurs in reaction to any type of bodily injury. Symptoms include rubor (redness), calor (heat), tumor (swelling), and dolor (pain).

Malaise: Discomfort, uneasiness, or indisposition, often indicative of infection.

Open-chain exercises: Distal end of extremity is not fixed and can move freely. For example, if you raise one foot off the ground, you can move the leg in any direction.

Proteoglycan: A glycoprotein that retains water therefore providing more absorptive properties to the cartilage.[2]

REFERENCES

1. American College of Sports Medicine: *ACSM's guidelines for exercise testing and prescription*, ed 6, Philadelphia, 2000, Lippincott Williams & Wilkins.
2. American Pain Society: *Guideline on the management of pain in osteoarthritis, rheumatoid arthritis, and juvenile chronic arthritis*, ed 2, Glenview, Ill., 2002, American Pain Society.
3. American Physical Therapy Association: *Guide to physical therapist practice*, Alexandria, Va., 2003, American Physical Therapy Association.
4. Andrews JR, Harrelson GL, Wilk KE: *Physical rehabilitation of the injured athlete*, ed 3, Philadelphia, 2004, Saunders.
5. Berger TG: Skin, hair, and nails. In Tierney LM, McPhee SJ, Papadakis MA, editors: *Current medical diagnosis and treatment*, New York, 2006, Lange.
6. Bolten WW: Differential analgesic treatment in arthrosis and arthritis, *MMW Fortschr Med* 146(13):40–42, 2004.
7. Brinker MR, Miller MD: *Fundamentals of orthopaedics*, Philadelphia, 1999, Saunders.
8. Burckhardt CS: Fibromyalgia. In Robbins L, Burckhardt CS, Hannan MT, et al: *Clinical care in the rheumatic diseases*, Atlanta, 2001, Association of Rheumatology Health Professionals.
9. Dunkin MA: *The Arthritis Foundation's guide to managing your arthritis*, Atlanta, 2001, Arthritis Foundation.
10. Ettinger WH, Burns R, Messier SP, et al: A randomized trail comparing aerobic exercise and resistance exercise with a health education program in older adults with knee osteoarthritis. The fitness arthritis and seniors trial (FAST), *JAMA* 277:25–31, 1997.
11. Foley RA: Transcutaneous electrical nerve stimulation. In Hayes KW, editor: *Manual for physical agents*, Saddle River, N.J., 2000, Prentice Hall.
12. Gabriel SE, Crowson CS, O'Fallon WM: Comorbidity in arthritis, *J Rheumatol* 26:2475–2479, 1999.
13. Goodman CC: *Pathology: implications for the physical therapist*, ed 2, St Louis, 2009, Saunders.
14. Gornisiewicz M, Moreland LW: Rheumatoid arthritis. In Robbins L, Burckhardt CS, Hannan MT, et al: *Clinical care in the rheumatic diseases*, Atlanta, 2001, Association of Rheumatology Health Professionals.
15. Hannan MT: Epidemiology of rheumatic diseases. In Robbins L, Burckhardt CS, Hannan MT, et al: *Clinical care in the rheumatic diseases*, Atlanta, 2001, Association of Rheumatology Health Professionals.
16. Harrell PB: Splinting of the hand. In Robbins L, Burckhardt CS, Hannan MT, et al: *Clinical care in the rheumatic diseases*, Atlanta, 2001, Association of Rheumatology Health Professionals.
17. Hayes KW: Physical modalities. In Robbins L, Burckhardt CS, Hannan MT, et al: *Clinical care in the rheumatic diseases*, Atlanta, 2001, Association of Rheumatology Health Professionals.
18. Helewa A, Stokes B: Spondylarthropathies. In Robbins L, Burckhardt CS, Hannan MT, et al: *Clinical care in the rheumatic diseases*, Atlanta, 2001, Association of Rheumatology Health Professionals.
19. Hellmann DB, Stone JH: Arthritis and musculoskeletal disorders. In Tierney LM, McPhee SJ, Papadakis MA, editors: *Current medical diagnosis and treatment*, New York, 2006, Lange.
20. Horstman J: *Arthritis Foundation's guide to alternative therapies*, Atlanta, 1999, Arthritis Foundation.
21. Kelly J, Devonshire R: *Taking charge of fibromyalgia: a self-management program for your fibromyalgia syndrome*, Wayzata, Minn., 2001, Fibromyalgia Educational Systems.
22. Kishiyama JL, Adelman DC: Allergic and immunologic disorders. In Tierney LM, McPhee SJ, Papadakis MA, editors: *Current medical diagnosis and treatment*, New York, 2006, Lange.
23. Koopman WJ: *Arthritis and allied conditions: a textbook of rheumatology*, Philadelphia, 2001, Lippincott Williams & Wilkins.
24. Lozada CJ, Altman RD: Osteoarthritis. In Robbins L, Burckhardt CS, Hannan MT, et al: *Clinical care in the rheumatic diseases*, Atlanta, 2001, Association of Rheumatology Health Professionals.
25. Luggen AS, Meiner SE: *Care of arthritis in the older adult*, New York, 2002, Springer.
26. Lundon K: *Orthopedic rehabilitation science: principles for clinical management of bone*, Boston, 2000, Butterworth-Heinemann.
27. Magee DJ: *Orthopedic physical assessment*, ed 5, St Louis, 2009, Saunders.
28. Mannerkorpi K, Iverson MD: The use of exercise and rehabilitation regimens. In Wallace DJ, Clauw DJ, editors: *Fibromyalgia and other central pain syndromes*, Philadelphia, 2005, Lippincott Williams & Wilkins.
29. Maricic MJ: Osteoporosis. In Robbins L, Burckhardt CS, Hannan MT, et al: *Clinical care in the rheumatic diseases*, Atlanta, 2001, Association of Rheumatology Health Professionals.
30. McAlindon TE, Lavalley MP, Gulin JP, et al: Glucosamine and chondroitin for treatment of osteoarthritis: a systematic quality assessment and analysis, *JAMA* 283:1469–1475, 2000.

31. Miller DR: Pharmacologic interventions in the 21st century. In Robbins L, Burckhardt CS, Hannan MT, et al: *Clinical care in the rheumatic diseases*, Atlanta, 2001, Association of Rheumatology Health Professionals.

32. Miller MD: *Review of orthopaedics*, ed 3, Philadelphia, 2000, Saunders.

33. Minor MA: Exercise in the treatment of osteoarthritis, *Rheum Dis Clin North Am* 25:387–415, 1999.

34. Minor MA, Westby MD: Rest and exercise. In Robbins L, Burckhardt CS, Hannan MT, et al: *Clinical care in the rheumatic diseases*, Atlanta, 2001, Association of Rheumatology Health Professionals.

35. Moldofsky H, MacFarlane JG: Sleep and its potential role in chronic pain and fatigue. In Wallace DJ, Clauw DJ, editors: *Fibromyalgia and other central pain syndromes*, Philadelphia, 2005, Lippincott Williams & Wilkins.

36. Nichols LA: History and physical assessment. In Robbins L, Burckhardt CS, Hannan MT, et al: *Clinical care in the rheumatic diseases*, Atlanta, 2001, Association of Rheumatology Health Professionals.

37. Ramsey-Goldman R: Connective tissue diseases. In Robbins L, Burckhardt CS, Hannan MT, et al: *Clinical care in the rheumatic diseases*, Atlanta, 2001, Association of Rheumatology Health Professionals.

38. Rayman M, Callaghan A: *Nutrition and arthritis*, Danvers, Mass, 2006, Blackwell.

39. Rhoades RA, Tanner GA: *Medical physiology*, Baltimore, 2003, Lippincott Williams & Wilkins.

40. Richy F, Bruyere O, Ethgen O, et al: Structural and symptomatic efficacy of glucosamine and chondroitin in knee osteoarthritis, *Arch Intern Med* 163:1514–1522, 2003.

41. Rodenburg RJ, Ganga A, vanLent PL, et al: The antiinflammatory drug sulfasalazine inhibits tumor necrosis factor alpha expression in macrophages by inducing apoptosis, *Arthritis Rheum* 43(9): 1941–1950, 2000.

42. Schumacher RH, Gall EP: *Rheumatoid arthritis: an illustrated guide to pathology, diagnosis, and management*, Philadelphia, 1988, JB Lippincott.

43. Sherwood L: *Human physiology from cells to systems*, ed 2, Independence, Ky, 2010, Brooks Cole.

44. Taylor J, Erlandson D: Pediatric rheumatic disorders. In Robbins L, Burckhardt CS, Hannan MT, et al: *Clinical care in the rheumatic diseases*, Atlanta, 2001, Association of Rheumatology Health Professionals.

45. Van Vugt RM, Derksen RH, Kater J, et al: Deforming arthropathy or lupus and rhupus hands in systemic lupus erythematosus, *Ann Rheum Dis* 57:540–544, 1998.

46. Wang TJ, Belza B, Thompson EF, et al: Effects of aquatic exercise on flexibility, strength, and aerobic fitness in adults with osteoarthritis of the hip or knee, *J Adv Nurs* 57(2):141–152, 2007.

REVIEW QUESTIONS

Short Answer

1. Name at least five characteristics that can predispose someone to arthritis.
2. Discuss at least seven differences between OA and RA.
3. List two examples from each of these types of drugs: analgesics, NSAIDs, corticosteroids, DMARDs, and biological response modifiers.
4. List the three types of juvenile rheumatoid arthritis and how many joints are affected by each disease.
5. List five risk factors for septic arthritis.
6. List four diagnosis criteria for systemic lupus erythematosus.

True/False

7. OA is the most common form of arthritis.
8. Arthritis is more common in women.
9. Closed-chain exercises are more encouraged than open-chain exercises for patients with OA.
10. Extraarticular manifestations of RA can affect the heart, lungs, and eyes.
11. Patients with RA can stretch aggressively when tissues are inflamed.
12. Patients should perform isometric exercises during an acute exacerbation.
13. During the acute phase of arthritis patients should rest and not stretch or exercise.
14. When performing isometric exercises the joint should be placed at midrange.
15. Patients older than the age of 50 years should perform three sets of five repetitions when strengthening.
16. Strength training can be performed every day.
17. The intensity of exercise should be 50% of the patient's maximum heart rate.
18. Water temperature for patients with arthritis should range from 78° F to 84° F.
19. Corticosteroids usually provide the fastest and most effective antiinflammatory response.
20. Chondroitin sulfate is a glycosaminoglycan.
21. Non–weight-bearing exercise is recommended for patients with osteoporosis.
22. Pain and stiffness will increase with rest and will decrease with activity in patients with ankylosing spondylitis.
23. A prone program is recommended for a patient diagnosed with ankylosing spondylitis.
24. Reactive arthritis is usually asymmetrical and involves the weight-bearing joints.
25. Psoriatic arthritis is usually asymmetrical and involves the small joints of hands and feet.
26. The sacroiliitis in psoriatic arthritis is usually bilateral.
27. The metatarsophalangeal joint of the great toe is the most common site of gout.
28. Patients with fibromyalgia should avoid exercise.
29. Gonococcal arthritis usually takes months to respond to drug therapy.
30. Jaccoud arthropathy is ulnar deviation of the second to fifth fingers and subluxation of the interphalangeal joints.
31. Patients with systemic lupus erythematosus should be cautioned against prolonged sun exposure.

25 Pain

Michelle H. Cameron

LEARNING OBJECTIVES

1. Define the different types of pain.
2. Provide clinical implications for physical therapy regarding the different types of pain.
3. Describe the components and mechanisms of pain reception and transmission.
4. Explain the role of the sympathetic nervous system and substance P in pain reception and modulation.
5. Describe the theories associated with pain modulation and control.
6. Outline various clinical methods to measure and document pain perception.
7. Explain the role of physical agents in managing a patient's pain.
8. Describe the purpose and components of a multidisciplinary treatment program for pain management.

KEY TERMS

Afferent nerves
Allodynia
Analgesia
Autonomic nervous system
Central sensitization
Complex regional pain syndrome (CRPS)

Efferent innervation
Endogenous opiate theory
Enkephalins
Hyperalgesia
Nociception
Opiopeptins
Pain

Pain-spasm-pain cycle
Peripheral sensitization
Referred pain
Sensitization
Sympathetic nervous system
Synapse
Transduction

CHAPTER OUTLINE

This chapter appears in a modified form from Cameron MH: *Physical agents in rehabilitation: from research to practice,* ed 3, St Louis, 2009, Saunders.

423

Pain is an experience based on a complex interaction of physical and psychological processes. It has been defined as an unpleasant sensory and emotional experience associated with actual or potential tissue damage or described in terms of such damage.[16,108,150] Pain usually acts as a warning to protect the body from damage and thus serves an essential function in survival.[163] It is important to realize that pain is not just the activation of receptors of noxious stimuli, known as *nociception,* but also the sensory experiences, suffering, and alterations in behavior associated with such activation.

Pain is the most common symptom prompting patients to seek medical attention and is a predominant symptom leading patients to receive rehabilitation.[162] Many patients with musculoskeletal or neurological impairments report pain, and most of these individuals consider pain control or relief to be the primary goal of treatment.[72] Pain may alter body structure and function, limiting participation in home, work, and recreational activities. Pain symptoms encountered by rehabilitation professionals are generally related to inflammation of musculoskeletal or neurological structures caused by injury, trauma, or degenerative disease. These structures can be sources of pain and can increase the responsiveness of peripheral pain receptors to other painful stimuli.[49,141,145]

The goals of pain management include resolving the underlying condition causing the pain, when possible; modifying the patient's perception of the discomfort; and maximizing function within the limitations imposed by the source of pain, whether that source can or cannot be modified. Even when the source of pain is identified and can be modified, pain control during recovery is important. Limiting pain helps the patient fully participate in rehabilitation and reach goals of increased activity and participation. Examples include pain caused by structural malalignment from poor posture or imbalanced muscle length, or a self-limiting condition such as inflammation after an acute soft tissue injury. When the pain is caused by a condition that cannot be directly modified, such as phantom limb pain or rheumatoid arthritis, pain control may facilitate increased participation in a rehabilitation program and increased patient activity and participation.

TYPES OF PAIN

Pain can be categorized according to its duration or source as acute, chronic, or referred. Acute pain is generally defined as pain of less than 6 months duration for which an underlying pathology can be identified.[17] Acute pain is felt in response to actual or potential tissue damage that resolves when tissue damage or the threat of damage passes. Chronic pain persists beyond the normal time for tissue healing.[49] Chronic pain conditions are usually the result of activation of dysfunctional

neurologic or psychological responses that cause the individual to continue to experience the sensation of pain even when no damaging or threatening stimulus is present. **Referred pain** is the experience of pain in one area when the actual or potential tissue damage is in another area. Knowing whether a patient's pain is acute, chronic, or referred will help the clinician determine the mechanisms and processes that may be contributing to the sensation and facilitate selection of the most appropriate intervention to control or relieve this symptom.

Acute Pain

Acute pain is a complex combination of unpleasant sensory, perceptual, and emotional experiences with associated autonomic, psychological, emotional, and behavioral reactions that occur in response to a noxious stimulus provoked by acute injury or disease.[15,161] Acute pain is generally viewed as biologically meaningful, useful, and time-limited. Acute pain is mediated through rapidly conducting pathways and is associated with increases in muscle tone, heart rate, blood pressure, skin conductance, and other manifestations of increased **sympathetic nervous system** activity.[106] The intensity and location of the pain are usually related to the degree of tissue inflammation, damage, or destruction in the area in which the pain is felt. Acute pain is generally well-localized and defined, although its degree of localization varies to some extent with the type of tissue involved. Acute pain lasts as long as the noxious stimulation persists. Acute pain serves a protective function after an injury by limiting activity to prevent further damage and promote tissue healing and recovery; however, it may also adversely affect an individual's quality of life and impair the ability to function. For example, when a patient sustains a rotator cuff injury while playing racquetball, he or she will feel acute pain in the shoulder. This pain will probably cause the patient to restrict shoulder motion and thereby avoid further injury. This acute pain will likely prevent the patient from playing racquetball for a number of days or weeks but will gradually resolve as the injured tissues heal, allowing return to full activity.

Treatment of acute pain resulting from musculoskeletal injury generally attempts to resolve the underlying disorder, reduce inflammation, and modify the transmission of pain from the periphery to the central nervous system (CNS).

Chronic Pain

Chronic pain may start as acute pain related to a chronic disease as with peripheral polyneuropathy, poststroke, or spinal cord injury pain syndrome, and fibromyalgia, or it may have no identifiable cause. Chronic pain is usually defined as pain that does not resolve in the usual time it takes for the disorder to heal or that continues beyond the duration of noxious stimulation.[13]

Some authors and organizations use time-based definitions, defining chronic pain as any pain lasting longer than 3 months or 6 months.[28,63] Whatever its precise definition, chronic pain is an ongoing condition that is difficult to manage. It has been estimated that approximately one third of the United States population has chronic pain, and 14% of the U.S. population suffers from chronic pain related to the joints and the musculoskeletal system.[95,117] Other disease states, such as cancer, are also commonly associated with chronic pain. A study of pain in 13,625 elderly and minority nursing home residents with cancer found that more than 25% reported daily pain.[9]

Chronic pain may be classified according to pathophysiology.[1,36,42] Nociceptive pain is caused by the stimulation of pain receptors by noxious mechanical, chemical, or thermal stimuli and associated with ongoing tissue damage. Conditions associated with chronic nociceptive pain include arthritis, ischemia, cancer, and chronic pancreatitis. Neuropathic pain is the result of peripheral or CNS dysfunction without ongoing tissue damage. Neuropathic pain is seen in diabetic neuropathy, postherpetic neuralgia, and phantom limb pain. Mixed pain syndromes are those with multiple or uncertain pathophysiology. Examples include recurrent headache and some vasculitic syndromes. Psychological pain syndromes are those in which psychological processes play a large role. This kind of pain may be seen in somatoform disorders and conversion reactions. Although this classification of pain can be helpful for systematically approaching a patient with pain, the pathophysiology of chronic pain in an individual patient is often only partially understood. In addition, chronic pain may have more than one cause. The pain associated with arthritis, for example, may be caused by inflammation, joint distortion, strain on muscles and connective tissue, and microfracture from eroded cartilage or bone. This pain may also be magnified by psychological distress related to loss of function.[36]

Chronic pain may be the result of changes in sympathetic nervous system and adrenal activity, reduced production of endogenous opioids, or **sensitization** of primary afferent **(peripheral sensitization)** and spinal cord neurons. Decreased levels of **enkephalins** and increased numbers and sensitivity of nociceptors have been observed in individuals with chronic pain.[87] These individuals frequently have increased sensitivity to both noxious **(hyperalgesia)** and innocuous **(allodynia)** stimuli.[113] These changes in pain perception may in part be the result of a process known as *wind-up*, or *central sensitization*, in which the pathways that transmit pain continue to discharge after the discontinuation of intense or repeated stimulation. Then, even a small additional stimulus exceeds the threshold that is perceived as painful.[29,30,122,178] Thus, for an individual with a painful condition that is severe or long-lasting, the noxious stimulation may result in increased pain receptor activity and a consequent reduced tolerance for noxious or innocuous stimuli. Understanding of this sensitization mechanism has led to increased study and use of preemptive **analgesia** before procedures that are known to be painful in an attempt to reduce postprocedural pain and reduce recovery time.[22,47,68]

Although many patients with chronic pain have found ways to adapt and cope with their condition, there are some who catastrophize or perceive their symptoms to be debilitating. These patients are more likely to have difficulties with social function and employment. Some individuals, such as those with preexisting affective or anxiety disorders, or chemical dependence, are predisposed to becoming more dysfunctional in the face of chronic pain. Psychological and social factors associated with chronic pain include depression; catastrophizing; decreased function, quality of life, and ability to work; and increased dependence on others. In a study of 5,800 patients, 41% of those with depression reported disabling chronic pain compared with 10% of those without depression.[2] Patients with concurrent depression and disabling chronic pain had significantly poorer health-related quality of life, greater somatic symptom severity, and higher prevalence of panic disorder than other patients.[2] A study of 1800 depressed older adults also found that patients with coexisting arthritis (56%) who were treated for depression not only had decreased depressive symptoms but also had reduced pain and improved function and quality of life.[92] Catastrophizing has been positively correlated with the reported severity of pain, affective distress, muscle and joint tenderness, pain-related disability, poor outcomes of pain treatment, and possibly inflammatory disease activity.[32] These associations exist even after controlling for depression. Proposed effects of catastrophizing range from maladaptive influences on the social environment to direct amplification of the processing of pain by the CNS.[32] Although most studies have found a correlation between chronic pain and psychological factors, no studies have confirmed this relationship, making this an area in need of further research.[71]

Chronic pain can decrease a person's participation in normal activities. A study in Europe found that more than half of a group of patients with chronic pain were less able or unable to work outside the home, 19% had lost their jobs, and 13% had changed jobs because of their pain.[19] Chronic pain also impacts a person's relationship to others, particularly those in the caregiving role. In an enmeshed or solicitous relationship, the patient assumes a sick role that is unknowingly reinforced by the caregiver through "checking" behaviors and excessively supportive responses. It is important to note that although health care professionals may suspect that a patient is using chronic pain for secondary gain, to play the sick role, or to justify certain behaviors, this attitude may obstruct a patient's adjustment to chronic pain, prolong sick leave, and hinder rehabilitation.[52]

Ideally, the development of chronic pain should be prevented by early identification of individuals at risk. Patients with prolonged, severe, or disabling acute pain are at increased risk of developing chronic pain. To reduce this risk, pain-controlling interventions, such as physical agents or medications, should be applied during the acute stage of an injury and during the later recovery phases, when pain is still the result of pain receptor activation.[14] The prevention of chronic pain in patients who have had surgery should include avoiding nerve damage while in surgery and effective pain control immediately after surgery, because the intensity of acute postoperative pain correlates with the risk of developing chronic pain.[78]

If chronic pain develops, successful treatment usually requires that all components of the dysfunction be addressed. Multidisciplinary treatment programs based on a biopsychosocial model of pain have been specifically developed to address these problems.[163] These treatment programs are described in the section on pain management.

Referred Pain

Referred pain is felt at a location distant from its source. Pain may be referred from one joint to another, from a peripheral nerve to a distal area of innervation, or from an internal organ to an area of musculoskeletal tissue (Fig. 25-1). For example, hip joint pathology

occasionally refers pain to the knee, particularly in children, and compression of the spinal nerve roots at the L5 to S1 level as they exit through the spinal foramen may cause pain in the lateral leg because this is the area of sensory innervation.[81,153] Common referral patterns from internal organs to musculoskeletal tissue include the pain associated with myocardial infarction or angina caused by cardiac ischemia that is felt in the upper chest, left shoulder, jaw, and arm, and pain originating from the central portion of the diaphragm that is frequently felt in the lateral tip of either shoulder. The gallbladder also frequently refers pain to the right shoulder or the inferior angle of the right scapula, and the spleen refers pain to the left shoulder.

It is proposed that pain is referred in one of three ways: from a nerve to its area of innervation, from one area to another derived from the same dermatome, or from one area to another derived from the same embryonic segment. The peripheral neural pathways from these different areas converge on the same or similar areas of the spinal cord and **synapse** with the same second-order neurons to ascend the spinal cord and reach the central cortex.[175] For example, pain is referred from the diaphragm to the tip of the shoulder because both of these areas initially develop in the neck region during embryonic development, causing them both to have **efferent innervation** from the phrenic nerve and afferent innervation to the second through fourth levels of the cervical spine. When pain that may be of either visceral

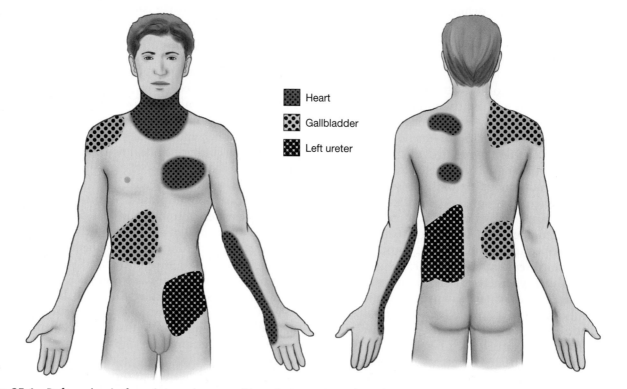

	Heart
	Gallbladder
	Left ureter

Fig. 25-1 Referred pain from internal organs. (From Cameron MH: *Physical agents in rehabilitation: from research to practice,* ed 3, St Louis, 2009, Saunders.)

or musculoskeletal origin converges on the same neuron in the spinal cord, it is usually interpreted to be of musculoskeletal origin. This may be because musculoskeletal injury and pain are so much more common that the brain "learns" that activity arriving along that pathway is associated with pain stimulus in a particular musculoskeletal area.

Clinicians who treat neuromusculoskeletal dysfunction must be aware of the potential for pain referral and be familiar with common pain referral patterns to determine the source of a patient's complaints and select appropriate treatment methods. Therefore, when a patient with pain in a musculoskeletal area seeks treatment, the clinician should first determine if the source of the pain is located in the area of this sensation. Pain of musculoskeletal origin generally varies with position or movement of the painful area, whereas pain caused by dysfunction in other systems generally varies with stress on those systems. For example, shoulder pain that is aggravated by raising the arm is likely to originate in the shoulder, whereas left shoulder pain that is aggravated by all forms of strenuous exercise may be caused by a cardiac condition. When assessing pain that is determined to be of musculoskeletal origin, it is also important to accurately determine the structure(s) at fault to provide the most effective treatment. This can be done by performing provocative tests to reproduce the patient's chief complaint. Physical agents may effectively relieve referred pain; however, they should not be used as a substitute for determining the true source of the pain or for treating its underlying cause. They may be used for pain relief while the source of the pain is being investigated, during the recovery process, and for controlling referred pain in which the underlying cause cannot be directly treated.

MECHANISMS OF PAIN RECEPTION AND TRANSMISSION

Pain is generally felt in response to stimulation of peripheral nociceptive structures. The stimulus is transmitted along peripheral nerves to the CNS, from where it can reach the cortex and consciousness. The sensation of pain and the individual's response to the sensation are influenced by a variety of factors, including the physiologic mechanisms of the pain receptors, the anatomy of pain-transmitting structures, neurotransmitter levels, and the motivation, behavior, and physiologic and emotional state of the individual. Variations in any of these factors can alter the individual's perception of pain severity, type, location, and duration.

Specific nerve endings called *nociceptors* respond to all painful stimuli, and specific nerve types, small myelinated A-delta fibers and unmyelinated C fibers, transmit the sensation of pain from these nerve endings to the spinal cord and then, within specific tracts, to the brain.

The quality of the pain depends on the type of tissue from which the stimulus originates and which of the two nerve types transmits the pain; the intensity of the pain is related to the firing rate of the nerves. Pain from cutaneous noxious stimulation is usually perceived as sharp, pricking, or tingling and is easy to localize, whereas pain from musculoskeletal structures is usually dull, heavy, or aching and is harder to localize.[155] Visceral pain has an aching quality similar to that of musculoskeletal pain but tends to refer superficially rather than deeply.[80]

Pain transmitted by C fibers is usually dull, long-lasting, and aching, whereas pain transmitted by A-delta fibers is generally sharp. The intensity of the pain and the responses to it are thought to be more severe when the intensity of nociceptive receptor stimulation is greater than that of nonnociceptive receptor stimulation, when levels of endogenous opioids are low, and with certain variations in the individual's psychological state.[182]

Pain Receptors

Nociceptors are free, noncorpuscular peripheral nerve endings consisting of a series of spindle-shaped, thick segments linked by thin segments to produce a "string-of-beads" appearance. The beads and end bulbs contain mitochondria, glycogen particles, vesicles, and bare areas of axolemma that are not covered by Schwann cell processes.[59] Nociceptors are present in almost all types of tissue. For example, low back pain is thought to be transmitted from free nerve endings that have been found in facet joints, discs, ligaments, nerve roots, and muscles.[23] In damaged discs, nerves also penetrate areas where they would normally not be present, such as the inner annulus fibrosus and the nucleus pulposus, thus contributing to discogenic pain.[119]

Nociceptors can be activated by intense thermal, mechanical, or chemical stimuli from exogenous or endogenous sources. For example, intense mechanical stimulation, such as that caused by a brick falling on someone's foot or a piece of broken bone compressing a nociceptor, will result in nociceptor activation. Chemical stimulation by exogenous substances, such as acid or bleach, or by endogenously produced substances, such as bradykinin, histamine, and arachidonic acid, which are released as part of the inflammatory response to tissue damage, can also activate nociceptors. Because these chemical mediators remain after the initial physical stimulus has passed, they generally cause pain to persist beyond the duration of the initial noxious stimulation. It is important to note that chemical mediators of inflammation also sensitize nociceptors, reducing their activation threshold to other stimuli.[5,8] This is the reason that clinically many activities and stimuli to recently injured areas are perceived as painful even when they are not damaging.

When nociceptors are activated, they release a variety of neuropeptides from their peripheral terminals,

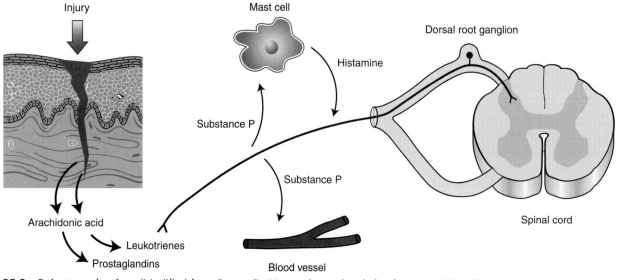

Fig. 25-2 **Pain transduction.** (Modified from Purves D: *Neuroscience*, Sunderland, Mass., 2004, Sinauer Associates; In Cameron MH: *Physical agents in rehabilitation: from research to practice*, ed 3, St Louis, 2009, Saunders.)

including substance P and a number of breakdown products of arachidonic acid, such as prostaglandins and leukotrienes.[87] Nociceptors also convert the initial stimulus into electrical activity, in the form of action potentials, by a process known as *transduction* (Fig. 25-2). It is thought that the released neuropeptides may initiate or participate in transduction because they sensitize nociceptors.[174] The action potentials resulting from the process of transduction propagate from the nociceptors along **afferent nerves** toward the spinal cord.

Peripheral Nerve Pathways

Nociceptors give rise to two types of first-order afferent nerve fibers, C fibers and A-delta fibers. The activity in both types of fibers increases in response to peripheral noxious stimulation, including that associated with acute inflammation or muscle ischemia.* Eighty percent of afferent pain-transmitting fibers are C fibers, and the remaining 20% are A-delta fibers.[38] Generally, about 50% of the sensory fibers in a cutaneous nerve have nociceptive functions.[182]

C fibers, also known as *group IV afferents*, are small, unmyelinated nerve fibers that transmit action potentials quite slowly, at the rate of 1.0 to 4.0 m/sec.[33] They respond to noxious levels of mechanical, thermal, and chemical stimulation, causing pain that is generally described as dull, throbbing, aching, or burning and may also be reported as tingling or tapping (Fig. 25-3).[115,154] The pain sensations transmitted by these fibers have a slow onset after the initial painful stimulus, are long-lasting, emotionally difficult for the individual to tolerate, and tend to be diffusely localized, particularly when the stimulus is intense.[54,97] They can be accompanied by autonomic responses such as sweating, increased heart rate and blood pressure, or nausea.[177] The pain associated with C fiber activation can be reduced by opiates, and this pain relief is blocked by the opiate antagonist naloxone.[167]

A-delta fibers, also known as *group III afferents*, are also small-diameter fibers; however, they transmit more rapidly than C fibers, at a rate of about 30 m/sec, because they are myelinated.[33,58] They are most sensitive to high-intensity mechanical stimulation, although they can also respond to stimulation by heat or cold and are capable of transmitting innocuous information.[114] The sensations associated with A-delta fiber activity are generally described as sharp, stabbing, or pricking.[182] The pain sensations transmitted by these fibers have a quick onset after the painful stimulus, last only for a short time, are generally localized to the area from which the stimulus arose, and are not generally associated with emotional involvement. The pain associated with A-delta fiber activation is generally not blocked by opiates.[48]

Mechanical trauma usually activates both C and A-delta fibers. Take the example of a brick landing on someone's foot. Almost immediately the individual feels a sharp sensation of pain. The initial pain is followed by a deep ache that may last for several hours or days. The initial sharp pain is transmitted by the A-delta fibers and is produced in response to the high-intensity mechanical stimulation of the nociceptors as a result of the impact of the brick. The later, deep ache is transmitted by the C fibers and is produced in response to stimulation by chemical mediators of inflammation released by the tissue after the initial injury.

A-beta nerve fibers can also be involved in abnormal pain transmission and perception. A-beta fibers,

*See references 5, 8, 23, 40, 44, 46, 55, 56, 59, 107, 119, 121, 147, 148, 155, 182.

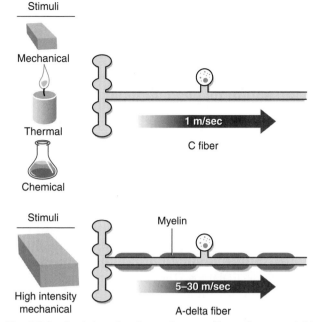

Fig. 25-3 Peripheral pain pathways. (From Cameron MH: *Physical agents in rehabilitation: from research to practice,* ed 3, St Louis, 2009, Saunders.)

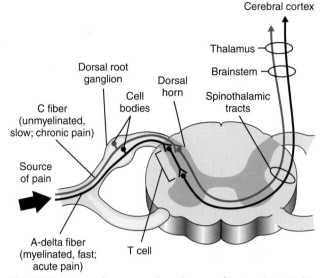

Fig. 25-4 Ascending neural pathway of pain via A-delta and C fibers. (From Cameron MH: *Physical agents in rehabilitation: from research to practice,* ed 3, St Louis, 2009, Saunders.)

or wide dynamic-range neurons, have relatively large myelinated axons that conduct impulses more quickly than A-delta and C fibers. Their receptors are located in the skin, bones, and joints. Normally, they transmit sensation related to vibration, stretching of skin, and mechanoreception and do not transmit pain. However, in states such as neuropathic pain and central sensitization, these neurons alter their transduction so that normal stimuli result in pain. There are three theories on how A-beta fibers contribute to pain.[132] The first theory states that firing of A-beta fibers activates spinal neurons that have undergone central sensitization. The second theory posits that A-beta fibers might sprout into spinal cord layers normally targeted by C-fibers and when activated, stimulate the wrong neurons.[179] A third theory states that intact A-beta nerve fibers near damaged nociceptive nerves begin firing abnormally.[180] This alteration in nerve function is key in prolonged pain.

Central Pathways

The peripheral first-order C and A-delta afferents project from the periphery to the grey matter of the spinal cord. The C and A-delta fibers synapse, either directly or via interneurons, with second-order neurons in the superficial dorsal horn of the gray matter (the substantia gelatinosa).[33,85,89-91] Some A-delta fibers penetrate more deeply into the dorsal horn to terminate at the normal termination sites of A-beta afferents. The interneurons in the dorsal horn are also known as *transmission cells,* or *T cells* (Fig. 25-4).

T cells make local connections within the spinal cord, either with efferent neurons as part of spinal cord reflexes

or with afferent neurons that project toward the cortex. Continued or repetitive C-fiber activation can sensitize the T cells, causing them to fire more rapidly and to increase their receptor field size, and input from other interneurons originating in the substantia gelatinosa of the spinal cord or from descending fibers originating in higher brain centers can inhibit T-cell activity.[10] Inhibitory interneurons in the substantia gelatinosa are activated by input from large-diameter, myelinated, low-threshold sensory neurons (primarily A-beta nerves) that respond to nonpainful stimuli.[60,103] These inhibitory interneurons release various neurotransmitters, including norepinephrine, serotonin, and enkephalins, to modulate the flow of the afferent pain pathways.[6,39,157] Thus the transmission cells receive excitatory input from the C fibers and A-delta nociceptor afferents and inhibitory input from large-diameter, nonnociceptor sensory afferents and from descending fibers from higher brain centers (Fig. 25-5).[182]

The balance of these excitatory and inhibitory inputs influences whether the individual feels pain and how severe the pain sensation is.[103] The inhibition of pain by inputs from nonnociceptor afferents is known as *pain gating* and is discussed in greater detail in the section on pain modulation and control theories.

Transmission cell activation can increase muscle spasm via a spinal cord reflex in which the transmission cell synapses with anterior horn cells to cause muscle contractions. The ongoing muscle contractions can cause accumulation of fluid and tissue irritants. The contracting muscles may also initiate further nociceptive impulses by mechanically compressing the nociceptors. In this way the combination of ongoing chemical and mechanical stimuli can set up a self-sustaining cycle of pain causing muscle spasm, which then causes more

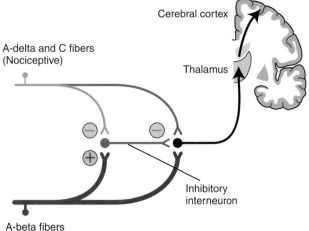

Fig. 25-5 Simplified diagram of the gate control mechanism of pain modulation. (From Cameron MH: *Physical agents in rehabilitation: from research to practice,* ed 3, St Louis, 2009, Saunders.)

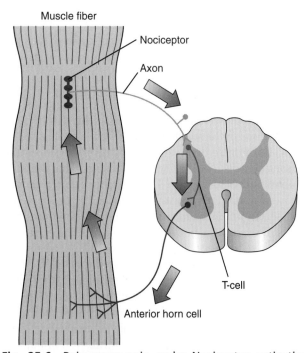

Fig. 25-6 Pain-spasm-pain cycle: Nociceptor activation resulting in T-cell activation stimulating an anterior horn cell to cause a muscle fiber to contract, resulting in accumulation of fluid and tissue irritants and mechanical compression of the nociceptor and increasing nociceptor activation. (From Cameron MH: *Physical agents in rehabilitation: from research to practice,* ed 3, St Louis, 2009, Saunders.)

pain. This is known as the *pain-spasm-pain cycle* (Fig. 25-6). Many interventions indirectly reduce pain, even after their direct analgesic effect has passed, because they reduce muscle spasms and thereby interfere with this self-perpetuating cycle.

Ascending second-order nerves carry stimuli within the spinal cord toward the higher brain centers (Fig. 25-7). The second-order pathways that carry pain stimuli are located primarily in the anterolateral aspect of the cord.[173] This area of the spinal cord also transmits information about temperature and touch. Most axons in the anterolateral system cross midline in the spinal cord to ascend contralaterally. Information regarding pain is transmitted within the anterolateral cord via both the lateral spinothalamic tract and the larger anterospinothalamic tract to project to the thalamus. The lateral spinothalamic tract projects directly to the medial area of the thalamus, whereas the anterospinothalamic tract separates from the lateral spinothalamic tract in the brain stem to synapse with neurons in the reticular formation and the hypothalamic and limbic systems, to then project to lateral, ventral, and caudal areas of the thalamus. The anterospinothalamic tract also relays information to the periaqueductal gray matter, which has a large concentration of opiate receptors and is thought to be associated with pain modulation. Impulses relayed via the lateral spinothalamic tract are involved in transmission of sharp pain and in localization of the painful stimulus, whereas those sent via the anterospinothalamic tract are involved in transmission of more prolonged, aching pain and are thought to have stronger association with the disturbing emotions that accompany the pain sensation. The second-order neurons synapse in the thalamus with third-order neurons to project to the cortex, from which the sensation of pain can reach consciousness.

Sympathetic Nervous System Influences

The sympathetic nervous system is a component of the **autonomic nervous system.** The autonomic nervous system consists of the sympathetic and parasympathetic systems and is concerned with the activities of smooth and cardiac muscles and with glandular secretion. This contrasts with most of the nervous system, which is concerned with voluntary activation of the skeletal muscles or with transmission of sensory impulses from the periphery (Fig. 25-8).[45,64] The sympathetic nervous system is considered to be primarily involved in producing effects that prepare the body for "fight or flight," such as increasing heart rate and blood pressure, constricting cutaneous blood vessels, and increasing sweating in the palms of the hands. Although it is normal for the sympathetic nervous system to be activated by acute pain or injury, stimulation of the sympathetic nervous system efferents does not usually cause pain.[65] However, abnormal sympathetic activation, caused by a hyperactive response of the sympathetic nervous system to an acute injury or by a failure of its response to subside, can increase pain severity and cause exaggerated signs and symptoms of sympathetic activity, such as excessive vasomotor or sweating reactions. In patients with these

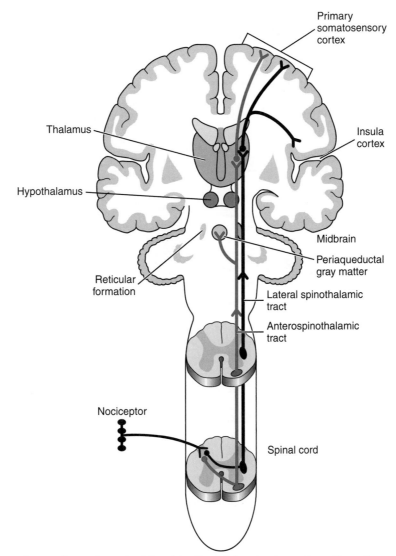

Fig. 25-7 Central pain pathways from the spinal level to the higher brain centers. (From Cameron MH: *Physical agents in rehabilitation: from research to practice,* ed 3, St Louis, 2009, Saunders.)

signs and symptoms, pain relief can often be achieved by interrupting sympathetic nervous system activity by chemical or surgical means.[18,21,84] In addition, stimuli that evoke sympathetic discharges, such as the startle reflex or emotional events, frequently exacerbate pain. It has therefore been proposed that excessive sympathetic nervous system activation may increase or maintain pain.[45,64] Although anesthetic blockade of the sympathetic nervous system is widely used to reduce pain in **complex regional pain syndrome (CRPS)**, its effectiveness has not yet been proven.[24,25]

Pain that is believed to involve sympathetic nervous system overactivation has a variety of names, including causalgia, reflex sympathetic dystrophy (RSD), shoulder-hand syndrome, posttraumatic dystrophy, Sudeck atrophy, and sympathetically maintained pain.[123] Currently, the International Association for the Study of Pain (IASP) recommends the use of the term *complex regional pain syndrome.*[90] CRPS involving tissue damage

without nerve damage is categorized as type I, and CRPS associated with nerve involvement is categorized as type II.[90] In addition, pain that is reduced with sympathetic blockade may be called *sympathetically maintained pain* (SMP), whereas pain that does not respond to sympathetic blockade may be called *sympathetically independent pain* (SIP).[90]

CRPS generally includes the following signs and symptoms: severe pain that is out of proportion to the inciting injury or disease, hyperesthesia (excessive reaction to painful stimuli), and allodynia (the sensation of pain in response to stimuli that are not usually painful). CRPS frequently also includes trophic changes such as skin atrophy and hyperhidrosis, edema, stiffness, increased sweating, and decreased hair growth.[90] These symptoms generally result in decreased function and if the syndrome is prolonged, spotty osteoporosis in the affected area.[37] Other sensory, vasomotor, and skeletal motor abnormalities have also been associated with this

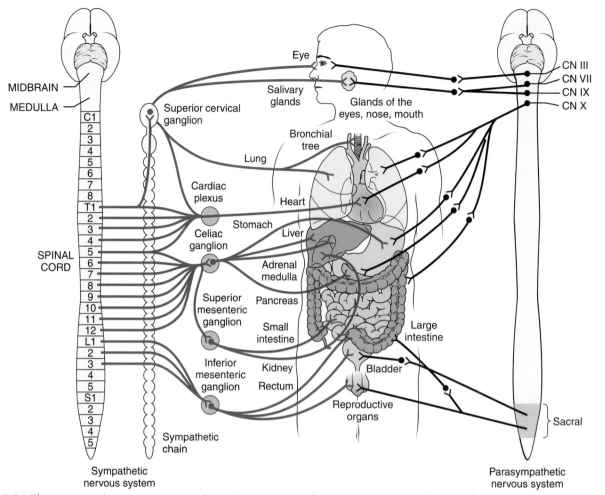

Fig 25-8 The autonomic nervous system. (From Cameron MH: *Physical agents in rehabilitation: from research to practice,* ed 3, St Louis, 2009, Saunders.)

syndrome.[135] CRPS can occur in any area of the body but is most common in the hand and in such cases, is frequently associated with ipsilateral restriction of shoulder motion. CRPS may develop as a consequence of major or minor trauma, after visceral disease or CNS lesions, or without any known antecedent event.

The Role of Substance P

Substance P is a neurotransmitter thought to be involved in the transmission of neuropathic and inflammatory pain. Substance P is present in both the central and peripheral nervous systems. In the CNS, it is found in approximately 20% of C fibers.[168] It is also released from peripheral nociceptors and has been detected in inflammatory exudate.[41,86,98] Substance P release can excite pain-transmitting neurons in the dorsal horn of the spinal cord and is involved in nociceptive processing at the spinal cord level.* Although less than 5% of the neurons in the dorsal horn express substance P receptors,

the majority of pain-transmitting neurons express these receptors. Substance P levels in the spinal cord increase in response to induction of joint inflammation and in response to movement of inflamed joints. Elevated levels of substance P in both the cerebrospinal fluid (CSF) and blood of fibromyalgia patients correlate with elevated inflammatory markers in the blood.[94] Substance P receptor activation appears to be involved in the sensitization of pain-transmitting neurons and in the development of hyperalgesia.[94,116,130,146,159] Substance P release and receptor activation is thought to be a response to tissue injury and stress.

A number of mechanisms have been proposed for the action of substance P on pain transmission. Substance P may facilitate excitation of afferent pain fibers by activating the neurokinin-1 receptors in the spinal cord.[126,140] Substance P may also contribute to localized inflammation by causing mast cells to release proinflammatory and neurosensitizing molecules.[94,134] When released into the periphery, substance P increases the production of the inflammatory mediator prostaglandin E_2 (PGE_2) and the release of cytokines from macrophages and

---

*See references 18, 21, 24, 25, 37, 41, 45, 64, 65, 84, 86, 98, 112, 123, 127, 135, 143, 146, 157, 168, 173.

neutrophils.[83] Both prostaglandins and cytokines sensitize primary afferent nociceptors.[160]

Treatments to control pain based on inhibiting substance P release or using substance P receptor antagonists seem promising but have shown poor results thus far. Although certain substances have been found to inhibit the release of substance P in rats,[109] it is uncertain if these substances would affect pain in humans. Substance P receptor antagonists have not been found to decrease pain in human subjects[43] or relieve depression, another condition associated with elevated levels of substance P.[79] Opiates may in part exert an analgesic effect by inhibiting the release of substance P from peripheral nerves, although substance P receptor–expressing neurons are not the major site of action of opiates.[67,116] One study found that opiates reduced the sensation of pain related to substance P by inhibiting its effects both presynaptically and postsynaptically.[166] By activating the μ opioid receptor, morphine may also impact the neurokinin-1 receptor and substance P, impacting immune responses in the CNS.[165] Noradrenalin may be the link between opiate-induced pain relief and substance P. In mice without noradrenaline, morphine was not effective and levels of substance P and pain were elevated; this effect was reversed with administration of noradrenaline or substance P receptor antagonists.[66] Substance P has also been linked to the paradoxical increased pain seen with high-dose opiates in animals.[131]

PAIN MODULATION AND CONTROL

Pain transmission and perception are subject to inhibition and modification. For example, rubbing or shaking an area that hurts can relieve pain in that area, and stress can cause pain not to be felt at the time an injury occurs. Several mechanisms have been proposed to explain pain control and modulation. These proposed mechanisms attempt to correlate what is known regarding the experience of pain with the structures and physiologic processes thought to be involved in pain transmission. According to the gate control theory, pain is modulated at the spinal cord level by inhibitory effects of innocuous afferent input. According to the theory of endogenous opiates, pain is modulated at the peripheral, spinal cord, and cortical levels by endogenous neurotransmitters that have the same effects as opiates. Psychological central control mechanisms are also thought to affect pain perception and control.

Various physical, chemical, and psychological interventions have been developed based on the current understanding of the mechanisms underlying pain modulation. For example, transcutaneous electrical nerve stimulation (TENS) devices were developed based on the gate control theory of pain modulation. Also, the efficacy of a number of established treatment approaches is now better understood because the underlying mechanisms of pain control have become clearer. For example,

it is now thought that thermal agents, which have been used to control pain for centuries, may be effective for this purpose because they gate pain transmission at the spinal cord.

Gate Control Theory

The gate control theory of pain modulation was first proposed by Melzack and Wall[103] in 1965. According to this theory, severity of the pain sensation is determined by the balance of excitatory and inhibitory inputs to the T cells in the spinal cord. These cells receive excitatory input from C and A-delta nociceptor afferents and inhibitory input via the substantia gelatinosa from large-diameter A-beta nonnociceptor sensory afferents. Increased activity of the nonnociceptor sensory afferents causes presynaptic inhibition of the T cells and thus effectively closes the spinal gate to the cerebral cortex and decreases the sensation of pain (see Fig. 25-5).

Many physical agents and interventions are thought to control pain in part by activating nonnociceptive sensory nerves, thereby inhibiting activation of pain transmission cells and closing the gate to the transmission of pain.[111,164] For example, electrical stimulation (ES), traction, compression, and massage can all activate low-threshold, large-diameter, nonnociceptive sensory nerves and therefore may inhibit pain transmission by closing the gate to pain transmission at the spinal cord level.

Although the gate control theory explains many observations regarding pain control and modulation, it fails to account for the finding that descending controls from higher brain centers, in addition to ascending input from sensory afferents, can affect pain perception.[82,110] Therefore the gate theory has been modified to include influences from descending neurons from the limbic system, the raphe nucleus, and the reticular systems, which affect pain perception, the emotional aspects of pain, and motor responses to pain.[105]

The Endogenous Opioid System

Pain perception is also modulated by endogenous opiate-like peptides. These peptides are called *opiopeptins* (previously known as *endorphins*). Opiopeptins control pain by binding to specific opiate receptors in the nervous system.

An endogenous system of analgesia was first discovered by three independent groups of researchers who were investigating the mechanisms of morphine-induced analgesia. In 1973, they discovered specific opiate-binding sites in the CNS.[120,138,151] In 1975, two peptides, met-enkephalin (methionine-enkephalin) and leu-enkephalin (leucine-enkephalin), which were isolated from the CNS of a pig, were shown to produce physiologic effects similar to those of morphine.[62] These peptides also bind specifically to the opiate receptors, and their action and binding are blocked by naloxone, an opiate antagonist.[99] These findings demonstrated that these endogenous peptides are similar to exogenous opiates such as morphine. Consequently, researchers identified and isolated other similar-acting endogenous peptides, such as beta-endorphin and dynorphin A and B.[139]

Opiopeptins and opiate receptors have been found in many peripheral nerve endings and in neurons in several regions of the nervous system.[170] Concentrations of opiopeptins and opiate receptors have been identified in various areas of the brain, including the periaqueductal gray matter (PAGM) and the raphe nucleus of the brain stem, which are structures that induce analgesia when electrically stimulated, and in various areas of the limbic system. Opiopeptins are also found in high concentrations in the superficial layers of the dorsal horn of the spinal cord (layers I and II) and in the enteric nervous system, as well as in the nerve endings of C fibers. It has been proposed that opiate receptors inhibit the release of substance P from C-fiber terminals because local opiate application to C-fiber terminals depresses pain transmission at the spinal cord level.[96]

Opioids and opiopeptins always have an inhibitory action. They cause presynaptic inhibition by suppressing the inward flux of calcium and cause postsynaptic inhibition by activating an outward potassium current. In addition, opiopeptins indirectly inhibit pain transmission by inhibiting the release of gamma-aminobutyric acid (GABA) in the PAGM and the raphe nucleus.[57] GABA inhibits the activity of various pain-controlling structures, including A-beta afferents, the PAGM, and the raphe nucleus, and can thus increase pain transmission in the spinal cord. The concentration of opiate receptors and opiopeptins in the limbic system, an area of the brain largely associated with emotional phenomena, also provides an explanation for the emotional responses to pain and for the euphoria and relief of emotional stress associated with the use of morphine and the release of opiopeptins.[142]

The release of opiopeptins is thought to play an important role in the modulation and control of pain during times of emotional stress. Levels of opiopeptins in the brain and CSF become elevated, and pain thresholds increase in both animals and humans when stress is induced experimentally by the anticipation of pain.[152,171] Experimentally, animals have been shown to experience a diffuse analgesia when placed under stress. Humans demonstrate a naloxone-sensitive increase in pain threshold and a parallel depression of the nociceptive flexion reflex when subjected to emotional stress.[171,172] These findings indicate that pain suppression by stress is most likely caused by increased opiopeptin levels at the spinal cord and higher CNS centers.

The **endogenous opiate theory** also provides an explanation for the paradoxical pain-relieving effects of painful stimulation and acupuncture. Bearable levels of painful stimulation, such as topical preparations that cause the sensation of burning, or noxious TENS that causes the sensation of pricking or burning, have been shown to reduce the intensity of less bearable preexisting pain in the area of application and in other areas.[172] Painful stimuli have also been shown to reduce the nociceptive flexion reflex of the lower limb in animals.[156] Because these effects of painful stimulation are blocked by naloxone, they are thought to be mediated by opiopeptins.[4,100,171,172] Pain may be relieved because the applied painful stimulus causes neurons in the PAGM regions of the midbrain and thalamus to produce and release opiopeptins.[4]

Placebo analgesia is also thought to be mediated in part by opiopeptins. This claim is supported by the observation that the opiate antagonist naloxone can reverse placebo analgesia and that placebos can also produce respiratory depression, a typical side effect of opioids.[7,88]

MEASURING PAIN

To determine the most appropriate treatment for a patient's pain and to assess the efficacy of such treatment, it is helpful to assess the nature and severity of the patient's pain. Such an assessment should attempt to ascertain the causes and sources of pain, the intensity and duration of pain, and the degree to which the pain affects body function, activity, and participation.

Various methods and assessment tools have been developed to quantify and qualify both experimentally induced and clinical pain. These methods are based on patients rating their pain on a visual analog or numeric scale; comparing their present pain with that experienced in response to a predefined, quantifiable pain stimulus; or selecting words from a list to describe their present experience of pain. In cases where a person cannot express their pain by one of these methods, as with infants, observational scales are used. These tools provide different amounts and types of information and require varying amounts of time and cognitive ability to complete.

Visual Analog and Numeric Scales

Visual analog and numeric scales assess pain severity by asking the patient to indicate the present level of pain on a drawn line or to rate the pain numerically on a scale of 0 to 10 or 0 to 100.[31] With a visual analog scale, the patient marks a position on a horizontal or vertical line, where one end of the line represents no pain and the other end represents the most severe pain possible or the most severe pain the patient can imagine (Fig. 25-9). With a numeric rating scale, 0 is no pain and 10 or 100, depending on the scale used, is the most severe pain possible or the most severe pain the patient can imagine.

Scales similar to the visual analog or numeric scales have been developed for use with individuals who have difficulty using numeric or standard visual analog scales. For example, children who understand words or pictures but are too young to understand numeric representations of pain can use a scale with faces with different expressions to represent different experiences of pain, as shown in Fig. 25-10. This type of scale can also be used to assess pain in patients with limited comprehension because of language barriers or cognitive deficits. For example, patients with dementia can reliably use self-assessment pain scales, and this self-assessment is more accurate than observing the patient for signs of pain according to an observational pain scale.[118] Pain scales based on a child's expression and behavior are used to rate pain in very young children and infants (Table 25-1).

These types of scales are frequently used to assess the severity of a patient's clinical pain because they are quick and easy to administer and easily understood and provide readily quantifiable data.[31] However, visual analog and numeric scales reflect only the intensity of pain

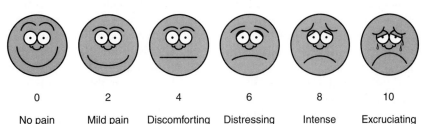

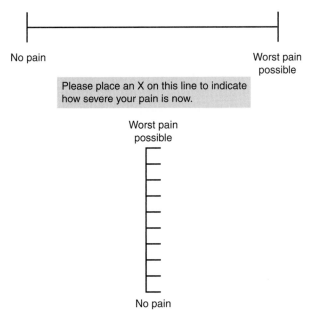

Fig. 25-9 Visual analog scales for rating pain severity. (From Cameron MH: *Physical agents in rehabilitation: from research to practice,* ed 3, St Louis, 2009, Saunders.)

and lack information about the patient's response to pain or the effect of the pain on function and activity. Sometimes, combining a visual analog scale with quality of life questions can be an effective way to obtain more information about the impact of pain on a person's life.[158] The reliability of visual analog and numeric rating varies between individuals and with the patient group examined, although the two scales have a high degree of agreement between them.[50] These types of measures are most useful in the clinical setting for a quick estimate of a patient's perceived progress or change in symptoms over time or in response to different activities or interventions.

Semantic Differential Scales

Semantic differential scales consist of word lists and categories that represent various aspects of the patient's pain experience. The patient is asked to select from these lists words that best describe his or her present experience of pain. These types of scales are designed to collect a broad range of information about the patient's pain experience and to provide quantifiable data for intrasubject and intersubject comparisons. The semantic differential scale included in the McGill Pain Questionnaire, or variations of this scale, are commonly used to assess pain (Fig. 25-11).[20,104,124] This scale includes descriptors of sensory, affective, and evaluative aspects of the patient's pain and groups the words into various categories within each of these aspects. The categories include temporal, spatial, pressure, and thermal to describe the sensory aspects of the pain; fear, anxiety, and tension to describe the affective aspects of the pain; and the cognitive experience of the pain based on past experience and learned behaviors to describe the evaluative aspects of the pain. The patient circles the one word in each of the applicable categories that best describes his or her present pain.[104,124]

Semantic differential scales have a number of advantages and disadvantages compared with other types of pain measures. They allow assessment and quantification of the pain's scope, quality, and intensity. Counting the total number of words chosen provides a quick gauge of the pain severity. A more sensitive assessment of pain

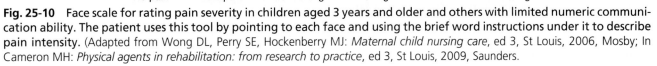

0	2	4	6	8	10
No pain	Mild pain	Discomforting	Distressing	Intense	Excruciating

Fig. 25-10 Face scale for rating pain severity in children aged 3 years and older and others with limited numeric communication ability. The patient uses this tool by pointing to each face and using the brief word instructions under it to describe pain intensity. (Adapted from Wong DL, Perry SE, Hockenberry MJ: *Maternal child nursing care,* ed 3, St Louis, 2006, Mosby; In Cameron MH: *Physical agents in rehabilitation: from research to practice,* ed 3, St Louis, 2009, Saunders.

Table 25-1	*Neonatal Infant Pain Scale Operational Definitions*	
Parameter	**Behavior and Score**	**Description**
Facial expression	0: Relaxed muscles	Restful face, neutral expression
	1: Grimace	Tight facial muscles, furrowed brow, chin, jaw (negative facial expression—nose, mouth, and brow)
Cry	0: No cry	Quiet, not crying
	1: Whimper	Mild moaning, intermittent
	2: Vigorous cry	Loud screams, rising, shrill, continuous (Note: Silent cry may be scored if baby is intubated, as evidenced by obvious mouth, facial movement.)
Breathing patterns	0: Relaxed	Usual pattern for this baby
	1: Change in breathing	Indrawing, irregular, faster than usual, gagging, breath holding
Arms	0: Relaxed/restrained	No muscular rigidity, occasional random arm movements
	1: Flexed/extended	Tense, straight arms, rigid or rapid extension, flexion
Legs	0: Relaxed/restrained	No muscular rigidity, occasional random leg movements
	1: Flexed/extended	Tense, straight legs, rigid or rapid extension, flexion
State of arousal	0: Sleeping/awake	Quiet, peaceful, sleeping, or alert and settled
	1: Fussy	Alert, restless, and thrashing

Score 0 = no pain likely; maximum score 7 = severe pain likely.
From Neonatal Infant Pain Scale, Children's Hospital of Eastern Ontario, Ottawa, Canada.

severity can be obtained by adding the rank sums of all the words chosen to produce a pain rating index (PRI). For greater specificity with regard to the most problematic area, an index for the three major categories of the questionnaire can also be calculated.[124] The primary disadvantages of this scale are that it is time-consuming to administer and requires the patient to have an intact cognitive state and a high level of literacy. Given these advantages and limitations, the most appropriate use for this type of scale is when detailed information about a patient's pain is needed, such as in a chronic pain treatment program or in clinical research. For example, in patients with chronic wounds, the McGill Pain Questionnaire was more sensitive to pain experience than a single rating of pain intensity and positively correlated with wound stage, affective stress, and symptoms of depression.[129]

Other Measures

Other measures or indicators of pain that may provide additional useful information about the individual's pain complaint and clinical condition include daily activity/pain logs indicating which activities ease or aggravate the pain, body diagrams on which the patient can indicate the location and nature of the pain (Fig. 25-12), and open-ended, structured interviews.[125,128] Physical examination that includes observation of posture and assessment of strength, mobility, sensation, endurance, response to functional activity testing, and soft tissue tone and quality can also add valuable information to the evaluation of the severity and cause(s) of a patient's pain complaint.

In selecting the measures to assess pain, consider symptom duration, the patient's cognitive abilities, and the time needed to assess the patient's report of pain. Often, a simple visual analog scale may be sufficient, as when evaluating a progressive decrease in pain as a patient recovers from an acute injury. However, in more complex or prolonged cases, detailed measures such as semantic differential scales or a combination of several measures are more appropriate.

DOCUMENTING PAIN

To most clearly document pain, it is best to be as thorough as possible. Documentation should note the pain's location, quality, severity, and timing, as well as the factors that make it better or worse, the setting in which it occurs, and associated manifestations.[11,125] The pain should be quantified, and there should be an assessment of how the pain has affected a person's function, activities, and participation. An example of the documentation of pain follows:

JS reports 7/10 aching central low back pain when sitting for more than 15 minutes that improves to 5/10 with movement or ibuprofen. The pain began 1 week ago after bending to lift a heavy box, and since then JS has been unable to lift anything heavier than 10 pounds and has been unable to work in his construction job.

PAIN MANAGEMENT APPROACHES

Once the severity and nature of an individual's pain has been evaluated and ideally its source and nature determined, the goals of treatment include eliminating

What does your pain feel like?

Some of the words below describe your *present* pain. Indicate which words describe it best. Leave out any word group that is not suitable. Use only a single word in each appropriate group—the one that applies *best.*

1	2	3	4
1 Flickering	1 Jumping	1 Pricking	1 Sharp
2 Quivering	2 Flashing	2 Boring	2 Cutting
3 Pulsing	3 Shooting	3 Drilling	3 Lacerating
4 Throbbing		4 Stabbing	
5 Beating		5 Lancinating	
6 Pounding			

5	6	7	8
1 Pinching	1 Tugging	1 Hot	1 Tingling
2 Pressing	2 Pulling	2 Burning	2 Itchy
3 Gnawing	3 Wrenching	3 Scalding	3 Smarting
4 Cramping		4 Searing	4 Stinging
5 Crushing			

9	10	11	12
1 Dull	1 Tender	1 Tiring	1 Sickening
2 Sore	2 Taut	2 Exhausting	2 Suffocating
3 Hurting	3 Rasping		
4 Aching	4 Splitting		
5 Heavy			

13	14	15	16
1 Fearful	1 Punishing	1 Wretched	1 Annoying
2 Frightful	2 Gruelling	2 Blinding	2 Troublesome
3 Terrifying	3 Cruel		3 Miserable
	4 Vicious		4 Intense
	5 Killing		5 Unbearable

17	18	19	20
1 Spreading	1 Tight	1 Cool	1 Nagging
2 Radiating	2 Numb	2 Cold	2 Nauseating
3 Penetrating	3 Drawing	3 Freezing	3 Agonizing
4 Piercing	4 Squeezing		4 Dreadful
	5 Tearing		5 Torturing

Fig. 25-11 Semantic differential scale from the McGill Pain Questionnaire. (From Melzack R: The McGill Pain Questionnaire: major properties and scoring methods, *Pain* 1(3):277-299, 1975.)

the cause of pain, controlling the nociceptor input, and improving patient function. A wide range of pain management approaches may help achieve these goals. These approaches are based on our current understanding of pain transmission and control mechanisms. They may act by controlling inflammation, altering nociceptor sensitivity, increasing binding to opiate receptors, modifying nerve conduction, modulating pain transmission at the spinal cord level, or altering higher-level aspects of pain perception. Some treatment approaches also address the psychological and social aspects of pain. Different approaches are appropriate for different situations and clinical

presentations and are frequently most effective when used together.

The primary intervention used to alleviate pain is the administration of pharmacologic agents. Although pharmacologic agents often provide effective pain relief, they can also produce a variety of adverse effects. Therefore the use of physical agents, which also effectively control pain in many cases and produce fewer adverse effects, may be more appropriate. Some patients, particularly those with persistent pain, may need integrated multidisciplinary treatment, which includes psychological and physiologic therapies, to achieve pain relief or return to a more normal functional activity level.

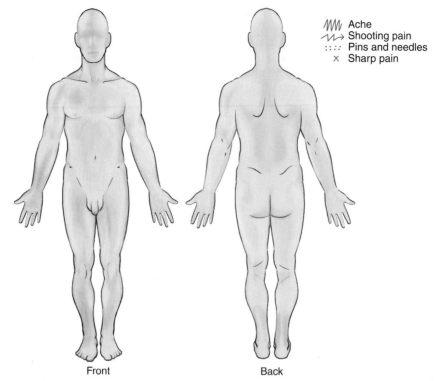

$\wedge\wedge\wedge$	Ache
$\wedge\wedge\rightarrow$	Shooting pain
: : : :	Pins and needles
×	Sharp pain

Front   Back

Fig. 25-12 Body diagrams for marking the location and nature of pain. (From Cameron MH, Monroe, LG: *Physical rehabilitation: evidence-based examination, evaluation, and intervention,* St Louis, 2007, Saunders.)

Pharmacologic Approaches

Pharmacologic analgesic agents control pain by modifying inflammatory mediators at the periphery, altering pain transmission from the periphery to the cortex, or altering the central perception of pain. The selection of a particular pharmacologic analgesic agent depends on the cause of the pain, the length of time the individual is expected to need the agent, and the side effects of the agent. Pharmacologic agents may be administered systemically by mouth, injection, transdermally, or locally by injection into structures surrounding the spinal cord or into painful or inflamed areas. These different routes of administration allow concentration of the drug at different sites of pain transmission to optimize the control of symptoms with varying distributions. Pharmacologic agents used to control pain fall into the following categories: nonsteroidal antiinflammatory drugs (NSAIDs), acetaminophen, opiates and opioids, and antidepressants.

Physical Agents

Physical agents are one of the primary pain control interventions utilized in physical therapy and can relieve pain directly by moderating the release of inflammatory mediators, modulating pain at the spinal cord level, altering nerve conduction, or increasing opiopeptin levels. They may indirectly reduce pain by decreasing the sensitivity of the muscle spindle system, thereby reducing muscle spasms, or by modifying vascular tone

and the rate of blood flow, thereby reducing edema or ischemia.[27,34,181] In addition, physical agents may reduce pain by helping resolve the underlying cause of the painful sensation.

Different physical agents control pain in different ways. For example, cryotherapy, the application of cold, controls acute pain in part by reducing the metabolic rate and thus reducing the production and release of inflammatory mediators such as serotonin, histamine, bradykinin, substance P, and prostaglandins.[102] These chemicals cause pain directly by stimulating nociceptors and indirectly by impairing the local microcirculation; they can damage tissue and impair tissue repair. Reducing the release of inflammatory mediators can thus directly relieve pain caused by acute inflammation and may indirectly limit pain by controlling edema and ischemia. These short-term benefits can also optimize the rate of tissue healing and recovery.

Cryotherapy (Fig. 25-13, *A*), thermotherapy (Fig. 25-13, *B*), ES, and traction (Fig. 25-13, *C*), which provide thermal, mechanical, or other nonnociceptive sensory stimuli, are thought to alleviate pain in part by inhibiting pain transmission at the spinal cord. Physical agents that act by this mechanism can be used for the treatment of acute and chronic pain because they do not generally produce significant adverse effects or adverse interactions with drugs and do not produce physical dependence with prolonged use. They are also

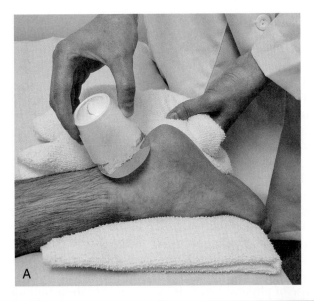

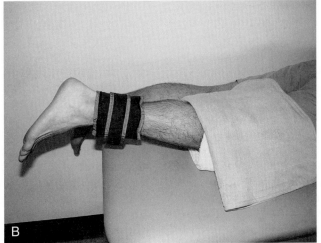

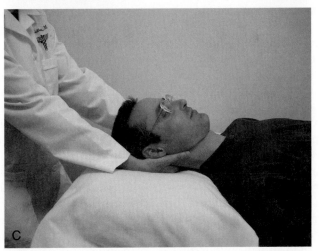

Fig. 25-13 Examples of several physical agents useful in rehabilitation. **A,** Application of ice massage (cryotherapy). **B,** Low-load prolonged stretch with heat (thermotherapy). **C,** Manual cervical traction. (From Cameron MH: *Physical agents in rehabilitation: from research to practice,* ed 3, St Louis, 2009, Saunders.)

effective and appropriate for pain caused by conditions that cannot be directly modified, such as pain caused by malignancy or a recent fracture, and for pain caused by peripheral nervous system pathology, such as phantom limb pain and peripheral neuropathy.[61]

ES is also thought to control pain in part by stimulating the release of opiopeptins at the spinal cord and at higher levels.[4] Studies have shown that pain relief by certain types of ES is reversed by naloxone.[4]

Physical agents have many advantages over other pain-modifying interventions. They are associated with fewer and generally less severe side effects than pharmacologic agents. The adverse effects of physical agents used to control pain are generally localized to the area of application and are easily avoided with care in applying the treatment. When used appropriately, attending to all contraindications and dose recommendations, the risk of further injury from the use of physical agents is minimal. For example, an excessively warm hot pack may cause a burn in the area of application, but this risk can be minimized by carefully monitoring the hot pack's temperature, using adequate insulation between the hot pack and the patient, not applying hot packs to individuals with impaired sensation or an impaired ability to report pain, and by checking with the patient for any sensation of excessive heat. Patients also do not develop dependence on physical agents, although they may wish to continue to use them even after they are no longer effective because they enjoy the sensation or attention associated with their application. For example, patients may wish to continue to be treated with ultrasound even though they have reached a stage of recovery where they would benefit more from active exercise. Physical agents also do not generally cause a degree of sedation that would impair an individual's ability to work or drive safely.

Many physical agents can be used independently by patients to treat themselves. For example, a patient can learn to apply a pain-controlling agent, such as heat, cold, or ES, when needed, and so become more independent of the health care practitioner and pharmacologic agents. The application of such physical agents at home can be an effective component of the treatment of both acute and chronic pain.[176] This type of self-treatment can also help contain the costs of medical care.

Physical agents used either alone or in conjunction with other interventions, such as pharmacologic agents, manual therapy, or exercises, can also help remediate the underlying cause of pain while controlling the pain itself. For example, cryotherapy applied to an acute injury controls pain; however, this treatment also controls inflammation, limiting further tissue damage and pain. In this case, the use of NSAIDs, rest, elevation, and compression in conjunction with cryotherapy could also prove beneficial, although it may make assessment of the benefits of any one of these interventions more difficult.

Multidisciplinary Pain Treatment Programs

Over the past two to three decades, multidisciplinary programs have been developed specifically for the treatment of chronic pain.[12,163] These programs are based on a biopsychosocial model of pain and attempt to address the multiple facets of chronic pain with a multidisciplinary, coordinated program of care.[3,163] These programs attempt to address not only the physical and physiologic aspects of the patient's pain but also the behavioral, cognitive-affective, and environmental factors contributing to their symptoms by the use of medical, psychological, and physical interventions. Examples of interventions that might be part of a multidisciplinary program include exercise, physical agents, education, counseling, occupational therapy, and cognitive behavioral therapy. Physical therapy is often a component of these multidisciplinary programs.

Psychological intervention is focused on improving the coping skills of patients and modifying their behavior, whereas physical activities are focused on reversing the adverse effects of the sedentary lifestyle adopted by most patients with chronic pain. Coping skills can be improved with relaxation training, activity pacing, distraction techniques, cognitive restructuring, and problem solving.[26,73] Behavior modification using the principles of operant conditioning can also alter the patient's perception of and response to pain.[77] Cognitive-behavioral therapy can be tailored to address concerns, such as pain, disability, fatigue, negative mood, and social relationships, and has been highly effective at reducing fatigue and depression in some patients with chronic pain.[169] Graded activation and exercise programs, in which the patient learns the difference between hurt and harm, can help patients with chronic pain return to a more functional, active lifestyle.[35] The patient's family members are generally involved in these programs by learning appropriate coping skills for themselves and the patient. Such involvement can assist family members to help individuals with chronic pain more effectively rather than reinforce pain-related behaviors.

In contrast with traditional treatment approaches to acute pain, in which the goal of care is to eliminate the sensation of pain, the goals of care in most multidisciplinary pain treatment programs also include learning to cope and function with pain that may not resolve, although frequently patients also report a reduction in pain after completing these programs.[75,93] Goals of treatment also generally include decreasing dependence on health care personnel and pain-relieving medications, particularly habit-forming opioids; increasing physical activities; and returning patients to their usual social roles. If necessary, opioid medications are replaced with non–habit-forming drugs or with nonchemical modes of pain relief such as exercise or physical agents.[163] These programs have also been shown to be cost effective.[76,136,149]

Studies have shown that multidisciplinary pain treatment programs do result in increased functional activity levels while reducing pain behaviors and the use of medical interventions in patients with chronic pain.[51,74,101,144] Various types of pain may be successfully treated with a multidisciplinary approach. In patients with chronic back pain, multidisciplinary programs have been found to improve function and pain, although they may or may not affect a patient's return to the workplace.[137] In patients with subacute back pain, multidisciplinary programs that include workplace visits can help patients to return to work faster, result in fewer sick leaves, and alleviate subjective disability.[53] One trial comparing multidisciplinary treatment with standard biomedical treatment of subacute low back pain found that although both approaches had a positive short-term effect, at 6 months the patients in the multidisciplinary program showed further improvement, whereas those on standard therapy were back to where they had started. During the 2 years after therapy, far fewer patients in the multidisciplinary program required sick leave.[69] A review of studies on neck and shoulder pain showed no evidence that a multidisciplinary approach helps, although few studies were included in this review and most studies were of poor quality.[133] Chronic musculoskeletal disorders, such as fibromyalgia, are often treated with multidisciplinary programs. Although high-quality studies are lacking, overall the evidence does suggest that behavioral treatment and stress management can help patients with chronic pain and that education combined with physical training has some positive long-term effects.[70]

❖ GLOSSARY

Acute pain: Pain of less than 6 months duration for which an underlying pathology can be identified.

A-beta fibers: Relatively large myelinated nerve fibers with receptors located in the skin, bones, and joints that transmit sensation related to vibration, stretching of skin, and mechanoreception. When working abnormally, can contribute to the sensation of pain; also called *wide dynamic-range neurons.*

A-delta fibers: Small, myelinated nerve fibers that transmit pain quickly to the CNS in response to high-intensity mechanical stimulation, heat, or cold; pain transmitted by these fibers usually has a sharp quality; also called *group III afferents.*

Afferent nerves: Nerves that conduct impulses from the periphery toward the CNS.

Allodynia: Pain in response to stimuli that do not usually produce pain.

Analgesia: Insensibility to pain, as in the effect of pain killers.

Autonomic nervous system: The division of the nervous system that controls involuntary activities of smooth and cardiac muscles and glandular secretion. Composed of the sympathetic and parasympathetic systems.

C fibers: Small, unmyelinated nerve fibers that transmit pain slowly to the CNS in response to noxious levels of mechanical, thermal, and chemical stimulation. Pain transmitted by these fibers is usually dull, long-lasting, and aching; also called *group IV afferents.*

Central sensitization: Lowering of the firing threshold of spinal cord pain-transmitting neurons caused by increased input from peripheral nociceptors; central sensitization amplifies the response to both noxious (hyperalgesia) and innocuous (allodynia) inputs, causes neurons to fire after the initiating input has ceased, and expands sensitivity so that pain is experienced beyond the original site of damage. Central sensitization is also called *wind-up.*

Chronic pain: Pain that persists beyond the usual amount of time for tissue healing; also called *persistent pain.*

Complex regional pain syndrome (CRPS): Pain believed to involve sympathetic nervous system over-activation; previously called *reflex sympathetic dystrophy* and *sympathetically maintained pain.*

Efferent innervation: Nerves that conduct impulses from the CNS to the periphery.

Endogenous opiate theory: A theory of pain control and modulation that states that pain is modulated at the peripheral, spinal cord, and cortical levels by endogenous neurotransmitters that have the same effect as opiates.

Endorphins: See Opiopeptins.

Enkephalins: Pentapeptides that are naturally occurring in the brain and that bind to opiate receptors producing analgesic and other opiate-like effects.

Gamma-aminobutyric acid (GABA): An inhibitory neurotransmitter, GABA increases pain by inhibiting the activity of pain-controlling structures, including A-beta afferents, and neurons in the periaqueductal gray matter and the raphe nucleus.

Gate control theory of pain modulation: A theory of pain control and modulation that states that pain is modulated at the spinal cord level by inhibitory effects of innocuous afferent input.

Hyperalgesia: Increased sensitivity to a noxious stimuli.

Neurotransmitter: A substance released by presynaptic neurons that activates postsynaptic neurons.

Nociception: The sensory component of pain.

Nociceptors: Nerve endings that are activated by noxious stimuli, contributing to a sensation of pain.

Noxious stimulus: Anything that activates a nerve to cause pain.

Opiopeptins: Endogenous opiate-like peptides that reduce the perception of pain by binding to opiate receptors in the nervous system; previously called *endorphins.*

Pain: An unpleasant sensory and emotional experience associated with actual or threatened tissue damage.

Pain gating: The inhibition of pain by inputs from non-nociceptor afferents.

Pain-spasm-pain cycle: A cycle in which nociceptor activation results in transmission cell activation that stimulates anterior horn cells to cause muscles to contract. This produces compression of blood vessels and thus accumulation of fluid and tissue irritants and mechanical compression of the nociceptor, which then further increases nociceptor activation.

Peripheral sensitization: Lowering of the nociceptor firing threshold in response to the release of various substances, including substance P, neurokinin A, and calcitonin gene–related peptide (CGRP), from nociceptive afferent fibers; also causes an increased magnitude of response to stimuli, an increase in spontaneous activity, and an increase in the area from which stimuli can evoke action potentials.

Referred pain: Pain that is experienced in one area when the actual or threatened tissue damage is in another area.

Sensitization: A lowering of the pain threshold that increases the experience of pain.

Substance P: A chemical mediator thought to be involved in the transmission of neuropathic and inflammatory pain.

Sympathetic nervous system: The part of the autonomic nervous system involved in the fight-or-flight reaction of the body that causes increased heart rate, blood pressure, and sweating and dilation of the pupils.

Synapse: The site of functional connection between neurons where an impulse is transmitted from one neuron (the presynaptic neuron) to another (the postsynaptic neuron), usually by a chemical neurotransmitter.

Transduction: A process by which a chemical or mechanical stimulus is converted into electrical activity (i.e., action potentials).

Transmission cells (T cells): Second-order neurons located in the dorsal horn of the spinal cord that receive signals from pain fibers and make connections with other neurons in the spinal cord.

REFERENCES

1. AGS Panel on Chronic Pain in Older Persons: The management of chronic pain in older persons, *J Am Geriatr Soc* 46:635–651, 1998.
2. Arnow BA, Hunkeler EM, Blasey CM, et al: Comorbid depression, chronic pain, and disability in primary care, *Psychosom Med* 68(2):262–268, 2006.
3. Aronoff AM: *Pain centers: a revolution in health care*, New York, 1988, Raven Press.
4. Bassbaum AI, Fields HL: Endogenous pain control mechanisms: review and hypothesis, *Ann Neurol* 4:451–462, 1978.
5. Beck PW, Handwerker HO: Bradykinin and serotonin effects on various types of cutaneous nerve fibers, *Pflugers Arch* 347:209–222, 1974.
6. Belcher G, Ryall RW, Schaffner R: The differential effects of 5-hydroxytryptamine, noradrenaline, and raphe stimulation on nociceptive and non-nociceptive dorsal horn interneurons in the cat, *Brain Res* 151:307–321, 1978.
7. Bendetti F, Amanzio M, Baldi S, et al: Inducing placebo respiratory depressant responses in humans via opioid receptors, *Eur J Neurosci* 11:625–631, 1999.
8. Berberich P, Hoheisel U, Mense S: Effects of a carrageenan-induced myositis on the discharge properties of group III and IV muscle receptors in the cat, *J Neurophysiol* 59:1395–1409, 1988.
9. Bernabei R, Gambassi G, Lapane K, et al: Management of pain in elderly patients with cancer. SAGE Study Group. Systematic assessment of geriatric drug use via epidemiology, *JAMA* 279:1877–1882, 1998.
10. Besson JM, Charouch A: Peripheral and spinal mechanisms of nociception, *Physiol Rev* 67(1):67–186, 1988.
11. Bickley LS, Hoekelman RA: *JG Bates' guide to physical examination and history taking*, ed 7, Philadelphia, 1999, Lippincott Williams & Wilkins.
12. Bigos S, Bowyer O, Braen G, et al: *Acute low back problems in adults, clinical practice guideline no 14. AHCPR Publication No. 95-0642*, Rockville, Md., 1994, Agency for Health Care Policy and Research, Public Health Service, US Dept of Health and Human Services.
13. Black RG: Evaluation of the pain patient, *J Disabil* 1:85–97, 1990.
14. Blackwell B, Galbraith JR, Dahl DS: Chronic pain management, *Hosp Community Psychiatry* 35:999–1008, 1984.
15. Bonica JJ: Importance of the problem. In Aronoff GM, editor: *Evaluation and treatment of chronic pain*, Baltimore, 1985, Urban & Schwarzenberg.
16. Bonica JJ: Pain: what is science doing about it? *Pain* 2:12–15, 1975.
17. Bonica JJ: *The management of pain*, ed 2, Philadelphia, 1990, Lea & Febiger.
18. Bonica JJ, Liebeskind JC, Albe-Fessard DG: *Advances in pain research and therapy, vol. 3*, New York, 1979, Raven Press.
19. Breivik H, Collett B, Ventafridda V, et al: Survey of chronic pain in Europe: prevalence, impact on daily life, and treatment, *Eur J Pain* 10(4):287–333, 2006.
20. Byrne M, Troy A, Bradley LA, et al: Cross-validation of the factor structure of the McGill Pain Questionnaire, *Pain* 13(2):193–201, 1982.
21. Campbell JN, Raja SN, Selig DK, et al: Diagnosis and management of sympathetically maintained pain. In Fields HL, Liebeskind JC, editors: *Pharmacological approaches to the treatment of chronic pain: new concepts and critical issues: progress in pain research and management*, vol. 1 Seattle, 1994, IASP Press.
22. Carr DB: Preempting the memory of pain, *JAMA* 279:1114–1115, 1998.
23. Cavanaugh JM, Ozaktay AC, Yamashita T, et al: Mechanisms of low back pain: a neurophysiologic and neuroanatomic study, *Clin Orthop Relat Res* 335:166–180, 1997.
24. Cepeda MS, Carr DB, Lau J: Local anesthetic sympathetic blockade for complex regional pain syndrome, *Cochrane Database Syst Rev* (4):CD004598, 2005.
25. Cepeda M, Soledad, Lau J, et al: Defining the therapeutic role of local anesthetic sympathetic blockade in complex regional pain syndrome: a narrative and systematic review, *Clin J Pain* 18(4):216–223, 2002.
26. Cicala RS, Wright H: Outpatient treatment of patients with chronic pain: an analysis of cost savings, *Clin J Pain* 5:223–226, 1989.
27. Crockford GW, Hellon RF, Parkhouse J: Thermal vasomotor response in human skin mediated by local mechanisms, *J Physiol* 161:10–15, 1962.
28. Crue BL, editor: *Pain: research and treatment*, New York, 1974, Academic Press.
29. Dickenson AH: NMDA receptor agonists as analgesics. In Fields HL, Liebeskind JC, editors: *Pharmacologic approaches to the treatment of chronic pain: new concepts and critical issues: progress in pain research*, vol. 1 Seattle, 1994, IASP Press.

30. Dickenson AH, Sullivan AF: Evidence for a role of the NMDA receptor in the frequency dependent potentiation of deep rat dorsal horn nociceptive neurones following C fibre stimulation, *Neuropharmacology* 26:1235–1238, 1987.

31. Downie W, Leatham PA, Rhind VM, et al: Studies with pain rating scales, *Ann Rheum Dis* 37:378–388, 1978.

32. Edwards RR, Bingham CO III, Bathon J, et al: Catastrophizing and pain in arthritis, fibromyalgia, and other rheumatic diseases, *Arthritis Rheum* 55(2):325–332, 2006.

33. Elliott KJ: Taxonomy and mechanisms of neuropathic pain, *Semin Neurol* 14(3):195–205, 1994.

34. Ernst E, Fialka V: Ice freezes pain? A review of the clinical effectiveness of analgesic cold therapy, *J Pain Symptom Manage* 9(1):56–59, 1994.

35. Evers AW, Kraaimaat FW, van Riel PL, et al: Tailored cognitive-behavioral therapy in early rheumatoid arthritis for patients at risk: a randomized controlled trial, *Pain* 100:141–153, 2002.

36. Ferrell B: Acute and chronic pain. In Cassel C, editor: *Geriatric medicine: an evidence based approach*, ed 4, New York, 2003, Spring-Verlag.

37. Fields HL: *Pain: mechanisms and management*, New York, 1987, McGraw Hill.

38. Fields HL, Levine JD: Pain—mechanisms and management, *West J Med* 141:347–357, 1984.

39. Fleetwood-Walker SM, Mitchell R, Hope PJ, et al: An A2 receptor mediates the selective inhibition by noradrenaline of nociceptive responses of identified dorsal horn neurons, *Brain Res* 334:243–354, 1985.

40. Freeman MA, Wyke B: The innervation of the knee joint: an anatomical and histological study in the cat, *J Anat* 101:505–532, 1967.

41. Gamse R, Holzer P, Lembeck F: Decrease of substance P in primary afferent neurons and impairment of neurogenic plasma extravasation by capsaicin, *Br J Pharmacol* 68:207–213, 1980.

42. Garcia J, Altman RD: Chronic pain states: pathophysiology and medical therapy, *Semin Arthritis Rheum* 27:1, 1997.

43. Gerspacher M: Selective and combined neurokinin receptor antagonists, *Prog Med Chem* 43:49–103, 2005.

44. Gilfoil TM, Klavins I: 5-Hydroxytryptamine, bradykinin and histamine as mediators of inflammatory hyperesthesia, *J Physiol* 208:867–876, 1965.

45. Gilman AG, Goodman L, Rall TW, et al: *Goodman and Gilman's the pharmacologic basis of therapeutics*, ed 7, New York, 1985, Macmillan.

46. Goldscheider A: *Veber den schmertz in physiologischer und klinischer hensicht*, Berlin, 1894, Hirschwald.

47. Gottschalk A, Smith DS, Jobes DR, et al: Preemptive epidural analgesia and recovery from radical prostatectomy: a randomized controlled trial, *JAMA* 279:1076–1082, 1998.

48. Grevert P, Goldstein A: Endorphins: naloxone fails to alter experimental pain or mood in humans, *Science* 199:1093–1095, 1978.

49. Grigg P, Stubble HG, Schmidt RF: Mechanical sensitivity of group III and IV afferents from posterior articular nerve in normal and inflamed cat knee, *J Neurophysiol* 55:635–643, 1986.

50. Grossman SA, Shudler VR, McQuire DB, et al: A comparison of the Hopkins Pain Rating Instrument with standard visual analogue and verbal description scales in patients with chronic pain, *J Pain Symptom Manage* 7:196–203, 1992.

51. Guck TP, Skultety FM, Meilman DW, et al: Multidisciplinary pain center follow-up study: evaluation with no-treatment control group, *Pain* 21:295–306, 1985.

52. Gullacksen AC, Lidbeck J: The life adjustment process in chronic pain: psychosocial assessment and clinical implications, *Pain Res Manag* 9(3):145–153, 2004.

53. Guzmán J, Esmail R, Karjalainen K, et al: Multidisciplinary bio-psycho-social rehabilitation for chronic low back pain, *Cochrane Database Syst Rev* (1):CD000963, 2002.

54. Gybels J, Handwerker HO, Van Hees J: A comparison between the discharges of human nociceptive fibers and the subject's rating of his sensations, *J Physiol (Lond)* 186:117–132, 1979.

55. Halata Z, Badalamente ME, Dee R, et al: Ultrastructure of sensory nerve endings in monkeys' knee joint capsule, *J Orthop Res* 2:218–226, 1984.

56. Halata Z, Groth HP: Innervation of the synovial membrane of the cat's joint capsule, *Cell Tissue Res* 169:415–418, 1976.

57. Hao JX, Xu XJ, Yu YX, et al: Baclofen reverses the hypersensitivity of dorsal horn wide dynamic range neurons to mechanical stimulation after transient spinal cord ischemia: implications for a tonic GABAergic inhibitory control of myelinated fiber input, *J Neurophysiol* 68:392–396, 1992.

58. Heppleman B, Heuss C, Schmidt RF: Fiber size distribution of myelinated and unmyelinated axons in the medial and posterior articular nerves of the cat's knee joint, *Somatosens Res* 5:267–275, 1988.

59. Heppleman B, Meslinger K, Neiss WF, et al: Ultrastructural three-dimensional reconstruction of group III and IV sensory nerve endings ("free nerve endings") in the knee joint capsule of the cat: evidence for multiple receptive sites, *J Comp Neurol* 292:103–116, 1990.

60. Hillman P, Wall PD: Inhibitory and excitatory factors influencing the receptive fields of lamina 5 spinal cord cells, *Exp Brain Res* 9:161–171, 1969.

61. Hocutt JE, Jaffe R, Ryplander CR: Cryotherapy in ankle sprains, *Am J Sports Med* 10:316–319, 1982.

62. Huges J, Smith TW, Kosterlitz HW, et al: Identification of two related pentapeptides from the brain with potent opiate agonist activity, *Nature* 258:577–579, 1975.

63. International Association for the Study of Chronic Pain: Subcommittee on Taxonomy: Classification of chronic pain, *Pain Suppl* 3:S1–S225, 1986.

64. Janig W, Kollmann W: The involvement of the sympathetic nervous system in pain, *Drug Res* 34(2):1066–1073, 1984.

65. Janig W, McLachlan EM: The role of modification in noradrenergic peripheral pathways after nerve lesions in the generation of pain. In Fields HL, Liebeskind JC, editors: *Pharmacologic approaches to the treatment of chronic pain: new concepts and critical issues: progress in pain research and management*, vol. 1 Seattle, 1994, IASP Press.

66. Jasmin L, Tien D, Weinshenker D, et al: The NK1 receptor mediates both the hyperalgesia and the resistance to morphine in mice lacking noradrenaline, *Proc Natl Acad Sci USA* 99:1029–1034, 2002.

67. Jessell TM, Iversen LL: Opiate analgesics inhibit substance P release from rat trigeminal nucleus, *Nature* 268:549–551, 1977.

68. Ji RR, Baba H, Brenner GJ, et al: Nociceptive-specific activation of ERK in spinal neurons contributes to pain hypersensitivity, *Nat Neurosci* 2:1114–1119, 1999.

69. Karjalainen KA, Malmivaara A, van Tulder MW, et al: Multidisciplinary biopsychosocial rehabilitation for neck and shoulder pain among working age adults, *Cochrane Database Syst Rev* (2):CD002194, 2003.

70. Karjalainen KA, Malmivaara A, van Tulder MW, et al: Multidisciplinary biopsychosocial rehabilitation for subacute low back pain among working age adults, *Cochrane Database Syst Rev* (2):CD002193, 2003.

71. Kato K, Sullivan PF, Evengard B, et al: Chronic widespread pain and its comorbidities: a population-based study, *Arch Intern Med* 166:1649–1654, 2006.

72. Kazis LE, Meenan RF, Anderson JJ: Pain in the rheumatic diseases. Investigations of a key health status component, *Arthritis Rheum* 26(8):1017–1022, 1983.

73. Keefe FJ, Beaupre PM, Gil KM: Group therapy for patients with chronic pain. In Turk DC, Gatchel RJ, editors: *Psychological factors in pain: critical perspectives*, New York, 1999, Guildford Press.

74. Keefe FJ, Caldwell DS, Queen KT, et al: Pain coping strategies in osteoarthritis patients, *J Consult Clin Psychol* 55:208–212, 1987.

75. Keefe FJ, Caldwell DS, Williams DA, et al: Pain coping skills training in the management of osteoarthritic knee pain: a comparative study, *Behav Ther* 21:449–462, 1990.

76. Keefe FJ, Caldwell DS, Williams DA, et al: Pain coping skills training in the management of osteoarthritic knee pain: follow-up results, *Behav Ther* 21:435–448, 1990.

77. Keefe FJ, Kashikar-Zuck S, Opiteck J, et al: Pain in arthritis and musculoskeletal disorders: the role of coping skills training and exercise interventions, *J Orthop Sport Phys Ther* 24(4):279–290, 1996.

78. Kehlet H, Jensen TS, Woolf CJ: Persistent postsurgical pain: risk factors and prevention, *Lancet* 367(9522):1618–1625, 2006.

79. Keller M, Montgomery S, Ball W, et al: Lack of efficacy of the substance p (neurokinin1 receptor) antagonist aprepitant in the treatment of major depressive disorder, *Biol Psychiatry* 59(3):216–223, 2006.

80. Kellgren JH: Observations on referred pain arising from muscle, *Clin Sci* 3:175–190, 1938.

81. Kendall FP, McCreary EK: *Muscles, testing and function*, ed 3, Baltimore, 1983, Williams & Wilkins.

82. Kerr FW: Pain: a central inhibitory balance theory, *Mayo Clin Proc* 50:685–690, 1975.

83. Khalil Z, Hleme RD: Sequence of events in substance P mediated plasma extravasation in rat skin, *Brain Res* 500:256–262, 1989.

84. Kleinert HE, Norberg H, McDonough JJ: Surgical sympathectomy: upper and lower extremity. In Omer GE, editor: *Management of peripheral nerve problems*, Philadelphia, 1980, Saunders.

85. Lamotte C: Distribution of the tract of Lissauer and the dorsal root fibers in the primate spinal cord, *J Comp Neurol* 72:529–561, 1977.

86. Larsson J, Ekblom A, Henriksson K, et al: Concentration of substance P, neurokinin A, calcitonin gene-related peptide, neuropeptide Y and vasoactive intestinal polypeptide in synovial fluid from knee joints in patients suffering from rheumatoid arthritis, *Scand J Rheumatol* 20:326–335, 1991.

87. Leavitt F, Garron DC: Psychological disturbance and pain report differences in both organic and non-organic low back pain patients, *Pain* 7:65–68, 1979.

88. Levine JD, Gordon NC, Fields HL: The mechanism of placebo analgesia, *Lancet* 2:654–657, 1978.

89. Light AR, Perl ER: Differential termination of large-diameter and small-diameter primary afferent fibers in the spinal dorsal gray matter as indicated by labeling with horseradish peroxidase, *Neurosci Lett* 6:59–63, 1977.

90. Light AR, Perl ER: Re-examination of the dorsal root projection to the spinal dorsal horn including observations on the differential termination of course and fine fibers, *J Comp Neurol* 186:117–132, 1979.

91. Light AR, Perl ER: Spinal termination of functionally identified primary afferent neurons with slowly conducting myelinated fibers, *J Comp Neurol* 186:133–150, 1979.

92. Lin EH, Katon W, Von Korff M, et al: Effect of improving depression care on pain and functional outcomes among older adults with arthritis: a randomized controlled trial, *JAMA* 290:2428–2429, 2003.

93. Linton LJ, Bradley LA, Jensen I, et al: The secondary prevention of low back pain: a controlled study with follow up, *Pain* 36:197–207, 1989.

94. Lucas HJ, Brauch CM, Settas L, et al: Fibromyalgia–new concepts of pathogenesis and treatment, *Int J Immunopathol Pharmacol* 19(1):5–10, 2006.

95. Magni G, Caldieron C, Luchini SR, et al: Chronic musculoskeletal pain and depressive symptoms in the general population: an analysis of the 1st national health and nutrition examination survey data, *Pain* 43:299–307, 1990.

96. Mao J, Price DD, Mayer DJ: Mechanisms of hyperalgesia and morphine tolerance: a current view of their possible interactions: review article, *Pain* 62:259–274, 1995.

97. Marchettini P, Cline M, Ochoa JL: Innervation territories for touch and pain afferents of single fascicles of the human ulnar nerve, *Brain* 113:1491–1500, 1990.

98. Marshall KW, Chiu B, Inman RD: Substance P and arthritis: analysis of plasma and synovial fluid levels, *Arthritis Rheum* 33:87–90, 1990.

99. Mayer DJ, Price DD: Central nervous system mechanisms of analgesia, *Pain* 2:379–404, 1976.

100. Mayer DJ, Price DD, Barber J, et al: Acupuncture analgesia: evidence for activation of a pain inhibitory system as a mechanism of action. In Bonica JJ, Albe-Fessard D, editors: *Advances in pain research and therapy*, New York, 1976, Raven Press.

101. Mayer TG, Gatchel RJ, Mayer H, et al: A prospective two-year study of functional restoration in industrial low back injury—an objective assessment procedure, *JAMA* 258:1763–1767, 1987.

102. McMaster WC, Liddie S: Cryotherapy influence on posttraumatic limb edema, *Clin Orthop Relat Res* 150:283–287, 1980.

103. Melzack JD, Wall PD: Pain mechanisms: a new theory, *Science* 150:971–979, 1965.

104. Melzack R: The McGill Pain Questionnaire: major properties and scoring methods, *Pain* 1:277–299, 1975.

105. Melzack R, Casey KL: Sensory, motivational, and central control determinants of pain. In Kenshalo DR, editor: *The skin senses*, Springfield, Ill, 1968, Charles C Thomas.

106. Melzack R, Dennis SG: Neurophysiological foundations of pain. In Sternbach RA, editor: *The psychology of pain*, New York, 1978, Raven Press.

107. Mense S, Stahnke M: Responses in muscle afferent fibres of slow conduction velocity to contraction and ischemia in the cat, *J Physiol (Lond)* 342:383–387, 1983.

108. Merskey H: Classification of chronic pain: description of chronic pain syndromes and definition of pain terms, *Pain Suppl* 3:S1, 1986.

109. Nakae K, Saito K, Yamamoto N, et al: A prostacyclin receptor antagonist inhibits the sensitized release of substance P from rat sensory neurons, *J Pharmacol Exp Ther* 315(3):1136–1142, 2005.

110. Nathan PW, Rudge P: Testing the gate control theory of pain in man, *J Neurol Neurosurg Psychiatry* 3:645–657, 1974.

111. Nathan PW, Wall PD: Treatment of post-herpetic neuralgia by prolonged electrical stimulation, *Br Med J* 3:645–657, 1974.

112. Neugebauer V, Wieretter F, Stubble HG: Involvement of substance P and neurokinin-1 receptors in hyperexcitability of dorsal horn neurons during development of acute arthritis in rat's knee joint, *J Neurophysiol* 73:1574–1583, 1995.

113. Nichols ML, Allen BJ, Rogers SD, et al: Transmission of chronic nociception by spinal neurons expressing the substance P receptor, *Science* 286:1558–1561, 1999.

114. Nolan MF: Anatomic and physiologic organization of neural structures involved in pain transmission, modulation, and perception. In Echternach JL, editor: *Pain*, New York, 1987, Churchill Livingstone.

115. Ochoa JL, Torebjork HE: Sensations by intraneural microstimulation of single mechanoreceptor units innervating the human hand, *J Physiol (Lond)* 342:633–654, 1983.

116. Oku R, Satoh M, Tagaki H: Release of substance P from the spinal dorsal horn is enhanced in polyarthritic rats, *Neurosci Lett* 74:315–319, 1987.

117. Osterweis M, Kleinman A, Mechanic D, editors: *Pain and disability: clinical, behavioral, and public policy perspective*, Washington, DC, 1987, National Academies Press.

118. Pautex S, Herrmann F, Le Lous P, et al: Feasibility and reliability of four pain self-assessment scales and correlation with an observational rating scale in hospitalized elderly demented patients, *J Gerontol A Biol Sci Med Sci* 60(4):524–529, 2005.

119. Peng B, Wu W, Hou S, et al: The pathogenesis of discogenic low back pain, *J Bone Joint Surg Br* 87:62–67, 2005.

120. Pert CB, Pasternak G, Snyder SH: Opiate agonists and antagonists discriminated by receptor binding in the brain, *Science* 182(119):1359–1361, 1973.

121. Polacek P: Receptors of joints: their structure, variability and classification, *Acta Facultat Med Univesitat Brunensis* 23:1–107, 1966.

122. Price DD, Hayes RL, Ruda M, et al: Spatial and temporal transformation of input to the spinothalamic tract neurons and their relationship to somatic sensations, *J Neurophysiol* 41:933–947, 1978.

123. Price DD, Long S, Huitt C: Sensory testing of pathophysiological mechanisms of pain in patients with reflex sympathetic dystrophy, *Pain* 49:163–173, 1992.

124. Prieto EJ, Hopson L, Bradley LA, et al: The language of low back pain: factor structure of the McGill Pain Questionnaire, *Pain* 8(1):11–19, 1980.

125. Quinn L, Gordon J: *Functional outcomes documentation for rehabilitation,* St Louis, 2003, Saunders.

126. Radharkrishnan V, Henry JL: Antagonism of nociceptive responses of cat spinal dorsal horn neurons in vivo by the NK-1 receptor antagonists CP-96,345 and CP-99,994, but not by CP-96,344, *Neuroscience* 64:943–958, 1995.

127. Randic M, Miletic V: Effect of substance P in cat dorsal horn neurons activated by noxious stimuli, *Brain Res* 128:164–169, 1977.

128. Ransford AO, Cairns D, Mooney V: The pain drawing as an aid to the psychological evaluation of patients with low-back pain, *Spine* 1(2):127–134, 1976.

129. Roth RS, Lowery JC, Hamill JB: Assessing persistent pain and its relation to affective distress, depressive symptoms, and pain catastrophizing in patients with chronic wounds: a pilot study, *Am J Phys Med Rehabil* 83(11):827–834, 2004 Nov.

130. Russell IJ, Orr MD, Littman B, et al: Elevated cerebrospinal fluid levels of substance P in patients with the fibromyalgia syndrome, *Arthritis Rheum* 37(11):1593–1601, 1994.

131. Sakurada T, Komatsu T, Sakurada S: Mechanisms of nociception evoked by intrathecal high-dose morphine, *Neurotoxicology* 26(5):801–809, 2005.

132. Schaible HG, Richter F: Pathophysiology of pain, *Langenbecks Arch Surg* 389:237–243, 2004.

133. Schiltenwolf M, Buchner M, Heindl B, et al: Comparison of a biopsychosocial therapy (BT) with a conventional biomedical therapy (MT) of subacute low back pain in the first episode of sick leave: a randomized controlled trial, *Eur Spine J* 15(7):1083–1092, 2006.

134. Schinkel C, Gaertner A, Zaspel J, et al: Inflammatory mediators are altered in the acute phase of posttraumatic complex regional pain syndrome, *Clin J Pain* 22(3):235–239, 2006.

135. Selkowitz DM: The sympathetic nervous system in neuromotor function and dysfunction and pain: a brief review and discussion, *Funct Neurol* 7:89–95, 1992.

136. Seres JL, Newman RI: Results of treatment of chronic low-back pain at the Portland Pain Center, *J Neurosurg* 45:32–36, 1976.

137. Simmons JW, Avant WS Jr, Demski J, et al: Determining successful pain clinic treatment through validation of cost effectiveness, *Spine* 13:342–344, 1988.

138. Simon EJ: In search of the opiate receptor, *Am J Med Sci* 266(3):160–168, 1973.

139. Simon EJ, Hiller JM: The opiate receptors, *Annu Rev Pharmacol Toxicol* 18:371–377, 1978.

140. Slake KA, Milton MA, Westlund KN, et al: Involvement of neurokinin receptors in the joint inflammation and heat hyperalgesia following acute inflammation in unanesthetized rats, *J Physiol (Lond)* 483P:152–153, 1995.

141. Sluka KA: Pain mechanisms involved in musculoskeletal disorders, *J Orthop Sports Phys Ther* 24(4):240–254, 1996.

142. Snyder SH: Opiate receptors and internal opiates, *Sci Am* 240(3):44–56, 1977.

143. Stanton-Hicks M, Janig W, Hassenbusch S, et al: Reflex sympathetic dystrophy: changing concepts and taxonomy, *Pain* 63:127–133, 1995.

144. Stieg RL, Williams RC, Timmermans-Williams G, et al: Cost benefits of interdisciplinary chronic pain treatment, *Clin J Pain* 1:189–193, 1986.

145. Stubble HG, Grubb BD: Afferent and spinal mechanisms of joint pain, *Pain* 55:5–54, 1993.

146. Stubble HG, Jarrott B, Hope PJ, et al: Release of immunoreactive substance P in the spinal cord during development of acute arthritis in the knee joint of the cat: a study with antibody microprobes, *Brain Res* 529:214–223, 1990.

147. Stubble H, Schmidt RF: Effects of an experimental arthritis on the sensory properties of fine articular afferent units, *J Neurophysiol* 54:1109–1122, 1985.

148. Stubble H, Schmidt RF: Time course of mechanosensitivity changes in articular afferents during a developing experimental arthritis, *J Neurophysiol* 60:2180–2194, 1988.

149. Swanson DW, Swenson WM, Maruta T, et al: Program for managing chronic pain. Program description and characteristics of patients, *Mayo Clin Proc* 51:401–408, 1976.

150. Sweet WH: Neurophysiology. In Field J, Magoun HW, Hall VE, editors: *Handbook of Physiology. Section 1: Neurophysiology,* vol. I, Washington, DC, 1959, American Physiological Society.

151. Terenius L: Characteristics of the "receptor" for narcotic analgesics in synaptic plasma membrane fraction from rat brain, *Acta Pharmacol Toxicol (Copenh)* 33(5):377–384, 1973.

152. Terman GW, Shavit Y, Lewis JW, et al: Intrinsic mechanisms of pain inhibition: activation by stress, *Science* 226:1270–1277, 1984.

153. Tippett SR: Referred knee pain in a young athlete: a case study, *J Orthop Sports Phys Ther* 19(2):117–120, 1994.

154. Torebjork HE, Ochoa JL, Schady W: Referred pain from intraneuronal stimulation of muscle fascicles in the median nerve, *Pain* 18:145–156, 1984.

155. Torebjork HE, Schady W, Ochoa J: Sensory correlates of somatic afferent fibre activation, *Hum Neurobiol* 3:15–20, 1984.

156. Tricklebank MD, Curzon G: *Stress-induced analgesia,* Chichester, England, 1984, Wiley.

157. Unnerstall JR, Kopajtic TA, Kuhar MJ: Distribution of A2 agonist binding sites in the rat and human central nervous system: analysis of some functional autonomic correlates of the pharmacologic effects of clonidine and related adrenergic agents, *Brain Res* 319:69–101, 1984.

158. Ushijima S, Ukimura O, Okihara K, et al: Visual analog scale questionnaire to assess quality of life specific to each symptom of the International Prostate Symptom Score, *J Urol* 176(2):665–671, 2006.

159. Vaeroy H, Helle R, Forre O, et al: Elevated CSF levels of substance P and high incidence of Raynaud phenomenon in patients with fibromyalgia: new features for diagnosis, *Pain* 32:21–26, 1988.

160. Vasko MR, Campbell WB, Waite KJ: Prostaglandin E2 enhances bradykinin-stimulated release of neuropeptides from rat sensory neurons in culture, *J Neurosci* 14:4987–4997, 1994.

161. Vasudevan SV: Management of chronic pain: what have we achieved in the last 25 years? In Ghia JN, editor: *The multidisciplinary pain center: organization and personnel functions for pain management,* Boston, 1988, Kluwer.

162. Vasudevan SV: Rehabilitation of the patient with chronic pain: is it cost effective? *Pain Digest* 2:99–101, 1992.

163. Vasudevan SV, Lynch NT: Pain centers: organization and outcome, *West J Med* 154(5):532–535, 1991.

164. Wall PD, Sweet WH: Temporary abolition of pain in man, *Science* 155:108–109, 1967.

165. Wang X, Douglas SD, Commons KG, et al: A non-peptide substance P antagonist (CP-96,345) inhibits morphine-induced NF-kappa B promoter activation in human NT2-N neurons, *J Neurosci Res* 75(4):544–553, 2004.

166. Watanabe H, Nakayama D, Yuhki M, et al: Differential inhibitory effects of mu-opioids on substance P- and capsaicin-induced nociceptive behavior in mice, *Peptides* 27(4):760–768, 2006.

167. Watkins LR, Mayer D: Organization of endogenous opiate and nonopiate pain control systems, *Science* 216:1185–1192, 1982.

168. White DM, Helme RD: Release of substance P from peripheral nerve terminals following electrical stimulation of the sciatic nerve, *Brain Res* 336:27–31, 1985.

169. Wickramaskerra I: Biofeedback and behavior modification for chronic pain. In Echternach HL, editor: *Pain*, New York, 1987, Churchill Livingstone.

170. Willer JC: Endogenous, opioid, peptide-mediated analgesia, *Int Med* 9(8):100–111, 1988.

171. Willer JC, Dehen H, Cambrier J: Stress-induced analgesia in humans: endogenous opioids and naloxone-reversible depression of pain reflexes, *Science* 212:689–691, 1981.

172. Willer JC, Roby A, Le Bars D: Psychophysical and electrophysiological approaches to the pain-relieving effects of heterotopic nociceptive stimuli, *Brain Res* 107:1095–1112, 1984.

173. Willis WD: Control of nociceptive transmission in the spinal cord. In Autrum H, Ottoson D, Perl ER, et al: *Progress in sensory physiology vol. 3*, Berlin, 1982, Springer-Verlag.

174. Willis WD: *The pain system: the neural basis of nociceptive transmission in the mammalian nervous system*, Basel, 1985, Karger.

175. Willis WD, Coggeshall RE: *Sensory mechanisms of the spinal cord*, New York, 1991, Plenum Press.

176. Winnem MF, Amundsen T: Treatment of phantom limb pain with transcutaneous electrical nerve stimulation, *Pain* 12:299–300, 1982.

177. Wood L: Physiology of pain. In Kitchen S, Bazin S, editors: *Clayton's electrotherapy*, ed 10, London, 1996, Saunders.

178. Woolf CJ: Evidence for a central component of post-injury pain hypersensitivity, *Nature* 41:686–688, 1983.

179. Woolf CJ, Shortland P, Coggeshall RE: Peripheral nerve injury triggers central sprouting of myelinated afferents, *Nature* 355:75–78, 1992.

180. Wu G, Ringkamp M, Hartke TV, et al: Early onset of spontaneous activity in uninjured C-fiber nociceptors after injury to neighboring nerve fibers, *J Neurosci* 21:1–5, 2001.

181. Zhang WY: Li Wan Po A: The effectiveness of topically applied capsaicin. A meta-analysis, *Eur J Clin Pharmacol* 46(6):517–522, 1994.

182. Zimmerman M: Basic concepts of pain and pain therapy, *Drug Res* 34(2):1053–1059, 1984.

REVIEW QUESTIONS

Short Answer

1. A common pain referral pattern is from the diaphragm to _____.

2. The transmission of pain at the spinal cord may be inhibited by increased activity of _____.

3. Which pain measurement tool is most appropriate for quickly estimating a patient's perceived progress or change in severity of symptoms over time?

4. Which pain measurement tool is most appropriate for obtaining detailed quantifiable information about a patient's pain?

5. Which pain measurement tool is most appropriate for localizing the area and nature of a patient's symptoms?

6. Naloxone reverses the effects of _____.

7. Multidisciplinary pain treatment programs generally focus on _____.

8. Which structure frequently refers pain to the right shoulder or the inferior angle of the right scapula?

True/False

9. Pain is an unpleasant sensory and emotional experience associated with actual or potential tissue damage or described in terms of such damage.

10. Features of chronic pain include all of the following: (1) pain different from that associated with the initial injury; (2) substantial psychosocial changes; and (3) pain that persists beyond normal time for tissue healing.

11. Acute pain is generally of less than 6 months duration, well localized, and mediated through slowly conducting pathways.

12. The pain transmitted by C fibers is generally long lasting.

13. The pain transmitted by A-delta fibers generally (1) has fast onset and offset after the initial painful stimulus, (2) is well localized, and (3) is sharp in nature.

14. A hyperactive sympathetic nervous system response to a painful stimulus or injury can cause exaggerated sweating.

15. Physical agents can be an effective component of the treatment of both acute and chronic pain.

16. Physical agents should not be used by patients to treat themselves.

26 Introduction to Orthotics and Prosthetics

Leslie K. King

LEARNING OBJECTIVES

1. Define the terms orthotics and prosthetics.
2. Obtain basic understanding of materials.
3. Learn the nomenclature—the naming of orthoses and prostheses in relation to the joint they support or replace.
4. Describe the key differences when off-the-shelf orthoses can be chosen instead of custom fabricated.
5. Have a general understanding of orthotic options for supporting major joints in the body.
6. List levels of amputation sites as well as the reasons for amputation.
7. Develop an understanding of basic prosthetic componentry and how the selection of componentry relates to patient function and outcome.

KEY TERMS

Brace
Componentry
Doff
Don

Foot drop
Liner
Orthosis
Packing out

Prosthesis
Splint

CHAPTER OUTLINE

When it comes to selecting an appropriate **orthosis** or **prosthesis** for a patient there are numerous options available for either prefabricated or custom fabricated devices. The plethora of possible manufacturers makes it increasingly difficult to select the best device simply because of the number of optimal choices. The proper selection of each device, then, is based upon diagnosis, functional goals, and the patient's cognitive and physical abilities to properly **don** and **doff** these devices.

The process developed for naming orthoses and prostheses is a fairly simple technique. The International Standards Organization (ISO) recognizes common descriptors for orthoses and prostheses, based on the acronyms from the body joint or joints that are supported or replaced (Table 26-1). This method of nomenclature is both effective and easily learned.

ORTHOTICS

An orthosis is a product or device that supports a body part or joint. These devices provide the patient with stability, support, positioning, and protection.

Orthoses range from a prefabricated wrist **splint** to a custom fabricated reciprocating gait orthosis. Orthoses are tools used to help the patient become more independent and functional with tasks such as activities of daily living (ADLs) and ambulation. Selecting the proper device is crucial in providing the patient with optimal support, results, care, and outcome results.

There are two key terms commonly used when discussing orthotics: splinting and bracing. Splinting is a term used today and most often refers to an orthosis that will immobilize a joint, such as a finger splint used to hold a broken phalange immobile or a hip spica splint fitted to a patient postsurgical hip repair or replacement, and that will allow only a specific range of motion as rehabilitation protocol requires. Bracing is a term that is still used today by the lay population; it is a dated term for clinicians. The term *orthotic* is derived from the Greek *ortho*, meaning to straighten. Today, when speaking of orthotics, it relates to the biomechanical, musculoskeletal support, and correction of abnormalities within the human body.

Table 26-1	*ISO Naming Conventions for Orthoses and Prostheses*		
Device Type		**Amputation Level**	**Nomenclature**
Orthoses	Upper extremity	Finger orthosis	FO
		Hand orthosis	HO
		Wrist-hand orthosis	WHO
		Wrist orthosis	WO
		Elbow orthosis	EO
		Elbow-wrist-hand orthosis	EWHO
		Shoulder orthosis	SO
	Spinal	Cervical-thoracic-lumbosacral orthosis	CTLSO
		Cervical orthosis	CO
		Thoracic-lumbosacral orthosis	TLSO
		Lumbosacral orthosis	LSO
		Sacroiliac orthosis	SIO
	Lower extremity	Foot orthosis	FO
		Knee orthosis	KO
		Ankle-foot orthosis	AFO
		Knee-ankle-foot orthosis	KAFO
		Hip-knee-ankle-foot orthosis	HKAFO
Prostheses	Upper extremity	Shoulder disarticulation	SD
		Trans-humeral	TH
		Elbow disarticulation	ED
		Trans-radial	TR
		Wrist disarticulation	WD
	Lower extremity	Hip disarticulation	HD
		Trans-femoral	TF
		Knee disarticulation	KD
		Trans-tibial	TT
		Ankle disarticulation	Symes
		Trans-metatarsal amputation	TMA

From Shurr DG, Michael JW: *Prosthetics and orthotics*, ed 2, Upper Saddle River, NJ, 2002, Prentice Hall, p 16.

PROSTHETICS

A prosthesis is any device that replaces a body part. This group consists of arms, legs, partial feet, hands, ears, breasts, and so on. The goal for each prosthesis is to provide function, body balance, ease of use, and optimal cosmesis in order to restore self image, quality of life, and independence (Table 26-2). Prostheses are custom fabricated and require adjustments and realignment on a regular basis.

The amount of **componentry,** or parts of a prosthesis, is dependent upon the involved level of amputation. For an upper extremity prosthesis, the components may include a socket, shoulder joint, pylon, elbow joint, wrist unit, and a hand, depending upon where the amputation site is located along the arm. For a lower extremity prosthesis, the components are similar to upper extremity, but the hands and wrists are replaced by feet, knees, and hip joints. Each of the components (for both upper- and lower-extremity prostheses) play a specific role in whether the prosthesis is ultimately used successfully by the patient. The socket, for example, is the custom fabricated portion created from a mold of the patient's residual limb. This mold is obtained by casting the patient or by computer-aided manufacturing (CAM), a process during which the residual limb is scanned using a computer-aided design (CAD) program. Proper fit of the socket is crucial, and intimacy of the fit is directly related to the patient's end result for use and wear time. The rest of the prosthetic componentry is carefully selected from the vast list of products available from manufacturers. Hands, elbows, and shoulder joints are chosen by the prosthetist in order to assemble the most appropriate and functional prosthesis.

All prostheses use prosthetic socks for optimal fit. Prosthetic socks are available in different thicknesses

Table 26-2	*Specifications for the Ideal Prosthesis/Orthosis*
Need	**Definition**
Function	Meets the user's needs, simple, easily learned, dependable
Comfort	Fits well, easy to don/doff, lightweight, adjustable
Cosmesis	Looks, smells, sounds "normal," cleans easily, stain-resistant
Fabrication	Fast, modular, readily and widely available
Economics	Affordable, worth cost of monetary investment

From Shurr DG, Michael JW: *Prosthetics and orthotics,* ed 2, Upper Saddle River, NJ, 2002, Prentice Hall, p 29.

referred to as *ply.* As the amputee retains or loses fluid throughout the course of the day, adding or removing a sock is done in order to maintain the optimal fit of the socket. This process is referred to as *sock management.* Prostheses may also incorporate silicone **liners** for suspension and cushion. Liners are fabricated out of materials such as silicone, polyurethane, and gel elastomers. These materials are chosen because of their ease of use for donning or doffing, quality of hygiene, and durability. To obtain proper limb length, a pylon, which is an aluminum or stainless steel tube, is fitted between the foot and the socket or knee unit.

Fitting for Orthoses or Prostheses

As each orthosis or prosthesis is being fabricated or fitted, the functional goals of each patient are key to making the most appropriate selection for componentry. The patient's weight, age, activity level, and potential to regain independence and agility are the factors used to determine which type of orthosis or type of material to choose.

When selecting orthotic or prosthetic components it is important to consider what devices may be necessary for safety and transferring from one seated position to another. This particular use offers the patient something to support the lower extremity or provide a prosthetic leg on which to stand, or use for weight bearing to assist themselves or care givers.

Material Selection

When fabricating orthoses and prostheses, the material selection is the first consideration of the process. There are multiple types of thermoplastics, metals, carbon fiber composites, and interface materials to choose from. Each type of material will have certain desirable characteristics or properties that will best suit each patient's needs. Body weight, activity level, amount of rigidity needed, flexibility of material, energy storing properties, amount of cushioning required, and patient strength are all variables to consider when selecting fabrication materials (Table 26-3).

Plastic

Plastics used in orthoses and prostheses are copolymer, thermoplastic polyethylene, polypropylene, and acrylics. Plastics used for custom orthoses such as ankle-foot orthoses (AFOs), knee-ankle-foot orthoses (KAFOs), and upper extremity bracing are chosen for thermal properties and level of rigidity or flexibility and weight of material. When fabricating a lower extremity **brace,** a thicker, stronger plastic should be chosen over a thin plastic that may be used for an upper extremity splint. The heaviness, strength, and rigidity necessary for supporting one's body weight would not be necessary for an upper extremity brace.

Table 26-3	*Important Characteristics of Prosthetic and Orthotic Materials*
Need	**Definition**
Strength	Maximum external load that can be withstood
Stiffness	Stress/strain or force-to-displacement ratio
Durability	Ability to withstand repeated loading
Density	Weight per unit volume
Corrosion resistance	Resistance to chemical degradation
Ease of fabrication	Equipment and techniques needed to shape it

From Shurr DG, Michael JW: *Prosthetics and orthotics*, ed 2, Upper Saddle River, NJ, 2002, Prentice Hall, p 29.

Metal

Metals most commonly used in orthoses are aluminum and steel alloys, titanium, copper, and bronze. These metals are used when designing and fabricating short leg braces or AFOs and KAFOs, and for pylons in prostheses. They are strong, lightweight, and noncorrosive. Metals are also used in knee orthoses and casings for prosthetic knees and torsion units.

Carbon Fiber Composites

Carbon fiber composites are being used more commonly in custom and prefabricated orthoses. Floor reaction, anterior tibial shell AFOs, foot plates, knee bracing, and KAFOs all use varying layers and pattern designs of carbon composites. The patterns create varying degrees of strength, flexibility, weight, and energy storing properties. This advancement has been beneficial to all users: the ability to provide a support that is lightweight and conserves energy. Reduced energy output for ambulation during the day is a tangible benefit. The potential of wearing a less cumbersome device under clothing is a cosmetic advantage, and also provides a more optimal, intimate fit of the device. Lastly, the energy storing property provides each patient with the ability to work and walk for longer periods of time, thus resulting in a more productive and happier individual. This same technology of layering carbon fiber in multiple, pattern specific directions is utilized in the production of prostheses feet in order to produce the same lightweight, yet strong, energy return benefit.

Interface Material

Interface material is used for cushioning an orthosis or prosthesis for comfort and fit, and for fabricating custom arch supports. Varying durometers of firmness, as well as multiple thicknesses and color options (which is a bonus when working with children) make obtaining the best option available possible. Plastazote, PPT, and pelite are some of the most commonly used interface materials. These product properties include vacuum molding, closed or open cell, and whether the material is subject to **packing out,** will resist packing out, or will not pack out. Packing out is what happens to the material over time and use, and the result is the material compresses and eventually collapses.

DEVICE SELECTION

According to information gathered from the patient and the prescription ordered by the physician, a decision must be made by the physical therapist (PT) to determine whether to fit the patient with a prefabricated orthosis or a custom fabricated device. A prefabricated orthosis is designed with a high percentage of the general population's size and measurements taken into account. The first choice is to fit the patient with a prefabricated orthosis as long as the patient's measurements fit into the measurement guidelines provided by the manufacturer, and proper fit and function are not compromised. The prefabricated orthosis can be an appropriate and cost-saving selection. When the patient's size and/or skeletal deformities will not allow for proper fit of a prefabricated orthosis, then the patient will be casted, scanned, and measured as needed to custom fabricate the orthotic device. Custom fabricated orthoses include wrist splints, knee orthoses, and diabetic shoes.

The advancements made in prefabricated orthoses have created a wide range of readily available prefabricated products. Therefore a large percentage of the general population can be fitted with these new devices. However, there are adjustments and changes necessary for a custom fit and optimal patient benefit. There are certain indications, diseases, and deformities that require custom fabricated splints, including progressive, dynamic, and static varieties. A progressive splint is one that can be modified as the patient's rehabilitation progresses so that it will accommodate those changes and still provide the necessary support from a greater to lesser support and allow for increases in range of motion (ROM). Dynamic splinting uses springs or tension rod joints to apply a constant resistance or assistance for flexion or extension. The amount of tension is adjustable and can be set to meet rehabilitation protocols. Lastly, static splinting holds the joint or joints in a specific position.

All prosthetic devices are fabricated by combining a custom made socket designed from a mold or scanned file taken of the residual limb and selected componentry for the rest of the prosthesis that will be replacing the amputated body part. Depending upon patient size, measurements, and deformity, items such as liners can be custom fabricated if a prefabricated item does not fit properly. Patients who exceed the recommended weight limit for prefabricated prosthetic feet and knee units can also be fitted with a custom fabricated component.

Orthoses

Upper Extremity

Fingers, hand, and wrist

A splint for the fingers and hand should only support the affected joint or joints and allow the unaffected joints free ROM. There are single joint splints for the fingers available, such as proximal interphalangeal (PIP) and distal interphalangeal (DIP) splints which maintain or promote active range of motion (AROM) in the phalanges after sprains, fractures, or contractures. Some splints maintain or hold the joint in a fixed position, whereas dynamic splints that are spring-loaded allow the patient some movement of flexion or extension while applying constant force in the desired direction (Fig. 26-1). One particular type of wrist-hand-finger orthosis (WHFO) is the Thomas suspension splint. The function of this splint is to apply tension to the wrist joint and thumb in order to dorsiflex the wrist for diagnoses such as radial palsy. The long opponens splint is often used for flexion contractures, nerve or tendon damage due to traumatic accidents, or rheumatoid arthritis. These splints offer dynamic finger extension and allow the patient to use flexors needed for gripping.

Another example of a functional custom fabricated WHFO is the tenodesis splint (also known as a *wrist action splint*) (Fig. 26-2). This splint is used to increase functional levels and independence mainly for quadriplegia. The design is ultra lightweight and uses the available ability to flex the wrist to accentuate the natural movement of opposition for gripping objects by using the three-jaw chuck pinch position. The wrist-driven wrist/hand orthosis employs the flexor hinge principle. The fingers and thumb are stabilized in the position

of function. A small amount of wrist extensor strength will create flexion motion in the metacarpal phalangeal (MP) joints to produce adequate pinch for a variety of daily activities. Because it is custom fabricated, this style of splint requires a cast of the hand and forearm and measurements for fabrication.

There are multiple orthotic options available when supporting the hand and wrist, depending on the diagnosis and desired limitations for movement. For diagnoses such as carpal tunnel syndrome, tendonitis, or a sprain, a cock-up wrist splint, which holds the wrist in a neutral position is the most common choice (Fig. 26-3, *A*). This splint is a prefabricated brace that is readily available in varying sizes. For diagnoses such as a contracture secondary to a cerebral vascular accident (CVA) or rheumatoid arthritis (RA), a prefabricated malleable wrist-hand-finger orthosis will suffice. This orthosis is progressive in design because the wrist joint and finger platform is easily flexed or extended to accommodate gains made by stretching protocols in physical therapy sessions. These prefabricated, lightweight splints are called *platform* or *resting splints* and provide static positioning (Fig. 26-3, *B*). Some of the soft versions of these splints are more skin-friendly because they offer the option of a cover that can be removed and washed, which promotes good hygiene.

Elbow

Fitting choices for elbow orthoses can usually be prefabricated. A lateral epicondylitis splint (a band with a silicone or air pocket), is used to disperse the pressure placed on the tendon caused by use over a greater area, thus decreasing the point of high stress and pain (Fig. 26-4). ROM splints that limit AROM or provide pressure to increase ROM can also be purchased as prefabricated orthoses. The Flex POP Elbow Orthosis by RCAI

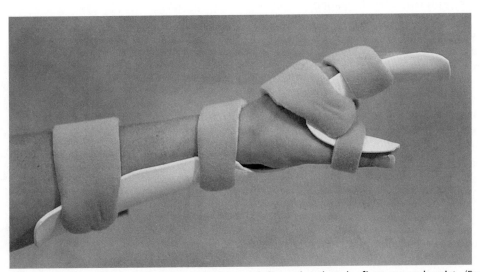

Fig. 26-1 Static immobilization splint. This static splint immobilizes the thumb, fingers, and wrist. (From Coppard BM, Lohman H: *Introduction to splinting: a clinical reasoning and problem-solving approach,* ed 3, St Louis, 2008, Mosby.)

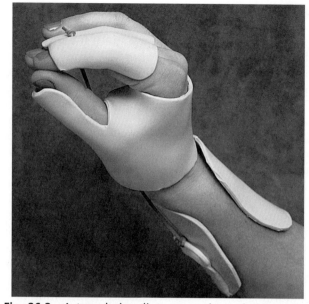

Fig. 26-2 A tenodesis splint uses active wrist extension to aid passive finger flexion. (From Coppard BM, Lohman H: *Introduction to splinting: a clinical reasoning and problem-solving approach,* ed 3, St Louis, 2008, Mosby.

(St. Petersburg, Fla.), for example, provides rehabilitation for joint stiffness and contractures, instabilities, strains, sprains, and ligament repairs. This ROM elbow orthosis offers flexion/extension stop sets at 5-degree increments, which allows changes to be made in therapy sessions as the patient progresses. Dynamic elbow splints can be used when the function desired is to gain ROM by applying a constant stretch to the elbow joint tendons and muscles. Protocols are set for wear time and when the tension placed upon the joint can be increased. Static splints can be set to a designated degree of flexion or extension and depending upon the style or brand, may or may not be adjustable. The physician's prescription, rehabilitation protocols, and the patient's level of compliance and tolerance all contribute to the decision-making process when fitting these types of elbow splints. Elbow contractures can be caused by a variety of injuries or diseases, such as cerebral palsy and CVA.

Shoulder

Shoulder splinting for immobilization can use a sling and swath or a shoulder immobilizer that will support the shoulder joint. One commonly used design utilizes a chest band, upper arm cuff, and a forearm cuff that is adjustable and positions the arm securely against the body (Fig. 26-5). If the required position is abduction, then an airplane splint can be fitted.

Specialized orthoses for the upper extremity

ADLs require a multitude of orthoses to promote independence for individuals who have suffered a stroke or debilitating injury. There are hand and wrist splints

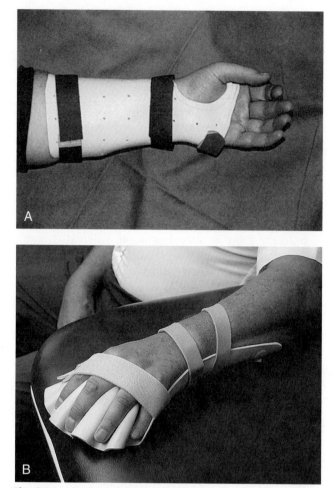

Fig. 26-3 **A,** Completed radial bar cock-up splint. **B,** Positional resting splint. (**A,** From Early MB: *Physical dysfunction practice skills for the occupational therapy assistant,* ed 2. St Louis, 2007, Mosby. **B,** From Pierson FM, Fairchild S: *Principles & techniques of patient care,* ed 4, St Louis, 2008, Saunders.)

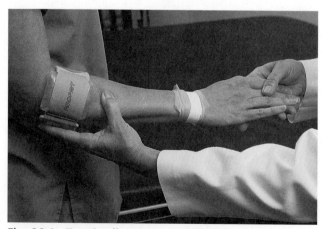

Fig. 26-4 Tennis elbow strap applied. (From Pierson FM, Fairchild S: *Principles & techniques of patient care,* ed 4, St Louis, 2008, Saunders.)

that are used to assist with feeding oneself, holding an ink pen, using a brush, and so on (Fig. 26-6). There are many types of foam available to place around utensils and items with handles to increase their circumference, therefore decreasing the grip strength and ROM needed to hold and use such items.

Fracture splinting uses a compression method for stabilization of the fracture site. The compression of fluid and soft tissue around the fracture site is key when providing a femoral, humeral, radial, or ulnar splint. These splints can be modified to a custom fit by heating and/or adding a soft interface material to provide added comfort. The fracture splint is a bivalve, two-piece orthosis and uses adjustable hook and loop strapping (Fig. 26-7). The splint will allow movement of the unaffected joints such as elbow and wrist for the ulnar fracture. The technique and principles used in splinting for upper extremity fractures is the same for lower extremity fractures.

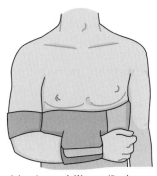

Fig. 26-5 Shoulder immobilizer. (Redrawn from Beare PG, Meyers JL: *Principles and practice of adult health nursing*, ed 3, 1998, Mosby; In Elkin MK: *Nursing interventions & clinical skills*, ed 4, St Louis, 2008, Mosby.)

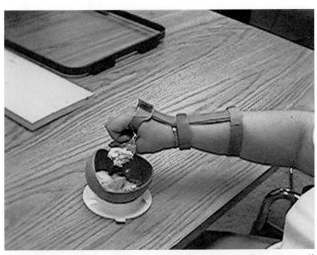

Fig. 26-6 Eating using a special splint with a utensil holder fitted to the hand. (From Early MB: *Physical dysfunction practice skills for the occupational therapy assistant*, ed 2, St Louis, 2007, Mosby.)

Spine and Trunk
Cervical spine

Cervical orthoses are fitted for the purpose of supporting the cervical muscles; limiting rotation, flexion, and extension; or immobilization of the cervical spine. A soft cervical collar can be fitted for lesser injuries such as sprains and strains. The soft collar is a prefabricated orthosis made of foam with a cotton cover and has a hook and loop closure in the back (Fig. 26-8). They are available in different heights and lengths. A cervicothoracic orthosis is a semirigid, two-piece brace that can be fitted for whiplash, degenerative joint disease, arthritis,

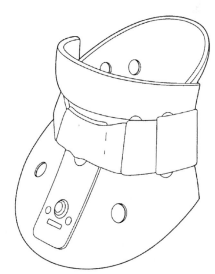

Fig. 26-7 Designed to facilitate adjustments as edema diminishes, this two-piece metacarpal fracture splint has excellent contiguous fit. (Courtesy Lin Beribak, OTR/L, CHT, Chicago, Ill. In Fess EE, Gettle K, Philips C, et al: *Hand and upper extremity splinting: principles and methods*, ed 3, St Louis, 2005, Mosby.)

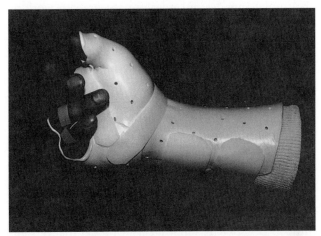

Fig. 26-8 The Philadelphia collar, with an anterior opening for tracheostomy care. (From Shurr DG: Prosthetics, orthotics and orthopaedic rehabilitation. In Clark CR, Bonfiglio M, editors: *Orthopaedics: essentials of diagnosis and treatment*, New York, 1994, Churchill Livingstone.)

and presurgical or postsurgical repairs. These collars are adjustable in height, circumference, and rigidity, but, as with all bracing, the therapist must always check pressure points to make sure that there is no skin breakdown.

Lumbosacral spine

When supporting the spine, there are numerous custom and off-the-shelf products available. The severity of the injury, pain, or disease determines the amount of support that should be fitting to each individual. The more that an individual wears the support, the more dependant he or she becomes upon the support because the abdominal muscles are now not required to work as when unsupported. With this concept in mind, the least amount of support necessary is always the best option.

Trunk support encompasses abdominal binders, rigid panel supports, hyperextension braces, and custom fabricated scoliosis orthoses. Each orthosis will require certain specific circumferential measurements, length measurements, width measurements, and for custom bracing, casting of the torso. When making a custom spinal orthosis, material selection becomes very important. Selecting the necessary amount of rigidity with the least amount of weight is crucial.

The most flexible and therefore the least rigid lumbosacral orthosis (LSO) is the abdominal binder. This orthosis is a stretchy surgical elastic binder that is available in varying widths and lengths to provide optimal fit to a wide range of sizes. The LSO provides support and compression to the abdominal muscles, which in turn support the lower back. The abdominal binder is most often fitted for low back pain.

Pregnancy supports are abdominal binders and are available for use during pregnancy. They provide relief to the lumbar spine as well as support and assistance with unloading the abdomen while compressing the hip complex.

There are numerous styles of rigid back panel LSOs. Depending upon where the injury or disease is in the lumbar region, there are two choices for which orthosis style to fit. If the region lies between L1 and L5, there are supports that fit and support this narrow region. This type of orthosis limits motion in the sagittal plane. This support is created by intracavity pressure to reduce the intervertebral load on the discs. The Aspen QuickDraw RAP is an example of a prefabricated orthosis that falls into this category. This LSO is easy to don and doff, which contributes to the compliance of the patient in wearing the support. It is fabricated of a material that is made to be worn next to the skin. This decreases the occurrence of migration. The fabric is lightweight and breathable, which makes cleaning easier and prolongs the life of the orthosis and increases the patient's hygiene. The back panel has a pocket in which to insert the customizable rigid panel, and a hot or cold pack can

be placed in the pocket for therapeutic benefit. This LSO uses effective compression and leverage to give strong support and immediate pain relief.[3]

An LSO can be transformed into a thoracolumbosacral orthosis (TLSO) by adding shoulder straps, chest panel, and the torso straps. With the additional strapping and pads, the region of support now includes the posterior side from the sacrococcygeal junction to just inferior to the scapular spine. The anterior section of the TLSO extends from the symphysis pubis to the sternal notch, restricting motion in the transverse and sagittal planes and therefore restricting gross trunk movement (Fig. 26-9). TLSOs also provide intracavity pressure to the lumbar and lower thoracic region. Typically, using the least software and hardware necessary makes it easier to don and doff the orthosis. Therefore a higher level of compliance by the wearer is required when adding more componentry (or pieces) to the orthosis.[2]

Hyperextension TLSOs are worn on the anterior side of the body. They operate and function by using a three-point pressure system to maintain full extension and allow for healing of stress fractures. Two pads are used on the anterior portion of the trunk: a sternal pad that sits below the sternal notch and a pubis pad that sits just superior to the symphysis pubis. A third pad is on the posterior side attached to the strap, and it applies pressure in the center of the spine. This orthosis is typically indicated for stress fractures due to osteoporosis, and therefore it is commonly used by elderly women. Since the design of the TLSO is to hold the wearer in good

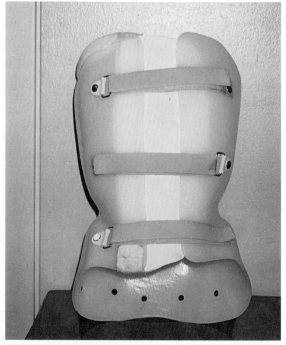

Fig. 26-9 The Wilmington brace is a custom-molded, total-contact thoracolumbosacral orthosis. (From Campbell S: *Physical therapy for children*, ed 3, St Louis, 2007, Saunders.)

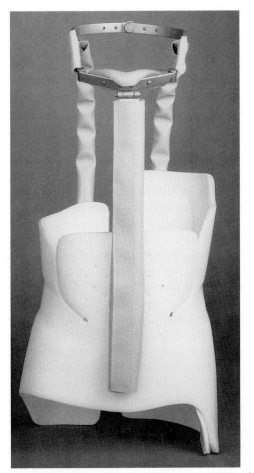

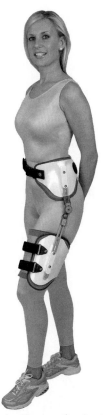

Fig. 26-11 Hip abduction orthosis. (Courtesy of Ortho-america Products, Orlando, Fla.)

Fig. 26-10 Milwaukee brace. Note the tightly fitting pelvic section and the superstructure with its ringlike chin and occipital supports. (From Lusardi MM, Nielson CC: *Orthotics and prosthetics in rehabilitation*, ed 2, St Louis, 2007, Saunders.)

posture, compliance is often an issue with wearing this support, because good posture often decreases with age.

In order to provide complete spinal support throughout the cervical to lumbar vertebrae, a cervicalthoracolumbosacral orthosis (CTLSO) should be fitted. A CTLSO has a mandibular piece on which the chin rests (Fig. 26-10). A forehead strap is also incorporated to assist in controlling the rotation on the head. This type of orthosis is very rigid and therefore immobilizing. These devices are usually fitted for degenerative diseases, fractures, or after spinal surgeries.

Lower Extremity

Sprains, fractures, torn ligaments, arthritis, foot drop, and paralysis all require specific orthoses depending upon the diagnosis. Similar to upper extremity orthoses, lower extremity orthoses also have prefabricated and custom options. Necessary support, varying degrees of immobilization, and function are all required criteria to be met in each fitting.

Hip orthoses

The realm of splinting for the hip joint encompasses immobilization during injury, presurgical and postsurgical intervention, and limited ROM control to meet rehabilitation protocols. When splinting for hip dislocations, subluxations, or postsurgical hip replacement, a hip spica abduction orthosis is often selected (Fig. 26-11). The hip orthosis provides hip stability and proper hip alignment, limits unwanted motion, and reduces stress on the hip. The hip orthosis is prefabricated and offers hip joint options to provide the best orthosis to meet individual rehabilitation protocols. Hip joints will have settings for flexion, extension, abduction, and adduction. The pelvic section and the thigh cuff section can be ordered individually for optimum fit. The interface is soft and can be removed for cleaning. Depending upon the need, there can be either one or two hip joint hinges and thigh cuffs attached to the pelvic section, making the orthosis adaptable for one or two leg spica supports.[12]

Certain neuromuscular disorders, especially cerebral palsy, are associated with pronounced instability and poor balance due to spastic hip adduction. This hip adduction creates a very narrow base of support when sitting and standing, causing crouched posture, genu valgum, foot pronation, and poor gait. One hip orthosis on the market today that may be helpful for these conditions is called the *S.W.A.S.H.* (Standing, Walking And Sitting Hip Orthosis) by Allard (Rockaway, NJ) (Fig. 26-12). This orthosis is designed for children with neuromuscular diagnoses, such as spastic hemiplegia, quadriplegia, low trunk tone, or cerebral palsy, or who have a risk of hip displacement. This orthosis should not be fit to patients with chronic hip dislocation or fixed hip flexion contracture greater than 20°. The S.W.A.S.H. is designed to reduce hip adduction, promote hip abduction, and allow for better control in gait and sitting. This product has been shown to reduce hip adduction and tone, improve hip alignment and ambulation, and create greater independence for patients over time. Maximum success can be achieved with ongoing therapy while wearing this device. S.W.A.S.H. also allows for greater interaction during play and rehabilitation since it frees the patient's hands.[1]

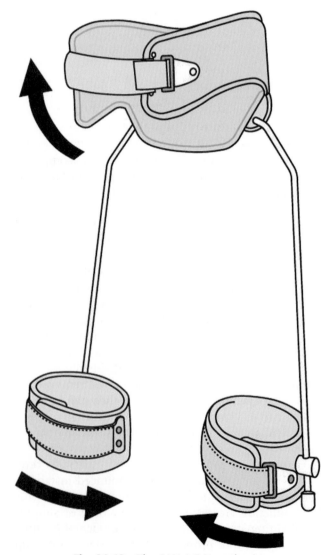

Fig. 26-12 The S.W.A.S.H. orthosis.

Knee orthoses

Knee orthoses range from a neoprene sleeve to a structured combined instability orthosis that has a rigid frame and is hinged at the knee joint. A knee sleeve can be selected when the knee instability is not significant. Reasons to select a knee sleeve may be that heat is desired to relieve pain in an arthritic joint, or to provide proprioceptive cues. Diagnoses such as knee pain or mild osteoarthritis (OA) can be qualified for the fitting of the knee sleeve.

Patella tracking knee orthoses are usually fit for someone with patellofemoral syndrome, patella tracking problems, or patella dislocations. The main symptom for these diagnoses is knee pain in front of the knee exacerbated during squatting or climbing steps. Patella tracking orthoses are usually a neoprene fabric with an additional strap that presses against the patella to promote normal tracking during ambulation and prevent further dislocations or injury. Increasing quadriceps strength is also beneficial.

A hinged knee orthosis may be indicated when more significant knee pain or some mild instabilities are involved. A knee sprain or strain or possible meniscal tear is indicated for the fitting of a hinged knee brace. By adding the hinges to the knee orthosis, medial and lateral stability is gained; therefore the hinged splint provides more stability. Hinged knee orthoses may be neoprene with hinges, a single upright hinge with strapping for placement and support, or a more structured combined instability brace (Fig. 26-13). Combined instability orthoses are used for anterior cruciate ligament (ACL) tears, posterior cruciate ligament (PCL) tears, medial collateral ligament (MCL) tears, or meniscal tears. These orthoses are also fit for prophylactic needs for athletes to prevent ligament injuries or instabilities. Combined instability knee orthoses can be either prefabricated or custom-made depending upon the size and deformity of the knee. These braces provide protection against hyperextension and medial and lateral shifting.

For the diagnosis of OA with medial or lateral compartment failure involved, there are OA knee braces to be fitted. This particular style of knee orthosis is designed to assist with realigning the skeleton to unload the compressed side of the knee joint. By decreasing the load on the compressed compartment, pain will be decreased and the degeneration will be slowed in the joint. By providing proper support and correction to the compromised joint, the likelihood of increasing the patient's quality of life and mobility is the main goal to maintain a healthy lifestyle. These knee braces are available in prefabricated or custom sizes. Custom knee orthoses require casting and measuring.

Postoperative knee orthoses use a knee hinge with adjustable ROM settings that can be changed as the rehabilitation protocols are met and changed. The knee brace can be set to hold a certain position or allow

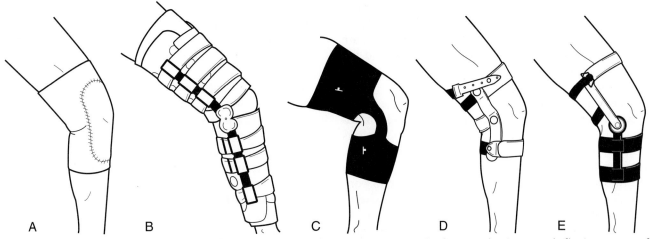

Fig. 26-13 Various knee orthoses. **A,** Soft neoprene knee sleeve. **B,** Postoperative knee orthosis controls flexion range of motion and extension range of motion with adjustable joints. **C,** Prophylactic knee orthosis with lateral joint. **D,** Rehabilitative design to control knee hyperextension. **E,** Custom knee orthosis to stabilize injured knee. (From Coppard BM, Lohman H: *Introduction to splinting: a clinical reasoning & problem-solving approach,* ed 3, St Louis, 2008, Mosby.)

only desired ROM as prescribed by the physician, or reassessed by the PT or the physical therapist assistant (PTA). This type of knee orthosis is generally not meant for long term use and the patient will either graduate out of a knee orthosis altogether or move into a knee orthosis that is less bulky, is more durable, and has a more specific design depending on the diagnosis.

Ankle orthoses

When providing an orthosis for an ankle sprain, there are two common choices available. The stirrup splint will allow free dorsiflexion and plantar flexion to occur while providing limitations to inversion and eversion to prevent the sprain from recurring. This splint is often used for patients who chronically sprain their ankles. The other variety is the ankle gauntlet. This splint provides more immobilization in all planes of motion and is also easily worn inside a tennis shoe. Therefore, depending upon the diagnosis, physician's prescription, and the patient's history, assessments will be made as to which orthosis to provide.

Boot walkers or cam walkers are appropriate selections when treating fractures or severe sprains or for immobilizing the foot or ankle after surgery. These orthoses are removable for bathing and sleeping. The sole of the boot walker incorporates a rocker bottom to assimilate a more natural gait. The length of time worn is dependent upon the patient's required healing time.

Foot orthoses

Custom foot orthoses are another means of obtaining proper foot position and protecting areas of great pressure in the foot. The transverse arch and the medial and lateral longitudinal arches can then be supported. By creating pocketed areas of relief for the plantar surface of the foot, we can slow down degenerative processes and correct skeletal alignment of the foot. Prominent bony landmarks in the anatomy of the foot, such as the metatarsal heads, navicular, talus, and cuneiform bones, can be supported or relieved depending upon the condition of the foot. Diagnoses such as diabetes, plantar fasciitis, heel spurs, pronation, ulcerations, and collapsed arches all benefit from the use of custom made arch supports to correct the position of the foot and assist with a better gait pattern. There are numerous materials available to use to meet the needs of each individual patient, including but not limited to carbon fiber, cork, pelite, Plastazote, and elastomer gel offering a wide range of firmness from rigidity to softness. Individual needs can be met by combining two or more materials to obtain forgiveness and cushion in portions of the foot requiring soft support and firm support to align the foot in the best position possible.

Shoe wear. When treating a patient for foot problems, proper shoe wear is pertinent. The shoe becomes an integral part of the brace when the AFO or KAFO is a metal upright attached to the shoe as well as when the shoe is necessary to properly seat the plastic or carbon fiber AFO in it for stable ambulation. If the patient is not diabetic, then a high quality walking shoe or tennis shoe is recommended for use. If the patient is diabetic, insurance companies will cover the cost of the shoes, and there are numerous options for diabetic shoe brands and styles. Each manufacturer must meet set guidelines to qualify for diabetic shoes status. Diabetic shoes are as seamless as possible and have extra depth in order to accommodate custom arch supports and custom AFOs. Most brands also incorporate a hidden rocker bottom to decrease pressure on the metatarsal heads. For the patient who has such deformity that an off-the-shelf pair of shoes will not fit, custom shoes can be fabricated. Custom shoes are made from a cast or scanned file of the patient's feet. Numerous options are available so that any needed design is possible and the fit is intimate and protective.

Combination orthoses

Ankle-foot orthoses. Diagnoses such as CVA, multiple sclerosis (MS), spinal cord injury (SCI), and various neuropathies can cause a condition known as ***foot drop.*** This condition causes the patient to lose the ability to fire the peroneal nerve, thus losing the ability to contract the anterior tibialis muscle. The patient is essentially unable to pick the toe up by dorsiflexing the ankle complex. When this happens the frequency of dragging the toe during the gait cycle increases and can cause the patient to fall. AFOs can help this condition by holding the ankle foot complex at 90°. The AFO will allow dorsiflexion as the patient rolls over the foot during the stance phase of the gait cycle.

All AFOs limit inversion and eversion and place the foot in subtalar neutral position if obtainable. A pelite liner can also be molded into the AFO as a soft interface, creating a more comfortable, padded support for the patient. The diabetic patient population especially needs custom AFOs to decrease the potential for developing sores or ulcers that may not heal because of rubbing or areas of high pressure. When a custom AFO is fabricated, areas of relief are built into the orthosis. These areas accommodate heavy callused areas, ulcerations, and provide support and relief for collapsed arches that cannot be corrected. Plastic AFOs are in complete contact with the patient's foot and calf and are fitted inside a shoe, causing the shoe to be an integral part of the orthosis. Shoe wear is limited to mostly lace or hook and loop attachments because this feature of the shoes seats the heel of the AFO into the shoe. Slip-on shoes do not work as well because they allow the heel to slip in and out of the shoe too easily.

There are several types of AFO, including leaf spring, solid ankle, free ankle, and dorsi-assist (Fig. 26-14). These orthoses fall into two categories, static or dynamic, with both types consisting of either prefabricated or custom fabricated devices. AFOs can be classified either as static orthoses (prohibiting motion at the ankle) or dynamic orthoses (permitting ankle motion, primarily in the sagittal plane). The solid ankle AFO, the anterior floor reaction brace, and the patellar tendon-bearing (PTB) AFO are examples of static AFOs. Those in the dynamic group include posterior leaf spring and hinged-ankle (articulating) AFO designs.[9] Dynamic AFOs are contraindicated in patients with severe edema, nonhealing diabetic ulcers, and severe foot deformity.

The most simple and cost-effective AFO is the leaf spring. The leaf spring AFO fits under the plantar surface of the foot and into the shoe. It extends up the posterior portion of the calf and has a single strap just distal to the fibula head. It is lightweight, streamlined, and effective, especially if no other instabilities or weaknesses are present. The leaf spring is available in a wide variety of sizes of foot length, foot width, and height of the upright portion.

The solid ankle AFO provides the highest level of support and immobilization. The dorsi-assist ankle joint allows and assists dorsiflexion, while plantar flexion can be limited to stopping at 90° or free plantar flexion. A free ankle AFO allows free plantar and dorsi flexion.

Prefabricated Versus Custom Ankle-Foot Orthoses. If a prefabricated AFO does not fit properly under the foot or have proper contouring around the malleoli, a custom AFO can be made. Fabricating a custom AFO will provide a more intimate fit and thus creates an orthosis that the patient can wear for longer periods of time, which increases compliance and quality of life. The custom AFO will incorporate areas of relief for bony prominences such as malleoli; dropped or collapsed bones of the foot, such as the navicular or talus; and dropped, callused, or ulcerated metatarsal heads. When fabricating a custom AFO, the design of the orthosis is dependent upon patient requirements as well as the practitioner's expertise in componentry selection. If minimal support is required, the trim lines can be very narrow, therefore allowing more movement and flexibility and it is less limiting. If the trim lines are wide and encompassing of the malleoli, then the AFO is more rigid and immobilizing, thus providing increased levels of ankle stability and immobilization.

Plastic Versus Metal Ankle-Foot Orthoses. The plastic AFO is total contact and this feature is not an option for certain patient populations. For patients who suffer from edema in their lower extremities, the metal AFO is a good choice because it does not touch the patient except for the one strap that is just distal to the fibula head. This allows for edema accumulation during the day without rubbing along all of the trim lines that the plastic AFO has. Another reason to select a metal AFO is that it enables incorporation of a custom arch support into the shoe. There would not be enough depth in a shoe for a plastic AFO and a custom arch support. A metal AFO, more commonly known as a *short leg brace,* consists of metal uprights contoured specifically to each patient and attached to the shoe using a metal stirrup that is riveted into the sole of the shoe. The options of solid ankle, limited motion, or dorsi-assist apply to metal bracing as well as plastic. Metal AFOs are heavier and less cosmetic, but when the patient is not a candidate for a plastic total contact AFO, then a metal brace must be fabricated. Metal ortheses are most commonly fit for diagnoses of post-polio syndrome, CVAs, spinal cord injuries, cerebral palsy, and multiple sclerosis patients. Making the proper selection for metal type

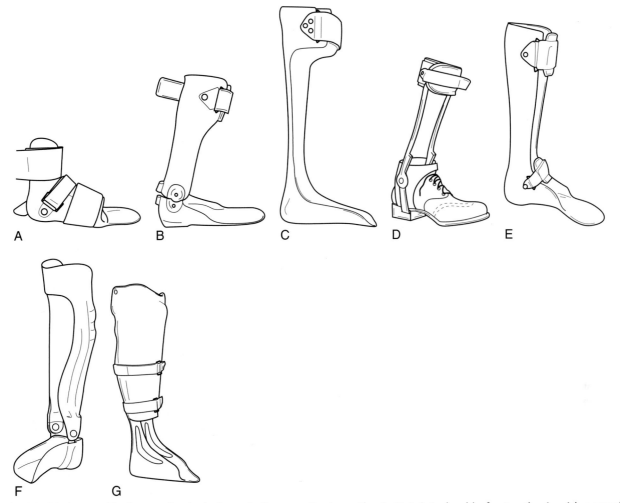

Fig. 26-14 Various ankle-foot orthosis designs. **A,** Supramalleolar orthosis. **B,** Jointed ankle-foot orthosis with posterior plantar-flexion stop and full-length foot plate. **C,** Posterior leaf spring. **D,** Double-upright design with medial T-strap and dorsiflexion-assist ankle joints. **E,** Solid ankle-foot orthosis with instep strap. **F,** Laminated ankle-foot orthosis with double-action ankle joints and pretibial shell. **G,** Patellar tendon-bearing orthosis for load-bearing relief of the foot and ankle complex with carbon fiber reinforcements at ankle. (From Coppard BM, Lohman H: *Introduction to splinting: a clinical reasoning & problem-solving approach,* ed 3, St Louis, 2008, Mosby.)

used for the uprights in a lower extremity brace is crucial for optimal patient outcome. For instance, if the patient is of small stature, experiencing weakness, or fairly inactive, choosing aluminum uprights for the patient's bracing allows the practitioner to provide a material with required strength and adequate support for ambulation without fabricating a brace that would be too heavy for the patient to use. The consideration of patient ability is a crucial factor in choosing fabrication materials. Providing a patient with an orthosis that is too heavy for use will lead to nonuse of the orthosis and noncompliance of the patient, therefore increasing the likelihood of injury and further progression of the deformity. The shoe attached to the orthosis is considered to be a part of the orthosis. Shoe selection is limited to walking shoes and other closed heel and toe shoes. Please refer to the previous section on shoe wear for more information about shoes.

Specialized Ankle-Foot Orthoses. Certain conditions may not respond to commonly used types of AFOs and may require the use of specialized ortheses. The ToeOFF, an orthosis to aid gait manufactured by Allard USA (Rockaway, NJ), and the Charcot restraint orthotic walker (CROW) are two types of specialized custom AFOs.

The CROW is one form of a custom fabricated boot using a clam shell two-piece design and a rocker bottom sole. The function of the CROW is to provide a custom, intimate fit to eliminate friction, shear forces, and motion inside the boot to promote the healing process for nonhealing decubitus ulcers or fractures of the foot, or Charcot deformities. Since it is removable, the boot helps to promote proper hygiene. Often patients who are fitted with a CROW are also receiving wound care treatment. The CROW has an anterior/posterior bivalve construction and is fabricated using a mold of

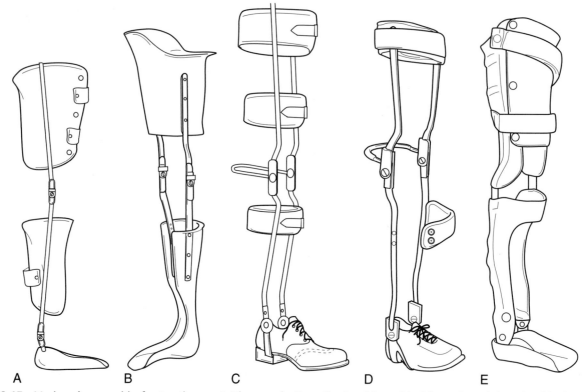

Fig. 26-15 Various knee-ankle-foot orthoses. **A,** Thermoplastic orthosis with molded foot plate, jointed ankle, long anterior tibial shell, drop locks, and circumferential thigh shell. **B,** Thermoplastic orthosis with molded foot plate, solid ankle, drop locks, and quadrilateral thigh shell. **C,** Double-upright orthosis attached to shoe, with jointed ankle, posterior calf band, bail lock knee, and two posterior thigh bands. **D,** Scott-Craig orthosis with double-action ankle joints, pivot anterior tibial band, bail lock knee, and posterior thigh band. **E,** Laminated orthosis with molded foot plate, double-action ankle, pretibial shell, free knee, and posterior thigh shell with long anterior tongue. (From Coppard BM, Lohman H: *Introduction to splinting: a clinical reasoning & problem-solving approach,* ed 3, St Louis, 2008, Mosby.)

the patient's lower leg. The closure for the CROW uses a butterfly chafe design with hook and loop for ease of don and doff.

Knee-ankle-foot orthoses. When instability, deformity or both are present in the knee as well as the foot and ankle, a KAFO can be fabricated. The KAFO will extend from just distal of the femur head and extend to the foot. Oftentimes fitting both a knee orthosis and an AFO is tried but is not always successful or optimal for patient outcomes. Because of the difficulty in trying to fit a patient with the two components of a knee orthosis and an AFO, the fit is compromised where the two orthoses meet or overlap. Frequently, there will be rubbing and pinching at this junction. The knee orthosis would have to extend down past the proximal edge of the AFO causing the purchase of the knee orthosis to be sacrificed.

Types of Knee-Ankle-Foot Orthoses. For the KAFO, there are options for different types of knee joints in order to accommodate varied levels of instabilities (Fig. 26-15). Locked knee joints hold the patient in full extension to prevent knee buckling during ambulation. The patient must use hip hiking or circumduction to progress the

limb forward during ambulation, thus providing supported and secure ambulation. The use of drop locks enables the patient to release the locked position and allow knee flexion for sitting. The drop locks can be unlocked by simply grasping with the hands and pulling up until the joint is cleared, or by the use of a trigger release mechanism attached to the upper, lateral portion of the KAFO. If quadriceps strength is adequate, a free knee joint can be used to allow full ROM and a more natural gait for ambulation. This type KAFO will not lock during heel strike, and therefore will not protect against knee buckling. For patients with a disease such as OA or deformity, this type of orthosis provides adequate support for ambulation due to the patient having adequate quadriceps strength while still providing medial and lateral support.

In the last few years the benefits of technology have become substantial in the realm of KAFOs. New knee joint designs that allow a locked knee at heel strike and/or full knee extension and a free knee swing during the swing phase of the gait cycle are becoming more widely prescribed and fitted. The mechanism for locking and unlocking the knee unit is determined by the manufacturer, and therefore each design will have a slightly different patient population selection.

The Free Walk KAFO by Otto Bock (Minneapolis, Minn.) helps achieve a more natural gait by locking during the stance phase and unlocking during the swing phase. The automatic lock is initiated by knee extension moment, and is only released to swing freely when a knee extension moment and dorsiflexion occur simultaneously in terminal stance. The KAFO joint requires the simultaneous extension moment and 10° of dorsiflexion to release the lock, making it safe for descents and ascents. The Free Walk has an open frame design that uses only one upright instead of two (Fig. 26-16, *A*). The upright is on the lateral side of the leg. The locking mechanism control cable is contained in the tubular stainless steel sidebar. The Free Walk is a custom fabricated orthosis, but the patient must be able to obtain a knee extension moment and dorsiflexion of ankle and foot to operate this device.[7]

Fillauer Company (Chattanooga, Tenn.) has designed a dynamic KAFO called the *Swing Phase Lock* (SPL). The SPL KAFO utilizes a simple internal pendulum mechanism to lock and unlock the knee depending upon the angle of the joint in the sagittal plane (Fig. 26-16, *B*). During the gait cycle, the knee joint will lock just before heel strike for support during stance and unlock the knee at heel off in preparation for swing phase. The SPL KAFO has three modes of operation controlled by a proximal remote push-button switch: automatic lock and unlock, manual unlock, and manual lock. These three modes allow the patient to select automatic lock for walking, unlock for sitting, or lock for standing. Candidate selections for this KAFO are patients with post-polio syndrome, spinal involvement, CVA, peripheral paresis or paralysis, nerve inflammations, neurological failures, myopathies, and MS or similar diseases. Contraindications are knee flexion contractures greater than 10°, central paralysis, hip flexion contractures, hip musculature involvement, poor balance/coordination, and knee hyperextension greater than 10°.[7]

Both of these KAFOs eliminate the need for circumduction or hip hiking as seen in the traditional KAFOs.

Hip-knee-ankle-foot orthoses. The HKAFO is a hip-knee-ankle-foot orthosis that supports all of the joints that it crosses. There are different styles, materials, and componentry to choose from to design every orthosis specifically to each individual's needs (Fig. 26-17). Some styles of HKAFO can be heavy and cumbersome simply because of the bulk of the orthosis and the number of anatomical joints that it crosses, creating a steep learning curve for the patient as well as the PT and PTA. Practicing the donning and doffing process, focusing rehabilitation sessions on upper body strength, ROM, and developing a successful gait pattern are a few of the hurdles that face the patient, PT, PTA, and family members and caregivers. In addition to the physical demands, the emotional stressors should also be addressed by setting clear, concise, attainable goals and ensuring that each individual has the patience needed to fulfill the physical therapy sessions and protocols. Indications are spina bifida, traumatic paraplegia, muscular dystrophy, and osteogenesis imperfecta. The patient must have plantigrade feet, knees should not have flexion contractures greater than 5° to 10°, hips should be free of contractures and flexible (not rigid or spastic), upper extremity strength should be good, the patient should be well motivated and have a supportive family, and goals and expectations should be realistic.

Contraindications are severe contractures, spasticity or other involuntary movements, obesity, and poor upper extremity strength. The reciprocating gait orthosis (RGO) provides excellent walking function and hands-free standing, and the use of the orthosis helps to stretch the hip flexors to prevent contractures. With every step,

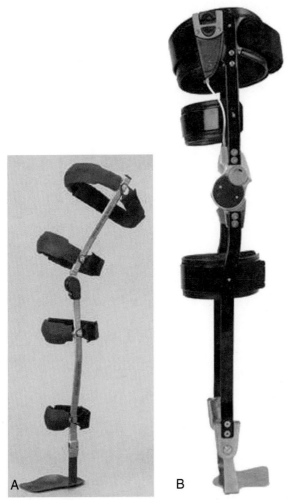

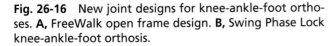

Fig. 26-16 New joint designs for knee-ankle-foot orthoses. **A,** FreeWalk open frame design. **B,** Swing Phase Lock knee-ankle-foot orthosis.

as one leg flexes, the other leg must extend and thus stretch the hip flexors. The age one can be fitted with the isocentric RGO is as young as 17 months, giving them a better chance for walking and standing and therefore enjoying earlier the physiologic, skeletal, and psychological benefits of being upright. In order to ambulate, the patient must be able to use forearm crutches to provide upper body support. A tripod gait is often used when covering a greater distance is required, such as when outdoors. When using the isocentric RGO inside one's house or indoors, the patient can use a normal ambulation pattern with their crutches. The RGO is a custom-made device in which measurements and a cast of the torso and hip portion of the patient is required. There are two styles available. One is an open design in which the wearer will don the device by slipping into the open posterior side. It fits over all clothing including shoes. The second will fit more intimately to the patient and the ankle-foot portion will fit into a shoe.[6]

Prostheses

As discussed in the beginning of this chapter, a prosthesis replaces a body part. The process for fabricating a custom prosthesis has several steps:

■ Evaluation to determine the type of prosthesis to be fabricated based upon activity level, strength, amputation site, personal goals set, and, of course, insurance guidelines

■ Casting or scanning of the patient's affected body area; manufacture of a check socket to assess fit

■ Fabrication of the permanent socket and assembly of the prosthesis

■ Fitting of the prosthesis, and delivery of all necessary componentry and accessories

The patient also has the option of a protective, cosmetic covering on the prosthesis. This covering is custom-made and matches the existing limb in color and shape as closely as possible. The patient will return as necessary for follow-up appointments.

Reasons for Amputations

There are numerous reasons for amputations, including traumatic injury, cancer, infections, and diabetes. Many amputees are born with congenital deformities in which the limb did not develop, or the limb deformity is so great that it must be amputated. The younger the amputee, the better the outcome for most cases because there is a longer period of time available to learn coping skills, compensation techniques, and ways to adapt physically to their environment. The younger the amputee, the greater the likelihood that they will have higher levels of flexibility, strength, and balance, and have marked improvements at a faster rate. For the congenital amputee, whether upper or lower extremity, they will learn many ways to compensate for the absence of the limb, thus becoming very efficient

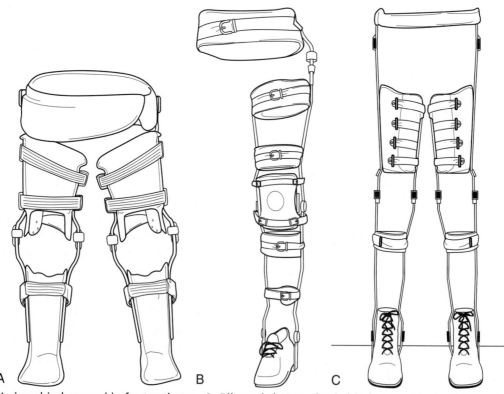

Fig. 26-17 Various hip-knee-ankle-foot orthoses. **A,** Bilateral thermoplastic hip-knee-ankle-foot orthosis. **B,** Unilateral double-upright hip-knee-ankle-foot orthosis. **C,** Bilateral double-upright hip-knee-ankle-foot orthosis. (From Coppard BM, Lohman H: *Introduction to splinting: a clinical reasoning & problem-solving approach,* ed 3, St Louis, 2008, Mosby.)

in ambulation or tasks that require upper extremity involvement and dexterity. The psychological involvement can also be lessened for the congenital or very young amputee for issues such as self image if the family maintains a positive attitude. Experts in the pediatric prosthetics field believe that as long as the parents, extended family, and support team maintain a positive attitude toward the missing limb or deficiency whether acquired or congenital, then the child will also have a positive attitude and outlook on life. If the parents do not handle the limb deficiency well, it is likely that the child will also not cope well with the limb loss. When the patient or family begins to have difficulty coping with the limb loss, then referring them to a psychologist, a peer group, or both becomes essential. The earlier the intervention and support for the family and the child, the better the outcome.[4]

In a recent study done by National Limb Loss Information Center, revised in 2008, there are approximately 1.7 million people living in the United States with limb loss.[10] An average of one out of every 200 people in the United States has had an amputation. Table 26-4 lists the possible causes for amputation.

Suspension Methods

Suspension of a prosthesis refers to the manner in which the prosthesis is held onto the residual limb. Locking pins, suction valves, patella straps, harnesses, and simply the pure design of the socket are all means by which the prosthesis is suspended. Proper suspension of the prosthesis is a key factor in fit, function, and usability of the prosthesis.

Locking pins

Many prostheses, whether upper or lower extremity, are suspended by the use of a liner with a locking pin. The pin is located on the distal end of the liner and slips into a locking mechanism that is housed within the distal end of the socket (Fig. 26-18). A liner is a means of interface that lies between the skin and the socket. Liners are made of silicone, polypropylene, elastomer gels, or urethane blends. The liners act as a cushion for shock absorbency, prevent abrasions, and protect against shearing forces and skin breakdown of the residual limb. This type of suspension provides a secure attachment, and because of the visual and audible cues made as the pin engages into the lock, this type of suspension provides a

Table 26-4	Causes of Amputation
Cause	**Rationale**
Dysvascular-related amputations	Problems associated with the blood vessels: 38.30 per 100,000 in 1988 increased to 46.19 per 100,000 in 1996 Lower-limb amputations: 97% In all age groups, the highest risks were for males and African-Americans
Trauma-related amputations	Upper extremity accounts for 68.6% Males were at slightly higher risk For both males and females, risk of traumatic amputation increased steadily with age, reaching its highest level among people aged 85 years and older
Cancer-related amputations	Most common occurrence in the lower limb accounting for 36% No notable differences found between sexes and races, and lower occurrence rate found in African-Americans
Congenital-related incidences	Rates for newborns were 26 per 100,000 live births, relatively unchanged over the study period Upper limb accounted for 58.5%

From National Limb Loss Information Center. Amputation Statistics by Cause: Limb Loss in the United States. Published by the National Limb Loss Information Center. Available online: http://www.amputee-coalition.org/fact_sheets/limbloss_us.html.

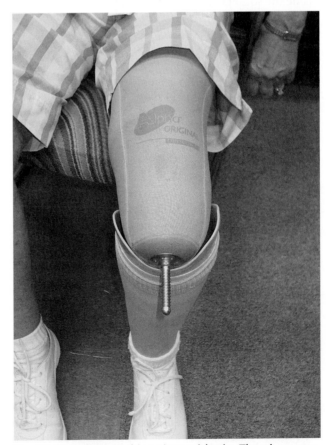

Fig. 26-18 Alpha Locking Liner with pin. The pin engages the lock in the distal socket.

factor of emotional security that the prosthesis is donned correctly. There is a release button to press that will disengage the lock and allow the prosthesis to be removed.

The Alpha Liner, for example, is composed of a unique, mineral oil–based, thermoplastic, elastomer gel with durable fabric covering that makes the liner last longer. The mineral oil within the liner seeps into the skin, creating a skin friendly environment. This gel liner also conforms to the shape of the residual limb providing a custom fit. The Alpha Liner is available in prefabricated and custom-made variations for pediatric, transfemoral, transtibial, and upper extremity amputees. Liners are also available without the distal umbrella for pin attachment and provide an interface between the socket and the limb.[11]

Suction/vacuum suspension

Suction is also a viable and desirable way to suspend a prosthesis. Suction creates an airtight socket through the use of an expulsion valve. At the distal end of the prosthesis there is a valve that the wearer pulls a thin sock through, which pulls the residual limb completely into the socket, and then the valve cap is placed back into the opening to create a closed environment (Fig. 26-19). The top cap of the valve uses an expulsion valve that the amputee can press to release air that may get trapped inside the socket to regain optimal fit.

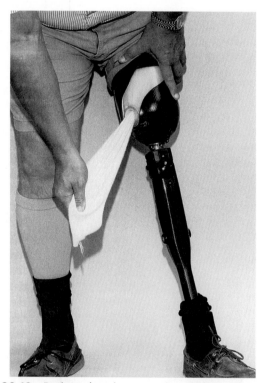

Fig. 26-19 Patient donning a suction socket using a pull sock. The air expulsion valve has been removed so that the sock can be pulled completely out of the socket. (From Lusardi MM, Nielsen CC, editors: *Orthotics and prosthetics in rehabilitation*, ed 2, St Louis, 2006, Butterworth-Heinemann.)

The use of a vacuum system within the socket provides multiple benefits to the amputee. Fluid fluctuation throughout the course of the day is better managed, less pistoning occurs, and circulation is enhanced, thus contributing to a healthier residual limb. One of the main problems that amputees experience on a daily basis is the control of volume change within the socket during the length of the day. The more active the amputee, the more volume loss the individual will experience throughout the day. Traditionally the way to control volume changes inside the socket is to add prosthetic socks as the residual limb volume decreases. If the amputee does not use sock management effectively, then chaffing and pistoning become a problem and cause skin breakdown.

Patella straps

A patella strap can be added to a transtibial prosthesis to provide suspension above the femoral condyles while still allowing full flexion and extension. This strap can be made out of leather or other strapping materials and secured with buckles or hook and loop closures.

Supracondylar suspension is obtained by the design of the socket. By creating a snug, intimate fit just superior to the femoral or humeral condyles, this design creates a suspension that is easy to use, maintains appropriate fit, and allows for full ROM.

Harnesses

For upper extremity prostheses, the use of a harness for suspension is widely used. The harness not only suspends the prosthesis, but also acts as a mechanism for control of the terminal device (TD) or hand for opening and closing the hand for grip (Fig. 26-20). The hand can be one of several types of hooks or a hand that has more cosmesis and looks like a real hand. By elevating or depressing the shoulder or scapular manipulations, the cables that connect to the hand are tightened, and this tension on the cable opens the hand. The harness will also operate the elbow unit for the transhumeral amputee. There are separate cables, controls, and body movements necessary to lock and unlock the elbow joint.

There are many designs for harnesses. The style desired is the most simple that will provide the amputee with the ability to control the TD. Harnessing uses the body's movements and transmits them to the cable portion of the harness and causes movement of the TD. The movements necessary for TD control are glenohumeral forward flexion, biscapular abduction, shoulder depression and elevation and chest expansion. Depending upon the level of amputation and the amputee's strength and ROM, the correct harness can be chosen. Different motions can be used to control the TD or the elbow joint. Each movement must be mastered to efficiently use the prosthesis.[16]

There are advantages and disadvantages to using a harness. These can be found in Box 26-1.

Limb design

One more technique used to suspend a prosthesis is a joint and corset. This type of suspension is usually reserved for transtibial amputees who also have knee conditions such as OA, ligament or meniscal damage, or other instabilities on the amputated side. A pair of metal knee joints is incorporated into the socket, making sure to maintain the knee center alignment. The upper thigh portion called the *corset* is commonly fabricated from leather and is attached to the upper half of the knee joint encompassing the thigh. The corset portion is then laced up because this technique provides suspension for the prosthesis as well as a functional knee brace. Another advantage of the corset is that it helps to unload the residual limb by transferring the weight of the prosthesis to the thigh portion of the limb, preventing further injury or degeneration of the involved knee.

Upper Extremity Prostheses

Body powered versus myoelectric

The difference between a body powered prosthesis and a myoelectric prosthesis is that the body powered prosthesis operates by the amputee actually moving a body part to elicit the movement of the TD. A myoelectric prosthesis is controlled by the ability to stimulate the antagonist and agonist muscle group. The electrodes

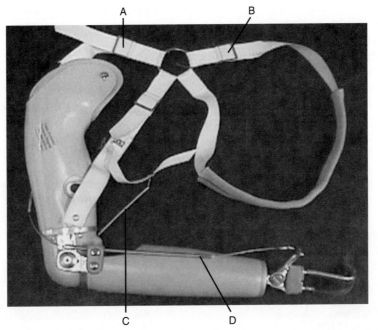

Fig. 26-20 The figure-of-eight harness with posterior ring and cable control systems used in a conventional (body-powered) transhumeral prosthesis includes an anterior suspension loop *(A)*, the contralateral axillary loop *(B)*, a cable to control locking and unlocking of the elbow mechanism *(C)*, and a cable that will lift the forearm if the elbow unit is unlocked or operate the terminal device if the elbow unit is locked *(D)*. (From Lusardi MM, Nielsen CC, editors: *Orthotics and prosthetics in rehabilitation*, ed 2, St Louis, 2006, Butterworth-Heinemann.)

BOX 26-1

Advantages and Disadvantages of Using a Harness

ADVANTAGES
- Harness generates enough power and excursion (length of movement) to open/close the terminal device
- Harness can be worn under clothing
- Ease of donning and doffing
- Easy to learn
- Patient gets immediate biofeedback when movement is elicited

DISADVANTAGES
- Movements can be unnatural
- Harness may be cumbersome (it may require a waist belt)
- Depending upon level of amputation a harness may not generate enough power and excursion. Nerve impingement syndrome can occur over time from the axilla pressure applied to the contralateral limb or both sides if the amputee is bilateral

Data from Uellendahl JE, Uellendahl EN: Body-powered upper-limb, prosthetic designs. In Carroll K, Edelstein JE, editors: *Prosthetics and patient management: a comprehensive clinical approach*, Thorofare, N.J., 2006, Slack.

seated within the socket wall directly receive the stimuli to produce movement. This type of prosthesis does not require a harness for suspension or TD control. As with any device fitted to a patient, the patient must have the cognitive ability to use the device, the physical ability to operate the device, and clearly understood goals and limitations for use of the device. The learning curve for using myoelectric components is greater than the learning curve for body powered components. Software packages are available that can be used during a physical therapy session to assist with learning control of the speed and the strength of the muscle contractions needed for different tasks, whether the desired motion is opening or closing the TD (hand) or rotating the wrist unit.

Prosthetic shoulders

Shoulder joints do not have as many options as elbows and hands. Most shoulder components are friction controlled, allowing for movements of abduction, flexion, and extension of the humeral joint. The amount of friction can be changed depending upon tasks and need. Some shoulder components also provide an extension stop with full humeral flexion.

Prosthetic elbows

Body powered elbow components are controlled by friction or locking positions. The elbows with locking positions have as many as 11 positions in which to place the elbow and can also assist in lifting. The units that are friction controlled can be manually placed in desired flexion or extension. The elbows are available in adult or pediatric sizes (Fig. 26-21).

Myoelectric elbow units are also a consideration to make. One such type is the DynamicArm, a myoelectric prosthetic elbow unit by Otto Bock. This unit lifts loads up to 13 pounds and offers a feature called *Automated Forearm Balance (AFB)*. AFB stores energy when the arm is extended and reuses it for flexion, which results in a smooth, natural swing during walking. The DynamicArm unlocks easily, even when under load. It can be positioned without having to send an unlocking signal, which enables the user to make fewer compensatory movements while providing a more natural appearance.[14]

Prosthetic wrists

Wrist units provide a connection between the hand and the prosthetic forearm or socket. Some wrists can be manually twisted against a constant friction to allow for

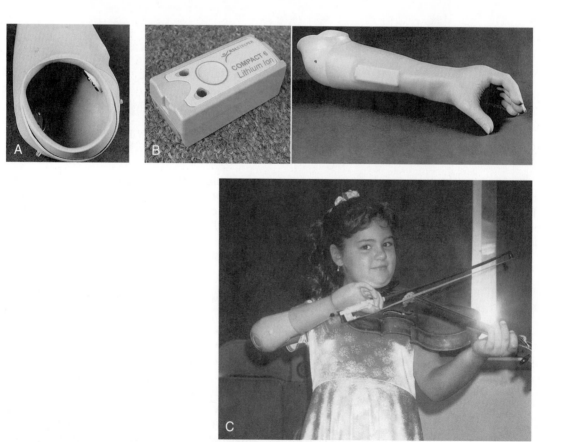

Fig. 26-21 Myoelectric transradial prosthesis. **A,** Electrode placement within the socket. **B,** The battery pack is positioned in the forearm. **C,** Playing the violin with a myoelectric prosthesis. (**A** and **B,** From Zenie J: Prosthetic options for persons with upper extremity amputation. In Lusardi MM, Nielsen CC, editors: *Orthotics and prosthetics in rehabilitation*, ed 2, St Louis, 2006, Butterworth-Heinemann. **C,** Courtesy of MH Mandelbaum Orthotic & Prosthetic Services.)

positioning of the hand. Other wrist units are myoelectric and a cocontraction of both the agonist and antagonist muscle groups is required to control the wrist unit to achieve pronation or supination of the hand. Quick disconnect wrist units can be fabricated into the distal end of the socket for ease of changing out the prosthetic hand.

Prosthetic hands

There are two main types of TDs or hands offered: hooks and hands (Fig. 26-22). They can both be either body powered, where the hand is controlled by a cable system through a harness, or myoelectrically powered, where the hand is controlled by muscle stimulus received by sensors placed within the socket.

Hooks come in a variety of shapes and sizes to accommodate children and adults. The various shapes are offered to make different tasks easier to accomplish. Hooks can be body powered or myoelectric. The body powered hooks are opened by pulling the cable and closed automatically under spring or rubber band tension. Multiple rubber bands can be placed on the TD to increase the grip strength for different tasks. Hooks also

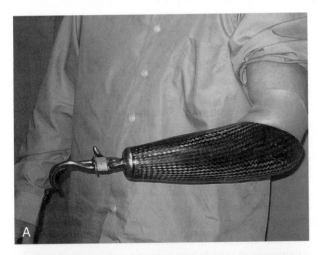

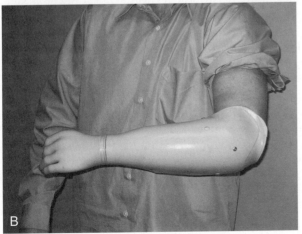

Fig. 26-22 Two types of prosthetic hands. **A**, Hook. **B**, Hand.

have varieties available for specific recreational tasks, such as designs for fishing, bowling, and wearing a baseball glove. Assistive TDs are also available that attach to the wrist unit. These TDs include saws, knives, gardening tools, spoons, and kitchen tools.

Prosthetic hands can be body powered or myoelectric. The hands can use a protective glove, which provides cosmesis. They are many sizes and designs. A passive hand has a gripping function that is opened by the sound hand and closes automatically. This type of hand is used by a wearer who possibly cannot cognitively understand how to operate a hand, is physically unable to operate a hand, or quite simply does not wish to learn how to use one and still has the need for body balance and symmetry. Voluntary opening and voluntary closing hands are controlled by a cable-activated prosthesis. The voluntary opening hand opens when the cable is pulled and then closes under a spring tension. The voluntary closing hand uses the opposite technique.

Mastectomy products

Today, there are numerous options available for the postmastectomy patient. There are prefabricated silicone breast forms that range in size, shape, and color. This selection variance makes it possible to fit most patients with a prefabricated breast form. For times when the heaviness of a silicone form is not desired, there are also foam filled forms that are very lightweight but not as shapely. External garments or camisoles are also offered as an alternative to a bra, which is an especially nice offering for use during or after radiation because it fits loosely and does not rub against the already compromised skin tissue. There are also many mastectomy bras available, varying in size and color. For the patient who has difficulty with the prosthesis slipping inside the bra or chaffing the skin, or for the patient who has more radical scar tissue or severe chest wall deformity, there are custom fabricated breast forms. The chest wall must be either casted or scanned for the fabrication of the form. The goal for mastectomy forms and products is to balance the body with weight distribution and cosmesis.

Lower Extremity Prostheses
Componentry selection guidelines

When selecting the appropriate foot or knee for each patient, there are set medical guidelines for levels of ambulation to direct the prosthetist's choice. Depending upon the activity and ambulation abilities or potential of each amputee, the Medicare chart found in Box 26-2 can be adhered to when selecting the foot or knee for each prosthesis. Careful consideration and evaluation for this potential to regain ambulatory ability is a crucial step in determining appropriate componentry. The PTA in conjunction with the prosthetist can make optimal decisions as a team and create better outcomes for the patient.

Activity Guidelines K0 through K4

- K0 does not have the ability or potential to ambulate or transfer safely with or without assistance and a prosthesis does not enhance their quality of life or mobility.
- K1 has the ability or potential to use a prosthesis for transfers or ambulation on level surfaces at a fixed cadence. Typical of the limited household ambulatory.
- K2 has the ability or potential for ambulation with the ability to traverse low level environmental barriers such as curbs, stairs or uneven surfaces. Typical of the limited community ambulatory.
- K3 has the ability or potential for ambulation with variable cadence. Typical of the community ambulatory who has the ability to transverse most environmental barriers and may have vocational, therapeutic, or exercise activity that demands prosthetic utilization beyond simple locomotion.
- K4 has the ability or potential for prosthetic ambulation that exceeds the basic ambulation skills, exhibiting high impact, stress, or energy levels, typical of the prosthetic demands of the child, active adult, or athlete.

From DMERC Medicare Advisory Bulletin. Columbia, S.C.: DMERC, 1994. pp. 95-145.

An additional tool that can be used when evaluating the activity level of the amputee is the Amputee Mobility Predictor Questionnaire and the Amputee Mobility Predictor (AMP) Testing Methodology.[8] These evaluation tools where developed by Robert Gailey, PhD, PT, and are widely used in the clinical setting to determine the functional level of each amputee. By gathering qualitative data, the PT, PTA, and the prosthetist can have shared data to use while collaborating on treatment plans for shared patients.

Prosthetic knees

Types of knees. A prosthetic knee functions as a means of support and ambulation. Providing the proper combination of stability, shock absorption, and agility is the key to selecting and fitting the right knee to each patient.

Locking Knee. A locking knee is inherently the most stable and safe knee. This knee will have a manual switch or button that will unlock the knee and allow flexion for sitting. During ambulation the knee will remain locked throughout the gait cycle. This feature allows the amputee to ambulate and roll over the knee without fear of buckling, and thus decreasing the percentage of falls. Since the knee does not bend during swing phase, hip hiking or circumduction may be used to propel the prosthesis.

Weight Activated Knee. A weight activated or stance control knee unit will provide some limited locked knee moments and also allow free swing during the swing phase of the gait. In order to lock the knee for a safe stance phase, the knee must reach full extension at heel strike. Most weight activated knees have a built-in angle of flexion of approximately 15° before breaking and releasing the knee for swing phase. As the amputee rolls over the foot and the knee begins to break, the knee will release the locked, safe position and flex, then swing forward freely. This swing phase of the knee units is adjustable and can be set to meet each individual's cadence requirements. The use of hydraulics or pneumatics controls the rate of swing by increasing or decreasing the viscosity or pressure of fluids or air within the knee component.

Microprocessor Knee. Current technology has added some very important control features that have not been offered until the past few years. The use of computerized componentry to control swing and stance phase has provided transfemoral amputees with a new type of freedom. The C-Leg, Rheo Knee, Plié MPC Knee, and Smart Adaptive are all examples of microprocessor (MPC) knee components (Fig. 26-23). Each knee works on a slightly different mechanism of gait, but this freedom of cadence change without the fear of falling and less use of mental focus required by traditional knee units provides huge gains for the transfemoral amputees.[13]

Prosthetic feet

Prosthetic feet types are best described by the function that each provides, and there are three general types of feet: solid ankle cushion heel (SACH), single axis, and dynamic (Fig. 26-24).

The SACH foot does not allow any motion. This foot is most commonly used on a temporary prosthesis or for an amputee who will be using the prosthesis for transfers only. The SACH foot provides stability and shock absorption at heel strike.

The single axis foot allows motion for dorsiflexion and plantar flexion. Single axis feet use bumpers in the forefoot and hindfoot for shock absorption. These bumpers come in a variety of durometers or stiffness to make the amount of cushion as customized as possible. Single axis feet are fitted to transfemoral or transtibial amputees with low activity level who traverse uneven ground on a daily basis, traveling between their homes and their vehicles, but who are still relatively low activity amputees.

The next type of prosthetic foot is the multiaxial, dynamic foot. This type of foot is most commonly selected because of the ability to mimic the natural foot and ankle's complex ROM, rotation, stability and shock absorption. Any lower extremity amputee can be fitted with this type foot. It is usually selected for more active amputees, such as community ambulators, people who like to go hiking or walking for exercise or therapy. The dynamic feet allow motion in all directions as well as provide energy return to the amputee. As the heel of the foot strikes the ground and some form of compression is acquired at the heel and ankle portion of the foot,

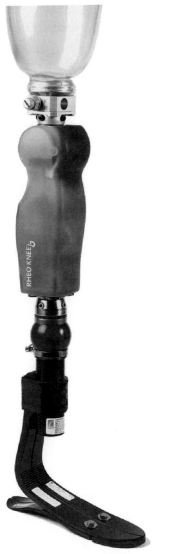

Fig. 26-23 Microprocessor-controlled knee unit. (Photo of Rheo Knee courtesy of Össur, Aliso Viejo, Calif.)

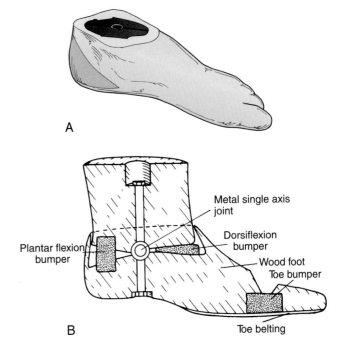

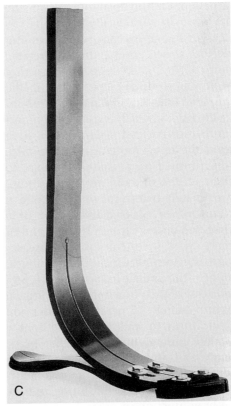

Fig. 26-24 Types of prosthetic feet. **A,** Solid ankle cushion heel (SACH) foot. **B,** Single axis foot. **C,** Flex-foot. (**A,** From Cameron MH, Monroe LG: *Physical rehabilitation: evidence-based examination, evaluation, and intervention*, St Louis, 2008, Saunders. **B,** From Fergason J: Prosthetic feet. In Lusardi MM, Nielsen CC, editors: *Orthotics and prosthetics in rehabilitation*, St Louis, 2000, Butterworth-Heinemann. **C,** Photo courtesy Össur North America, Aliso Viejo, Calif.)

energy is retained in the material that the foot keel is fabricated from. As the amputee rolls over the midfoot and forefoot section this stored energy is then returned at toe off and acts springlike to help propel the amputee forward just as the sound limb foot and ankle complex functions. Restoring normal ROM, function, and shock absorption is the goal for this type of foot. The Pathfinder Foot, manufactured by Ohio Willow Wood, is a dynamic foot with great stability that is indicated for high activity amputees. The Pathfinder has a unique construction of a toe spring, foot plate, and an adjustable pneumatic heel spring in a triangular configuration providing high energy return, rotation, and inversion and eversion motion.

Other Prosthetic Products

The replacement of body parts such as ears, noses, fingers, and toes falls within the realm of prosthetics. This process consists of making an impression of the existing ear or finger and duplicating it as closely as possible in size and color. These prostheses are functional and assist with tasks such as typing, hearing, and walking. The prosthesis will be suspended in a variety of manners depending upon the available site for attachment. Adhesive glues and suction are often utilized for suspension. These prostheses are made of vinyl or silicone and are custom fabricated.

Summary

This introduction to orthotics and prosthetics has provided a brief overview of products and indications for use of the orthotic or prosthetic componentry. There are many considerations involved with each patient, and familiarizing oneself can be time consuming and ongoing throughout one's career. When fitting an orthosis, the main concerns are finding a proper fit, not compromising the patient's function, using as little orthotic support as required, and supporting only the joint or joints that are deficient in strength or ROM or have deformity. Prosthetic componentry for lower extremity amputees should be selected based upon the patient's ability to ambulate using the Activity Guidelines chart to gauge the selection process (see Box 26-2). For upper extremity amputees, the choice can be decided based upon ability to operate the TD, the patient's AROM, and strength. Preprosthetic therapy is beginning to be discussed in the medical field among professionals. According to the American Geriatrics Society (AGS), which is composed of more than 6800 health care professionals who are focused on the issues of the aging, more than 75% of all amputations are performed on persons older than 65 years. Approximately 90% of those involved are lower limb, and approximately two thirds of lower-limb amputations are transtibial. More than 65% of all amputations performed on people age 50 years and older are due to diabetes or peripheral vascular disease (PVD), according to the Amputee Coalition of America (ACA). What can help the patient to have a satisfying quality of life and achieve their functional goals after amputation? "Approximately 75 percent of older adults can regain their ability to walk with or without assistive devices if they undergo the proper rehabilitation program before and after they receive...a prosthesis."[8] The physical therapy program should address the patient's strength, stamina, flexibility, and improved heart and lung function in order to be optimally prepared before the amputation surgery. Wearing a prosthesis for ambulation requires an increased level of energy consumption of about 60%. Providing a team approach to each patient, including a PT, physician, physiatrist, counselor, and a prosthetist, enables the patient to be better prepared mentally and physically and more educated about the process and the answer to the question of exactly what is a prosthesis.[5]

❖ GLOSSARY

Brace: A term, now mostly used outside of a clinical setting, referring to a splint.

Componentry: The parts of a prosthesis.

Doff: The removal of a residual limb.

Don: The fastening of a residual limb onto the body.

Foot drop: A condition in which the foot drags during gait as a result of a loss of function in the peroneal nerve. This loss of nerve function can be caused by conditions such as CVA, MS, SCI, or various neuropathies.

Liner: An interface that lies between the skin and the socket. The liner acts as a cushion for shock absorbency and to protect against abrasions, shear forcing, and skin breakdown of the residual limb.

Orthosis: A device that provides biomechanical, musculoskeletal support, and correction of abnormalities within the human body.

Packing out: What happens to the material lining a prosthesis over time. Through general wear and tear during device usage, the material compresses and eventually collapses.

Prosthesis: A device that replaces a body part. This group consists of arms, legs, partial feet, hands, ears, breasts, and so on.

Splint: An orthosis that will immobilize a joint and will allow only a specific range of motion as rehabilitation protocol requires.

REFERENCES

1. Allard USA: S.W.A.S.H. (website): www.allardusa.com. Accessed April 18, 2010.
2. Aspen Medical Products, Inc.: Aspen TLSO LumboSacral Bracing System (website): www.aspenmp.com. Accessed September 21, 2008.
3. Aspen Medical Products, Inc.: QuickDraw RAP LumboSacral Bracing (website): www.aspenmp.com. Accessed September 21, 2008.
4. Fairley M: Early Prosthetic Fitting—Yes or No? *The O & P EDGE* 7(4):26–34, 2008.
5. Fairley M: Preprosthetic Therapy: Is It Needed? Does It Help? *The O & P EDGE* 7(10):34–40, 2008.
6. Fillauer Companies: *Continuing the Climb*, Chattanooga, Tenn., 2001, The Isocentric RGO (website): www.fillauer.com.
7. Fillauer Companies: Swing Phase Lock (SPL), Chattanooga, Tenn., 2004 (website): www.fillauer.com.
8. Gailey RS, Roach KE, Applegate EB, et al: The amputee mobility predictor: an instrument to assess determinants of the lower-limb amputee's ability to ambulate, *Arch Phys Med Rehabil* 83(5):613–627, 2002.
9. Lusardi, MM: *Orthotics and prosthetics in rehabilitation*, ed 2, St Louis, 2008, Butterworth-Heinemann.
10. National Limb Loss Information: Amputation statistics by cause (website): www.amputee-coalition.org/fact_sheets/amp_stats_cause.html. Accessed April 18, 2010.
11. Ohio Willow Wood: Liners and suspension (online PDF): www.owwco.com/pdf/catalog/B/oww%20catalog%20sec%20B_006.pdf. Accessed April 18, 2010.
12. Otto Bock HealthCare: ABD LockSystem Hip Abduction Orthosis (website): www.ottobock.ca. Accessed September 21, 2008.

13. Otto Bock HealthCare: C-Leg Clinical and Technical Information (website): www.ottobockus.com. Accessed June 20, 2008.
14. Otto Bock HealthCare: DynamicArm 12K100 (website): www.ottobockus.com. Accessed October 26, 2008.
15. Otto Bock HealthCare: FreeWalk Stance Control System (website): www.ottobockus.com. Accessed May 13, 2008.
16. Uellendahl JE, Uellendahl EN: Body-powered upper-limb, prosthetic designs. In Carroll K, Edelstein JE, editors: *Prosthetics and patient management: a comprehensive clinical approach*, Thorofare, N.J., 2006, Slack.

REVIEW QUESTIONS

Short Answer

1. Describe the difference between custom fitted and custom fabricated.
2. Describe how a SACH foot varies from a single axis foot.
3. Discuss the desired features for an orthosis/prosthesis.
4. Describe the differences in a body powered upper extremity prosthesis and a myoelectric prosthesis.
5. When splinting an injured joint, explain why you would or would not brace more than the injured joint.

True/False

6. A prosthesis supports a body joint or joints.
7. Nomenclature for prostheses and orthoses is based upon the person who invented the device.
8. A floor reaction AFO has energy return properties.
9. Ears can be considered to be a prosthesis.
10. The Reciprocating Gait Orthosis is designed to benefit people suffering from a stroke.
11. Splinting only the affected joint is recommended.
12. There is no knee brace available to prevent knee buckling.
13. Custom arch supports should not be fitted unless there is a specific diagnosis of deformity.
14. The stirrup splint prevents inversion and eversion.
15. A CROW and a boot walker are the same device.
16. Some KAFOs can provide free swing and a locked knee at full knee extension.
17. Nerve impingement syndrome can affect upper extremity amputees who use a harness.

Commonly Used Medications in Orthopedics

LaDonna S. Hale

This is not an all inclusive list. Please consult an appropriate drug information resource for full information regarding therapeutic uses, side effects, and precautions.

Type of Medication	Generic Name	Trade Name	Important Rehabilitation Information
Nonsteroidal antiinflammatory drugs (NSAIDs) Treat mild to moderate acute or chronic pain and inflammation	Aspirin	Bayer, Anacin and others	• Available over-the-counter. • Not appropriate for all patients and should not be used by children or for pain or inflammation treatment by adults with difficult to control hypertension, congestive heart failure, kidney disease, stomach ulcers, bleeding disorders, alcoholism, and persons prescribed warfarin. • A few important side effects include: rash, increased risk of bleeding, stomach upset, and stomach ulcers. • Low dosages (81-325 mg/day) are used for antiplatelet benefits.
	Diclofenac	Cataflam, Voltaren	• Ibuprofen, naproxen, and ketoprofen are available over-the-counter. Ketorolac and ibuprofen are also available in injection form. NSAIDs are not appropriate for all patients and should not be used by persons with difficult to control hypertension, congestive heart failure, kidney disease, stomach ulcers, bleeding disorders, alcoholism, and persons prescribed warfarin. • A few important side effects include: rash, increased risk of bleeding, stomach upset, and stomach ulcers.
	Etodolac	Lodine	
	Fenoprofen	Nalfon	
	Ibuprofen	Advil, Motrin, and others	
	Indomethacin	Indocin	
	Ketoprofen	Orudis	
	Ketorolac	Toradol	
	Meloxicam	Mobic	
	Nabumetone	Relafen	
	Naproxen	Aleve, Anaprox, Naprosyn, and others	
	Oxaprozin	Daypro	
	Piroxicam	Feldene	
	Sulindac	Clinoril	
	Tolmetin	Tolectin	
Selective COX-2 inhibitor Treat mild to moderate acute or chronic pain and inflammation	Celecoxib	Celebrex	• Celecoxib is not appropriate for all patients and should not be used by persons with difficult to control hypertension, congestive heart failure, or kidney disease. • Safer than NSAIDs in persons with stomach ulcers, bleeding disorders, alcoholism, and persons prescribed warfarin. • Should not be taken by persons allergic to sulfonamide antibiotics.

Type of Medication	Generic Name	Trade Name	Important Rehabilitation Information
Nonnarcotic analgesic Treat mild to moderate, acute or chronic noninflammatory pain	Acetaminophen	Tylenol and others	• Available over-the-counter. • Does not treat inflammatory type pain. • Generally considered safe for most patients; the most problematic side effect is liver toxicity. • Accidental overdoses are common. To reduce the risk of liver failure, adult dosages should not exceed 4 g/day. • Should not be used by persons who chronically consume alcohol.
Opioid analgesics and combination products Treat mild to severe, acute or chronic pain	Codeine + acetaminophen Hydrocodone + acetaminophen Hydromorphone Fentanyl Methadone Meperidine Morphine Oxycodone Oxycodone + acetaminophen Oxymorphone Pentazocine + aspirin Propoxyphene Propoxyphene + acetaminophen Tramadol	Tylenol #3 and others Lortab, Lorcet, Vicodin, and others Dilaudid Duragesic patch Dolophine Demerol MS Contin, Oramorph, Roxanol and others OxyContin Percocet, Tylox, and others Opana Talwin Darvon Darvocet Ultram	• Opioid selection is based upon level and intensity of pain. • Physical dependence can occur with chronic use; however, physical dependence does not necessarily indicate addiction. • Possibility of addiction exists. • A few important side effects include: stomach upset, rash, sedation, drowsiness, dizziness, constipation, low blood pressure, orthostatic hypotension, slowed respirations, and impaired judgment. Tolerance will develop to most of these side effects except constipation. • Many opioids contain acetaminophen (see acetaminophen section for additional precautions)
Bisphosphonates Treat and prevent osteoporosis	Alendronate Risedronate Ibandronate Zoledronic Acid	Fosamax Actonel Boniva Reclast	• Osteoporosis treatment will not be effective without adequate calcium and vitamin D intake. • Oral bisphosphonates may be prescribed orally once daily, weekly, or monthly. Injection bisphosphonates may be administered annually. • Important patient instructions: Tablets should be taken on an empty stomach with a full glass of water. Patient must remain upright for at least 30 minutes after the dose. • A few important side effects include: bone and muscle pain, heartburn, and esophageal ulcers when patient instructions are not followed.
Other osteoporosis medications Treat and prevent osteoporosis	Raloxifene Calcitonin Teriparatide	Evista Miacalcin Forteo	• Estrogen agonist/antagonist. • Generally used in female patients only. • Calcitonin hormone. • Administered daily as a nasal spray. • Recombinant human parathyroid hormone. • Injected subcutaneously daily. • FDA approved for short-term use only (less than 2 years)

Continued

Type of Medication	Generic Name	Trade Name	Important Rehabilitation Information
Corticosteroids/ glucocorticoids Suppress and reduce inflammation	Betamethasone Cortisone Dexamethasone Fludrocortisone Hydrocortisone Methylpredniso-lone Prednisolone Prednisone Triamcinolone	Celestone and others Decadron Florinef various Solu-Medrol Prelone and others Deltasone Kenalog and others	• Most are available oral and/or injection. • Betamethasone, dexamethasone, prednisone, and triamcinolone may be administered intraarticularly and intradermally. • Betamethasone and triamcinolone may be administered intrasynovially. • A few important side effects include: increased risk of osteoporosis and infection; high blood glucose level; muscle weakness; abnormal fat distribution to abdomen, face, and upper back; edema; cataracts; glaucoma; stomach ulcers; high blood pressure; impaired wound healing; insomnia; mood changes; and even serious psychiatric disturbances. • A few important side effects of intraarticular injection include: same as those just listed plus osteonecrosis, tendon rupture, and skin atrophy at injection site.

COX-2, Cyclooxygenase-2; *FDA,* U.S. Food and Drug Administration.

REFERENCES

1. DiPiro JT, Talbert RL, Yee GC, et al: *Pharmacotherapy: a pathophysiologic approach,* ed 7, New York, 2008, McGraw-Hill.
2. Lacy CF, Armstrong LL, Goldman MP, et al: *Drug information handbook 2008 – 2009,* ed 17, Hudson, Ohio, 2008, Lexi-Comp.

B

Reference Ranges for Commonly Used Tests

APPENDIX

Jaime C. Paz
Gary A. Shankman

For the reference ranges that follow, be aware that each laboratory in respective facilities may have different reference ranges based on their testing procedures and standards. Therefore likely variances are specified.

The lab tests are categorized into their more commonly associated diagnostic category. Please note however, that there is overlap with certain tests into other diagnostic categories not specified in the tables. For example the metabolic panel covers both the endocrine and renal system. The specific indication for the use of a test is ultimately determined by the physician.

Additionally, any lab value that falls outside of reference range should result in consultation with the supervising physical therapist and medical team to decide on the appropriateness of proceeding with physical therapy intervention.

Metabolic Panel Test(s)	Reference Range
Blood glucose	60-115 mg/dL (fasting finger stick)
Glycated hemoglobin (Hb A1c or A1C)	<7% of total hemoglobin over a 2-3 month period in well-controlled diabetes
Calcium (Ca^{2+})	8.5-10.5 mg/dL Panic: <6.5 or >13.5 mg/dL
Chloride (Cl^-)	98-107 mEq/L
Osmolality	285-293 mOsm/kg H_2O
Sodium (Na^+)	135-145 mEq/L
Potassium (K^+)	3.5-5 mEq/L
Blood urea nitrogen (BUN)	8-20 mg/dL
Creatine (Cr)	0.6-1.2 mg/dL

Hematologic Panel Test(s)	Reference Range
Erythrocyte count (RBC count)	Male: 4.7-6.1 million/μL Female: 4.2-5.4 million/μL
Hematocrit (Hct)	Male: 39%-49% Female: 35%-45% (age-dependent)
Hemoglobin, total (Hb)	Male: 13.6-17.5 g/dL Female: 12.0-15.5 g/dL
Leukocyte (white blood cell) count, total (WBC count)	5,000-10,000/μL
Erythrocyte sedimentation rate	Male: <10 mm/h Female: <15 mm/h (laboratory-specific)
Erythropoietin (EPO)	5-20 mIU/mL
Ferritin	Male: 16-300 ng/mL Female: 4-161 ng/mL
Folic acid (red cells)	165-760 mg/mL
Iron (Fe^{2+})	50-175 μg/dL
Iron-binding capacity, total (TIBC)	250–460 μg/dL
Mean corpuscular hemoglobin (MCH)	26-34 pg
Mean corpuscular hemoglobin concentration (MCHC)	31-36 g/dL
Mean corpuscular volume (MCV)	80-100 fL

Coagulation Profile Test(s)	Reference Range
Fibrin D-dimers	Negative
International normalized ratio (PT/INR)	0.9-1.1 (ratio)
Ratio = Patient value/reference value	
Prothrombin time (PT)	11-15 seconds
Partial thromboplastin time (PTT)	60-70 seconds
Activated partial thromboplastin time (aPTT)	30-40 seconds
Platelet count (Plt)	150,000 -450,000/µL

Cardiac Panel Test(s)	Reference Range
Creatine kinase (CK)	32-267 IU/L (method-dependent)
CK-MB	0%-3%
Troponin T (cTnT)	<0.2 pg/L
Troponin I (cTnI)	<3.1 pg/L
Brain natriuretic peptide (BNP)	<100 pg/mL
	>500 pg/mL positive for heart failure
High sensitivity C-reactive protein (hs-CRP)	<1.0 mg/L = low risk for developing heart disease
	1.0-3.0 mg/L = average risk for developing heart disease
	>3.0 mg/L = high risk for developing heart disease

Arterial Blood Gases Test(s)	Reference Range
pH	Arterial 7.35-7.45
	Venous 7.31-7.41
Oxygen, partial pressure (Po_2)	83-108 mm Hg
Carbon dioxide, partial pressure (Pco_2)	35-45 mm Hg
Bicarbonate (total)	22-28 mEq/L

Liver Panel Test(s)	Reference Range
Alanine aminotransferase (ALT, SGPT, GPT)	0-35 IU/L (laboratory-specific)
Alkaline phosphatase	41-133 IU/L (method- and age-dependent)
Aspartate aminotransferase (AST, SGOT, GOT)	0-35 IU/L (laboratory-specific)
Gamma-glutamyl transpeptidase (GGT)	9-85 U/L (laboratory-specific)
Bilirubin (total)	0.3-1.2 mg/dL

REFERENCES

1. Goodman CC, Snyder TE: *Differential diagnosis for physical therapists: screening for referral*, St Louis, 2007, Saunders.
2. Paz JC, West MP: *Acute care handbook for physical therapists*, ed 3, St Louis, 2009, Saunders.
3. Tierney LM, McPhee SJ, Papadakis M: *Current medical diagnosis and treatment*, Norwalk, Conn., 1995, Appleton and Lange.

Units of Measurement and Terminology for the Description of Exercise and Sport Performance

C

APPENDIX

Jaime C. Paz
Gary A. Shankman

UNITS FOR QUANTIFYING HUMAN EXERCISE[2]

Mass: kilogram (kg)
Distance: meter (m)
Time: second (s)
Force: newton (N)
Work: joule (J)
Power: watt (w)
Velocity: meters per second (m·s-1)
Torque: newton-meter (N·m)
Acceleration: meters per second2 (m·s-2)
Angle: radian (rad)
Angular velocity: radians per second (rad·s-1)
Amount of substance: mole (mol)
Volume: liter (L)

TERMINOLOGY

Concentric action: One in which the ends of the muscle are drawn closer together.[2]

Eccentric action: One in which a force external to the muscle overcomes the muscle force and the ends of the muscle are drawn further apart.[2]

Endurance: The ability to perform low intensity, repetitive, or sustained activities over a prolonged period of time without fatigue (SI unit: second).[3-5]

Energy: The capability of producing force, performing work, or generating heat (SI unit: joule).[2]

Exercise: Any and all activity involving generation of force by the activated muscle(s). Exercise can be quantified mechanically as force, torque, work, power, or velocity of progression.[2]

Exercise intensity: A specific level of muscular activity that can be quantified in terms of power (energy expenditure or work performed per unit of time), the opposing force (e.g., by free weight of weight stack), isometric force sustained, or velocity of progression.[2]

Force: That which changes or tends to change the state of rest or motion in matter. A muscle generates force in a muscle action (SI unit: newton).[2]

Free weight: An object of known mass, not attached to a supporting or guiding structure, which is used for physical conditioning and competitive lifting.[2]

Isometric: One in which the ends of the muscle are prevented from drawing closer together, with no change in length.[2]

Isokinetic: A form of assessing muscular force production (concentric or eccentric) at a constant velocity. The force of rotation of the body segment about its joint axis is measured as torque (newton-meters, N·m).[1]

Mass: The quantity of matter of an object that is reflected in its inertia (SI unit: kilogram).[1]

Muscle action: The state of activity of muscle.[2]

Power: The rate of performing work; the product of force and velocity. The rate of transformation of metabolic potential energy to work or heat (SI unit: watt).[2]

Strength: The maximal force or torque a muscle or muscle group can generate at a specified or determined velocity. Maximal muscular strength is typically quantified by directly assessing the maximal weight an individual can lift in a specific exercise, the amount of force generated in an isometric contraction or the amount of torque generated during an isokinetic contraction.[1,2]

Torque: The effectiveness of a force to overcome the rotational inertia of an object. The product of force and the perpendicular distance from the line of action of the force to the axis of rotation (SI unit: newton-meter).[2]

Weight: The force exerted by gravity on an object (SI unit: newton; traditional unit: kilogram of weight) (Note: mass = weight/acceleration due to gravity).[2]

Work: Force expressed through a displacement but with no limitation on time (SI unit: joule; note: 1 newton × 1 meter = 1 joule).[2]

REFERENCES

1. Hoffman J: *Norms for fitness, performance and health*, Champaign, Ill., 2006, Human Kinetics.
2. Komi PV, editor: *Strength and power in sport: the encyclopaedia of sports medicine*, ed 2, Malden, Mass., 2003, Blackwell Science.
3. McCardle WD, Katch FI, Katch VI: *Exercise physiology: energy, nutrition, and physical human performance*, ed 4, Baltimore, 1996, Lippincott Williams & Wilkins.
4. Powers SK, Howley ET: *Exercise physiology: theory and application*, Boston, 2001, McGraw-Hill.
5. Wilmore JH, Costill DL: *Physiology of sports and exercise*, ed 2, Champaign, Ill., 1992, Human Kinetics.

D Fracture Eponyms[1]

APPENDIX

Jaime C. Paz
Gary A. Shankman

This appendix provides a descriptive list of commonly encountered terms associated with fractures. Eponyms are labels that provide two kinds of information: the pattern of a complex injury or pathologic problem and the name of an individual who has been closely identified with that problem.[2]

Aviator's astragalus: Implies a variety of fractures of the talus; described after World War I as "rudder bar is driven into foot during plane crash."

Barton fracture: Displaced articular lip fracture of the distal radius; may be associated with carpal subluxation. Fracture configuration may be in a dorsal or volar direction. Dorsal fracture is the most common fracture dislocation.[3]

Bennett fracture: Oblique intraarticular fracture of the first metacarpal base separating a small triangular fragment of the volar lip from the proximally displaced metacarpal shaft.

Bosworth fracture: Fracture of the distal fibula with fixed displacement of the proximal fragment posteriorly behind the posterolateral tibial ridge. Posterior displacement of the talus also occurs.

Boxer's fracture: Fracture of the fifth metacarpal neck with volar displacement of the metacarpal head.

Burst fracture: Fracture of the vertebral body from axial load, usually with anterior and posterior displacement of the fragments. May occur in the cervical, thoracic, or lumbar spine.

Chance fracture: Distraction (transverse) fracture of the thoracolumbar vertebral body with horizontal disruption of the spinous process, neural arch, and vertebral body.

Chauffeur's fracture (Hutchinson fracture): Oblique fracture of the radial styloid initially attributed to the starting crank of an engine being forcibly reversed by a backfire. Ulnar deviation and supination are the forces involved in creating this fracture.

Chopart fracture and dislocation: Fracture or dislocation involving Chopart joints (talonavicular and calcaneocuboid) of the foot.

Clay-shoveler's (coal-shoveler's) fracture: Fracture at the base of the spinous process, typically of the lower cervical or upper thoracic vertebrae. Injury initially attributed to workers attempting to throw a full shovel of clay upward, but the clay, adhering to the shovel, caused a sudden flexion force opposite to the neck musculature.

Colles fracture: General term for nonarticular fractures of the distal radius with dorsal displacement, with or without an ulnar styloid fracture.

Cotton fractures: Trimalleolar ankle fracture with fractures of both malleoli and the posterior lip of the tibia.

Die-punch fracture: Intraarticular fracture of the distal radius with impaction of the dorsal aspect of the lunate fossa.

Dupuytren fracture: Fracture of the distal fibula, above the lateral malleolus, with rupture of the distal tibiofibular ligaments and lateral displacement of the talus. The medial malleolus may be fractured as well.

Duverney fracture: Fracture of the iliac wing without disruption of the pelvic ring.

Essex-Lopresti fracture: Fracture of the radial head with associated dislocation of the distal radioulnar joint. Radial head is generally comminuted and displaced.

Galeazzi fracture: Fracture of the radius in the middle to distal third of the radial shaft associated with dislocation of the distal radioulnar joint.

Greenstick fracture: Incompletely fractured bone in a child, with a portion of the cortex and periosteum remaining intact on the compression side of the fracture.

Hangman's fracture: Fracture through the neural arch of the second cervical vertebra (axis) occurring from hyperextension, with or without concurrent cervical distraction.

Hill-Sachs fracture: Posterolateral humeral head compression fracture caused by anterior glenohumeral dislocation and impaction of the humeral head against the anterior glenoid rim.

Holstein-Lewis fracture: Fracture of the distal third of the humerus with entrapment of the radial nerve.

Hutchinson fracture: See *Chauffeur's fracture.*

Jefferson fracture: Comminuted fracture of the ring of the atlas caused by axial compressive forces. Fractures usually occur anterior and posterior to the lateral facet joints.

Jones fracture: Diaphyseal fracture of the base of the fifth metatarsal distal to the metatarsal tuberosity.

Lisfranc fracture dislocation: Fracture and/or dislocation involving Lisfranc (tarsometatarsal) joint of the foot. Typically the second to the fifth joints are involved. Lisfranc was one of Napoleon's surgeons. He described traumatic foot amputation through the level of the tarsometatarsal joint.

Maisonneuve fracture: Spiral fracture of the proximal fibula with syndesmosis rupture and associated fracture of the medial malleolus or rupture of the deltoid ligament. External rotation is typically the mechanism of fracture.

Malgaigne fracture: Unstable pelvic fracture with vertical fractures anterior and posterior to the hip joint. Associated dislocation of the sacroiliac joint and/or pubic symphysis may also be present.

Mallet finger: Flexion deformity of the distal interphalangeal joint caused by separation of the extensor tendon from the distal phalanx. The deformity may be secondary to direct injury of the extensor tendon or an avulsion fracture from the dorsum of the distal phalanx, where the tendon inserts.

Monteggia fracture: Fracture of the proximal third of the ulna with associated anterior dislocation of the radial head.

Nightstick fracture: Isolated fracture of the ulna secondary to direct trauma.

Posadas fracture: Transcondylar humeral fracture with displacement of the distal fragment anteriorly, and dislocation of the radius and ulna from the bicondylar fragment.

Pott fracture: Fracture of the fibula 2 to 3 inches above the lateral malleolus with rupture of the deltoid ligament and lateral subluxation of the talus.

Rolando fracture: A comminuted Y- or T-shaped intraarticular fracture of the thumb metacarpal with resultant disruption in the articular surface of the first metacarpal.

Segond fracture: Avulsion fracture of the lateral tibial condyle from the bony insertion of the iliotibial band. It is frequently associated with anterior cruciate ligament and meniscal injuries.

Shepherd fracture: Fracture of the lateral tubercle of the posterior talar process.

Smith fracture: Fracture of the distal radius with palmar displacement of the distal fragment. Also referred to as a reverse Colles fracture, a reverse Barton fracture, or a Goyrand fracture. The palmar displacement of the fragment may also be referred to as a "garden spade" deformity.

Stieda fracture: Avulsion fracture of the medial femoral condyle at the origin of the medial collateral ligament.

Straddle fracture: Bilateral fractures of the superior and inferior pubic rami.

Teardrop fracture: Flexion fracture or dislocation of the cervical spine with associated triangular anterior fragment of the involved vertebrae. Injury complex is unstable, with posterior ligamentous disruption. Hyperextension may also cause a teardrop fracture.

Tillaux fracture: Fracture of the lateral half of the distal tibial physis during differential closure of the growth plate. The medial part of the tibial physis has already fused. Occurs in adolescents between the ages of 12 and 15 years.

Torus fracture: Impaction fracture of childhood as the bone buckles instead of fracturing completely. The lower forearm of young children tends to be most often injured.

Walther's fracture: Ischioacetabular fracture that passes through the pubic rami and extends toward the sacroiliac joint. The medial wall of the acetabulum is displaced inward.

REFERENCES

1. Hart RG, Rittenberry TJ, Uehara DT: *Handbook of orthopaedic emergencies*, Philadelphia, 1999, Lippincott-Raven.
2. Hunter TB, Peltier LF, Lund PJ: Radiologic history exhibit. Musculoskeletal eponyms: who are those guys? *Radiographics* 20:819–836, 2000.
3. Wheeless CR III: *Wheeless' Textbook of Orthopaedics* (website): www.wheelessonline.com. Accessed April 20, 2010.

Major Movements of the Body and the Muscles Acting on the Joints Causing the Movement

Jaime C. Paz
Gary A. Shankman

THE MUSCLES ACTING AT THE JOINTS CAUSING THE MOVEMENT

Please note that specific muscle activation is dependent upon the patient's posture and skeletal alignment, along with the starting position of the joint.

Joint	Joint Movement	Description	Muscles
Ankle	Inversion (supination) of the ankle	Sole of foot turns inward	Tibialis anterior Tibialis posterior Flexor digitorum longus Flexor hallucis longus Gastrocnemius Soleus
	Eversion (pronation) of the ankle	Sole of foot turns outward	Peroneus longus Peroneus brevis Peroneus tertius Extensor digitorum longus
	Dorsiflexion of the ankle	Toes move toward shin	Tibialis anterior Extensor digitorum longus Peroneus tertius Extensor hallucis longus
	Plantar flexion of the ankle	Toes move away from the shin	Gastrocnemius Soleus Peroneus longus Peroneus brevis Tibialis posterior Flexor digitorum longus Flexor hallucis longus Peroneus longus
Knee	Knee flexion	Bend at the knee, making the angle smaller	Biceps femoris Semitendinosus Semimembranosus Sartorius Gracilis Popliteus Gastrocnemius
	Knee extension	Straighten the knee, making the angle larger	Vastus lateralis Vastus intermedius Vastus medialis Rectus femoris Tensor fasciae latae

Joint	Joint Movement	Description	Muscles
Hip	Medial (internal) rotation of the knee	Knee turns inward (knee must be bent)	Semitendinosus Semimembranosus Sartorius Gracilis Popliteus
	Lateral (external) rotation of the knee	Knee turns outward (knee must be bent)	Biceps femoris Tensor fasciae latae
	Hip flexion	Bend at the hip, which reduces the angle	Iliopsoas Pectineus Rectus femoris Sartorius Gluteus maximus Tensor fasciae latae Adductor brevis Adductor longus
	Hip extension	Straighten at the hip, which increases the angle	Biceps femoris Semitendinosus Semimembranosus Gluteus maximus Adductor magnus
	Hip abduction	Leg moves away from the body at the hip	Gluteus medius Gluteus minimus Gluteus maximus Tensor fasciae latae Rectus femoris Sartorius
	Hip adduction	Leg moves toward the body at the hip	Gracilis Pectineus Adductor magnus Adductor longus Adductor brevis Gluteus maximus
	Medial (internal) rotation of the hip	Leg rotates inward at the hip	Gluteus minimus Gluteus medius Gluteus maximus Semitendinosus Semimembranosus Pectineus Gracilis Adductor brevis Tensor fasciae latae
	Lateral (external) rotation of the hip	Leg rotates outward at the hip	Rectus femoris Iliopsoas Sartorius Biceps femoris Adductor magnus Gluteus maximus Gluteus medius Gluteus minimus Piriformis Obturator internus/externus Quadratus femoris Gemelli superior/inferior

Continued

Joint	Joint Movement	Description	Muscles
	Transverse pelvic girdle rotation*	Twisting movement at the hip and waist	External oblique Internal oblique Erector spinae (sacrospinalis)
	Posterior pelvic girdle rotation†	Posterior pelvic tilt or "suck and tuck"	External oblique Internal oblique Rectus abdominis
Spine	Lumbar flexion†	With hips locked, bend forward at the lumbar vertebrae	External oblique Internal oblique Rectus abdominis
	Lumbar extension†	With hips locked, bend backward at the lumbar vertebrae	Erector spinae (sacrospinalis)
Neck	Cervical flexion†	Chin moves toward the chest	Sternocleidomastoid Longus capitis and colli Scalenes
	Cervical extension†	Chin moves away from the chest	Rectus capitis lateralis Rectus capitis posterior Obliquus capitis superior Semispinalis capitis Splenius capitus and cervicis Levator scapulae Sternocleidomastoid Upper trapezius
	Cervical rotation†	Head rotates from side to side	Sternocleidomastoid Obliquus capitis superior and inferior Semispinalis capitis Splenius capitus and cervicis Rectus capitis posterior Upper trapezius Scalenes
	Lateral bending* (flexion) of the cervical spine	Ear moves toward the shoulder	Levator scapulae Rectus capitis lateralis Longissimus capitis and cervicis Obliquus capitis superior Rectus capitis posterior Upper trapezius Sternocleidomastoid Scalenes
	Lateral bending* (flexion) of the trunk	Trunk moves side to side (no movement at the hip)	External oblique Internal oblique Erector spinae (sacrospinalis, quadratus lumborum)

Joint	Joint Movement	Description	Muscles
Shoulder	Shoulder elevation	Shoulder shrug	Levator scapulae Upper trapezius Rhomboids
	Shoulder depression	Shoulders move downward	Pectoralis minor Trapezius
	Scapular abduction (protraction)	Scapulas move further apart	Pectoralis minor Serratus anterior Rhomboids
	Scapular adduction (retraction)	Scapulas move closer together	Levator scapulae Trapezius Rhomboids
	Upward rotation of the scapula	Left (from rear) scapula rotates clockwise and right scapula, counterclockwise	Serratus anterior Trapezius
	Downward rotation of the scapula	Right (from rear) scapula rotates clockwise and left scapula counterclockwise	Rhomboids Pectoralis minor Levator scapulae
	Shoulder adduction	Arms move sideways inward toward the body	Latissimus dorsi Teres major & minor Pectoralis Subscapularis
	Shoulder abduction	Arms move sideways away from the body	Deltoid (middle) Supraspinatus Trapezius Serratus anterior Rhomboids Infraspinatus Subscapularis Biceps brachii
	Shoulder flexion	Arms straight up in front of the body	Deltoid (anterior) Pectoralis (clavicular) Deltoid (posterior) Serratus anterior Biceps brachii
	Shoulder extension	Arms move from straight up in front of body to the anatomic position	Pectoralis (sternal) Latissimus dorsi Teres major Deltoid (posterior)
	Shoulder hyperextension	Arms move from anatomic position to behind the body	Deltoid (posterior)
	Medial rotation of the shoulder	Humerus rotates inward at the shoulder	Latissimus dorsi Teres major Pectoralis major Supraspinatus Subscapularis
	Lateral rotation of the shoulder	Humerus rotates outward at the shoulder	Infraspinatus Supraspinatus Teres minor
	Horizontal shoulder adduction	With arm straight at shoulder height to the side, move arm toward the midline	Pectoralis
	Horizontal shoulder abduction	With arm straight at shoulder height at the midline, move arm toward the side of the body	Deltoid (middle and posterior) Infraspinatus Teres minor

Continued

Joint	Joint Movement	Description	Muscles
Elbow	Elbow flexion	Bend elbow, making the angle smaller	Biceps brachii Brachialis Brachioradialis Pronator teres
	Elbow extension	Straighten elbow, making the angle larger	Triceps brachii (long, lateral, and medial)
Wrist	Supination of radioulnar joint	Palm is turned upward	Biceps brachii Brachioradialis Supinator Extensor carpi radialis
	Pronation of radioulnar joint	Palm is turned downward	Pronator teres Brachioradialis Extensor carpi radialis
	Wrist flexion	Wrist bends toward volar surface of forearm, making angle between the hand and the forearm	Flexor carpi radialis Flexor carpi ulnaris Palmaris longus Flexor digitorum superficialis Abductor pollicis longus Extensor pollicis brevis
	Wrist extension	Wrist bends toward the dorsal surface of the forearm, making angle between the hand and the forearm	Extensor carpi radialis Extensor carpi ulnaris Extensor digitorum Abductor pollicis longus Extensor pollicis brevis Extensor pollicis longus

*Muscles listed are active unilaterally to create motion.
†Muscles listed are active bilaterally to create motion.
Data from Oatis CA: *Kinesiology: the mechanics & pathomechanics of human movement,* ed 2, Baltimore, 2009, Lippincott Williams & Wilkins; Levangie PK, Norkin CC: *Joint structure & function: a comprehensive analysis,* Philadelphia, 2005, FA Davis.

ANALYSIS OF BASIC WEIGHT TRAINING EXERCISES*

Chin-Up

Exercise description: Using a horizontal bar suspended above the head, grasp the bar with the palms toward the body. Pull the body vertically upward until the chin passes the bar, and then return downward in a controlled manner to the initial hanging position.

Segment Movement	Joint Movement	Primary Muscles Involved	Phase of Isotonic Contraction
Upward motion	Elbow flexion	Biceps brachii Brachialis Brachioradialis	Concentric
	Shoulder extension	Latissimus dorsi Teres major Deltoid (posterior) Pectoralis	Concentric

*A more detailed description of the proper lifting technique for these basic weight training exercises can be found in most weight training textbooks (e.g., Sandler D: *Weight training fundamentals,* Champaign, Ill., 2003, Human Kinetics; Nyland J: *Clinical decisions in therapeutic exercise: planning and implementation,* Upper Saddle River, NJ, 2005, Prentice Hall). Further information on structural kinesiology and the analysis of other weight training exercises can be found in Thompson CW, Floyd RT: *Manual of structural kinesiology,* ed 14, Boston, 2001, McGraw-Hill.

Segment Movement	Joint Movement	Primary Muscles Involved	Phase of Isotonic Contraction
Downward motion	Scapula adduction	Trapezius Rhomboids Levator scapulae	Concentric
	Shoulder depression	Trapezius Pectoralis minor	Concentric
	Elbow extension	Biceps brachii Brachialis Brachioradialis	Eccentric
	Shoulder flexion	Latissimus dorsi Teres major Deltoid (posterior) Pectoralis	Eccentric
	Scapula abduction	Trapezius Rhomboids Levator scapulae	Eccentric
	Shoulder elevation	Trapezius Pectoralis	Eccentric

Latissimus Pull-Down

Exercise description: Gasp the bar suspended over the head with palms facing away from the body. Pull the bar downward until the bar touches the shoulders behind the head, and then return upward in a controlled manner to the initial position.

Segment Movement	Joint Movement	Primary Muscles Involved	Phase of Isotonic Contraction
Downward motion	Elbow flexion	Biceps brachii Brachialis Brachioradialis	Concentric
	Shoulder adduction	Latissimus dorsi Teres major Pectoralis minor	Concentric
	Scapular adduction	Trapezius Rhomboids Levator scapulae	Concentric
	Shoulder depression	Trapezius Pectoralis minor	Concentric
Upward motion	Elbow extension	Biceps brachii Brachialis Brachioradialis	Eccentric
	Shoulder abduction	Latissimus dorsi Teres major Pectoralis	Eccentric
	Scapular abduction	Trapezius Rhomboids Levator scapulae	Eccentric
	Shoulder elevation	Trapezius Pectoralis	Eccentric

Bent Knee Sit-Up

Exercise description: While lying on your back with knees bent, arms across the chest, and feet on the floor, curl upward until the elbows touch the thighs, and then return downward in a controlled manner to the initial supine position.

Segment Movement	Joint Movement	Primary Muscles Involved	Phase of Isotonic Contraction
Upward motion	Lumbar flexion	Rectus abdominis External oblique Internal oblique	Concentric
Downward motion	Lumbar extension	Rectus abdominis External oblique Internal oblique	Eccentric

Squat

Exercise description: With a bar across the shoulders behind the head, bend at the knees and waist, moving downward to a position where the thighs are parallel with the floor, and then return upward in a controlled manner to the standing position.

Segment Movement	Joint Movement	Primary Muscles Involved	Phase of Isotonic Contraction
Downward motion	Hip flexion	Gluteus maximus Biceps femoris Semitendinosus Semimembranosus	Eccentric
	Knee flexion	Rectus femoris Vastus lateralis Vastus medialis Vastus intermedius	Eccentric
	Ankle dorsiflexion	Gastrocnemius Soleus	Eccentric
Upward motion	Hip extension	Gluteus maximus Biceps femoris Semitendinosus Semimembranosus	Concentric
	Knee extension	Rectus femoris Vastus lateralis Vastus medialis Vastus intermedius	Concentric
	Ankle plantar flexion	Gastrocnemius Soleus	Concentric

Leg Press

Exercise description: Using a leg press machine, position the feet about shoulder width apart. Push the foot pad forward until the knees are extended, and then return backward in a controlled manner to the initial position.

Segment Movement	Joint Movement	Primary Muscles Involved	Phase of Isotonic Contraction
Forward motion	Hip extension	Gluteus maximus Biceps femoris Semitendinosus Semimembranosus	Concentric

Segment Movement	Joint Movement	Primary Muscles Involved	Phase of Isotonic Contraction
	Knee extension	Rectus femoris Vastus lateralis Vastus medialis Vastus intermedius	Concentric
Backward motion	Hip flexion	Gluteus maximus Biceps femoris Semitendinosus Semimembranosus	Eccentric
	Knee flexion	Rectus femoris Vastus lateralis Vastus medialis Vastus intermedius	Eccentric

Bench Press

Exercise description: While lying on your back, grasp the bar with hands shoulder width apart and palms facing toward the feet. Lower the bar in a controlled manner to a position across the chest, and then push the bar upward to the initial position.

Segment Movement	Joint Movement	Primary Muscles Involved	Phase of Isotonic Contraction
Downward motion	Elbow flexion	Triceps brachii	Eccentric
	Shoulder extension	Pectoralis Deltoid (anterior)	Eccentric
	Scapular adduction	Serratus anterior Pectoralis	Eccentric
Upward motion	Elbow extension	Triceps brachii	Concentric
	Shoulder flexion	Pectoralis Deltoid (anterior)	Concentric
	Scapular abduction	Serratus anterior Pectoralis	Concentric

Shoulder Press

Exercise description: Grasp the bar at chest height with hands shoulder width apart and palms facing forward. Push the bar upward until the elbows are extended, and then lower the bar in a controlled manner to the initial position.

Segment Movement	Joint Movement	Primary Muscles Involved	Phase of Isotonic Contraction
Upward motion	Elbow extension	Triceps brachii	Concentric
	Shoulder flexion	Pectoralis Deltoid (anterior)	Concentric
	Shoulder elevation	Trapezius Rhomboids Levator scapulae	Concentric
Downward motion	Elbow flexion	Triceps brachii	Eccentric
	Shoulder extension	Pectoralis Deltoid (anterior)	Eccentric
	Shoulder depression	Trapezius Rhomboids Levator scapulae	Eccentric

Arm Curl

Exercise description: While standing holding the bar with palms facing forward, curl the bar upward while bending at the elbow until the bar reaches shoulder height, and then lower the bar in a controlled manner to the initial position.

Segment Movement	Joint Movement	Primary Muscles Involved	Phase of Isotonic Contraction
Upward motion	Elbow flexion	Biceps brachii Brachialis Brachioradialis	Concentric
Downward motion	Elbow extension	Biceps brachii Brachialis Brachioradialis	Eccentric

Triceps Push-Down

Exercise description: While standing holding the bar at chin level with palms facing down, push the bar downward until the elbows are extended, and then raise the bar in a controlled manner to the initial position.

Segment Movement	Joint Movement	Primary Muscles Involved	Phase of Isotonic Contraction
Downward motion	Elbow extension	Triceps brachii	Concentric
Upward motion	Elbow flexion	Triceps brachii	Eccentric

Leg Curl

Exercise description: While lying prone on the bench with your heels hooked under the pad, curl the weight forward until the pad reaches the buttocks, and then lower the weight backward in a controlled manner to the initial position.

Segment Movement	Joint Movement	Primary Muscles Involved	Phase of Isotonic Contraction
Forward motion	Knee flexion	Biceps femoris Semitendinosus Semimembranosus	Concentric
Backward motion	Knee extension	Biceps femoris Semitendinosus Semimembranosus	Eccentric

Knee Extension

Exercise description: While sitting on the bench with your feet hooked under the pad, extend the weight upward until the knees are extended, and then lower the weight in a controlled manner to the initial position.

Segment Movement	Joint Movement	Primary Muscles Involved	Phase of Isotonic Contraction
Upward motion	Knee extension	Rectus femoris Vastus lateralis Vastus medialis Vastus intermedius	Concentric
Downward motion	Knee flexion	Rectus femoris Vastus lateralis Vastus medialis Vastus intermedius	Eccentric

Heel Raise

Exercise description: While standing with a bar supported on your shoulders, raise your body upward until you are standing on your toes, and then lower your body in a controlled manner to the initial position.

Segment Movement	Joint Movement	Primary Muscles Involved	Phase of Isotonic Contraction
Upward motion	Plantar flexion	Gastrocnemius Soleus	Concentric
Downward motion	Dorsiflexion	Gastrocnemius Soleus	Eccentric

Index

Page numbers followed by *f* indicate figures; *t*, tables; *b*, boxes.